MODELL'S ESSENTIAL DRUGS IN CURRENT USE AND NEW DRUGS 2006

ABOUT THE EDITORS

Milagros Fernandez, PharmD, received her bachelor of science in pharmacy from Arnold and Marie Schwartz College of Pharmacy and Health Sciences of Long Island University and her doctor of pharmacy from St. John's University College of Pharmacy and Health Professions. Dr. Fernandez is currently the lead pharmacist for general medicine at New York-Presbyterian Hospital. Prior to her current position, Dr. Fernandez worked as a target drug monitoring/staff pharmacist specializing in renal dosing of antibiotics and histamine$_2$ receptor antagonists for 5 years. She is a member of the Education Committee, Medication Safety and Informatics Committee, and Quality Improvement Committee at New York-Presbyterian Hospital. Her professional affiliations include the American Society of Health-System Pharmacists and the New York State Council of Health System Pharmacists. Her primary areas of interest are infectious diseases, oncology, and ambulatory care.

Lydia Calix, BS Pharm, RPh, received her bachelor of science in pharmacy from Arnold and Marie Schwartz College of Pharmacy and Health Sciences of Long Island University. Ms. Calix is currently a staff pharmacist for the division of Neurology/Pulmonary at Texas Children's Hospital. Her professional affiliations include the American Society of Health-System Pharmacists.

FIFTY-SECOND EDITION

MODELL'S ESSENTIAL DRUGS IN CURRENT USE AND NEW DRUGS 2006

Milagros Fernandez, PharmD
Lydia Calix, BS Pharm, RPh
Editors

SPRINGER PUBLISHING COMPANY
NEW YORK

Copyright © 2006
SPRINGER PUBLISHING COMPANY, INC.
11 West 42nd Street   New York, New York 10036
ALL RIGHTS RESERVED.

Library of Congress Catalog Card Number: 72-622-911

International Standard Book Number: 0-8261-7096-X

International Standard Serial Number: 1044-0704

Printed in the United States by Banta Book Group.

Acquisitions Editor: Sally J. Barhydt

Production Editor: Sara Yoo

Cover design: Mimi Flow

Composition: Compset, Inc.

CONTENTS

PREFACE

The publication of the 52nd edition of *Modell's Essential Drugs in Current Use and New Drugs* continues the commitment to provide health care professionals with timely, concise drug information about the newest therapeutic agents.

In this edition, new drugs are listed in Part I, giving special attention to drugs recently introduced to the market, most within the past year, in the United States. These new drugs are described in greater detail to provide readers with more information about the most current medications. Among these 28 new therapeutic agents are telithromycin, a new drug in a new class of antibiotics known as ketolides, as well as three new drugs for overactive bladders, five new agents for cancer, new molecular entities for Parkinson's, depression, insomnia, alcohol withdrawal, pain, chronic obstructive pulmonary disease, pulmonary hypertension, macular degeneration, traveler's diarrhea, mesothelioma, mucositis, hyperphosphatemia, and hyperparathyroidism.

Part II consists of monographs of common drugs currently in use. The purpose of this section is to provide useful and concise information, including the primary trade names, uses, and preparations for each of the medications included. More detailed information, including precautionary statements regarding adverse reactions, is included for the agents that are most frequently used in current therapy, as well as for the relatively new drugs that have been introduced over the last several years.

Drugs in both Parts I and II are listed alphabetically by their generic names. Common trade names and synonyms are included, but the listing of the trade names of many of the medications available from multiple companies is not complete. Trade names are followed by the symbol® or ™.

To facilitate understanding of the side effects of drugs, a glossary of the most common side effects is provided in Part III.

Although the emphasis of *Drugs in Current Use* continues to be on the properties and uses of individual therapeutic agents, a number of combination products are also listed. The combination products selected for inclusion are the most frequently used and those about which questions are most frequently asked of health care professionals.

Dosage information is provided for the new drugs listed in Part I. However, in view of the many factors that influence dosage determinations for a particular patient, this information is not provided for the agents listed in Part II. Thus, the product labeling or other more comprehensive references should be consulted.

The focus of *Modell's Essential Drugs in Current Use and New Drugs* is on the agents used for therapeutic purposes. Thus, we have not included most agents used for diagnostic purposes, biological products such as vaccines, and ingredients in pharmaceutical formulations that are not pharmacologically active.

The primary purpose of this book is to provide instant access to what is considered to be the most pertinent information regarding the drugs used in current therapy. However, such a publication as this cannot be all-inclusive, so the product literature and/or more comprehensive references should be consulted for prescribing purposes or when additional information is needed by the health care professional.

As in previous editions, we welcome any comments or suggestions as to how we might improve future editions of this book.

MILAGROS FERNANDEZ, PharmD

LYDIA CALIX, BS Pharm, RPh

PART I

New Drugs

ACAMPROSATE—Campral®

DESCRIPTION/ACTIONS

Acamprosate is a GABA agonist/glutamate antagonist. Its mechanism of action is not completely understood. Chronic alcohol exposure is thought to alter the normal balance between neuronal excitation and inhibition. Evidence suggests that acamprosate may interact with glutamate and GABA neurotransmitter systems centrally, leading to restoration of this balance. Acamprosate, in conjunction with psychosocial support, helps patients with alcoholism to maintain abstinence following acute alcohol detoxification. It does not have an abuse potential, nor does tolerance or dependence occur over time.

PRECAUTIONS/ADVERSE REACTIONS

Acamprosate is contraindicated in persons hypersensitive to acamprosate or any of its components and in patients with severe renal impairment (creatinine clearance ≤30 mL/min). Caution should be used in patients with moderate renal impairment (CrCl 30–50 mL/min). Sulfites were used in the synthesis of acamprosate and traces of residual sulfites may be present in the product. **Warning**: Suicidal ideation, attempts and completed suicides have occurred; monitor for depression and/or suicidal thinking. Families and caregivers of patients being treated with acamprosate should be alerted to the need to monitor patients for the emergence of symptoms of depression or suicidality and to report such symptoms to the patient's physician. Safety and efficacy have not been established in pediatric patients. Pregnancy risk factor C. Teratogenic in animal studies. No adequate or well-controlled studies in pregnant women. Use only if potential benefit outweighs possible risk to the fetus. Most common adverse effects were diarrhea, nausea, vomiting, palpitations, peripheral edema, weight gain, anxiety, depression, dizziness, headache, and pruritis. Three patients had a serious adverse event of acute kidney failure. Acamprosate does not interact with benzodiazepines, anxiolytics, sedatives, hypnotics, or non-opioid analgesics.

ADMINISTRATION

Recommended: 666 mg three times a day. *Dosage in renal impairment:* Moderate renal impairment (CrCl 30–50 mL/min): 333 mg three times a day. Patients with severe renal impairment (CrCl < 30 mL/min) should not be given acamprosate. Treatment should be initiated as soon as possible after the period of alcohol withdrawal. Coadministration of naltrexone produced a 25% increase in AUC and a 33% increase in the C_{max} of acamprosate.

PATIENT CARE IMPLICATIONS

Swallow tablet whole. Do not chew or crush. May be taken without regard to meals. Maintain adequate hydration. Can cause drowsiness; use caution when driving or engaging in activities requiring alertness until response to drug is known. Report persistent diarrhea, respiratory difficulties, fainting or thoughts of suicide. Advise patients to continue acamprosate even in the event of relapse and discuss any renewed drinking with their physician.

PREPARATIONS

Tablet, enteric coated, 333 mg.

APOMORPHINE—Apokyn™
DESCRIPTION/ACTIONS

Apomorphine is a dopamine agonist; it is indicated for the acute, intermittent treatment of hypomobility, and "off" episodes in advanced Parkinson's disease. The precise mechanism of action of apomorphine is not known: it is believed to be due to the stimulation of postsynaptic dopamine D_2-type receptors within the caudate-putamen in the brain.

PRECAUTIONS/ADVERSE REACTIONS

Apomorphine is contraindicated in patients with a hypersensitivity to apomorphine or its ingredients (metabisulfite). The concomitant use of apomorphine with $5HT_3$ antagonist drugs (ondansetron, granisetron, dolasetron, palonosetron and alosetron) is contraindicated because of profound hypotension and loss of consciousness. **Warning:** Avoid intravenous administration; intravenous crystallization of apomorphine occurs, leading to thrombus formation and pulmonary embolism. Severe nausea and vomiting can be expected. Treat with the antiemetic, trimethobenzamide for 3 days prior to starting apomorphine and then continue for at least 6 weeks. Use caution in patients with risk factors for torsade de pointes. Dopamine agonists may cause orthostatic hypotension at any time, especially during dose escalation. Apomorphine causes dose-related decreases in systolic and diastolic blood pressure. Effects on blood pressure may be increased by the concomitant use of alcohol, antihypertensive medications and vasodilators. **Warning:** There have been reports of patients who suddenly fell asleep without prior warning of sleepiness while engaged in activities of daily living. If patient develops significant daytime sleepiness or episodes of falling asleep during activities that require active participation, apomorphine should be discontinued. **Warning:** Extra caution should be used in patients with known cardiovascular and cerebrovascular disease. Angina, myocardial infarction, cardiac arrest and/or sudden death have occurred. Apomorphine has been shown to reduce resting systolic and diastolic blood pressure and as such, has the potential to exacerbate coronary (and cerebral) ischemia. **Warning:** Apomorphine might increase the risk of falling by simultaneously lowering blood pressure and altering mobility. Pregnancy risk factor C. The most common adverse effects were yawning, dyskinesias, nausea, vomiting, somnolence, dizziness, rhinorrhea, hallucinations, edema, chest pain, increased sweating, flushing, and pallor.

ADMINISTRATION

Subcutaneous: Patients in an "off" state should be given a 0.2 ml (2 mg) test dose. If patient tolerates the test dose and responds, the starting dose should be 0.2 ml (2 mg) as needed. If needed, the dose can be increased in 0.1 ml (1 mg) increments every few days up to a maximum dose of 0.6 ml (6 mg). If patient tolerates the test dose of 0.2 ml but achieves no response, a dose of 0.4 ml (4 mg) may be administered at the next observed "off" period. If patient tolerates a test dose of 0.4 ml (4 mg), the starting dose should be 0.3 ml (3 mg) as needed to treat existing "off" episodes. If patient does not tolerate a 0.4 ml (4 mg) test dose, a test dose of 0.3 ml (3 mg) should be given. If patient tolerates the 0.3 ml (3 mg) test dose, the starting dose should be 0.2 ml (2 mg) used on an as-needed basis. If needed, and the 0.2 ml (2 mg) dose is tolerated, dose can be increased to 0.3 ml (3 mg) after a few days.

Mild to moderate renal impairment: Reduce test dose and starting dose to 0.1 ml (1 mg). *Severe renal impairment:* Has not been studied. The prescribed dose should always be expressed in ml. Doses greater than 0.6 ml are not recommended. Trimethobenzamide (300 mg tid orally) should be started 3 days prior to the initial dose and continued at least during the first 2 months of therapy.

PATIENT CARE IMPLICATIONS

Medical supervision is required for all test doses. Supine and standing blood pressure should be checked predose and at 20, 40, and 60 minutes post dose. Patients who develop clinically significant orthostatic hypotension in response to the initial 0.2 ml (2 mg) test dose should not be considered candidates for apomorphine treatment. If subsequent test doses are required, wait 2 hours before another test dose is given. The next test dose should be timed with another "off" episode. Avoid alcohol; may cause headache, drowsiness, or dizziness (use caution when climbing stairs, driving, or if engaged in potentially hazardous tasks). May cause postural hypotension; use caution when changing position from lying or sitting to standing. Report immediately any irregular or rapid heartbeat, chest pain, palpitations, shortness of breath, unusual or sudden sleepiness, unusual muscle or skeletal movements or weakness, altered gait, hallucinations, confusion, anxiety, or depression. Never reuse needles. Patients should be taught the correct way to inject apomorphine. Choose an injection site on your stomach, upper arm, or upper leg. Change injection site each time apomorphine is used. Do not inject into an area of skin that is sore, red, infected, or damaged.

PREPARATIONS

Injection, solution, 10 mg/ml (2 ml) ampule and 3 ml multidose glass cartridge. Multiple dose injector pen provided in a package with 6 needles and a carrying case.

AZACITIDINE—Vidaza™

DESCRIPTION/ACTIONS

Azacitidine is an antimetabolite, antineoplastic agent. It is believed to exert its antineoplastic effects by causing hypomethylation of DNA and direct cytotoxicity on abnormal hematopoietic cells in the bone marrow. Hypomethylation may restore normal function to genes that are critical for differentiation and proliferation. Azacitidine is indicated for the treatment of patients with the following myelodysplastic syndrome subtypes: refractory anemia or refractory anemia with ringed sideroblasts (if accompanied by neutropenia or thrombocytopenia or requiring transfusions), refractory anemia with excess blasts in transformation, and chronic myelomonocytic leukemia.

PRECAUTIONS/ADVERSE REACTIONS

Azacitidine is contraindicated in persons with a hypersensitivity to azacitidine, mannitol, or any component of the formulation. It is also contraindicated in patients with advanced malignant hepatic tumors. **Warning:** Progressive hepatic coma leading to death has been reported in patients with extensive tumor burden. **Warning:** Pregnancy Category D. Azacitidine might cause fetal harm when administered to a pregnant woman. Azacitidine has caused multiple fetal abnormalities and fetal death in rats. Potentially hepatotoxic in patients with severe preexisting hepatic impairment; use caution in patients with liver disease. Patients with renal impairment should be monitored closely for toxicity as azacitidine and its metabolites are primarily excreted by the kidneys. Treatment is associated with neutropenia and thrombocytopenia. Complete blood counts should be performed to monitor response and toxicity prior to each dosing cycle. The most common adverse reactions were anemia, thrombocytopenia, neutropenia, pyrexia, fatigue, headache, dizziness, hypotension, peripheral edema, bruising, petechiae, nausea, diarrhea, constipation, and injection site erythema. Nausea, vomiting, diarrhea, and constipation tended to increase in incidence with increased dose of azacitidine.

ADMINISTRATION

First treatment cycle: For all patients, regardless of baseline hematology values, 75 mg/m^2 subcutaneously daily for 7 days. Cycles should be repeated every 4 weeks. Dose may be increased to 100 mg/m^2 if no beneficial effect is seen after 2 treatment cycles and if no toxicity (other than nausea and vomiting) has occurred.

Dosage adjustment based on hematology lab values: For patients with baseline WBC $\geq 3.0 \times 10^9$/L, ANC $\geq 1.5 \times 10^9$/L, and platelets $\geq 75 \times 10^9$/L: adjust the dose based on nadir counts.

Nadir count: ANC $< 0.5 \times 10^9$/L and platelets $< 25 \times 10^9$/L: administer 50% of dose for next course.

Nadir count: ANC 0.5–1.5×10^9/L and platelets 25–50×10^9/L: administer 67% of dose for next course.

Nadir count: ANC $> 1.5 \times 10^9$/L and platelets $> 50 \times 10^9$/L: administer 100% of dose for next course.

For patients whose baseline counts are WBC $< 3.0 \times 10^9$/L, ANC $< 1.5 \times 10^9$/L or platelets $< 75 \times 10^9$/L, dose adjustments should be based on nadir counts and bone marrow biopsy cellularity at the time of the nadir, unless there is a clear improvement in differentiation at the time of the next cycle. In this case, the current dose should be continued.

WBC or platelet nadir decreased 50–75% from baseline and bone marrow biopsy cellularity at time of nadir 30–60%: Administer 100% of dose during next course.

WBC or platelet nadir decreased 50–75% from baseline and bone marrow biopsy cellularity at time of nadir 15–30%: Administer 50% of dose during next course.

WBC or platelet nadir decreased 50–75% from baseline and bone marrow biopsy cellularity at time of nadir <15%: Administer 33% of dose during next course.

WBC or platelet nadir decreased >75% from baseline and bone marrow biopsy cellularity at time of nadir 30–60%: Administer 75% of dose during next course.

WBC or platelet nadir decreased >75% from baseline and bone marrow biopsy cellularity at time of nadir 15–30%: Administer 50% of dose during next course.

WBC or platelet nadir decreased >75% from baseline and bone marrow biopsy cellularity at time of nadir <15%: Administer 33% of dose at next course.

If nadir as defined above has occurred, the next course of treatment should be given 28 days after the start of the preceding course, provided that both the WBC and the platelet counts are >25% above the nadir and rising. If a >25% increase above the nadir is not seen by day 28, counts should be reassessed every 7 days. If a 25% increase is not seen by day 42, then the patient should be treated with 50% of the scheduled dose.

Renal function adjustment: If unexplained BUN or serum creatinine elevations occur, the next cycle should be delayed until values return to normal or baseline. Dose should be reduced by 50% on the next treatment course.

Serum electrolytes dosage adjustment: If unexplained reductions in serum bicarbonate levels to <20 meq/L occur, dose should be reduced by 50% for the next course. Doses greater than 4 ml should be divided into 2 syringes. After reconstitution, drug must be administered within 1 hour. Reconstituted product may be refrigerated for up to 8 hours. After removal from refrigerator, the suspension should be allowed to come to room temperature for up to 30 minutes before administration.

PATIENT CARE IMPLICATIONS

Women should be advised to avoid becoming pregnant and men not to father a child while receiving azacitidine. Inform patient they may be susceptible to infections (to avoid crowds). Report palpitations, chest pain, unusual weakness, bruising, bleeding, and difficulty breathing.

PREPARATIONS

Injection, lyophilized powder: 100 mg. Store at 25°C (77°F).

BEVACIZUMAB—Avastin™

DESCRIPTION/ACTIONS

Bevacizumab is a recombinant monoclonal antibody that binds to and inhibits the biologic activity of human vascular endothelial growth factor (VEGF). VEGF binding to its receptors leads to endothelial cell proliferation and new blood vessel formation (angiogenesis). Bevacizumab's binding capability is believed to reduce microvascular growth and inhibit metastatic tissue progression. Bevacizumab is used in combination with intravenous 5-fluorouracil-based chemotherapy for first-line treatment of patients with metastatic carcinoma of the colon or rectum.

PRECAUTIONS/ADVERSE REACTIONS

Bevacizumab is contraindicated in patients hypersensitive to bevacizumab, murine products, or any component of the formulation. **Warning:** Gastrointestinal perforations and wound healing complications can result, causing fatality in some instances. The typical presentation was reported as abdominal pain with symptoms such as constipation and vomiting. Therapy should be discontinued permanently in patients with GI perforation or wound dehiscence requiring medical intervention. Bevacizumab should not be initiated for at least 28 days following major surgery. The surgical incision should be fully healed prior to initiation of bevacizumab because of the potential for impaired wound healing. **Warning:** Arterial thromboembolic events (cerebral infarction, transient ischemic attacks, myocardial infarction, and angina) occurred and were fatal in some instances. Permanently discontinue if serious arterial thromboembolic events occur. Use with caution in patients with cardiovascular disease; may cause CHF and/or potentiate cardiotoxic effects of anthracyclines. Bevacizumab may cause and/or worsen hypertension; discontinue in patients with hypertensive crisis. Temporary suspension is recommended in patients with severe hypertension that is not controlled with medical management. Use caution in patients with pre-existing hypertension, and monitor BP closely. Proteinuria and nephrotic syndrome occurred; discontinue therapy in patients with nephrotic syndrome. Pregnancy risk factor C. Bevacizumab has been shown to be teratogenic in rabbits. Angiogenesis is critical to fetal development, and the inhibition of angiogenesis is likely to result in adverse effects on pregnancy. There are no adequate or well-controlled studies in pregnant women. Use only if potential benefit justifies the potential risk to the fetus. The most common adverse events were asthenia, pain, abdominal pain, headache, hypertension, diarrhea, nausea, vomiting, anorexia, stomatitis, constipation, upper respiratory infection, epistaxis, dyspnea, and proteinuria.

ADMINISTRATION

Intravenous: 5 mg/kg as an IV infusion given once every 14 days until disease progression is detected. Discontinue permanently in patients who develop gastrointestinal perforation, wound dehiscence requiring medical intervention, serious bleeding, a severe arterial thromboembolic event, nephrotic syndrome, or hypertensive crisis.

Dosage adjustment for toxicity: Temporary suspension is recommended in moderate to severe proteinuria or in patients with severe hypertension which is not controlled with medical management. Initial dose should be diluted in a total volume of 100 ml of NS and infused over 90 minutes. If the first infusion is well tolerated, the second infusion may be administered over 60 minutes. If the 60-minute infusion is well tolerated, all subsequent infusions may be administered over 30 minutes. Solutions for infusion may be stored at 2–8°C (36–46°F) for up to 8 hours. Do not mix with dextrose solutions.

PATIENT CARE IMPLICATIONS

Monitor closely during the infusion for signs and symptoms of an infusion reaction. Monitor CBC with differential. Monitor for signs and symptoms of gastrointestinal perforation (abdominal pain, constipation, and vomiting). Monitor blood pressure every 2 to 3 weeks during treatment with bevacizumab. Monitor for constipation, changes in urinary pattern, and any unusual bleeding or unusual symptoms.

PREPARATIONS

Injection, preservative-free solution: 25 mg/mL (4 mL, 16 mL). Refrigerate at 2–8°C (36–46°F). Protect from light. Store in original carton until time of use. Do not freeze. Do not shake.

CETUXIMAB—Erbitux™

DESCRIPTION/ACTIONS

Cetuximab is an antineoplastic, recombinant monoclonal antibody that binds specifically to the epidermal growth factor receptor (EGFR) on both normal and tumor cells. It competitively inhibits the binding of epidermal growth factor, thus blocking phosphorylation and activation of receptor-associated kinases, resulting in inhibition of cell growth, induction of apoptosis, and decreased vascular endothelial growth factor production. Expression of EGFR is detected in many human cancers, including those of the colon and rectum. Cetuximab, used in combination with irinotecan, is indicated for the treatment of EGFR-expressing, metastatic colorectal carcinoma in patients who are refractory to irinotecan-based chemotherapy. It is used as a single agent in patients who are intolerant of irinotecan-based chemotherapy.

PRECAUTIONS/ADVERSE REACTIONS

Cetuximab is contraindicated in patients hypersensitive to cetuximab, murine proteins, or any component of the product. **Warning:** Severe infusion reactions have occurred, characterized by rapid onset of airway obstruction (bronchospasm, stridor, hoarseness), urticaria, and hypotension. Severe infusion reactions require immediate interruption of infusion and should be permanently discontinued. Interstitial lung disease has occurred; use caution in patients with pre-existing lung disease. Dermatologic toxicities have been reported. Acneform rash was reported in about 90% of patients receiving cetuximab. Sunlight may exacerbate skin reactions. Pregnancy risk factor C. There are no adequate and well-controlled studies in pregnant women. EGFR has been implicated in the control of prenatal development and may be essential for normal organogenesis, proliferation, and differentiation in the developing embryo. Cetuximab should only be given to a pregnant woman if the potential benefit justifies the potential risk to the fetus. Breast-feeding should be discontinued during treatment with cetuximab and for 60 days following the last dose of cetuximab. The most common adverse effects were acneform rash, malaise, abdominal pain, fever, pain, infusion reactions, infection, diarrhea, nausea, vomiting, anorexia, constipation, stomatitis, leukopenia, and cough.

ADMINISTRATION

Initial loading dose: In combination with irinotecan or as monotherapy: 400 mg/m^2 as an initial loading dose infused over 120 minutes. Maximum rate of 5 mL/min.

Weekly maintenance dose: 250 mg/m^2 infused over 60 minutes. Maximum rate of 5 mL/min. Diphenhydramine premedication recommended.

Dose modifications for infusion reactions: Mild or moderate infusion reaction: Reduce infusion rate by 50%. Severe infusion reactions: Discontinue permanently.

Dose modifications for severe acneform rash: First occurrence: Delay infusion 1–2 weeks; if improvement, continue at 250 mg/m^2. Discontinue if no improvement.

Second occurrence: Delay infusion 1–2 weeks; if improvement, reduce dose to 200 mg/m². Discontinue if no improvement.

Third occurrence: Delay infusion 1–2 weeks; if improvement, reduce dose to 150 mg/m². Discontinue if no improvement.

Fourth occurrence: Discontinue.

Infuse over 1–2 hours. Do not administer as IV push. Administer with the use of a low-protein binding 0.22 micrometer in-line filter. Once solution has been drawn up, preparation is stable for 12 hours at 2–8°C (36–46°F) and up to 8 hours at controlled room temperature.

PATIENT CARE IMPLICATIONS

Premedicate with an antihistamine. Vital signs should be monitored during infusion and for 1 hour post infusion. Report immediately unusual chest tightness, difficulty breathing or swallowing, itching or skin rash, redness, swelling or pain at infusion site.

PREPARATIONS

Injection, preservative-free solution: 100 mg (50 ml). Store vials under refrigeration at 2–8°C (36–46°F). Do not freeze.

CINACALCET HCL—Sensipar™

DESCRIPTION/ACTIONS

Cinacalcet is a calcimimetic agent. The calcium-sensing receptor on the surface of the parathyroid gland is the principal regulator of parathyroid hormone (PTH) secretion. Cinacalcet directly lowers PTH levels by increasing the sensitivity of the calcium-sensing receptor to extracellular calcium. The reduction in PTH is associated with a concomitant decrease in serum calcium levels. Sensipar™ is indicated for the treatment of secondary hyperparathyroidism in patients with chronic kidney disease on dialysis and for the treatment of hypercalcemia in patients with parathyroid carcinoma.

PRECAUTIONS/ADVERSE REACTIONS

Cinacalcet is contraindicated in patients with a known hypersensitivity to it or to any component of the formulation. Monitor serum calcium levels closely in patients with a seizure disorder. Sensipar™ lowers serum calcium and therefore, patients should be carefully monitored for the occurrence of hypocalcemia. Potential manifestations of hypocalcemia include paresthesias, myalgias, cramping, tetany, and convulsions. Cinacalcet treatment should not be initiated if the serum calcium is below the lower limit of the normal range. Serum calcium should be measured within 1 week of initiation of therapy or dose adjustment. Once a maintenance dose has been established, calcium levels should be monitored monthly. If symptoms of hypocalcemia develop during treatment, calcium-containing phosphate binders and or vitamin D can be used to raise calcium levels. If symptoms of hypocalcemia persist and the dose of vitamin D cannot be increased, withhold administration of Sensipar™. Treatment should be re-initiated using the next lowest dose of cinacalcet. Adynamic bone disease may develop if intact PTH (iPTH) levels are suppressed below 100 pg/mL. If iPTH levels decrease below the recommended target range (150–300 pg/mL) in patients treated with Sensipar™, the dose of Sensipar™ and/or vitamin D sterols should be reduced or therapy discontinued. Cinacalcet is metabolized by CYP3A4, CYP2D6, and CYP1A2, and is a strong inhibitor of CYP2D6. Co-administration of cinacalcet and amitriptyline resulted in increased levels of amitriptyline and nortriptyline. Pregnancy Category C. No adequate and well- controlled studies in pregnant women. Excretion in human breast milk is unknown. Safety and efficacy in pediatric patients have not been established. Most common adverse effects observed in patients treated with cinacalcet include nausea, vomiting, diarrhea, myalgia, dizziness, hypertension, asthenia, anorexia, chest pain (noncardiac), and access infection.

ADMINISTRATION

Adults: oral. *Secondary hyperparathyroidism in patients with chronic kidney disease on dialysis:* 30 mg once daily. Serum calcium and serum phosphorus levels should be measured within 1 week, and iPTH should be measured 1–4 weeks after initiation or dose adjustment. Dose should not be titrated more frequently than every 2–4 weeks.

Parathyroid carcinoma: 30 mg twice daily. Dose should be titrated every 2–4 weeks.

Dosage adjustment for renal impairment: no adjustment necessary. *Dosage adjustment for hepatic impairment (moderate and severe):* PTH and serum calcium levels should be monitored closely.

PATIENT CARE IMPLICATIONS

Sensipar™ should be taken with food or shortly after a meal. Tablets should be taken whole and should not be divided. Calcium, phosphorus, and PTH levels should be closely monitored during therapy with cinacalcet.

PREPARATIONS

Tablets, 30 mg, 60 mg, and 90 mg.

CLOFARABINE—Clolar™

DESCRIPTION/ACTIONS

Clofarabine is a purine nucleoside anti-metabolite. Clofarabine competes with deoxycytidine kinase; it inhibits DNA synthesis by decreasing cellular deoxynucleotide triphosphate pools through the inhibition of ribonucleotide reductase. This results in termination of DNA chain elongation and inhibition of DNA repair. Clofarabine is approved for the treatment of pediatric patients, aged 1 to 21, with relapsed or refractory acute lymphoblastic leukemia after at least two prior regimens.

PRECAUTIONS/ADVERSE REACTIONS

Clofarabine is contraindicated in patients with a known hypersensitivity to clofarabine or any component of the formulation. **Warning:** Bone marrow suppression (neutropenia, anemia, and thrombocytopenia) should be anticipated. Patients are at an increased risk for severe opportunistic infections. Complete blood count and platelet count should be obtained. **Warning:** Rapid reduction in peripheral leukemia cells. Monitor for signs and symptoms of tumor lysis syndrome and for cytokine release (hypotension, tachycardia, tachypnea, pulmonary edema) that could develop into systemic inflammatory response syndrome (SIRS)/capillary leak syndrome and organ dysfunctions. Continuous IV fluids throughout treatment should be given to reduce the effects of tumor lysis and other adverse events. Allopurinol should be administered if hyperuricemia is expected. If significant signs and symptoms of SIRS/capillary leak syndrome occur, clofarabine should be discontinued immediately. When the patient is stable, clofarabine can be restarted, at a lower dose. Because clofarabine is primarily excreted renally and the liver is a target organ for toxicity, hepatic and renal function should be assessed prior to and during treatment. Clofarabine has not been studied in patients with hepatic or renal dysfunction; use with caution. Pregnancy category D. Clofarabine may cause fetal harm if administered to a pregnant woman. Teratogenic in rats and rabbits. There are no adequate and well-controlled studies in pregnant women. The most common adverse effects were hematologic (anemia, leukopenia, thrombocytopenia, neutropenia, febrile neutropenia), infection, gastrointestinal symptoms (vomiting, nausea, diarrhea, abdominal pain), headache, fatigue, and tachycardia. The most severe adverse reactions were renal and hepatic toxicities.

ADMINISTRATION

Intravenous: 52 mg/m^2, infused over 2 hours, for 5 consecutive days. Treatment is repeated following the return to baseline organ function, every 2 to 6 weeks. If patient shows early signs and symptoms of SIRS or capillary leak, clofarabine should be stopped. If there is an increase in creatinine or bilirubin, clofarabine should be stopped and reinstituted when the patient is stable and organ function has returned to baseline, possibly at a lower dose. If patient becomes hypotensive while receiving infusion, discontinue and retreat only if hypotension was transient, not requiring pharmacological intervention. Clofarabine should be filtered through a sterile 0.2 μm syringe filter and diluted with D5W or NS. Diluted clofarabine must be used within 24 hours. No other medications should be administered through the same line.

PATIENT CARE IMPLICATIONS

Respiratory, cardiac function, and blood pressure should be closely monitored during infusion. Advise patient to report dizziness, light-headedness, fainting spells, decreased urine output, signs of infection, chest pain, persistent GI upset, or other reactions. Avoid dehydration. Avoid drugs with known renal toxicity during the 5 days of administration. Monitor patients taking medications known to affect blood pressure or cardiac function closely. Patient should use effective contraceptive measures to prevent pregnancy. Complete blood counts and platelet counts should be monitored at regular intervals. Liver and kidney functions should be monitored during the 5 days of treatment. Use of prophylactic steroids may be of benefit in preventing signs and symptoms of SIRS or capillary leak.

PREPARATIONS

Injection, preservative-free solution: 1 mg/mL (20 mL). Store at 25°C (77°F).

DARIFENACIN—ENABLEX®
DESCRIPTION/ACTIONS

Darifenacin is a competitive muscarinic receptor antagonist. Darifenacin has greater affinity for the M_3 receptor. M_3 receptors are involved in contraction of the human bladder, gastrointestinal smooth muscle, saliva production, and iris sphincter function. Darifenacin is indicated for the treatment of overactive bladder with symptoms of urge urinary incontinence, urgency, and frequency.

PRECAUTIONS/ADVERSE REACTIONS

Darifenacin is contraindicated in patients with urinary retention, gastric retention, or uncontrolled narrow-angle glaucoma, and in patients who are at risk for these conditions. Use with caution in patients with clinically significant bladder outflow obstruction because of the risk of urinary retention. Use with caution in patients with gastrointestinal obstructive disorders because of the risk of gastric retention. Use with caution in patients with conditions such as severe constipation, ulcerative colitis, and myasthenia gravis. Use with caution in patients being treated for narrow-angle glaucoma and only where the potential benefits outweigh the risks. The most common adverse reactions were dry mouth, constipation, dyspepsia, abdominal pain, nausea, diarrhea, headaches, and urinary tract infections. Pregnancy risk factor C. There are no well-controlled studies in pregnant women; use only if potential benefit outweighs possible risk to fetus. Safety and efficacy have not been established in pediatric patients.

ADMINISTRATION

Starting dose: 7.5 mg daily. Dosage may be increased to 15 mg daily, after 2 weeks of starting therapy.

Moderate hepatic impairment or coadministration with potent CYP3A4 inhibitors: Daily dose should not exceed 7.5 mg. CYP3A4 inhibitors (such as ketoconazole, itraconazole, ritonovir, clarithromycin, and nefazadone).

Severe hepatic impairment: Subjects have not been studied; not recommended.

PATIENT CARE IMPLICATIONS

Take daily with liquid. May be taken with or without food. Swallow whole, do not chew, divide, or crush tablet. Patient should be informed of possibility of constipation, urinary retention, blurred vision, and heat prostration (due to decreased sweating). Because darifenacin may produce dizziness or blurred vision, advise patients to take caution in decisions to engage in potentially dangerous activities until the drug's effects have been determined.

PREPARATIONS

Extended-release tablets, 7.5 mg and 15 mg. Protect from light.

DIETHYLENE TRIAMINE PENTA-ACETIC ACID—Pentetate Calcium Trisodium

DESCRIPTION/ACTIONS

Trisodium calcium diethylene triamine penta-acetate is known as Ca-DTPA. Ca-DTPA forms stable chelates with metal ions by exchanging calcium for a metal of greater binding capacity. Radioactive chelates are then excreted into the urine. Ca-DTPA is indicated for the treatment of persons with known or suspected internal contamination with plutonium, americium, or curium. Ca-DTPA is not expected to be effective for uranium, iodine, and neptunium. Chelating capacity is greatest immediately and up to 24 hours after contamination, when the contaminant is still circulating and available for chelation. Effectiveness decreases with time because the transuranium elements become incorporated into tissues. A patient data form should be completed for all patients receiving treatment.

PRECAUTIONS/ADVERSE REACTIONS

Warning: Use with caution in persons with severe hemochromatosis; death has occurred. Ca-DTPA is associated with depletion of endogenous trace metals (zinc, magnesium, manganese). Depletion increases with split daily dosing, increasing dose, and increased duration of treatment. Monitor electrolytes and essential metals; vitamins plus mineral supplements containing zinc should be given. Nebulized therapy may be associated with asthma exacerbation. Ca-DTPA and its radioactive chelates are excreted by glomerular filtration. Impaired renal function may decrease their rates of elimination and increase the serum half-life of Ca-DTPA. Pregnancy Category C. Teratogenic based on animal studies. Ca-DTPA results in depletion of zinc, which is known to affect DNA and RNA synthesis in humans. Most common adverse reactions were headache, light-headedness, chest pain, allergic reaction, dermatitis, metallic taste, nausea, diarrhea, injection site reactions, and cough and wheezing (with nebulization treatment).

ADMINISTRATION

Initial: Adults and adolescents: A single 1 gm IV dose.

Pediatric (less than 12 years old): A single 14 mg/kg (max. 1 gm) IV dose.

Maintenance:

Adults and adolescents: 1 gm IV daily.

Pediatrics (less than 12 years old): 14 mg/kg IV daily.

Renal impairment: No dose adjustment needed. Renal impairment may reduce the rate at which radiocontaminants are eliminated. In heavily contaminated patients with renal impairment, dialysis may be used to increase the rate of elimination. A single dose of Ca-DTPA is recommended. If additional chelation therapy is needed, diethylene triamine penta-acetic acid (Zn-DTPA) is recommended. If Zn-DTPA is not available, chelation may continue with Ca-DTPA, but mineral supplements containing zinc should be given. The duration of treatment depends on the amount of internal contamination and individual response to treatment. Intravenous administration is recommended and should be used if the route of internal contamination is not known, or if multiple routes of internal contamination are likely. Ca-DTPA 1 gm in 5 ml by slow IV push over 3–4 minutes or diluted in 100–250 ml of either D5W, RL, or NS infused over 30 minutes. In individuals whose internal contamination is only by inhalation within the preceding 24 hours, Ca-DTPA can be administered by nebulized inhalation. Ca-DTPA should be diluted at a 1:1 ratio with sterile water or saline. Safety and effectiveness of the nebulized route has not been established in pediatrics.

PATIENT CARE IMPLICATIONS

Safety measures should be taken to minimize contaminations of others. Use a toilet instead of a urinal; flush several times after each use. Spilled urine or feces should be cleaned up completely and hands washed thoroughly. If blood or urine comes in contact with clothing or linens, they should be washed separately. Drink plenty of fluids and void frequently to promote dilution of the radioactive chelate. If a cough is present, any expectorant should not be swallowed and should be disposed of carefully. Nursing mothers should take precaution in disposing of breast milk. Precautions should be taken with dialysis fluid; it will become radioactive. During treatment, measure radioactivity in blood, urine, and fecal samples weekly. Monitor CBC with differential, BUN, serum chemistries, electrolytes, and urinalysis regularly. When possible, obtain baseline blood and urine samples.

PREPARATIONS

Injection, solution: 200 mg/mL (5 mL)

DIETHYLENE TRIAMINE PENTA-ACETIC ACID—Pentetate Zinc Trisodium

DESCRIPTION/ACTIONS

Trisodium zinc diethylene triamine penta-acetate is commonly referred to as Zn-DTPA. Zn-DTPA forms stable chelates with metal ions by exchanging zinc for a metal of greater binding capacity. Radioactive chelates are then excreted by glomerular filtration into the urine. Zn-DTPA is indicated for the treatment of individuals with known or suspected internal contamination with plutonium, americium, and curium. It is not expected to be effective for uranium and neptunium. Effectiveness of chelation decreases with time because the transuranium elements become incorporated into tissues. Treatment should be given as soon as possible. The manufacturer provides a patient data form that should be completed for all patients receiving treatment.

PRECAUTIONS/ADVERSE REACTIONS

Warning: Nebulized chelation therapy may be associated with exacerbation of asthma. Treatment over several months with Zn-DTPA could lead to depletion of magnesium and manganese. Monitor electrolytes and essential metals; vitamins and mineral supplements should be given. Pregnancy category B; no well-controlled human studies. Use only if clearly needed. The risk of toxicity from untreated internal radioactive contamination should be weighed against the risk of Zn-DTPA treatment. Radiocontaminants are known to be excreted in breast milk; breast-feeding is not recommended with Zn-DTPA. Most common adverse reactions were chest pain, headache, light-headedness, pelvic pain, injection site reaction, and diarrhea.

ADMINISTRATION

Initial: Adults and adolescents: Single 1 gm IV dose.

Pediatrics (less than 12 years old): Single 14 mg/kg IV dose (max. dose of 1 gm).

Maintenance: Adults and adolescents: 1 gm IV daily.

Pediatrics (less than 12 years old): 14 mg/kg IV daily (max dose of 1 gm).

Ca-DTPA is preferred, if available, as the initial dose because it is more effective than Zn-DTPA. Treatment of pregnant women should begin and continue with Zn-DTPA. Renal impairment may reduce the rate at which chelators remove radiocontaminants. In heavily contaminated patients with renal impairment, dialysis may be used to increase the rate of elimination. Duration of treatment depends on the amount of internal contamination and individual response to treatment. IV route is recommended and should be used if the route of contamination is not known or if multiple routes of contamination are likely. Administer 1 gm in 5 ml over 3–4 minutes or by infusion over 30 minutes. Dilute in 100–250 ml of D5W, RL, or NS. Persons whose contamination is by inhalation can be administered Zn-DTPA by nebulized inhalation. Dilute at a 1:1 ratio with sterile water or saline. Safety and effectiveness of nebulized route has not been established in pediatrics.

PATIENT CARE IMPLICATIONS

Safety measures should be taken to minimize contamination of others. A toilet should be used instead of a urinal, and it should be flushed several times after each use. Spilled urine or feces should be cleaned up completely and hands washed thoroughly. If blood or urine comes in contact with clothing or linens, they should be washed separately. Drink plenty of fluids and void frequently to promote dilution of radioactive chelate in urine and to minimize exposure to bladder. If cough is present, do not swallow expectorant, and dispose of the expectorant carefully. Nursing mothers should take precautions in disposing of breast milk. If possible, obtain baseline blood and urine samples. Measure radioactivity in blood, urine, and feces weekly. Monitor CBC with differential, BUN, serum chemistries, electrolytes, and urinalysis.

PREPARATIONS

Injection, solution: 200 mg/mL (5 mL)

DULOXETINE—Cymbalta®

DESCRIPTION/ACTIONS

Duloxetine has antidepressant and pain inhibitory actions that are related to its being a selective serotonin and norepinephrine reuptake inhibitor. Duloxetine is indicated for the treatment of major depressive disorder (MDD) and for the management of neuropathic pain associated with diabetic peripheral neuropathy (DPN). Safety and effectiveness in the pediatric population have not been established.

PRECAUTIONS/ADVERSE REACTIONS

Duloxetine is contraindicated in persons hypersensitive to duloxetine or any component of the formulation and in patients taking monoamine oxidase inhibitors (MAOIs) or within 2 weeks of use due to the risk of developing serious serotonin syndrome. Duloxetine is also contraindicated in patients with uncontrolled narrow-angle glaucoma due to increased risk of mydriasis. **Warning:** Antidepressants increased the risk of suicidal thinking and behavior in short-term studies in children and adolescents with MDD and other psychiatric disorders. Patients with MDD, both adult and pediatric, may experience worsening of their depression and/or the emergence of suicidal ideation or unusual changes in behavior, whether or not they are taking antidepressant medication. Patients started on therapy should be observed closely for clinical worsening, suicidality, or unusual changes in behavior, especially during the initial few months of therapy and at times of dose changes. Do not use in patients with hepatic impairment; duloxetine increases the risk of elevation of serum transamine levels. Because duloxetine is associated with increased risk of mydriasis, use caution in patients with controlled, narrow-angle glaucoma.

Duloxetine was associated with an increase in blood pressure; blood pressure should be measured prior to treatment and throughout treatment. Patients with seizure disorders were excluded from clinical studies; use with caution in patients with a history of a seizure disorder. Use cautiously in patients with a history of mania; activation of mania/hypomania has been reported in patients with mood disorders who were treated with other drugs effective in the treatment of MDD. Duloxetine is not recommended for patients with end-stage renal disease or severe renal impairment; there are increased plasma concentrations, especially metabolites. Serotonin syndrome may be caused with concurrent use of duloxetine and nefazodone, moclobemide, meperidine, SSRIs, sibutramine, serotonin agonists, tramadol, trazodone, venlaflaxine, MAOIs, linezolid, and buspirone. Pregnancy risk factor C. Animal studies showed adverse effects on embryo/fetal and postnatal development. Neonates exposed to SSRIs or serotonin and norepinephrine reuptake inhibitors (SNRIs) late in the third trimester have developed complications requiring prolonged hospitalization, respiratory support, and tube feeding. If treatment during pregnancy is required, consider tapering therapy during the third trimester. Excretion in breast milk is unknown; breast-feeding not recommended. Most common adverse reactions when used for diabetic peripheral neuropathic pain were nausea, dizziness, somnolence, constipation, and fatigue. Most common adverse reactions for MDD were nausea, dry mouth, constipation, decreased appetite, fatigue, somnolence, and increased sweating.

ADMINISTRATION

Initial dose: MDD: 40 to 60 mg/day; may be given once a day or as 30 mg bid, without regard to meals.

DPN pain: 60 mg/day; given once a day. Because diabetes is frequently complicated by renal disease, a lower starting dose and gradual increase in dose should be considered for patients with renal impairment.

Maintenance dose: MDD: Periodically reassess patient to determine need for maintenance.

DPN pain: Efficacy beyond 12 weeks has not been studied.

A gradual reduction in dose rather than abrupt cessation is recommended. If intolerable symptoms occur following a decrease in dose or upon discontinuation of treatment, then resuming the previously prescribed dose may be considered.

PATIENT CARE IMPLICATIONS

Med guides have been developed for all of the antidepressants to provide information about the risk of suicidality in children and adolescents for patients, their families, and caregivers. Med guides are to be distributed by the pharmacist with each prescription or refill. Patient's family or caregiver should closely monitor for clinical worsening, suicidality, or unusual changes in behavior. This should include weekly face-to-face contact with patients or family caregiver for the first 4 weeks of treatment. Avoid alcohol; heavy alcohol intake may be associated with severe liver injury. Swallow capsule whole. Do not open or crush. It may take 2–4 weeks to achieve results. Can cause dizziness; use caution when driving or engaging in activities requiring alertness until response to drug is known.

PREPARATIONS

Delayed-release capsules: 20 mg, 30 mg, and 60 mg.

ERLOTINIB—Tarceva™

DESCRIPTION/ACTIONS

Erlotinib is a human epidermal growth factor receptor type 1/epidermal growth factor receptor (HER1/EGFR) tyrosine kinase inhibitor. Erlotinib inhibits the intracellular phosphorylation of tyrosine kinase associated with the EGFR. EGFR is expressed on the cell surface of normal and cancer cells. Erlotinib is indicated for the treatment of patients with locally advanced or metastatic nonsmall cell lung cancer after failure of at least one prior chemotherapy regimen.

PRECAUTIONS/ADVERSE REACTIONS

Erlotinib is contraindicated in patients hypersensitive to erlotinib or any component of the formulation. **Warning:** Reports of infrequent serious interstitial lung disease (ILD), including fatalities, have occurred. If onset of new or progressive, unexplained pulmonary symptoms such as dyspnea, cough, or fever occur, therapy should be interrupted. If ILD is diagnosed, erlotinib should be discontinued. Pregnancy Category D. Erlotinib has been shown to cause maternal toxicity associated with embryo/fetal lethality and abortion in rabbits. Asymptomatic increases in liver transaminases have been observed; monitor periodic liver function. If changes are severe, dose reduction or interruption of erlotinib should be considered. Bleeding and international normalized ratio (INR) elevations have been reported; monitor patients taking warfarin or other coumarin-derivative anticoagulants regularly for changes in prothrombin time or INR. The safety and effectiveness in pediatric patients have not been studied. The most common adverse reactions were rash and diarrhea.

ADMINISTRATION

Initial dose: 150 mg/day. Take at least 1 hour before or 2 hours after the ingestion of food. Continue until disease progression or unacceptable toxicity occurs.

Dose modifications: Patients with severe diarrhea who are unresponsive to loperamide or who become dehydrated may require a dose reduction or temporary interruption of therapy. Patients with severe skin reactions and severe liver function changes may require a dose reduction or temporary interruption of therapy. Dose reductions should be made in 50 mg decrements.

PATIENT CARE IMPLICATIONS

Take on an empty stomach. Sedation is common. Patients should use caution when engaging in activities that require alertness. Patients should seek medical advice promptly if they have severe or persistent diarrhea, nausea, anorexia, or vomiting; if there is an onset or worsening of unexplained shortness of breath or cough and eye irritation. Women should be advised to have adequate contraceptive methods during treatment and for 2 weeks after treatment has been completed.

PREPARATIONS

Tablet, film coated: 25 mg, 100 mg, and 150 mg.

ESZOPICLONE—Lunesta™

DESCRIPTION/ACTIONS

Eszopiclone is a nonbenzodiazepine hypnotic agent. The precise mechanism of action as a hypnotic is unknown, but its effect is believed to result from its interaction with GABA-receptor complexes at binding domains located close to or allosterically coupled to benzodiazepine receptors. Eszopiclone is indicated for the treatment of insomnia, such as difficulty falling asleep, maintaining sleep during the night, and waking up too early in the morning. This hypnotic agent, unlike other sleeping medications, did not develop tolerance over 6 months of use.

PRECAUTIONS/ADVERSE REACTIONS

Eszopiclone is contraindicated in patients hypersensitive to eszopiclone or any component of the formulation. Because sleep disturbances may be the presenting manifestation of a physical and/or psychiatric disorder, symptomatic treatment of insomnia should be initiated only after a careful evaluation of the patient. Failure of insomnia to resolve after 7–10 days of treatment may indicate psychiatric and/or medical illness. Worsening of insomnia or the emergence of new thinking or behavior abnormalities may be the consequence of an unrecognized psychiatric or physical disorder. Administer with caution to patients exhibiting signs and symptoms of depression. Suicidal tendencies may be present in such patients, and protective measures may be required. Intentional overdose is more common in this group of patients. **Warning:** In primarily depressed patients, worsening of depression, including suicidal thinking, has been reported in association with the use of sedatives/hypnotics. Use caution in patients with a history of drug dependence; the risk increases with dose and duration of treatment. Use with caution with concomitant use of other psychoactive drugs and CNS depressants; effects of other sedative drugs or ethanol may be potentiated. Abrupt discontinuation may lead to withdrawal symptoms. Use caution in patients with respiratory compromise, hepatic dysfunction, or those taking strong CYP3A4 inhibitors. Safety and efficacy in children below the age of 18 have not been established. Pregnancy Category C. No adequate or well-controlled studies in pregnant women; use only if clearly needed. Most common adverse effects were headache, viral infections, dry mouth, nausea, somnolence, dizziness, unpleasant taste, rash, nervousness, vomiting, and urinary tract infection.

ADMINISTRATION

Adults, initial: 2 mg before bedtime. May be increased to 3 mg if indicated.

Concurrent use with strong CYP3A4 inhibitor: 1 mg before bedtime. If needed may be increased to 2 mg.

Elderly: *Difficulty falling asleep:* 1 mg before bedtime. May be increased to 2 mg.

Difficulty staying asleep: 2 mg before bedtime.

Dosage adjustment in severe hepatic impairment: 1 mg before bedtime.

PATIENT CARE IMPLICATIONS

Due to drowsiness or dizziness, and eszopiclone's rapid onset of action, eszopiclone should be taken right before bedtime to prevent accidental injuries. Taking a sedative/hypnotic while still up and about may result in short-term memory impairment, hallucinations, impaired coordination, dizziness, and light-headedness. Take immediately prior to bedtime or after patient has gone to bed and is having difficulty falling asleep. A person may not remember what has happened for several hours after taking the medicine. Memory problems can be avoided if you take eszopiclone only when you are able to have a full night of sleep.

Do not take with or following a high-fat meal; this slows absorption. Inform patients that they may have next-day sleepiness and to use extreme care while doing anything that requires complete alertness. Do not drink alcohol; alcohol can increase side effects. Inform patient withdrawal symptoms may occur when medication is stopped suddenly after being used daily for a long time. Some people using sleep medications have experienced unusual changes in their thinking and/or behavior. If you or your family notices any changes in your behavior, or if you have any unusual or disturbing thoughts, call your physician immediately. Do not increase the prescribed dose unless instructed by your doctor. You may have more sleeping problems the first night or two after stopping eszopiclone. Do not crush or break tablet.

PREPARATIONS

Tablets (film coated): 1 mg, 2 mg, and 3 mg.
Schedule IV controlled substance.

HYALURONIDASE BOVINE—Amphadase™
DESCRIPTION/ACTIONS

Hyaluronidase bovine is a preparation of purified bovine testicular hyaluronidase, a protein enzyme. Hyaluronidase bovine is a diffusing substance that modifies the permeability of connective tissue through the hydrolysis of hyaluronic acid, a polysaccharide found in connective tissue that resists diffusion of liquids through tissue. Hyaluronidase bovine hydrolyzes hyaluronic acid, decreasing the viscosity of the cellular cement, and promotes distribution and absorption of locally injected substances. Hyaluronidase bovine is approved to increase the absorption and dispersion of other injected drugs, and for hypodermoclysis and as an adjunct in subcutaneous urography for improving resorption of radiopaque agents. Hypodermoclysis is useful in dehydrated patients who have minimal oral intake and IV access is a problem.

PRECAUTIONS/ADVERSE REACTIONS

Hyaluronidase bovine is contraindicated in patients hypersensitive to hyaluronidase or any ingredient in the formulation. **Warning:** Do not use to enhance the absorption and dispersion of dopamine and/or alpha agonist drugs. Do not inject into or around an infected or acutely inflamed area due to the danger of spreading localized infection. Do not use to reduce swelling of bites or stings due to risk of spreading toxin, and venom from insect stings may include hyaluronidase allergens. Do not apply directly to the cornea. Do not use for intravenous injections because the enzyme is rapidly inactivated. When considering administration of any drug with hyaluronidase bovine, consult appropriate references to determine usual precautions for use of the other drug. Furosemide, benzodiazepines, and phenytoin have been found to be incompatible with hyaluronidase bovine. When hyaluronidase bovine is added to a local anesthetic agent, it hastens the onset of analgesia and tends to reduce the swelling caused by local infiltration. The wider spread of the local anesthetic solution increases its absorption; this shortens its duration of action and tends to increase the incidence of systemic reaction. Patients receiving large doses of salicyclates, cortisone, ACTH, estrogens, or antihistamines may require larger amounts of hyaluronidase bovine for equivalent dispersing effect, as these drugs render tissues partly resistant to the action of hyaluronidase bovine. Pregnancy Category C. No adequate and well-controlled studies have been conducted in women, or with animals. Use only if clearly needed. Most common adverse effects were local injection site reactions and edema (associated with hypodermoclysis).

ADMINISTRATION

Skin test: For hypersensitivity to hyaluronidase bovine. Intradermal injection of 0.02 mL (3 units) of a 150 unit/mL solution. A positive reaction consists of a wheal with pseudopods appearing within 5 minutes and persisting for 20–30 minutes and accompanied by localized itching.

Hypodermoclysis: Subcutaneous, 150 units will facilitate absorption of 1,000 mL or more of solution.

Premature infants and neonates: Do not exceed 25 mL/kg. Rate should not be >2 mL per minute.

Infants and children <3 years of age: Volume of a single clysis should be limited to 200 mL.

Children ≥3 years of age and adults: Rate and volume of a single clysis should not exceed those employed for intravenous infusion.

Subcutaneous urography: 75 units subcutaneously over each scapula, followed by injection of the contrast medium at the same sites.

PATIENT CARE IMPLICATIONS

Report immediately any unusual skin rash, pain, redness, or swelling at or around injection site, swelling of mouth or lips, difficulty breathing, or onset of sudden dizziness.

PREPARATIONS

Injection: 150 units/mL (2 mL) vial. Store at 2–8°C (36–46° F). Do not freeze. Not recommended for IV use.

HYALURONIDASE OVINE—VITRASE®

DESCRIPTION/ACTIONS

Hyaluronidase ovine is a preparation of purified ovine testicular hyaluronidase, a protein enzyme. Hyaluronidase ovine is a diffusing substance that modifies the permeability of connective tissue through the hydrolysis of hyaluronic acid, a polysaccharide found in connective tissue that resists diffusion of liquid through tissue. Hyaluronidase ovine decreases the viscosity of the cellular cement and promotes diffusion of injected fluids or of localized transudates, or exudates and facilitates their absorption. Hyaluronidase ovine is indicated as an adjuvant to increase absorption and dispersion of other injected drugs; for hypodermoclysis and as an adjunct in subcutaneous urography for improving resorption of radiopaque agents.

PRECAUTIONS/ADVERSE REACTIONS

Hyaluronidase ovine is contraindicated in persons hypersensitive to hyaluronidase ovine or any ingredient in the formulation. **Warning:** Hyaluronidase ovine should not be used to enhance the absorption and dispersion of dopamine and/or alpha agonist drugs. Do not inject into or around an infected or acutely inflamed area because of the danger of spreading a localized infection. Do not use to reduce the swelling of bites or stings. Do not apply directly to the cornea. Hyaluronidase ovine should not be used for IV injection because it is rapidly inactivated. Consult appropriate references first to determine usual precautions for the use of the other drug when considering the administration of another drug with hyaluronidase ovine. Furosemide, benzodiazepines, and phenytoin have been found to be incompatible. When added to a local anesthetic agent, it hastens the onset of analgesia and tends to reduce the swelling caused by local infiltration. The wider spread of the local anesthetic solution increases its absorption, but shortens its duration of action and tends to increase the incidence of systemic reactions. Patients receiving large doses of salicylates, cortisone, ACTH, estrogens, or antihistamines may require larger amounts of hyaluronidase ovine for equivalent dispersing effect because these drugs render tissues partly resistant to the action of hyaluronidase ovine. Pregnancy Category C. No adequate and well-controlled studies in pregnant women or animals; use only if clearly needed. Most common side effects were local injection site reactions.

ADMINISTRATION

Skin test: Intradermal 0.02 mL (3 units) of a 150 unit/mL solution. Positive reactions consist of a wheal with pseudopods appearing within 5 minutes and persisting for 20–30 minutes with localized itching.

Hypodermoclysis: Subcutaneous: 15 units added to each 100 mL of IV fluid to be administered.

Premature infants and neonates: Volume of a single clysis should not exceed 25 mL/kg. Rate should not exceed 2 mL/minute.

Children <3 years of age: Volume of a single clysis should not exceed 200 mL.

Children ≥3 years old and adults: Rate and volume of a single clysis should not exceed those used for IV infusion.

Subcutaneous urography: 75 units subcutaneously over each scapula, followed by injection of the contrast medium at the same sites.

Hyaluronidase ovine is reconstituted to a concentration of 1000 units/mL by adding 6.2 ml of NS to the vial. Prior to administration, the reconstituted solution should be further diluted to desired concentrations.

For 50 units/mL, draw up 0.05 mL of (1000 units/mL) and add 0.95 mL of NS.

For 75 units/mL, draw up 0.075 mL of (1000 units/mL) and add 0.925 mL of NS.

For 150 units/mL, draw up 0.15 mL of (1000 units/mL) and add 0.85 mL of NS.

For 300 units/mL, draw up 0.3 mL of (1000 units/mL) and add 0.7 mL of NS.

Compatible with D5W, NS, and LR.

PATIENT CARE IMPLICATIONS

Report immediately any unusual pain, redness, swelling at or around injection site, difficulty breathing, or any unusual symptoms.

PREPARATIONS

Lyophilized, powder for reconstitution: 6200 units/vial. Protect from light. Store unopened vial in refrigerator at 2–8°C (36–46°F). After reconstitution, store at room temperature and use within 6 hours.

ILOPROST—Ventavis®
DESCRIPTION/ACTIONS

Iloprost is a synthetic analogue of prostacyclin PGI_2. Iloprost dilates systemic and pulmonary arterial vascular beds. It also affects platelet aggregation. It is indicated for the treatment of pulmonary arterial hypertension (WHO Group 1) in patients with NYHA Class III or IV symptoms.

PRECAUTIONS/ADVERSE REACTIONS

Iloprost is contraindicated in patients with a known hypersensitivity to it or to any component of the formulation. Iloprost is intended for inhalation administration only via the Prodose® AAD® System. May cause syncope, so vital signs should be monitored while initiating iloprost. Therapy should not be initiated in patients with systolic blood pressure less than 85 mm Hg. If signs of pulmonary edema occur during treatment, treatment should be stopped immediately as this may be a sign of pulmonary venous hypertension. Iloprost has not been evaluated in patients with chronic obstructive pulmonary disease (COPD), severe asthma, or acute pulmonary infections. Iloprost has the potential to increase the hypotensive effects of vasodilators and antihypertensive agents. Because iloprost inhibits platelet aggregation there is a potential for increased risk of bleeding when coadministered with anticoagulants. Pregnancy Category C. No adequate and well-controlled studies in pregnant women. Excretion in human breast milk is unknown. Safety and efficacy in pediatric patients have not been established. Most common adverse events noted in patients treated with iloprost include vasodilation (flushing), cough, headache, trismus, insomnia, nausea, hypotension, vomiting, increased alkaline phosphatase, flu syndrome, back pain, tongue pain, palpitations, syncope, increased GGT, muscle cramps, hemoptysis, and pneumonia. Serious adverse events reported during treatment with iloprost include congestive heart failure, chest pain, supraventricular tachycardia, dyspnea, peripheral edema, and kidney failure.

ADMINISTRATION

Adults: Inhalation: Initial 2.5 mcg/dose. If tolerated, dose may be increased to 5 mcg/dose 6 to 9 times per day during waking hours (no more than every 2 hours). Maximum daily dose in clinical trials 45 mcg/day. Inhalation via Prodose® AAD® System. Mixing with other medications in the Prodose® AAD® System is not recommended. For each inhalation dose, the entire contents of one opened ampule of Ventavis® should be transferred into the Prodose® AAD® System. Dosage adjustment for hepatic impairment: use caution. *Dosage adjustment for renal impairment*: not necessary—use caution treating patients on dialysis.

PATIENT CARE IMPLICATIONS

Patients should be trained in the proper administration technique including dosing frequency, ampule dispensing, Prodose® AAD® System operation, and equipment cleaning. Patients should be advised that they might have a fall in blood pressure, and they might become dizzy or even faint. Patients should be instructed to stand up slowly when they get out of a chair or bed.

PREPARATIONS

Inhalation solution, 20 mcg iloprost per 2 mL ampule.

IMMUNE GLOBULIN INTRAVENOUS—Octagam®

DESCRIPTION/ACTIONS

Octagam® is a solvent/detergent-treated, sterile 5% liquid preparation of highly purified immunoglobulin G (IgG) derived from large pools of human plasma. Human plasma units used in the manufacture of Octagam® are provided by FDA-approved blood collection establishments, and are tested by FDA-licensed serological tests for HBsAg, antibodies to HCV and HIV-1, and Nucleic Acid Test (NAT) for HCV and HIV-1. Octagam® is indicated for the treatment of primary immune deficient diseases (congenital agammaglobulinemia and hypogammaglobulinemia, common variable immunodeficiency, Wiskoff-Aldrich syndrome, and severe combined immunodeficiencies.

PRECAUTIONS/ADVERSE REACTIONS

Octagam® is contraindicated in persons hypersensitive to immune globulin or any component of the formulation and in individuals who have intolerance to homologous immunoglobulins, especially in very rare cases of immunoglobulin A (IgA) deficiency, when the patient has IgE mediated antibodies to IgA. **Warning:** Immune Globulin Intravenous (IGIV) products have been known to be associated with renal dysfunction, acute renal failure, osmotic nephrosis, and death. Patients predisposed to acute renal failure include those with any degree of preexisting renal insufficiency, diabetes, older than 65 years of age, volume depletion, sepsis, paraproteinemia, or patients receiving known nephrotoxic drugs. IGIV products in these patients should be administered at the minimum concentration and the minimum rate of infusion. Periodic monitoring of renal function tests and urine output suggested. Immediate anaphylactic and hypersensitivity reactions are a possibility; epinephrine should be available. Because the product is made from human blood, it may carry a risk of transmitting infectious agents. All infections thought to have been transmitted by the product should be reported to Octapharma Pharmaceuticals. Aseptic meningitis syndrome (AMS) has been reported. Discontinuation of treatment has resulted in remission of AMS within several days after sequelae. AMS usually begins within several hours to 2 days following IGIV treatment with symptoms of severe headache, nuchal rigidity, drowsiness, fever, photophobia, painful eye movements, nausea, and vomiting. Patients exhibiting these signs and symptoms should receive a thorough neurological examination, including CSF studies, to rule out other causes of meningitis. IGIV products can contain blood group antibodies that may act as hemolysins and induce coating of red blood cells with immunoglobulin, causing a positive direct antiglobulin reaction and rarely hemolysis. Hemolytic anemia can develop subsequent to IGIV therapy; recipients should be monitored for signs and symptoms of hemolysis. Noncardiogenic pulmonary edema (Transfusion-Related Acute Lung Injury [TRALI]) has been reported. TRALI is characterized by severe respiratory distress, pulmonary edema, hypoxemia, normal L ventricular function, and fever. TRALI occurs within 1–6 hours after transfusion, and patients may be managed with oxygen therapy with adequate ventilatory support. Monitor patients for pulmonary adverse reactions. If TRALI is suspected, tests should be performed for the presence of anti-neutrophil antibodies in both the product and the patient's serum. Thrombotic events have been reported. Patients at risk may include those with a history of atherosclerosis, multiple cardiovascular risk factors, advanced age, impaired cardiac output, and/or suspected hyperviscosity. Baseline assessment of blood viscosity should be considered in patients at risk for hyperviscosity, including those with cryoglobulins, fasting chylomicronemia/markedly high triglycerides, or monoclonal gammopathies. Antibodies in Octagam® may interfere with the response to live viral vaccines, such as measles, mumps, and rubella. Administration of live vaccines should be given 3 or more months from the time of IGIV administration. Pregnancy Category C. No studies performed on animals. Give only if clearly needed. Most common adverse reactions were minor, such as headache, chills, backache, chest pain, fever, allergic reaction, arthralgia, dizziness, change in blood pressure, cutaneous reactions, and/or nausea and vomiting.

ADMINISTRATION

Primary immunodeficiency diseases: 300–600 mg/kg every 3–4 weeks. A 5% solution should initially be infused at a rate of 30 mg/kg/hr for the first 30 minutes; if tolerated, advance to 60 mg/kg/hr for the second 30 minutes; and if further tolerated, advance to 120 mg/kg/hr for the third 30 minutes. Thereafter, the infusion can be maintained at a rate up to, but not exceeding 200 mg/kg/hr. For patients at risk for developing renal dysfunction reduce infusion at a maximum rate less than 0.07 ml/kg/minute. Do not mix with IGIV from other manufacturers. Octagam® should be at room temperature when administered.

PATIENT CARE IMPLICATIONS

Patient to be monitored closely during infusion; report chills, chest pain, tightness, rapid heartbeat, acute back pain, respiratory difficulty, decreased urine output, sudden weight gain, and fluid retention.

PREPARATIONS

Injection, solution: 1 gm, 2.5 gm, 5 gm, and 10 gm single-use bottles. Store at 2–8°C (36–46°F) for 24 months or at temperature not exceeding 25°C (77°F) for 18 months from the date of manufacture.

LANTHANUM CARBONATE—Fosrenol™

DESCRIPTION/ACTIONS

Lanthanum (La) is a naturally occurring rare earth element. Fosrenol™ inhibits absorption of phosphate by forming highly insoluble lanthanum phosphate complexes, consequently reducing both serum phosphate and calcium phosphate product. It is indicated to reduce serum phosphate in patients with end-stage renal disease.

PRECAUTIONS/ADVERSE REACTIONS

Lanthanum is contraindicated in patients with a known hypersensitivity to it or to any component of the formulation. Caution should be used in using Fosrenol™ in patients with acute peptic ulcer, ulcerative colitis, Crohn's disease, or bowel obstruction as these patients were not included in clinical trials. Lanthanum is not metabolized and is not a substrate of the cytochrome P450 (CYP450) enzyme system. There is no evidence that Fosrenol™ forms insoluble complexes with warfarin, digoxin, furosemide, phenytoin, metoprolol, and enalapril. Compounds known to interact with antacids should not be taken within 2 hours of dosing with Fosrenol™. Pregnancy Category C. No adequate and well-controlled studies in pregnant women. Excretion in human breast milk is unknown. Not recommended for use in pediatric patients. Most common adverse effects observed in patients receiving lanthanum carbonate were nausea, vomiting, diarrhea, hypotension, rhinitis, headache, abdominal pain, constipation, bronchitis, and hypercalcemia.

ADMINISTRATION

Adults: oral 750–1500 mg daily in divided dosing, taken with meals. Tablets should be chewed completely before swallowing. Dosing changes should be made every 2–3 weeks until an acceptable serum phosphate level is reached. Doses are generally titrated in increments of 750 mg per day.

PATIENT CARE IMPLICATIONS

Monitor serum phosphorus levels. Tablets should be taken with or immediately after meals. Tablets should be chewed completely before swallowing. Whole tablets should not be swallowed.

PREPARATIONS

Tablets, 250 mg and 500 mg.

PALIFERMIN—Kepivance™

DESCRIPTION/ACTIONS

Palifermin is a human keratinocyte growth factor (KGF) produced by recombinant DNA technology in *Escherichia coli* (*E. Coli*). Endogenous KGF is produced in response to epithelial tissue injury. Palifermin differs from endogenous human KGF in that the first 23N-terminal amino acids have been deleted to improve protein stability. The binding of KGF to its receptor has been reported to result in proliferation, differentiation, and migration of epithelial cells in many tissues including, but not limited to, the tongue, buccal mucosa, esophagus, stomach, and intestines. Palifermin is indicated to decrease the incidence and duration of severe oral mucositis in patients with hematologic malignancies receiving myelotoxic therapy requiring hematopoietic stem cell support. Safety and efficacy have not been established in patients with non-hematologic malignancies.

PRECAUTIONS/ADVERSE REACTIONS

Palifermin is contraindicated in patients with known hypersensitivity to E. coli-derived proteins, palifermin, or any component of the formulation. **Warning:** Patients should be informed of the evidence of tumor growth and stimulation in animal models. Heparin has been shown to bind with palifermin in vitro. If heparin is used to maintain an IV line, saline should be used to rinse the line prior to and after palifermin. Administration within 24 hours of chemotherapy resulted in increased severity and duration of oral mucositis. Pregnancy Category C. Shown to be embryotoxic in rabbits and rats. No adequate and well-controlled studies in pregnant women; use only if the potential benefit to the mother justifies the potential risk to the fetus. Safety and effectiveness in pediatrics have not been established. Most common adverse reactions were skin rash, erythema, edema, pruritis, dysesthesia, tongue discoloration, tongue thickening, alteration of taste, pain, arthralgias, elevated serum lipase and amylase levels (reversible and didn't require treatment intervention). As with all therapeutic proteins there is a potential for immunogenicity. None of the samples had evidence of neutralizing activity in a cell-based assay.

ADMINISTRATION

Do not administer within 24 hours of chemotherapy.

Adults: IV: 60 mcg/kg/day for 3 consecutive days before and after myelotoxic therapy. Total of 6 doses. The third dose of premyelotoxic therapy should be given 24–48 hours before myelotoxic therapy begins. The first of the last 3 doses should be administered on the same day of (but after) hematopoietic stem cell infusion. Administer by IV bolus. Once vial is reconstituted with sterile water do not shake or vigorously agitate the vial. Do not filter. Use immediately once reconstituted. May be stored refrigerated in its carton for up to 24 hours. Allow to reach room temperature for a maximum of 1 hour and protect from light at this time. Discard if left at room temperature for more than 1 hour. Do not freeze reconstituted solution.

PATIENT CARE IMPLICATIONS

Inform of muco-cutaneous adverse effects and about the evidence of tumor growth and stimulation in animal studies.

PREPARATIONS

Injection, powder for reconstitution (preservative free): 6.25 mg. Refrigerate at 2–8°C (36–46°F). Keep vials in carton. Protect from light.

PEGAPTANIB—Macugen®
DESCRIPTION/ACTIONS

Pegaptanib is a vascular endothelial growth factor (VEGF) antagonist. VEGF induces angiogenesis and increases vascular permeability and inflammation, which are thought to contribute to the progression of the neovascular (wet) form of age-related macular degeneration (AMD). Pegaptanib binds to extracellular VEGF, which inhibits VEGF binding to its VEGF receptors, which then suppresses pathological ocular neovascularization. Pegaptanib is indicated for the treatment of neovascular (wet) age-related macular degeneration, a leading cause of blindness.

PRECAUTIONS/ADVERSE REACTIONS

Pegaptanib is contraindicated in persons hypersensitive to pegaptanib or any components of the formulation and in patients with ocular or periocular infections. **Warning:** Intravitreous injections have been associated with endophthalmitis. Proper aseptic injection technique should be used. Patients should be monitored during the week following injection. Increases in intraocular pressure (IOP) have been seen within 30 minutes of injection. IOP as well as the perfusion of the optic nerve head should be monitored. Pregnancy Category B. There are no studies in pregnant women. Use during pregnancy only if the potential benefit to the mother justifies the potential risk to the fetus. The most frequent adverse reactions were blurred vision, anterior chamber inflammation, cataract, conjunctival hemorrhage, corneal edema, eye discharge and irritation, eye pain, hypertension, increased IOP, reduced visual acuity, vitreous floaters, and vitreous opacities.

ADMINISTRATION

Adults: AMD: 0.3 mg every 6 weeks by intravitreous injection into the eye to be treated. The safety and efficacy of administration to both eyes concurrently have not been studied. Safety and efficacy have not been established with hepatic impairment or in patients requiring hemodialysis. Procedure should be carried out under controlled aseptic conditions. Adequate anesthesia and a broad-spectrum microbicide should be given prior to the injection.

PATIENT CARE IMPLICATIONS

Patients are at risk of endophthalmitis in the days following pegaptanib administration. Report immediately if eyes become red, sensitive to light, painful, or if a change in vision develops.

PREPARATIONS

Injection, solution (preservative free): 0.3 mg/90 μL (prefilled syringe). Store in refrigerator at 2–8°C (36–46°F). Do not freeze or shake vigorously.

PEMETREXED—ALIMTA®
DESCRIPTION/ACTIONS

Pemetrexed is an antifolate antineoplastic agent that exerts its action by disrupting folate-dependent metabolic processes essential for cell replication. Pemetrexed inhibits thymidylate synthase (TS), dihydrofolate reductase (DHFR), glycenamide ribonucleotide formyltransferase (GARFT), all folate-dependent enzymes involved in folate metabolism, and DNA synthesis. Pemetrexed in combination with cisplatin is indicated for the treatment of patients with malignant pleural mesothelioma whose disease is unresectable or who are otherwise not candidates for curative surgery. Pemetrexed as a single agent is indicated for the treatment of patients with locally advanced or metastatic nonsmall-cell lung cancer after prior chemotherapy.

PRECAUTIONS/ADVERSE REACTIONS

Pemetrexed is contraindicated in patients hypersensitive to pemetrexed or any component of the formulation. Skin rash reported frequently in patients not pretreated with a corticosteroid; pretreatment with dexamethasone has reduced the incidence and severity of cutaneous reaction. Pemetrexed suppresses bone marrow function; patients should be instructed to take folic acid and vitamin B_{12} as a prophylactic measure to reduce treatment-related hematologic and GI toxicity. Neutropenia, febrile neutropenia, and infection were reported less when folic acid and vitamin B_{12} pretreatment was administered. Pemetrexed is primarily eliminated unchanged by renal excretion; therefore, do not administer to patients whose creatinine clearance is <45 mL/minute. Concomitant administration of nephrotoxic drugs could result in delayed clearance of pemetrexed. Concomitant administration of drugs that are tubularly secreted (probenecid) could possibly result in delayed clearance of pemetrexed. Use caution when administering ibuprofen concurrently to patients with mild to moderate renal insufficiency. Patients with mild-to-moderate renal insufficiency should avoid taking NSAIDs with short elimination half-lives (ibuprofen, indomethacin, ketoprofen, ketorolac) for 2 days before, the day of, and 2 days following pemetrexed administration. All patients should stop taking NSAIDs with long half-lives (naproxen, piroxicam) 5 days before, the day of, and 2 days following pemetrexed. Pregnancy Category D; fetotoxic and teratogenic in mice. Most common adverse effects were hematologic effects, fever, infection, stomatitis, pharyngitis, and rash.

ADMINISTRATION

Malignant pleural mesothelioma with cisplatin: 500 mg/m², IV infusion over 10 minutes on day 1 of each 21-day cycle.

Nonsmall-cell lung cancer: 500 mg/m², IV infusion over 10 minutes on day 1 of each 21-day cycle.

Reconstitute and further dilute with NS. Incompatible with diluents containing calcium, LR, Ringers. Corticosteroids should be given twice a day, the day before, the day of, and the day after pemetrexed administration. To reduce toxicity, patients should take 400 μg of folic acid daily for 5 doses during the 7-day period preceding the first dose of pemetrexed and should continue during the full course of therapy and for 21 days after the last dose of pemetrexed. Patients should receive one IM injection of vitamin B_{12} during the week prior to the first dose of pemetrexed and every 3 cycles thereafter. Patients should not begin a new cycle unless the ANC is ≥1500 cells/mm³, the platelet count is ≥100,000 cells/mm³, and creatinine clearance is ≥45 mL/minute.

Dosage adjustment for toxicities:

Hematologic toxicity: Upon recovery, reinitiate.

If nadir ANC <500/mm³ and nadir platelets ≥50,000/mm³, give 75% of previous dose (both drugs).

If nadir platelets <50,000/mm3 regardless of nadir ANC, give 50% of previous dose (both drugs).

Nonhematologic toxicity (excluding neurotoxicity or ≥grade 3 transaminase elevations): Upon recovery, reinitiate therapy.

If grade 3 or 4 toxicity, except mucositis, give 75% of previous dose (both drugs).

If there is any diarrhea requiring hospitalization, give 75% of previous dose (both drugs).

If grade 3 or 4 mucositis, give 50% of previous pemetrexed dose and 100% of previous cisplatin dose.

Neurotoxicity:

If common toxicity criteria (CTC) grade 0–1, continue at previous dose of both drugs.

If CTC grade 2, continue at previous dose of pemetrexed and 50% of previous cisplatin dose.

Therapy should be discontinued if a patient experiences any hematologic or nonhematologic grade 3 or 4 toxicity after 2 dose reductions (except grade 3 transaminase elevations) or immediately if grade 3 or 4 neurotoxicity is observed.

Renally impaired patients: Do not give to patients whose creatinine clearance is <45 mL/minute.

PATIENT CARE IMPLICATIONS

Report immediately any burning, pain, itching, difficulty breathing, chest or back pain, fever, chills, diarrhea, and unusual fatigue. CBC, serum creatinine, bilirubin, ALT, and AST monitoring needed.

PREPARATIONS

Injection, powder for reconstitution: 500 mg. Reconstituted and infusion solutions stable for 24 hours after initial reconstitution, when stored refrigerated.

RIFAXIMIN—Xifaxan™

DESCRIPTION/ACTIONS

Rifaximin is a semi-synthetic, nonsystemic antibiotic. It is a structural analog of rifampin. It acts by binding to the beta-subunit of bacterial DNA–dependent RNA polymerase, resulting in inhibition of bacterial RNA synthesis. It is indicated for the treatment of patients (≥12 years of age) with traveler's diarrhea caused by noninvasive strains of *Escherichia coli* (enterotoxigenic and enteroaggregative strains).

PRECAUTIONS/ADVERSE REACTIONS

Rifaximin is contraindicated in patients with a known hypersensitivity to it, any of the rifamycin antimicrobial agents, or to any component of the formulation. Rifaximin is not suitable for treating systemic bacterial infections. Rifaximin is not effective in treating patients with diarrhea complicated by fever and/or blood in the stool or diarrhea due to pathogens other than *E. coli*. Rifaximin is not effective in treating traveler's diarrhea caused by *Campylobacter jejuni*. The effectiveness of rifaximin in treating traveler's diarrhea caused by *Shigella spp.* and *Salmonella spp.* has not been proven. Rifaximin should be discontinued if diarrhea symptoms get worse or persist more than 24–48 hours and alternative antibiotics should be considered. Pseudomembranous colitis may occur. Rifaximin was found to be an inducer of CYP450 3A4 (CYP3A4). Pregnancy Category C. No adequate or well-controlled studies in pregnant women. Excretion in human breast milk is unknown. Safety and efficacy in pediatric patients less than 12 years of age have not been established. Most common adverse events observed in patients treated with rifaximin include headache, abdominal pain, rectal tenesmus, constipation, pyrexia, and vomiting. Post marketing events noted include hypersensitivity reactions including allergic dermatitis, rash, angioedema, urticaria, and pruritis.

ADMINISTRATION

Oral: 200 mg three times a day for 3 days.

PATIENT CARE IMPLICATIONS

Tablets may be taken with or without food. Rifaximin should be discontinued and patients should seek medical care if diarrhea lasts more than 24–48 hours or worsens, or if they have fever and/or blood in the stool.

PREPARATIONS

Tablets, 200 mg.

SOLIFENACIN SUCCINATE—Vesicare®

DESCRIPTION/ACTIONS

Solifenacin is an anticholinergic agent; it competes with muscarinic receptors. Muscarinic receptors play a relevant role in contraction of urinary bladder smooth muscle and stimulation of salivary secretion. Solifenacin is used in the treatment of overactive bladder with symptoms of urinary frequency, urgency, or urge incontinence.

PRECAUTIONS/ADVERSE REACTIONS

Solifenacin is contraindicated in persons hypersensitive to solifenacin or any component of the formulation and patients with urinary retention, gastric retention, and uncontrolled narrow-angle glaucoma. Use with caution in patients with decreased gastrointestinal motility, reduced renal function, bladder outflow obstruction, and in patients with controlled, narrow-angle glaucoma. The most common adverse effects were dry mouth, constipation, urinary tract infections, and blurred vision. Pregnancy risk factor C. There are no adequate and well-controlled studies in pregnant women. Solifenacin should be used during pregnancy only if the potential benefit justifies the potential risk to the fetus. Safety and effectiveness in pediatric patients have not been established.

ADMINISTRATION

Dose: 5 mg once daily. If well tolerated, may increase to 10 mg/day.

Adjustment for renal impairment: For patients with severe renal impairment (Clcr <30 mL/minute), daily dose should not exceed 5 mg.

Adjustment in hepatic impairment: For patients with moderate hepatic impairment, dose not to exceed 5 mg. For severe hepatic impairment, use is not recommended.

Adjustment with CYP3A4 inhibitors: Ciprofloxacin, erythromycin, isoniazid, protease inhibitors, doxycycline, azole antifungals may increase levels/effects of solifenacin. Dose should not exceed 5mg/day.

Adjustment with CYP3A4 inducers: Carbamazapine, phenobarbital, phenytoin, nafcillin may decrease the levels/effects of solifenacin.

PATIENT CARE IMPLICATIONS

Swallow tablet whole. Take with liquids. May take without regard to food. Patient should be informed that solifenacin is associated with constipation and blurred vision. Patients should contact their physician if they experience severe abdominal pain or become constipated for 3 or more days. Advise patient to exercise caution in decisions to engage in potentially dangerous activities until the drug's effect on the patient's vision has been determined. Heat prostration due to decreased sweating can occur; use caution in hot weather, drink plenty of fluids, reduce exercise activity.

PREPARATIONS

Tablet, 5 mg and 10 mg.

TELITHROMYCIN—KETEK®

DESCRIPTION/ACTIONS

Telithromycin belongs to a new class of antibacterial agents known as ketolides which are structurally related to the macrolide class of antibiotics. In vitro, telithromycin has been shown to demonstrate concentration-dependent bactericidal activity against *Streptococcus pneumoniae* (including multidrug resistant isolates [MDRSP]). Telithromycin blocks protein synthesis by binding to domains II and μ of 23S rRNA of the 50S ribosomal subunit. Telithromycin has been shown to be active (both in vitro and in clinical settings) against *Staphylococcus aureus* (methicillin and erythromycin susceptible isolates only), *Streptococcus pneumoniae*, including MDRSP, *Haemophilus influenzae*, *Moraxella catarrhalis*, *Chlamydia pneumoniae*, and *Mycoplasma pneumoniae*. Telithromycin has been shown to be active against the following organisms in vitro: *Streptococcus pyogenes*, *Streptococci (Lancefield groups C and G)*, *Viridans group streptococci*, *Prevotella bivia*, *Prevotella intermedia*, *Peptostreptococcus spp.*, and *Legionella pneumophila*. However, the safety and efficacy of telithromycin in treating clinical infections due to these microorganisms have not been established. It is indicated for the treatment of infections caused by susceptible strains of the designated microorganisms in the following conditions: Acute bacterial exacerbations of chronic bronchitis due to *Streptococcus pneumoniae*, *Haemophilus influenzae*, or *Moraxella catarrhalis*; acute bacterial sinusitis due to *Streptococcus pneumoniae*, *Haemophilus influenzae*, *Moraxella catarrhalis* or *Staphylococcus aureus*; community acquired pneumonia due to *Streptococcus pneumoniae* (including *MDRSP*), *Haemophilus influenzae*, *Moraxella catarrhalis*, *Chlamydia pneumoniae*, or *Mycoplasma pneumoniae*.

PRECAUTIONS/ADVERSE REACTIONS

Telithromycin is contraindicated in patients with a known hypersensitivity to it, any macrolide antibiotic, or any component of the formulation. Concomitant administration of telithromycin with cisapride or pimozide is contraindicated. Pseudomembranous colitis has been reported with nearly all antibacterial agents. Telithromycin has the potential to prolong the QTc interval. QTc prolongation may lead to an increased risk for ventricular arrhythmias including torsades de pointes. Use of telithromycin should be avoided in patients with congenital prolongation of the QTc interval, and in patients with ongoing proarrhythmic conditions such as uncorrected hypokalemia or hypomagnesemia, clinically significant bradycardia, and in patients receiving class IA (e.g., quinidine and procainamide), or class III (e.g., dofetilide) antiarrhythmic agents. Exacerbations of myasthenia gravis have been reported in patients treated with telithromycin. Telithromycin is not recommended in patients with myasthenia gravis unless no other therapeutic alternatives are available. Telithromycin may cause visual disturbances, including blurred vision, difficulty focusing, and diplopia. Hepatic dysfunction, including increased liver enzymes and hepatitis with or without jaundice, has been reported with the use of telithromycin. Telithromycin is a strong inhibitor of the cytochrome P450 3A4 system. Use of simvastatin, lovastatin, or atorvastatin concomitantly with telithromycin should be avoided due to an increased risk of myopathy. Concomitant administration of telithromycin and rifampin should be avoided. Concomitant administration of telithromycin and CYP3A4 inducers such as phenytoin, carbamazepine, or phenobarbital is likely to result in subtherapeutic levels of telithromycin. Coadministration of telithromycin and metoprolol in patients with heart failure should be considered with caution. Digoxin serum levels and side effects should be monitored when coadministered with telithromycin. Concomitant administration of telithromycin and midazolam may lead to increased levels of midazolam. Dosage adjustments may be warranted. Coadministration of telithromycin and theophylline resulted in the worsening of gastrointestinal side effects such as nausea and vomiting. It is recommended to space the doses of telithromycin and theophylline by at least 1 hour to decrease the likelihood of gastrointestinal side effects. Coadministration of telithromycin and sotalol resulted in decreased absorption of sotalol. Post marketing reports suggest that the coadministration of telithromycin and oral anticoagulants may result in the potentiation of the anticoagulant effect. Prothrombin times and INR should be monitored. No specific drug interaction studies have been done with telithromycin and the following drugs: carbamazepine, cyclosporine, tacrolimus, sirolimus, hexobarbital, and phenytoin. However, these drug interactions have been observed with macrolide antibiotics. Coadministration of these drugs with telithromycin may result in increases or prolongation of the therapeutic and or adverse effects. Coadministration of ergot derivatives and macrolides results in acute ergot toxicity characterized by severe peripheral vasospasm and dysesthesia. Without further data, the coadministration of telithromycin and these drugs is not recommended. Pregnancy Category C. No adequate or well-controlled studies in pregnant women. Telithromycin may be excreted in human breast milk. Use caution when administering to a nursing mother. Safety and efficacy in pediatric patients have not been established. Most common adverse reactions observed in patients treated with telithromycin include diarrhea, nausea, headache, dizziness, vomiting, loose stools, and dysgeusia. Other reported side effects occurring in $\geq 0.2\%$ and $<2\%$ of patients include abdominal distention, dyspepsia, gastrointestinal upset, flatulence, constipation, gastroenteritis, gastritis, anorexia, oral candidiasis, glossitis, stomatitis, abnormal liver function tests, hepatitis with or without jaundice, dry mouth, somnolence, insomnia, vertigo, increased sweating, abdominal pain, fatigue, blurred vision, diplopia or difficulty focusing, vaginal candidiasis, vaginitis, vaginosis fungal, rash, and increased platelet count. Other reported side effects occurring in $<0.2\%$ of patients treated with telithromycin include anxiety, bradycardia, eczema, elevated bilirubin, erythema multiforme, flushing, hypotension, increased blood alkaline phosphatase, increased eosinophil count, paresthesia, pruritis, and urticaria. Post marketing adverse events reported include face edema, severe allergic reactions including angioedema and anaphylaxis, atrial arrhythmias, rare reports of palpitations and pancreatitis, hepatic dysfunction, hepatocellular and/or cholestatic hepatitis with or without jaundice, muscle cramps, rare reports of exacerbation of myasthenia gravis, and rare reports of syncope usually associated with vagal syndrome.

ADMINISTRATION

Adults: Oral.

Acute bacterial exacerbations of chronic bronchitis: 800 mg once daily ×5 days.

Acute bacterial sinusitis: 800 mg once daily ×5 days.

Community acquired pneumonia: 800 mg once daily ×7–10 days.

Dosage adjustment for hepatic impairment: not necessary.

Dosage adjustment for renal impairment (creatinine clearance <30 mL/min) or patients on dialysis: dose of telithromycin has not been established.

PATIENT CARE IMPLICATIONS

Telithromycin may cause problems with vision. If visual problems occur, patients should avoid driving a motor vehicle, operating heavy machinery, or engaging in hazardous activities. Patients should be informed to report any fainting occurring during drug treatment. Patients should inform their physician of any personal or family history of QTc prolongation or proarrhythmic conditions such as uncorrected hypokalemia or hypomagnesemia. Patients should inform their physician if they have myasthenia gravis. Patients should be advised that simvastatin, lovastatin, and/or atorvastatin should be avoided in patients receiving telithromycin. If telithromycin is prescribed, therapy with simvastatin, lovastatin, or atorvastatin should be stopped during the course of treatment.

PREPARATIONS

Tablets, 400 mg.

TINIDAZOLE—TINDAMAX™

DESCRIPTION/ACTIONS

Tinidazole is a synthetic nitroimidazole antiprotozoal agent. In trichomonas, the free nitro group appears to interact with and damage protozoal DNA. The mechanism by which tinidazole exhibits activity against *Giardia* and *Entamoeba* species is not known. Tinidazole is indicated in the treatment of trichomoniasis caused by *T. vaginalis*; treatment of giardiasis caused by *G. duodenalis* (*G. lamblia*); treatment of intestinal amebiasis and amebic liver abscess caused by *E. histolytica.*

PRECAUTIONS/ADVERSE REACTIONS

Tinidazole is contraindicated in persons hypersensitive to tinidazole, other nitroimidazole derivatives, or any component of the formulation. Tinidazole is contraindicated during the first trimester of pregnancy. **Warning:** Convulsive seizures and peripheral neuropathy (mainly numbness or paresthesia of an extremity) have been reported with nitroimidazole drugs. Use with caution in patients with CNS diseases. Use with caution in patients with current or a history of blood dyscrasias; tinidazole may produce transient leukopenia and neutropenia. Use caution in patients with hepatic impairment. Patients with severe hepatic disease metabolize nitroimidazoles slowly, resulting in accumulation of drug in plasma. Pregnancy risk factor C; benefits of use should outweigh possible risks. Tinidazole crosses the placenta and enters the fetal circulation. Breast-feeding should be discontinued during therapy and for 3 days after the last dose. The most common adverse effects were metallic/bitter taste, nausea, anorexia, dyspepsia, cramps, epigastric discomfort, weakness, and fatigue. Safety and effectiveness in pediatric patients younger than 3 years of age have not been established.

ADMINISTRATION

Trichomoniasis: Both female and males, a single 2 gm dose. Because trichomoniasis is a STD, with potentially serious sequelae, sexual partners should be treated simultaneously in order to prevent reinfection.

Giardiasis: Adults: A single 2 gm dose. Pediatrics older than 3 years of age: A single 50 mg/kg dose (up to 2 gm).

Amebiasis, intestinal: Adults, 2 gm per day for 3 days. Pediatrics older than 3 years of age: 50 mg/kg/day (up to 2 gm per day).

Amebic liver abscess: Adults: 2 gm per day for 3–5 days. Pediatrics older than 3 years of age: 50 mg/kg/day (up to 2 gm/day) for 3–5 days. Children should be closely monitored when treatment durations exceed 3 days.

Hemodialysis: During hemodialysis, tinidazole clearance is increased. Approximately 43% of the amount present in the body is eliminated during a 6–hour hemodialysis session. An additional dose of tinidazole equivalent to one-half of the recommended dose should be administered after the end of hemodialysis.

Hepatic impairment: Specific recommendations are not available; use with caution.

PATIENT CARE IMPLICATIONS

Take with food to minimize the incidence of epigastric discomfort and other side effects. Avoid ethanol during treatment and for 3 days after therapy is complete. Refrain from sexual intercourse, or use a barrier contraceptive if being treated for trichomoniasis. May cause headache, drowsiness, or dizziness; use caution while engaging in potentially hazardous tasks until response to drug is known. For pediatric patients unable to swallow tablets, tinidazole tablets may be crushed in artificial cherry syrup to be taken with food. There is a procedure for extemporaneous compounding for oral suspension. Report severe fatigue or weakness to your physician.

PREPARATIONS

Tablets, film coated: 250 mg, and 500 mg.

TIOTROPIUM BROMIDE—Spiriva®

DESCRIPTION/ACTIONS

Tiotropium is a long-acting, antimuscarinic agent, which is referred to as an anticholinergic. In the airways, it inhibits the M_3 receptors at the smooth muscle leading to bronchodilation. Tiotropium is indicated for the long-term, once daily maintenance treatment of bronchospasm associated with chronic obstructive pulmonary disease (COPD), such as bronchitis and emphysema. It is not indicated for the initial treatment of acute episodes of bronchospasms.

PRECAUTIONS/ADVERSE REACTIONS

Tiotropium is contraindicated in patients with a history of hypersensitivity to atropine or its derivatives, or to any components of the formulation. **Warning:** Immediate hypersensitivity reactions, including angioedema, may occur. Tiotropium is cleared by renal elimination; use caution in patients with moderate to severe renal impairment. Anticholinergics may potentially worsen signs and symptoms associated with narrow-angle glaucoma, prostatic hyperplasia, or bladder-neck obstruction. Patients with narrow-angle glaucoma, symptomatic prostatic hypertrophy, or bladder outlet obstruction were not included in studies. Pregnancy risk factor C. No adequate and well-controlled studies in pregnant women. Use only when expected benefit to the mother outweighs potential risk to the fetus. Most common adverse reactions were dry mouth, constipation, increased heart rate, blurred vision, glaucoma, urinary difficulty, urinary retention, epistaxis, and pruritis.

ADMINISTRATION

Inhalation: Contents of 1 capsule (18 mcg), once daily. Use HandiHaler® device.

PATIENT CARE IMPLICATIONS

Administer at the same time each day and only with the HandiHaler® device. For inhalation only. Not to be swallowed. HandiHaler® device should not be used to administer other drugs. Capsules should be stored in sealed blister packs and not stored in device. Expose one capsule at a time. Drug should be used immediately after being removed from blister pack. If not intended for immediate use, discard capsule because effectiveness is reduced. Take care to not allow powder to enter eyes, as this may cause blurring of vision and pupil dilation. Report eye pain, blurred vision, visual halos, or colored images; these may be signs of acute narrow-angle glaucoma. Do not use as an acute rescue bronchodilator.

PREPARATIONS

Capsules: 18 mcg, HandiHaler® device. Not to be exposed to extreme temperature or moisture.

TROSPIUM CHLORIDE—Sanctura™

DESCRIPTION/ACTIONS

Trospium is an antispasmodic, antimuscarinic agent. Trospium antagonizes the effect of acetylcholine on muscarinic receptors in cholinergically innervated organs. Its parasympatholytic action reduces the tonus of smooth muscle in the bladder. Sanctura™ is indicated for the treatment of overactive bladder with symptoms of urge urinary incontinence, urgency, and urinary frequency.

PRECAUTIONS/ADVERSE REACTIONS

Trospium is contraindicated in patients with a known hypersensitivity to it or to any component of the formulation. Trospium is contraindicated in patients with urinary retention, gastric retention, or uncontrolled narrow-angle glaucoma and in patients who are at risk for these conditions. Administer with caution in patients with clinically significant bladder outflow obstruction because of the risk of urinary retention. Sanctura™ may decrease gastrointestinal motility and should be used with caution in patients with ulcerative colitis, intestinal atony, and myasthenia gravis. In patients being treated for narrow-angle glaucoma, trospium should only be used if the potential benefits outweigh the risks and only with careful monitoring. Studies to assess drug-drug interactions with trospium have not been conducted. Sanctura™ may potentiate the anticholinergic side effects of other anticholinergic agents. Sanctura™ has the potential for interactions with other drugs that are eliminated via the kidneys by active tubular secretion such as digoxin, procainamide, pancuronium, morphine, vancomycin, metformin, and tenofovir due to competition for this elimination pathway. Patients should be monitored closely. Pregnancy Category C. No adequate and well-controlled studies in pregnant women. Excretion in human breast milk is unknown. Safety and efficacy in pediatric patients have not been established. Most common adverse effects observed in patients treated with trospium include dry mouth, constipation, abdominal pain, constipation aggravated, dyspepsia, flatulence, headache, fatigue, urinary retention, and dry eyes. Post marketing events noted include gastritis, palpitations, supraventricular tachycardia, chest pain, Stevens-Johnson syndrome, anaphylactic reaction, syncope, rhabdomyolysis, abnormal vision, hallucinations, delirium, and hypertensive crisis.

ADMINISTRATION

Adults: Oral, 20 mg twice daily 1 hour before meals or given on an empty stomach.

Dosage adjustment for renal impairment: (creatinine clearance <30 ml/min) 20 mg once daily at bedtime.

Dosage adjustment for hepatic impairment: no adjustment necessary. In geriatric patients ≥75 years of age, dose may be titrated down to 20 mg once daily based upon tolerability.

PATIENT CARE IMPLICATIONS

Patients should be informed of the anticholinergic side effects of Sanctura™. May cause heat prostration (fever and heat stroke due to decreased sweating) when used in a hot environment. May cause drowsiness; alcohol may enhance this effect. May produce dizziness and blurred vision; exercise caution.

PREPARATIONS

Tablets, 20 mg.

ZICONOTIDE—Prialt®

DESCRIPTION/ACTIONS

Ziconotide is an N-type calcium channel blocker, nonnarcotic analgesic. Ziconotide binds to N-type calcium channels located on the primary nociceptive afferent nerves in the superficial layers of the dorsal horn in the spinal cord. This is thought to block N-type calcium channels, which leads to a blockade of excitatory neurotransmitter release in the primary afferent nerve terminals and antinociception. Ziconotide is indicated for the management of severe chronic pain in patients where intrathecal (IT) therapy is warranted and who are intolerant of or refractory to other treatment.

PRECAUTIONS/ADVERSE REACTIONS

Ziconotide is contraindicated in patients with a hypersensitivity to ziconotide and any component of the formulation and in patients with a history of psychosis and IV administration. **Warning:** Severe psychiatric symptoms and neurological impairment may occur during treatment. Do not treat patients with a preexisting history of psychosis. Monitor all patients frequently for evidence of cognitive impairment, hallucinations, or changes in mood or consciousness. If reduced levels of unresponsiveness occur, ziconotide should be discontinued. Ziconotide can be discontinued abruptly without evidence of withdrawal effects in the event of serious neurological or psychiatric signs or symptoms. Patients taking concomitant antiepileptics, neuroleptics, sedatives, or diuretics may be at higher risk of depressed levels of consciousness. CNS-related adverse events such as psychiatric symptoms, cognitive impairment, and decreased alertness/unresponsiveness have occurred. Meningitis can occur due to inadvertent contamination of the IT device. Patients' caregivers and health care providers must be vigilant for the signs and symptoms of meningitis. Serious infection or meningitis can occur within 24 hours of a breach in sterility such as a disconnected catheter. Serum creatinine kinase (CK) levels above the upper limit of normal occurred. Elevated CKs were more often seen in patients being treated with antidepressants or antiepileptics or in patients treated with IT morphine. CK should be monitored every other week for the first month and then monthly. Clinical evaluation and CK measurements should be obtained if new neuromuscular symptoms (myalgias, myasthenia, muscle cramps, asthenia) appear or if there is a reduction in physical activity. Should these symptoms continue and CK levels remain elevated, the physician should consider reducing the dose or discontinuing ziconotide. The use of ziconotide with CNS depressants may be associated with an increased incidence of CNS adverse events such as dizziness and confusion. Pregnancy Category C; embryolethal in animal studies. Most common side effects were asthenia, headache, nausea, vomiting, diarrhea, dizziness, somnolence, confusion, ataxia, and abnormal vision.

ADMINISTRATION

IT: Chronic pain: Initial 2.4 mcg/day (0.1 mcg/hr). Doses may be titrated up by 2.4 mcg/day (0.1 mcg/hr) at intervals of no more than 2–3 times per week. Maximum dose of 19.2 mcg/day (0.8 mcg/hr) by day 21. Increments of less than 2.4 mcg/day (0.1 mcg/hr) and in frequency fewer than 2–3 times per week may be used. Administer by IT, using a programmable, implanted variable-rate microinfusion device or an external microinfusion device and catheter. Ziconotide is used undiluted (25 mcg/ml) or diluted (100 mcg/ml) with NS (preservative free). Saline solutions containing preservatives are not appropriate for IT administration and should not be used. After preparation of solution, refrigerate but do not freeze. Begin infusion within 24 hours. Only the undiluted 25 mcg/ml should be used for the first time pump priming. Dosage adjustment for toxicity or cognitive impairment: Reduce dose or discontinue; effects are generally reversible within 2 weeks of discontinuation.

PATIENT CARE IMPLICATIONS

Dizziness and sedation are common; caution against engaging in hazardous activity requiring mental alertness or coordination such as driving a vehicle. Contact physician immediately if there is a change in mental status (lethargy, confusion, disorientation, decreased alertness), a change in mood, perception (hallucinations, including unusual tactile sensations in the oral cavity), symptoms of depression or suicidal ideation, symptoms of meningitis, new or worsening muscle pain, soreness and weakness with or without darkened urine.

PREPARATIONS

Injection: solution, (preservative free): 100 mcg/mL (1 mL, 2 mL, 5 mL); 25 mcg/mL (20 mL). Store at 2–8°C (36–46°F). Do not freeze. Protect from light. Once diluted, may be stored at 2–8°C (36–46°F) for 24 hours.

PART II

Drugs in Current Use

A

A-200 PYRINATE®, see Pyrethrins

ABACAVIR—Ziagen®

Description/Actions: Indicated in the treatment of HIV-1 infection, in combination with other antiretroviral agents.

Precautions/Adverse Reactions: Abacavir is contraindicated in patients with a known sensitivity to the drug. Hypersensitivity reactions have been seen in about 5% of the adult and pediatric patients taking abacavir. Because these reactions are potentially fatal, patients developing symptoms of hypersensitivity (which may include fever, rash, fatigue, nausea, vomiting, diarrhea, or abdominal pain) should immediately discontinue the drug and seek medical attention. Abacavir should never be restarted after a hypersensitivity reaction because more severe symptoms will recur within hours and may include life-threatening hypotension and death. Hypersensitivity reactions may occur at any time during treatment, but usually appear in the first 6 weeks of use. Discontinue if clinical or lab findings of lactic acidosis or hepatotoxicity occur (risk is higher in women, in the obese, or with prolonged exposure to nucleosides). Use cautiously in liver disease and the elderly. Do not add as a single agent to a failing regimen. Not recommended in pregnancy (category C) or for nursing mothers. Adverse reactions may include nausea, vomiting, diarrhea, anorexia, insomnia, headache, fever, rash, hypersensitivity reactions including anaphylaxis (may be fatal), lactic acidosis, severe hepatomegaly with steatosis, mild hyperglycemia, and elevated triglycerides. Changes in body fat have been seen in some patients taking antiretroviral therapy. These changes may include increased amounts of fat in the upper back and neck, breast, and around the trunk. Loss of fat from legs, arms, and face may also occur.

Administration: Oral.

Patient Care Implications: Inform patients about the signs and symptoms of hypersensitivity reactions and the actions to take if they occur. Provide the patient with a Medication Guide and a Warning Card and instruct the patient to carry the card with him/her.

Preparations: Tablets, 300 mg. Oral solution, 20 mg/ml in strawberry-banana flavor.

ABACAVIR, LAMIVUDINE, AND ZIDOVUDINE—Trizivir™

Description/Actions: Trizivir™ is indicated for the treatment of HIV infection (either alone or in combination with other antiretroviral agents). This combination of antiretroviral is believed to act synergistically to inhibit reverse transcriptase through the incorporation of the nucleoside analogue and DNA chain termination.

Precautions/Adverse Reactions: Usage is contraindicated in patients with a hypersensitivity to abacavir, lamivudine, or any other formulation components. Do not restart patients who have had a hypersensitivity reaction to abacavir, a component of Trizivir™; life-threatening and fatal reactions have been reported. Patients must be monitored for possible fatal hypersensitivity reactions with abacavir. Patients exhibiting symptoms of fever, skin rash, fatigue, respiratory symptoms, and/or gastrointestinal symptoms should discontinue therapy immediately and call for medical attention. Trizivir™ should be permanently stopped if hypersensitivity cannot be ruled out, even when other diagnoses are possible. Do not restart following a hypersensitivity reaction to abacavir because more severe symptoms will recur within hours and may include life-threatening hypotension and death. Fatal hypersensitivity reactions have occurred following the reintroduction of abacavir in patients whose therapy was interrupted; serious reactions have occurred within hours. If Trizivir™ is to be restarted following an interruption in therapy, first evaluate the patient for previously unsuspected symptoms of hypersensitivity; therapy should not be reinstated if hypersensitivity is suspected or if hypersensitivity cannot be ruled out. Lactic acidosis and severe hepatomegaly with steatosis have been reported. Use caution in patients at risk for hepatomegaly and steatosis, such as patients with hepatic dysfunction, prior liver diseases, prolonged use with a nucleoside, and obesity. Use with caution in patients with bone marrow compromise, myopathy, and myositis; bone marrow suppression and myopathy have been associated with prolonged use of zidovudine. Pregnancy Category C. No well-controlled studies in pregnant women. Trizivir™ should be used during pregnancy only if the potential benefits outweigh the risks. Some components are excreted in breast milk and with the concomitant risk for postnatal HIV transmission, breast-feeding is not recommended. Not recommended for pediatric patients, in patients <40 kg, those requiring dosage adjustments or creatinine clearance ≤50 ml/minute. Should not be administered concomitantly with abacavir, lamivudine, or zidovudine. Some adverse effects are increased triglycerides, nausea, vomiting, diarrhea, loss of appetite/anorexia, insomnia, hypersensitivity, pancreatitis, and increased GGT. Changes in body fat have been seen in some patients taking antiretroviral therapy. These changes may include increased amounts of fat in the upper back and neck, breast, and around the trunk. Loss of fat from legs, arms, and face may also occur. Drug Interactions: Probenecid increases the effect of zidovudine. Ribavirin decreases the effect of zidovudine. Ganciclovir, interferon-alpha, and other bone marrow suppressive or cytotoxic agents may increase the hematologic toxicity of zidovudine.

Administration: Oral.

Patient Care Implications: Inform patient to take exactly as prescribed and educate patient of the potential hypersensitivity reactions associated with Trizivir™. Patient should carry the warning card that comes with this medicine.

Preparations: Tablet: Abacavir 300 mg, lamivudine 150 mg, and zidovudine 300 mg.

ABARELIX—Plenaxis™

Descriptions/Actions: Abarelix is a gonadotropin releasing hormone (GnRH) antagonist; it competes with naturally occurring GnRH for binding on receptors of the pituitary. It suppresses luteinizing hormone and follicle stimulating hormone secretion, thereby reducing the secretion of testosterone by the testes. Abarelix is indicated for the palliative treatment of advanced symptomatic prostate cancer, for patients in whom LHRH agonist therapy is not appropriate, and who refuse surgical castration and have one or more of the following due to metastases or local encroachment: (a) risk of neurological compromise, (b) ureteral or bladder outlet obstruction, or (c) severe bone pain that persists despite being on narcotic analgesia.

Precautions/Adverse Reactions: Abarelix is contraindicated in patients hypersensitive to abarelix or any component of the formulation. **Warning:** Associated with immediate-onset systemic allergic reactions, some resulting in hypotension and syncope. Reported to occur with initial and any dose following administration; risk increases with duration of treatment. Following each injection, patients should be observed for at least 30 minutes. Abarelix may prolong the QT interval. Physicians should carefully consider if risk outweighs benefits in patients with baseline QTc values >450 msec and in patients taking class IA or III antiarrhythmic medications. Strict monitoring of serum testosterone is warranted. Efficacy is monitored by suppression of serum testosterone

<50 ng/dL. Transaminase elevations were observed; serum transaminase levels should be obtained prior to treatment and periodically during treatment. Extended treatment may result in a decrease in bone mineral density. Pregnancy category X. May cause fetal harm if administered to a pregnant woman. Not known if abarelix is excreted in human milk, but not indicated for nursing mothers. Most common adverse reactions are hot flushes, sleep disturbance, pain, dizziness, headache, breast enlargement, nipple discharge/tenderness, constipation, diarrhea, back pain, and upper respiratory infections.

Administration: Intramuscular.

Patient Care Implications: Monitor serum testosterone (to identify treatment failure) just prior to abarelix on day 29 and every 8 weeks thereafter.

Preparations: Injection, powder for reconstitution (preservative free): 113 mg (provides 100 mg/2mL); packaged with NS diluent and 3cc syringe.

ABBOKINASE®, see Urokinase

ABCIXIMAB—ReoPro®

Description/Actions: Inhibits platelet aggregation by preventing binding of fibrinogen and other adhesive molecules to receptor sites on activated platelets. Indicated as an adjunct to percutaneous transluminal coronary angioplasty (PTCA) or arthrectomy for the prevention of acute cardiac ischemic complications in patients at high risk for abrupt closure of the treated coronary vessel. Is used in conjunction with heparin and aspirin.

Precautions/Adverse Reactions: Contraindicated in situations in which a significant risk of bleeding complications exists, when intravenous dextran is used before or during PTCA, and in individuals with known hypersensitivity to any component of the product or to murine proteins.

Administration: Intravenous.

Preparations: Vials (5 ml) 2 mg/ml. Vials should be stored in refrigerator but not frozen. Do not shake vials.

ABELCET®—Amphotericin B lipid Complex

ABILIFY®, see Aripiprazole

ABREVA®, see Docosanol 10% Cream

ACARBOSE—Precose®

Description/Actions: Reduces blood sugar by inhibiting alpha glucosidase enzymes in the GI tract, resulting in delayed glucose absorption. Indicated as an adjunct to diet in noninsulin-dependent diabetes mellitus (NIDDM). Administered alone or with sulfonylurea oral hypoglycemic agents, insulin, or metformin.

Precautions/Adverse Reactions: Risk of hypoglycemia is increased when used with oral hypoglycemic agents. Treat mild-to-moderate hypoglycemia with oral glucose (e.g., glucose tablets). Adverse reactions include flatulence, diarrhea, and abdominal pain. Contraindicated in ketoacidosis, cirrhosis, inflammatory bowel disease, chronic ulceration, partial or predisposition to intestinal obstruction, chronic intestinal disease with marked disorders of digestion or absorbency, and in conditions that may deteriorate from increased intestinal gas formation.

Administration: Oral. Take with first bite of each main meal.

Preparations: Scored tablets, 25, 50, and 100 mg.

ACCOLATE®, see Zafirlukast

ACCURETIC®, see Quinapril/Hydrochlorothiazide

ACCUPRIL®, see Quinapril Hydrochloride

ACCUTANE®, see Isotretinoin

ACEBUTOLOL HYDROCHLORIDE—Sectral®

Description/Actions: A cardioselective beta-adrenergic blocking agent possessing mild intrinsic sympathomimetic activity. Indicated for the treatment of hypertension, and may be used alone or in combination with other agents, usually a thiazide diuretic. Is also indicated in the management of ventricular premature beats.

Precautions/Adverse Reactions: Contraindicated in patients with persistently severe bradycardia, second- and third-degree heart block in the absence of a functioning artificial pacemaker, overt cardiac failure, and cardiogenic shock. Adverse reactions include fatigue, dizziness, headache, nausea, dyspepsia, arthralgias, and myalgias. Use is best avoided in patients with bronchospastic diseases, and therapy in diabetic patients must be closely monitored.

Administration: Oral. Patients should be cautioned about the interruption or discontinuation of therapy.

Preparations: Capsules, 200 and 400 mg.

ACETADOTE®, see Acetylcysteine

ACETAMINOPHEN—Panadol®, Tempra®, Tylenol®

Description/Actions: Analgesic/antipyretic used in the treatment of mild to moderate pain, and fever.

Precautions/Adverse Reactions: Overdosage may result in hepatotoxicity; acetylcysteine is used as the antidote.

Administration: Oral and rectal.

Preparations: Tablets/capsules/caplets, 80, 160, 325, 500, and 650 mg. Controlled-release caplets, 650 mg. Chewable tablets, 80 mg. Granules, 80 mg. Liquid, 160 mg/5 ml, 500 mg/15 ml, and 100 mg/ml. Drops, 100 mg/ml. Suppositories, 120, 325, and 650 mg.

ACETAZOLAMIDE—Diamox®

Description/Actions: Carbonic anhydrase inhibitor indicated in the treatment of glaucoma, edema, certain convulsive disorders, and for the prevention or relief of symptoms associated with acute mountain sickness.

Preparations: Tablets, 125 and 250 mg. Controlled-release capsules, 500 mg. Vials (sodium salt), 500 mg.

ACETIC ACID—VoSol®

Description/Actions: Anti-infective agent used as a bladder irrigant, for otic infections, and certain dermatologic conditions.

Preparations: Solution (bladder irrigation), 0.25%. Otic solution (Vo-Sol®), 2%.

ACETOHEXAMIDE—Dymelor®

Description/Actions: First-generation sulfonylurea hypoglycemic agent indicated in the treatment of noninsulin-dependent diabetes mellitus.

Preparations: Tablets, 250 and 500 mg.

ACETOHYDROXAMIC ACID—Lithostat®

Description/Actions: Adjunctive therapy in certain urinary tract infections. Inhibits the bacterial enzyme urease, thereby inhibiting the hydrolysis of urea and production of ammonia in urine infected with urea-splitting organisms.

Preparations: Tablets, 250 mg.

ACETOPHENAZINE MALEATE—Tindal®

Description/Actions: Phenothiazine antipsychotic agent indicated for psychotic disorders.

Preparations: Tablets, 20 mg.

ACETYLCARBROMAL—Paxarel®

Description/Actions: Central nervous system depressant used as a sedative and hypnotic.

Preparations: Tablets, 250 mg.

ACETYLCYSTEINE—Mucomyst®, Acetadote®

Description/Actions: Mucolytic agent indicated as adjunctive therapy in patients with abnormal or viscoid mucous secretions in various pulmonary disorders. Also indicated in the management of acetaminophen overdosage.

Preparations: Vials (solution of sodium salt), 10% and 20%. Administered by nebulization or direct instillation, or enterally. Usually administered via nasogastric tube as noxious taste causes regurgitation. Injection, 20% solution in 30 ml (200 mg/ml) single dose vials.

ACETYLSALICYLIC ACID, see Aspirin

ACHROMYCIN V®, see Tetracycline Hydrochloride

ACIPHEX®, see Rabeprazole

ACLOVATE®, see Alclometasone Diproprionate

ACRIVASTINE/PSEUDOEPHEDRINE HYDROCHLORIDE— Semprex-D®

Description/Actions: Antihistamine/decongestant combination indicated for the relief of symptoms associated with seasonal allergic rhinitis.

Precautions/Adverse Reactions: Contraindicated in patients with severe hypertension, severe coronary artery disease, and in patients taking a monoamine oxidase inhibitor. Adverse reactions preclude driving and operating machinery until response is ascertained. Avoid CNS acting drugs, including alcohol. Patients should be advised against the concurrent use with nonprescription antihistamines and/or decongestants.

Administration: Oral.

Preparations: Capsules, 8 mg of acrivastine and 60 mg of pseudophedrine hydrochloride.

ACTH, see Corticotropin

ACTHAR®, see Corticotropin

ACTIQ®, see Fentanyl

ACTIGALL®, see Ursodiol

ACTIMMUNE®, see Interferon gamma-1b

ACTINEX®, see Masoprocol

ACTISITE®, see Tetracycline Hydrochloride

ACTIVASE®, see Alteplase, Recombinant

ACTIVELLA™, combination of Norethindrone Acetate and Estradiol

ACTONEL®, see Risedronate

ACTOS®, see Pioglitazone

ACTRON®, see Ketoprofen

ACULAR®, see Ketorolac Tromethamine

ACULAR L5®, see Ketorolac Tromethamine

ACULAR PF®, see Ketorolac Tromethamine

ACYCLOVIR—Zovirax®

Description/Actions: Antiviral agent indicated in the treatment of genital herpes infections, varicella (chickenpox) infections, varicella zoster (shingles) infections, herpes simplex encephalitis, and mucosal and cutaneous herpes simplex (HSV-1 and HSV-2) infections in immunocompromised patients.

Preparations: Capsules, 200 mg. tablets, 800 mg. Suspension, 200 mg/5 ml.

Ointment, 5%. Vials (sodium salt), 500 and 1000 mg (administered by IV infusion). Cream, 5%.

ADAGEN®, see Pegademase Bovine

ADALAT®, see Nifedipine

ADALAT CC®, see Nifedipine

ADALIMUMAB—Humira™

Description/Actions: Adalimumab is a recombinant monoclonal antibody specific for tumor necrosis factor alpha (TNF-alpha). Adalimumab is indicated for reducing signs and symptoms, inhibiting the progression of structural damage, and improving physical function in adult patients with moderately to severely active rheumatoid arthritis who have had an inadequate response to one or more DMARDs. Humira™ can be used alone or in combination with methotrexate or other DMARDs.

Precautions/Adverse Reactions: Adalimumab is contraindicated in patients with a hypersensitivity to adalimumab or any component of the formulation. The needle cover of the syringe contains latex and should not be handled by persons sensitive to this substance. Serious infections and sepsis, including fatalities, have been reported. Patients should be evaluated for latent tuberculosis infection with a tuberculin skin test prior to therapy. Treatment with adalimumab may result in the formation of autoantibodies and, rarely, in the development of a lupus-like syndrome. If patient develops symptoms suggestive of a lupus-like syndrome, treatment should be discontinued. Pregnancy category B. The most serious adverse reactions were serious infections, neurologic events, and malignancies. The most common adverse reactions were injection site reactions, upper respiratory infection, sinusitis, nausea, headache, rash, and accidental injury.

Administration: Adults: subcutaneous.

Patient Care Implications: Patients may self-inject after proper training in injection technique. Do not use syringe if solution is cloudy, discolored, or contains particles.

Preparations: Injection, solution (preservative free): 40 mg/0.8 ml prefilled glass syringe.

ADAPALENE—Differin®

Description/Actions: A synthetic analogue, alcohol-free topical gel indicated in the treatment of *acne vulgaris.*

Precautions/Adverse Reactions: Do not use on cuts, abrasions, or broken eczematous or sunburned skin. Avoid contact with eyes, lips, angles of the nose, and mucous membranes. Minimize exposure to sun and UV light. Increased irritation may occur in extreme weather (e.g., wind, cold). Reduce frequency or discontinue if prolonged or severe irritation occurs. Do not use concomitantly with other topical irritants. Adverse reactions include erythema, scaling, dryness, pruritis, burning, and acne flares.

Administration: Apply a thin film to affected areas once daily at bedtime after washing.

Preparations: 0.1% gel, topical (alcohol free), 15, 45 g. 0.1% topical solution, 30 ml.

ADEFOVIR DIPIVOXIL—Hepsera™

Description/Actions: Adefovir is an acyclic nucleotide reverse transcriptase inhibitor that interferes with hepatitis B virus (HBV) viral RNA dependent DNA polymerase, resulting in inhibition of viral replication. Adefovir is indicated for the treatment of chronic hepatitis B in adults with evidence of active viral replication as well as either evidence of persistent elevations in serum aminotransferases or histologically active disease.

Precautions/Adverse Reactions: Adefovir is contraindicated in patients hypersensitive to the drug or any component of the formulation. Chronic administration of adefovir may result in nephrotoxicity in patients at risk of or having underlying renal dysfunction. Lactic acidosis and severe hepatomegaly with steatosis, including fatal cases, have been reported with the use of nucleoside analogs alone or in combination with other antiretrovirals. Caution should be exercised when administering nucleoside analogs to any patient with known risk factors for liver disease. Severe acute exacerbations of hepatitis have been reported in patients who have discontinued anti hepatitis-B therapy including Hepsera™. Hepatic function should be monitored closely. Pregnancy category C. Most common adverse effects were asthenia, headache, abdominal pain, and nausea.

Administration: Oral. May be taken without regard to food.

Preparations: Tablet: 10 mg

ADENOCARD®, see Adenosine

ADENOSINE—Adenocard®

Description/Actions: Slows conduction through the AV node of the heart and reestablishes normal heart rhythm. Has a rapid onset of action and a very short duration of action. Indicated for the conversion to sinus rhythm of paroxysmal supraventricular tachycardia (PSVT), including those associated with accessory bypass tracts (Wolff-Parkinson-White syndrome).

Precautions/Adverse Reactions: Contraindicated in second- or third-degree AV block (except in patients with a functioning artificial pacemaker), sick sinus syndrome (except in patients with a functioning artificial pacemaker), atrial flutter, atrial fibrillation, and ventricular tachycardia. Adverse reactions include myocardial conduction abnormalities, facial flushing, headache, shortness of breath/dyspnea, chest pressure, lightheadedness, and nausea. Action may be potentiated by dipyridamole. Caution must be exercised in patients concurrently receiving carbamazepine because a higher degree of heart block may be produced. Actions of adenosine may be competitively antagonized by methylxanthines such as theophylline and caffeine.

Administration: Administered as a rapid bolus IV injection over a 1- to 2-second period.

Preparations: Vials, 6 mg/2 ml. The product should not be refrigerated as crystallization may occur.

ADIPEX®, see Phentermine

ADRENALIN®, see Epinephrine

ADRIAMYCIN PFS®, see Doxorubicin

ADRIAMYCIN RDF®, see Doxorubicin

ADRUCIL®, see Fluorouracil

ADVAIR™ DISKUS®, combination of Fluticasone and Salmeterol

ADVICOR™, see Niacin and Lovastatin

ADVIL®, see Ibuprofen

AEROBID®, see Flunisolide

AEROSPORIN®, see Polymyxin B

AFRIN®, see Oxymetazoline

AFRINOL®, see Pseudoephedrine

AGGRASTAT®, see Tirofiban

AGRYLIN®, see Anagrelide

AKINETON®, see Biperiden

AKNE-MYCIN®, see Erythromycin Base (topical)

ALAMAST®, see Pemirolast

ALBAMYCIN®, see Novobiocin Sodium

ALBENZA®, see Albendazole

ALBENDAZOLE—Albenza®

Description/Actions: Anthelmintic indicated for treatment of cystic hydatid disease of the liver, lung, and peritoneum caused by the larval form of the dog tapeworm (*Echonococcus granulosus*) and for parenchymal neurocysticercosis from active lesions caused by larval forms of the pork tapeworm (*Taenia solium*). Also indicated in the treatment of ascariasis, hookworm, strongyloidiasis, giardiasis, and microsporidiosis in patients with HIV.

Precautions/Adverse Reactions: In treating neurocysticercosis, during the first week of therapy administer steroid and anticonvulsant therapy concurrently to prevent cerebral hypertension. The most common adverse drug reactions are alterations in LFTs, abdominal pain, and nausea and vomiting. Monitor LFTs prior to and during therapy. If enzymes significantly increase, discontinue the albendazole. Therapy can be reinstituted when enzymes have returned to pretreatment levels. Monitor white blood cells (WBC), as reversible reductions in total WBCs have been noted.

Administration: Oral.

Preparations: Tablets, 200 mg.

ALBUMIN (HUMAN)—Albuminar®, Buminate®, Plasbumin®

Description/Actions: Plasma protein fraction indicated as supportive treatment in patients in shock, or patients with burns, hepatic cirrhosis, nephrosis, and certain other conditions.

Preparations: Vials, 5% and 25%, administered by IV infusion.

ALBUMINAR®, see Albumin

ALBUTEROL—Proventil®, Proventil HFA Inhaler®, Ventolin®, Ventolin® HFA, Volmax®

Description/Actions: Stimulates beta 2-adrenergic receptors. Indicated for the relief of bronchospasm in patients with reversible obstructive airway disease and for the prevention of exercise-induced bronchospasm.

Precautions/Adverse Reactions: Adverse reactions include nervousness, tremor, headache, tachycardia, and palpitations. Should be used cautiously in patients with cardiovascular disorders. Concurrent use with other adrenergic (sympathomimetic) agents will have additive adrenergic effects. Must be used with caution in patients being treated with a tricyclic antidepressant or monoamine oxidase inhibitor because the action of albuterol may be increased. Beta-adrenergic blocking agents and albuterol may inhibit the effect of each other.

Administration: Oral and oral inhalation.

Preparations: Tablets, 2 and 4 mg. Controlled-release tablets, 4 and 8 mg. Capsules for inhalation, 200 ug. Syrup, 2 mg/5 ml. Metered-dose inhaler. (HFA inhaler is chloroflurocarbon free.) Solution for inhalation.

ALCLOMETASONE DIPROPIONATE—Aclovate®

Description/Actions: Topical corticosteroid indicated for relief of the inflammatory and pruritic manifestations of corticosteroid-responsive dermatoses.

Precautions/Adverse Reactions: Adverse reactions include itching, burning, erythema, dryness, irritation, and papular rashes. Children may absorb proportionally larger amounts of the drug and thus be more susceptible to the development of systemic effects.

Administration: Topical.

Preparations: Cream and ointment, 0.05%.

ALCOHOL—Ethyl alcohol

Description/Actions: Antiseptic, astringent, and solvent when applied topically. Also used intravenously as a source of calories.

Preparations: Solution (topical), 70%. Bottles (intravenous), 5% and 10% with 5% dextrose in water.

ALDACTONE®, see Spironolactone

ALDARA®, see Imiquimod

ALDESLEUKIN—Proleukin®

Description/Actions: A human recombinant interleukin-2 product (rIL-2) produced by recombinant DNA technology using a genetically engineered *E. coli* strain containing an analogue of the human interleukin-2 gene. Indicated for the treatment of adults (18 years of age and older) with metastatic renal cell carcinoma.

Precautions/Adverse Reactions: Contraindicated in patients with organ allografts and in patients who do not have normal cardiac and pulmonary functions as defined by thallium stress testing and formal pulmonary function testing. Many adverse reactions are associated with capillary leak syndrome, which results in hypotension and reduced organ perfusion. Pressor agents may be necessary to sustain blood pressure and the use of dopamine to help maintain organ perfusion. Other adverse reactions include renal dysfunction with oliguria/anuria, pulmonary congestion, dyspnea, respiratory failure, mental status changes, seizure, myocardial ischemia, myocarditis, gastrointestinal bleeding, intestinal perforation/ileus, sinus tachycardia, nausea, vomiting, diarrhea, anemia, thrombocytopenia, pruritus, erythema, fever and/or chills, pain, fatigue, and edema. It should be monitored closely. Hematologic tests (including CBC, differential, and platelet counts), blood chemistries (including electrolytes, renal and hepatic function tests), and chest X-rays should be conducted prior to beginning treatment and then daily during drug administration. Use is associated with an increased risk of disseminated infection, including sepsis and bacterial endocarditis; therefore, preexisting infections should be adequately treated prior to starting therapy. Patients with indwelling central lines should be evaluated for antibiotic prophylaxis against *staphylococcus aureus*.

Administration: Intravenous.

Preparations: Vials, 22 million units (1.3 mg).

ALDOMET®, see Methyldopa

ALDORIL® Combination of Methyldopa and Hydrochlorothiazide

ALEFACEPT—Amevive®

Description/Actions: Alefacept is a monoclonal antibody used in the treatment of moderate to severe plaque psoriasis in adults who are candidates for systemic therapy or phototherapy. Alefacept binds to CD2, a receptor on the surface of lymphocytes, inhibiting their interaction with leukocyte functional antigen 3(LFA-3). The interaction between CD2 and LFA-3 leads to the activation of T-lymphocytes, which secrete a number of inflammatory mediators that are involved in psoriasis.

Precautions/Adverse Reactions: Alefacept is contraindicated in patients hypersensitive to alefacept or any of its components. Patients receiving other immunosuppressants or phototherapy should not receive concurrent therapy with alefacept due to the possibility of excessive immunosuppression. Hypersensitivity reactions such as urticaria and angioedema were observed. **Warning:** Alefacept induces a decline in circulating T-lymphocytes (CD4+ and CD8+). Do not initiate therapy with a CD4+ T-lymphocyte count below normal. Withhold treatment in any patient who develops CD4+ a lymphocyte count <250 cell/mcL. Alefacept should be permanently discontinued if counts remain <250 cell/mcL for 1 month. May increase the risk of malignancies. Alefacept should not be administered to patients with a history of systemic malignancy. Discontinue treatment if patient develops a malignancy. Alefacept is an immunosuppressive agent and has the potential to increase the risk of infection and reactivate latent, chronic infections. Do not administer to patients with clinically important infections. Monitor for signs and symptoms of infection during or after a course of alefacept. New infections should be closely monitored; if a serious infection develops, discontinue medication. Pregnancy risk factor B. Effects in pregnancy are not known. Excretion in breast milk unknown; not recommended. Most common adverse effects were lymphopenia, local injection site reactions (pain, inflammation, bleeding, or edema), chills, nausea, and myalgia.

Administration: I.M.: 15 mg once weekly; usual duration of 12 weeks. I.V.: 7.5 mg once weekly; usual duration of 12 weeks. A second course of treatment may be initiated at least 12 weeks after completion of the initial course of treatment, provided CD4+ lymphocyte counts are within the normal range.

Patient Care Implications: Patients should be informed of regular, weekly monitoring of white blood cell counts. Report unusual feeling of fatigue or weakness, signs of infection, any pain, difficulty swallowing or breathing, or feeling of tightness in chest. Because the incidence of infections and certain malignancies is higher in the elderly, caution should be used in treating the elderly.

Preparations: Injection, powder for reconstitution: 7.5 mg (for I.V. administration; supplied with SWFI) Injection, powder for reconstitution: 15 mg (for I.M. administration; supplied with SWFI)

ALENDRONATE SODIUM—Fosamax®

Description/Actions: Inhibits resorption of bone by inhibiting osteoclast activity. Indicated in the prevention and treatment of osteoporosis in postmenopausal women and treatment of Paget's disease of the bone.

Precautions/Adverse Reactions: Should not be used in patients whose creatinine clearance is less than 35 ml/minute, or during pregnancy and lactation. Adverse reactions include headache, GI symptoms, rash, and musculoskeletal pain.

Administration: Oral. Administer first thing in the morning with 6–8 oz of plain water 30 minutes prior to other medication, beverages, or food. (Must also avoid lying down for at least 30 minutes after the dose is administered.)

Preparations: Tablets, 5, 10, 35, and 70 mg.

ALESSE®—Levonorgestrel/ethinyl estradiol

Low dose combination oral contraceptive containing 0.10 mg levonorgestrel and 0.02 mg of ethinyl estradiol.

ALEVE®, see Naproxen Sodium

ALFENTA®, see Alfentanil

ALFENTANIL HYDROCHLORIDE—Alfenta®

Description/Actions: Opioid analgesic/anesthetic. Indicated as an (a) analgesic adjunct given in incremental doses in the maintenance of anesthesia with barbiturate/nitrous oxide/oxygen, (b) as an analgesic administered by continuous infusion with nitrous oxide/oxygen in the maintenance of general anesthesia, and (c) as a primary anesthetic agent for the induction of anesthesia in patients undergoing general surgery in which endotracheal intubation and mechanical ventilation are required. Has an almost immediate onset of action and a short duration of action.

Precautions/Adverse Reactions: Skeletal muscle rigidity of the chest wall, trunk, and extremities is one of the most common adverse reactions; the incidence may be reduced by the appropriate use of a neuromuscular blocking agent. Respiratory depression including delayed respiratory depression and respiratory arrest have been reported, and the monitoring of the patient must be continued well after surgery. Caution must be exercised in patients with pulmonary disease or those with potentially compromised respiration. Other adverse reactions include cardiovascular effects (e.g., bradycardia, hypotension, arrhythmias), nausea, vomiting, and dizziness. When administered with other central nervous system depressants, the dose of one or both agents should be reduced. It can produce dependence and has the potential for being abused; is included in Schedule II under the provisions of the Controlled Substances Act.

Administration: Intravenous.

Preparations: Ampules (2, 5, 10, and 20 ml) containing the equivalent of 500 µg. of alfentanil base in each ml.

ALFERON N®, see Interferon alfa-n3

ALFUZOSIN—Uroxatral™

Description/Actions: Alfuzosin is an alpha$_1$ adrenergic antagonist, used in the treatment of functional symptoms of benign prostatic hyperplasia (BPH). Smooth muscle tone is regulated by alpha-adrenergic receptors in the lower urinary tract. Blockade of these adrenoreceptors can cause smooth muscles in the bladder neck and prostate to relax, resulting in an improvement in urine flow and a decrease of BPH symptoms. Alfuzosin is NOT indicated for the treatment of hypertension.

Precautions/Adverse Reactions: Alfuzosin is contraindicated in patients known to be hypersensitive to alfuzosin or any of its components. Alfuzosin should not be used in patients with moderate or severe hepatic insufficiency, as alfuzosin blood levels are increased in these patients. Alfuzosin should not be coadministered with potent CYP3A4 inhibitors (ketoconazole, itraconazole, ritonavir), as alfuzosin blood levels are increased. It should not be used in combination with other alpha blockers. Interactions have not been determined; however, interactions may be expected. Prior to initiating therapy, patients should be examined to rule out the presence of prostate cancer. These two diseases frequently coexist. If symptoms of angina pectoris should newly appear or worsen, alfuzosin should be discontinued. Bioavailability and maximum serum concentrations are increased approximately 50% with mild, moderate, or severe renal impairment: use with caution. **Warning:** May cause orthostasis, syncope, or dizziness. Use caution in patients with a history of QT prolongation or use with medications that may prolong the QT interval. The most common adverse reactions were dizziness, headache, fatigue, and upper respiratory tract infections. Post marketing adverse events reported were rash, tachycardia, chest pain, and priapism.

Administration: Oral.

Patient Care Implications: Inform patient it may cause drowsiness, impair judgment (use caution when driving or engaging in tasks that require alertness until response to drug is known). May cause postural hypotension (use caution when rising from sitting or lying position or when climbing stairs). Report unusual chest pain, respiratory difficulty, or any persistent adverse reactions. Advise patients not to take any new medication without consulting their physician.

Preparations: Tablet, extended-release, 10 mg.

ALGLUCERASE—Ceredase®

Description/Actions: Agent for Gaucher's disease. It is a modified form of the enzyme glucocerebrosidase. Indicated for use as long-term enzyme replacement therapy for patients with a confirmed diagnosis of type 1 Gaucher's disease who exhibit signs and symptoms that are severe enough to result in one or more of the following conditions: moderate to severe anemia, thrombocytopenia with bleeding tendency, bone disease, significant hepatomegaly or splenomegaly.

Precautions/Adverse Reactions: Adverse reactions include fever, chills, abdominal discomfort, nausea, vomiting, and discomfort, burning, and swelling at the site of venipuncture.

Administration: Intravenous. Is administered by IV infusion over 1–2 hours.

Preparations: Vials, 10 units/ml and 80 units/ml.

ALINIA™, see Nitazoxanide

ALITRETINOIN—Panretin®

Description/Actions: Alitretinoin is a retinoid indicated in the treatment of cutaneous AIDS-related Kaposi's sarcoma (KS) lesions. Whereas response may be seen in as little as 2 weeks, the average response time is 4–8 weeks, although some patients may need as many as 14 weeks before a response is seen.

Precautions/Adverse Reactions: Not indicated for use when systemic anti-KS therapy is needed. Do not place occlusive dressings over the lesions after applications of the medication. Use cautiously in the elderly and on T-cell lymphoma, as there is an increased risk of dermal toxicity. Minimize exposure to sun and UV light. Pregnancy category D. Instruct patients to use adequate contraception. Avoid concomitant use of DEET. May cause fetal harm if absorbed by a pregnant woman. Adverse reactions include rash (e.g., erythema, scaling), pain, pruritis, exfoliative dermatitis, skin disorders (e.g., excoriation, scab, eschar), paresthesia, edema, inflammation.

Administration: Topical.

Patient Care Implications: Instruct patients that a light dressing may be applied over the gel but not to place an occlusive dressing over it.

Minimize sun and UV light exposure and do not use insect repellants that contain DEET. Let patients know that local reactions are common and may improve with use as a tolerance develops.

Preparations: Gel, 0.1%.

ALKERAN®, see Melphalan

ALLEGRA®, see Fexofenadine Hydrochloride

ALLEGRA-D®—Combination Agent Fexofenadine Hydrochloride and Pseudoephredrine (Antihistamine and Sympathomimetic)

ALLOPURINOL—Aloprim™, Lopurin®, Zyloprim®

Description/Actions: A xanthine oxidase inhibitor indicated in the management of (a) gout; (b) patients with leukemia, lymphoma, and malignancies who are receiving cancer therapy that causes elevations of serum and urinary uric acid levels; and (c) patients with recurrent calcium oxalate calculi.

Precautions/Adverse Reactions: Adverse reactions include hypersensitivity reactions, and therapy should be discontinued at the first appearance of rash or other signs of an allergic response. Will increase the action of azathioprine and mercaptopurine, and the dosage of these agents should be reduced to one-third to one-quarter the usual dose when allopurinol is administered concomitantly.

Administration: Oral, intravenous.

Preparations: Injection, powder for reconstitution, 500 mg. Tablets, 100 and 300 mg.

ALMOTRIPTAN MALEATE—Axert™

Description/Actions: Almotriptan is indicated for the acute treatment of migraine with or without aura in adults.

Precautions/Adverse Reactions: Almotriptan should not be given to patients with risk factors for coronary artery disease until a thorough cardiovascular evaluation is performed. Significant elevations in blood pressure, including hypertensive crisis, have been reported on rare occasions in patients with and without a history of hypertension. Sensations of tightness, pain, pressure, and heaviness in the precordium, throat, neck, and jaw have been reported after treatment with Axert. If a patient does not respond to the first dose of almotriptan, the diagnosis of migraine headache should be reconsidered. Pregnancy category C. No adequate or well-controlled studies in pregnant women. Almotriptan should be used during pregnancy only if the potential benefit justifies the potential risk to the fetus. Excretion in human breast milk is unknown. Safety and efficacy in pediatrics have not been established. The most common adverse effects observed during treatment with almotriptan include nausea, somnolence, headache, paresthesia, and dry mouth. Serious and fatal cardiac events, including coronary artery vasospasm, transient myocardial ischemia, myocardial infarction, ventricular tachycardia, and ventricular fibrillation, have occurred. These events are extremely rare, and most have occurred in patients with risk factors predictive of coronary artery disease.

Administration: Oral.

Patient Care Implications: Patients should be instructed to report any sensations of tightness, pain, pressure, or heaviness in the chest, throat, neck, or jaw. If patient does not respond to the first dose of almotriptan, the diagnosis of migraine should be reconsidered.

Preparations: Tablets, 6.25 and 12.5 mg.

ALOCRIL®, see Nedocromil Sodium

ALOMIDE®, see Lodoxamide Tromethamine

ALOPRIM™, see Allopurinol

ALORA®, see Estradiol

ALOSETRON HYDROCHLORIDE—Lotronex®

Description/Actions: A potent and selective antagonist of the serotonin 5-HT3 receptor type indicated for the treatment of irritable bowel syndrome in women whose predominant bowel symptom is diarrhea.

Administration: Oral.

Preparations: Tablets. 1 mg.

ALPHAGAN®, see Brimonidine Tartrate

ALPHA1-ANTITRYPSIN, see Alpha1-Proteinase Inhibitor

ALPHA₁-PROTEINASE INHIBITOR (HUMAN)—Prolastin®

Description/Actions: Also known as alpha₁-antitrypsin, it is indicated for chronic replacement therapy in individuals having congenital deficiency of alpha$_1$-proteinase inhibitor with clinically demonstrable panacinar emphysema.

Precautions/Adverse Reactions: Preparation is purified from large pools of fresh human plasma obtained from many donors, and the presence of hepatitis viruses in such pools must be assumed. It is therefore recommended that patients be immunized against hepatitis B.

Administration: Intravenous.

Preparations: Vials, with the activity, in milligrams, stated on the label of each vial.

ALPRAZOLAM—Xanax®, Xanax® XR, Niravam™

Description/Actions: Benzodiazepine indicated for the management of anxiety disorders or the short-term relief of the symptoms of anxiety. Anxiety associated with depression is also responsive. Also indicated in the treatment of panic disorder.

Precautions/Adverse Reactions: Contraindicated in patients with acute narrow-angle glaucoma. Adverse reactions include drowsiness and other CNS effects. Patients should be cautioned regarding activities such as driving and operating machinery, as well as interactions with other CNS-acting drugs including alcohol. Can cause dependence and is included in Schedule IV.

Administration: Oral.

Preparations: Tablets, 0.25, 0.5, 1, and 2 mg. Extended release tablets, 0.5, 1, 2, and 3 mg. Orally disintegrating tablets, 0.25 mg, 0.5 mg, 1 mg, and 2 mg.

ALPROSTADIL—Caverject®, Edex®, Prostin VR Pediatric®, Prostaglandin E$_1$, PGE$_1$

Description/Actions: Prostaglandin indicated (Prostin VR Pediatric®) for palliative therapy to temporarily maintain the patency of the ductus arteriosus until corrective or palliative surgery can be performed in neonates who have congenital heart defects and who depend upon the patent ductus for survival. Also indicated (Caverject®) for the diagnosis and treatment of male erectile dysfunction due to neurologic, vascular, psychological, or mixed causes.

Administration: Intravenous infusion (Prostin VR Pediatric®) and into an area along the shaft of the penis known as the corpus cavernosum (Caverject®).

Preparations: Ampules, 500 mcg (Prostin VR Pediatric®). Vials, 5, 10, 20, and 40 mcg (Caverject®). 2 injection starter pack (1 inj. device and supplies edex.)

ALREX®, see Loteprednol Etabonate

ALTACE®, see Ramipril

ALTEPLASE, RECOMBINANT—Activase®, Cathflo™

Description/Actions: Is a form of the body's natural tissue plasminogen activator (TPA) that promotes the conversion of plasminogen to plasmin, which is fibrinolytic. Indicated for the management of acute myocardial infarction in adults for the lysis of thrombi obstructing coronary arteries, the improvement of ventricular function, and reduction of the incidence of congestive heart failure. Also indicated for the management of acute massive pulmonary embolism and acute ischemic stroke. Alteplase is also indicated to restore patency of occluded catheters.

Precautions/Adverse Reactions: Contraindicated in patients with active bleeding, history of cerebrovascular accident, recent (within 2 months) intracranial or intraspinal surgery or trauma, intracranial neoplasm, arteriovenous malformation or aneurysm, known bleeding diathesis, or severe uncontrolled hypertension. Serious bleeding reactions (i.e., internal and/or surface bleeding) may occur and appropriate precautions must be taken. Intramuscular injections should be avoided. Intracranial bleeding has occurred in some patients. The coronary thrombolysis produced by the drug may result in arrhythmias associated with reperfusion.

Administration: Intravenous infusion.

Preparations: Vials, 20 mg (11.6 million IU) and 50 mg (29 million IU). Powder for injection, 2 mg.

ALternaGEL®, see Aluminum Hydroxide Gel

ALTOPREV®, see Lovastatin

ALTRETAMINE—Hexalen®

Description/Actions: A synthetic cytotoxic agent that must be metabolized for its cytotoxic effect to develop. Indicated for use as a single agent in the palliative treatment of patients with persistent or recurrent ovarian cancer following firstline therapy with a cisplatin and/or alkylating agent-based combination.

Precautions/Adverse Reactions: Should not be used in patients with pre-existing severe bone marrow depression or severe neurologic toxicity. Adverse reactions include nausea, vomiting, peripheral neuropathy, and CNS symptoms (e.g., mood disorders, ataxia, dizziness, vertigo). Neurologic examinations should be performed regularly. May cause myelosuppression (e.g., leukopenia, thrombocytopenia), and peripheral blood counts should be monitored at least monthly prior to the initiation of each course of the drug. May cause fetal damage if administered during pregnancy. If a nursing mother is to be treated with the drug, it is recommended that breast-feeding be discontinued. Concurrent use with a monoamine oxidase inhibitor may cause severe orthostatic hypotension. Activity may be increased by the concurrent use of cimetidine.

Administration: Oral. The total daily dose should be given as 4 divided doses after meals and at bedtime.

Preparations: Capsules, 50 mg.

ALUDROX®, see Aluminum and Magnesium Hydroxide

ALUMINUM ACETATE

Description/Actions: Astringent used as a wet dressing (e.g., Burow's solution) for relief of inflammatory conditions of the skin.

Preparations: Solution.

ALUMINUM AND MAGNESIUM HYDROXIDE—Aludrox®, Maalox®

Description/Actions: Antacid indicated for hyperacidity associated with ulcers and other GI conditions.

Preparations: Liquid and tablets.

ALUMINUM CARBONATE GEL, BASIC—Basaljel®

Description/Actions: Antacid indicated for hyperacidity associated with ulcers and other GI conditions. Also indicated for the management of hyperphosphatemia or for use with a low phosphate diet to prevent formation of phosphate urinary stones.

Preparations: Capsules, tablets, and suspension.

ALUMINUM HYDROXIDE GEL—Amphojel®, ALternaGEL®

Description/Actions: Antacid indicated for hyperacidity associated with ulcers and other GI conditions.

Preparations: Capsules, tablets, suspension.

ALUMINUM PHOSPHATE GEL—Phosphaljel®

Description/Actions: Indicated to reduce fecal excretion of phosphates.

Preparations: Suspension.

ALUPENT®, see Metaproterenol Sulfate

ALURATE®, see Aprobarbital

AMANTADINE HYDROCHLORIDE—Symmetrel®

Description/Actions: Antiviral and antiparkinson agent indicated in the prevention and treatment of respiratory tract illness caused by influenza A virus strains. Also indicated for parkinsonism and drug-induced extrapyramidal reactions.

Precautions/Adverse Reactions: Adverse reactions include orthostatic hypotensive episodes, urinary retention, depression, psychosis, and congestive heart failure.

Administration: Oral.

Preparations: Capsules, 100 mg. Syrup, 50 mg/5 ml.

AMARYL, see Glimepiride

AMBENONIUM CHLORIDE—Mytelase®

Description/Actions: Anticholinesterase indicated for the treatment of myasthenia gravis.

Preparations: Tablets, 10 mg.

AMBIEN®, see Zolpidem Tartrate

AMCINONIDE—Cyclocort®

Description/Actions: Corticosteroid indicated in the topical treatment of corticosteroid-responsive dermatoses.

Preparations: Cream, ointment, and lotion, 0.1%.

AMERGE®, see Naratriptan

AMICAR®, see Aminocaproic Acid

AMIDATE®, see Etomidate

AMIFOSTINE—Ethyol®

Description/Actions: Cytoprotective agent for cisplatin. Reduces renal toxicity due to cumulative effects of cisplatin in patients being treated for ovarian cancer or nonsmall-cell lung cancer.

Precautions/Adverse Reactions: Allergic manifestations including anaphylaxis and severe cutaneous reactions have been associated rarely with amifostine administration. Serious cutaneous hypersensitivity reactions have included erythema multi-forme, Stevens-Johnson syndrome, toxic epidermal necrolysis, toxoderma, and exfoliative dermatitis, which have been reported more frequently when amifostine is used as a radioprotectant. Some of these reactions have been fatal or have required hospitalization and or discontinuance of therapy. Should not be used in patients with hypotension or dehydration. Adverse effects most commonly seen are hypotension, nausea, and vomiting.

Administration: Intravenous.

Preparations: Powder for injection, 500 mg/vial (with 500 mg mannitol).

AMIKACIN SULFATE—Amikin®

Description/Actions: Aminoglycoside antibiotic indicated in the treatment of serious infections caused by gram-negative bacteria, including *pseudomonas aeruginosa*. Is also effective in the treatment of staphylococcal infections.

Precautions/Adverse Reactions: May cause nephrotoxicity, ototoxicity, and neurotoxicity, and the concurrent or serial use of other nephrotoxic or ototoxic agents should be avoided.

Administration: Intravenous and intramuscular. Clinical response and dosage should be closely monitored.

Preparations: Vials, 100 and 500 mg, and 1 g. Syringes, 500 mg.

AMIKIN®, see Amikacin Sulfate

AMILORIDE HYDROCHLORIDE—Midamor®

Description/Actions: Potassium-sparing diuretic indicated as adjunctive treatment with thiazide or other potassium-depleting diuretics in patients with congestive heart failure or hypertension. Should be administered with food.

Preparations: Tablets, 5 mg.

AMINOACETIC ACID—Glycine

Description/Actions: Anti-infective for urological irrigation. Has also been used in conjunction with antacids.

Preparations: Solutions (for irrigation), 1.5%.

AMINOCAPROIC ACID—Amicar®

Description/Actions: Coagulant that inhibits fibrinolysis. Useful in enhancing hemostasis when fibrinolysis contributes to bleeding.

Preparations: Tablets, 500 mg. Syrup, 250 mg/ml. Vials (for IV use) 250 mg/ml.

AMINOLEVULINIC ACID HYDROCHLORIDE—Levulan Kerastick® for Topical Solution

Description/Actions: Used with BLU-U Blue Light Photodynamic Therapy Illuminator for treatment of nonhyperkeratotic actinic keratoses of the face or scalp.

Precautions/Adverse Reactions: Levulan Kerastick for Topical Solution plus blue light illumination is contraindicated in patients with cutaneous photosensitivity at wave lengths of 400–450 nm, porphyria or known allergies to porphyrins, and in patients with known sensitivity to any of the components of the Levulan Kerastick for Topical Solution. Transient local symptoms following photodynamic therapy include stinging and/or burning, itching, erythema, and edema. After application, patients should avoid exposure of the photosensitive treatment sites to sunlight or bright indoor light during the period prior to blue light treatment. Sunscreens will not protect the patient against photosensitivity reactions. Care should be taken not to apply Levulan Kerastick to perilesional skin.

Administration: The recommended treatment frequency is one application of Levulan Topical Solution and one dose of illumination per treatment site per 8-week treatment session. Application of the product to target lesions with Levulan Kerastick is followed 14–18 hours later by illumination with blue light using the BLU-U Blue Light Photodynamic Therapy Illuminator.

Patient Care Implications: This product is not intended for application by patients or unqualified medical personnel.

Preparations: Levulan Kerasticks for Topical Solution, 20%.

AMINOPHYLLINE—Theophylline Ethylenediamine, Phyllocontin®

Description/Actions: Bronchodilator indicated for the management of bronchial asthma, chronic bronchitis, and emphysema. Has been used as a diuretic and in certain cardiovascular disorders.

Preparations: Tablets, 100 and 200 mg. Controlled-release tablets, 225 mg. Liquid, 105 mg/5 ml. Suppositories, 250 and 500 mg. Ampules and vials, 250 mg.

AMINOSALICYLATE SODIUM—Para-aminosalicylate Sodium, PAS Sodium

Description/Actions: Antitubercular agent indicated for tuberculosis in combination with other antitubercular agents.

Preparations: Tablets, 500 mg. Powder.

AMINOSALICYLIC ACID, see Aminosalicylate Sodium

AMIODARONE HYDROCHLORIDE—Cordarone®

Description/Actions: A class III antiarrhythmic agent indicated for documented life-threatening, recurrent ventricular fibrillation and for recurrent, hemodynamically unstable ventricular tachycardia. Use when these conditions have not responded to treatment with other antiarrhythmic agents or when alternative drugs were not tolerated. Is often effective in patients with serious ventricular arrhythmias that are refractory to other agents.

Precautions/Adverse reactions: Contraindicated in patients with severe sinus-node dysfunction, causing marked sinus bradycardia; second- and third-degree AV block; and when episodes of bradycardia have caused syncope (except when used in conjunction with a pacemaker). Amiodarone is contraindicated in patients with a known hypersensitivity to the drug or to any component of the formulation including iodine. Amiodarone has several potential fatal toxicities including pulmonary toxicity, hepatic toxicity, and worsened arrhythmias. Cases of optic neuropathy and or optic neuritis usually resulting in visual impairment that may progress to permanent blindness have been reported in patients treated with amiodarone. Amiodarone can cause either hyperthyroidism or hypothyroidism. Thyroid function should be monitored prior to treatment and periodically thereafter, particularly in elderly patients, and in any patient with a history of thyroid nodules, goiter, or other thyroid dysfunction. Amiodarone-induced hyperthyroidism usually possesses a greater hazard to the patient than hypothyroidism because of the possibility of arrhythmia breakthrough or aggravation, which may result in death. Careful assessment of the potential risks versus benefits must be made when amiodarone is co-administered with other drugs known to prolong the QT_c interval. Adverse reactions include pulmonary toxicity that may be fatal, proarrhythmic events, GI effects, neurologic effects (e.g., fatigue, tremor), ocular effects (e.g., visual halos, blurred vision), hepatic dysfunction, hepatitis, cholestatic hepatitis, cirrhosis, epididymitis, vasculitis, pseudotumor cerebri, thrombocytopenia, angioedema, bronchiolitis obliterans organizing pneumonia (possibly fatal), pleuritis, pancreatitis, toxic epidermal necrolysis, myopathy, hemolytic anemia, aplastic anemia, pancytopenia, neutropenia, and dermatologic effects (e.g., photosensitivity reactions). May interact with and increase the activity of digoxin, warfarin, diltiazem, and other antiarrhythmic agents. Orally has variable absorption. Slow onset of action and long duration of action make dosing and monitoring of therapy difficult. IV administration results in complete bioavailability. Contains the preservative benzyl alcohol, which has been associated with a fatal "gasping syndrome" in neonates. Oral use during pregnancy has been associated with neonatal congenital goiter/hypothyroidism and hyperthyroidism.

Administration: Oral/IV.

Preparations: Tablets, 200 mg. Injection, 50 mg/ml in 3 ml ampules.

AMITRIPTYLINE HYDROCHLORIDE—Elavil®, Endep®

Description/Actions: Tricyclic antidepressant indicated for the relief of symptoms of depression.

Precautions/Adverse Reactions: Should not be given concomitantly with a monoamine oxidase inhibitor. Is not recommended for use during the acute recovery phase following myocardial infarction. Use cautiously in patients with history of seizure, urinary retention, glaucoma, cardiovascular disease, suicidal tendencies, surgery, ECT, psychosis, hyperthyroidism, diabetes, and liver dysfunction. Adverse reactions include CNS effects, so patients should be cautioned regarding activities such as driving and operating machinery, as well as interactions with other CNS-acting drugs including alcohol. Other adverse reactions include anticholinergic effects (e.g., dry mouth, blurred vision), GI effects (e.g., nausea, vomiting), and cardiovascular effects (e.g., orthostatic hypotension). Caution should be exercised in patients with cardiovascular disorders. May reduce the action of guanethidine and guanadrel.

Administration: Oral and intramuscular.

Preparations: Tablets, 10, 25, 50, 75, 100, and 150 mg. Vials, 10 mg/ml.

AMLEXANOX 5%—Aphthasol®

Description/Actions: Oral adhesive paste indicated in the treatment of canker sores.

Precautions/Adverse Reactions: Not for use in immunocompromised patients. Discontinue if rash or contact mucositis occurs. Pregnancy

Category B. Use cautiously in nursing mothers. Adverse reactions include transient local pain, burning, and/or stinging. Instruct patients to consult health care provider if ulcer does not heal after 10 days.

Administration: Topical.

Preparations: 5 g tubes of 5% adhesive oral paste.

AMLODIPINE BESYLATE—Norvasc®

Description/Actions: Is a calcium channel-blocking agent that causes a reduction in peripheral vascular resistance and a lowering in blood pressure. Indicated for the treatment of hypertension. Also indicated for the treatment of chronic stable angina and vasospastic angina (Prinzmetal's or variant angina).

Precautions/Adverse Reactions: Adverse reactions include edema, flushing, palpitation, dizziness, fatigue, somnolence, nausea, and abdominal pain.

Administration: Oral.

Preparations: Tablets, 2.5, 5, and 10 mg.

AMMONIA, AROMATIC SPIRIT—Aromatic Ammonia Spirit

Description/Actions: Respiratory stimulant used by inhalation to treat or prevent fainting.

Preparations: Inhalant and solution.

AMMONIATED MERCURY

Description/Actions: Anti-infective agent used for the topical treatment of certain skin infections and conditions such as psoriasis.

Preparations: Ointment, 5% and 10%.

AMMONIUM CARBONATE

Description/Actions: Respiratory stimulant used in the preparation of aromatic ammonia spirit and as a source of ammonia in smelling salts.

AMMONIUM CHLORIDE

Description/Actions: Expectorant, diuretic, and acidifying agent. Used orally as an expectorant, diuretic, and to acidify the urine, and intravenously in the treatment of certain hypochloremic states and metabolic alkalosis.

Preparations: Tablets, 500 mg and 1 g. Vials and bottles, 0.4 mEq/ml and 5 mEq/ml.

AMMONIUM LACTATE—Lac-Hydrin®

Description/Actions: Emollient indicated in treatment of dry skin and ichthyosis vulgaris. Transient stinging or burning, erythema, peeling, eczema, petechiae, dryness, and hyperpigmentation may occur.

Administration: Apply and rub into affected areas twice daily.

Preparations: Lotion and cream, 12%.

AMOBARBITAL SODIUM—Amytal Sodium®

Description/Actions: Barbiturate sedative-hypnotic indicated for the treatment of anxiety and convulsive disorders, for preanesthetic sedation, and in narcoanalysis and narcotherapy.

Preparations: Vials, 250 and 500 mg.

AMOXAPINE—Asendin®

Description/Actions: Antidepressant (dibenzoxazepine) indicated for the relief of symptoms of depression, and for depression accompanied by anxiety or agitation.

Preparations: Tablets, 25, 50, 100, and 150 mg.

AMOXICILLIN—Amoxil®, Dispermox®, Polymox®, Trimox®

Description/Actions: Is bactericidal and exhibits activity that is most similar to that of ampicillin. Indicated for the treatment of infections caused by susceptible strains of *Escherichia coli, Haemophilus influenzae, Proteus mirabilis, Neisseria gonorrhoeae, streptococci,* and *nonpenicillinase-producing staphylococci.* Is commonly used in the treatment of respiratory tract infections, otitis media, urinary tract infections, and uncomplicated gonorrhea.

Precautions/Adverse Reactions: Contraindicated in patients with a history of allergic reaction to any of the penicillins. Adverse reactions include hypersensitivity reactions, rash, urticaria, nausea, vomiting, and diarrhea.

Administration: Oral. May be administered without regard to meals.

Preparations: Capsules, 250 and 500 mg. Chewable tablets, 125, 250, and 875 mg. Tablets for oral suspension, 200 and 400 mg.

AMOXICILLIN/CLAVULANATE POTASSIUM—Augmentin®, Augmentin® XR

Description/Actions: Clavulanic acid inhibits beta-lactamase enzymes and protects amoxicillin from degradation by these enzymes; the spectrum of action of amoxicillin is extended to include many gram-positive and gram-negative bacteria, including *Moraxella catarrhalis.* Indicated for the treatment of lower respiratory infections, otitis media, sinusitis, skin and skin-structure infections, and urinary tract infections.

Precautions/Adverse Reactions: Contraindicated in patients with a history of allergic reaction to any of the penicillins. Adverse reactions include hypersensitivity reactions, rash, urticaria, nausea, vomiting, and diarrhea. Incidence of GI effects is higher than when amoxicillin is administered alone. Due to clavulanic acid component, 2 Augmentin 250 mg are not equivalent to 1 Augmentin 500 mg.

Administration: Oral. Administer with food.

Preparations: Tablets, 250, 500, and 875 mg with 125 mg potassium clavulanate, and 1g with 62.5 mg potassium clavulanate. Chewable tablets, 125 mg amoxicillin with 31.25 mg of clavulanic acid, 200 mg amoxicillin, with 28.5 mg clavulanic acid, 250 mg amoxicillin with 62.5 mg of clavulanic acid, and 400 mg amoxicillin with 57 mg of clavulanic acid. Powder for oral suspension, 125 mg amoxicillin with 31.25 mg clavulanic acid/5 ml; 200 mg amoxicillin with 28.5 mg clavulanic acid/5ml; and 400 mg amoxicillin with 57 mg clavulanic acid/5 ml; and 600 mg amoxicillin with 42.9 mg clavulanic acid/5 ml.

AMPHETAMINE SULFATE

Description/Actions: Central nervous system stimulant indicated in the treatment of narcolepsy, attention deficit disorder in children, and exogenous obesity.

Preparations: Tablets, 5 and 10 mg.

AMPHOJEL®, see Aluminum Hydroxide Gel

AMPHOTEC®—Amphotericin B Cholesteryl Sulfate

AMBISOME®—Amphotericin B Liposome for Injection

Description/Actions: Antifungal agent indicated in patients with aspergillosis who are intolerant of or refractory to conventional dosage form of Amphotericin B. Empiric treatment of presumed fungal infections in febrile neutropenic patients.

Administration: Intravenous

Preparations: Vials, 100 mg with single use filter needle.

AMPHOTERICIN B—Fungizone®

Description/Actions: Antifungal agent indicated for the intravenous treatment of systemic fungal infections, topical treatment of cutaneous candidal infections, and oral suspension for oral candidiasis.

Precautions/Adverse Reactionss: Be fully familiar with the use of this product. Administer under close supervision; cardiopulmonary resuscitation facilities should be available. Monitor serum creatinine, liver function, serum electrolytes (esp. magnesium and potassium), and CBC.

Preparations: Vials, 50 mg. Oral suspension, 100 mg/ml. Cream, ointment, and lotion, 3%.

AMPICILLIN—Omnipen®, Polycillin®, Principen®, Totacillin®

AMPICILLIN SODIUM

Description/Actions: Is bactericidal. Indicated for the treatment of infections caused by susceptible strains of *Escherichia coli, Haemophilus influenzae, Neisseria gonorrhoeae, Neisseria meningitidis, Proteus mirabilis, Salmonella* species, *Shigella, streptococci, and nonpenicillinase-producing staphylococci.* Is used in the treatment of urinary tract infections, respiratory tract infections, and uncomplicated gonorrhea. Used intravenously in the treatment of meningitis and septicemia caused by susceptible organisms.

Precautions/Adverse Reactions: Contraindicated in patients with a history of allergic reaction to any of the penicillins. Adverse reactions include hypersensitivity reactions, rash, urticaria, nausea, vomiting, and diarrhea.

Administration: Oral, intravenous, and intramuscular. When administered orally, it is best administered apart from meals.

Preparations: Capsules, 250 and 500 mg. Powder for oral suspension, 125, 250, and 500 mg/5 ml (when reconstituted). Vials, ampicillin sodium equivalent to 125, 500 mg, 1, 2, and 10 g of ampicillin per vial.

AMPICILLIN SODIUM/SULBACTAM SODIUM—Unasyn®

Description/Actions: A combination of ampicillin and a beta-lactamase inhibitor, sulbactam. By irreversibly binding to beta-lactamase enzymes that are produced by certain bacteria, sulbactam protects ampicillin against inactivation by these enzymes, thereby extending the spectrum of ampicillin to include many bacteria that are resistant to it when it is given alone. Indicated for intra-abdominal, gynecological, and skin-structure infections caused by susceptible bacteria. Among the bacteria that are susceptible are beta-lactamase producing strains of *Acinetobacter calcoaceticus, Bacteroides* species (including *B. fragilis*), *Enterobacter* species, *Escherichia coli, Klebsiella* species (including *K. pneumoniae*), *Proteus mirabilis,* and *Staphylococcus aureus.*

Precautions/Adverse Reactions: Contraindicated in patients with a known hypersensitivity to any of the penicillins. Adverse reactions include diarrhea, rash, pain at the intramuscular and intravenous injection sites, and thrombophlebitis. Should not be used in patients with mononucleosis because of the likelihood of a nonallergic skin rash developing.

Administration: Intravenous and intramuscular.

Preparations: Vials and piggyback bottles containing 1.5 g (1 g ampicillin sodium plus 0.5 g sulbactam sodium) and 3 g (2 g ampicillin sodium plus 1 g sulbactam sodium).

AMPRENAVIR—Agenerase®

Description/Actions: Amprenavir is an HIV protease inhibitor indicated as a combination agent with other antiretroviral agents in the treatment of HIV infection.

Precautions/Adverse Reactions: Amprenavir is contraindicated in concomitant use with several other drugs. Prescribers need to verify the patient's drug profile and consult product literature before prescribing. The capsules and solution are not interchangeable on a mg to mg basis. Use cautiously in patients with sulfa allergy and the elderly. Reduce the dose in patients with hepatic dysfunction. Monitor diabetics for hyperglycemia and fat redistribution and hemophiliacs for spontaneous bleeding. Pregnancy Category C. Use in nursing mothers not recommended. Adverse reactions include GI upset, rash (e.g., Stevens-Johnson), paresthesia, and depression.

Administration: Oral.

Patient Care Implications: Instruct patients to continue to use appropriate barrier precautions when engaging in sexual activity to prevent spread of the disease. Patients taking amprenavir should be instructed not to use hormonal contraceptives because some birth control pills have been found to decrease the concentration of amprenavir. Therefore, patients receiving hormonal contraceptives should be instructed to use alternative contraceptive measures during therapy with amprenavir. Let the patient know this drug is not a cure, but can keep the infection under control. Tell the patient to avoid taking the drug with a high fat meal. Do not take additional vitamin E supplements, as this drug supplies enough. Do not switch between capsules and oral solution without consulting the physician.

Preparations: Capsules, 50 and 150 mg (contain Vitamin E). Oral solution, 15 mg/ml grape-bubblegum-peppermint flavor (contains vitamin E).

AMYL NITRITE

Description/Actions: Antianginal agent administered by inhalation for the relief of acute angina pectoris.

Preparations: Inhalant, 0.18 and 0.3 ml.

AMYTAL®, see Amobarbital Sodium

ANADROL-50®, see Oxymetholone

ANAFRANIL®, see Clomipramine Hydrochloride

ANAGRELIDE—Agrylin®

Description/Actions: Indicated in the treatment of essential thrombocythemia. Reduces platelet counts at therapeutic doses and at higher doses inhibits platelet aggregation as well. Does not affect WBC counts or coagulation parameters at therapeutic doses, although it may have clinically insignificant effect on RBC parameters.

Precautions/Adverse Reactions: Anagrelide is contraindicated in patients with severe hepatic impairment. Exposure to anagrelide is increased 8-fold in patients with moderate hepatic impairment. In patients with moderate hepatic impairment, dose reduction is required and patients should be closely monitored for cardiovascular effects. Anagrelide should be used with caution in patients with known or suspected heart disease. A pre-treatment cardiovascular examination is recommended. Therapeutic doses of anagrelide may cause vasodilation, tachycardia, palpitations, and congestive heart failure. Adverse reactions include headache, palpitations, tachycardia, anorexia, edema, pain, dizziness, dyspnea, rash, paresthesia, tachycardia, anorexia, CHF, MI, malaise, cardiomyopathy, cardiomegaly, complete heart block, atrial fibrillation, CVA, pericarditis, pulmonary infiltrates/fibrosis, hypertension, pancreatitis, ulcer, and seizures. Instruct patients to report signs/symptoms of hepatic, renal, or cardiac dysfunction.

Administration: 0.5 mg 4 times daily or 1 mg twice daily for at least 1 week. Then adjust to the lowest effective dosage required to reduce and maintain platelet count <600,000/mcl.

Preparations: Capsules, 0.5 and 1 mg.

ANAKINRA—Kineret™

Description/Actions: Anakinra is indicated for the reduction in signs and symptoms and for slowing the progression of structural damage in moderately to severely active rheumatoid arthritis, in patients 18 years of age or older who have failed one or more disease modifying antirheumatic drugs (DMARDs). Anakinra can be used alone or in combination with DMARDs other than Tumor Necrosis Factor (TNF) blocking agents.

Precautions/Adverse Reactions: Anakinra is contraindicated in patients with a known sensitivity to *E. coli* derived proteins, to anakinra, or to any components of the drug. It has been associated with an increased incidence of serious infections. Administration should be discontinued if the patient develops a serious infection. Treatment should not be started in patients with active infections. Safety and efficacy in patients with chronic infections or immunosuppressed patients have not been evaluated. When used with tumor necrosis factor (TNF)–blocking agents, preliminary data suggest a higher rate of serious infections. When given with etanercept, neutropenia was observed. Anakinra interferes with normal immune response mechanisms to new antigens such as vaccines; therefore, vaccination may not be effective. Live vaccines should not be given concurrently with anakinra. Pregnancy Category B. No controlled trials in pregnant women. Use only if clearly needed. It is not known whether anakinra is secreted in breast milk; use caution in nursing women. Safety and efficacy in juvenile rheumatoid arthritis have not been established. The most common adverse reactions were injection site reactions (typically lasts 14–28 days), serious infection (stop drug), neutropenia, headache, nausea, diarrhea, sinusitis, and influenza-like symptoms.

Administration: Geriatrics and adults: 100 mg once a day by subcutaneous injection. Administer at same time each day.

Patient Care Implications: Rotate injection sites; injection should be given at least 1 inch away from previous site. Discard any unused portion; anakinra contains no preservative. Do not shake. Neutrophil counts should be obtained prior to treatment and repeated monthly for 3 months, and thereafter quarterly for a period up to 1 year. Instruct patient in the importance of proper disposal of syringe, and caution against reuse of needles, syringes, and drug. Should be stored in refrigerator. Do not freeze. Protect from light.

Preparations: Injection, prefilled 1 ml glass syringe with 27 gauge needle: 100 mg/0.67 ml.

ANAPROX®, see Naproxen Sodium

ANAPROX DS®, see Naproxen Sodium

ANASPAZ, see Hyoscyamine Sulfate

ANASTROZOLE—Arimidex®

Description/Actions: Antiestrogen that exerts antineoplastic effect and is indicated for the treatment of advanced breast cancer in postmenopausal women with disease progression after tamoxifen therapy and for the adjuvant treatment of postmenopausal women with hormone receptor positive early breast cancer.

Precautions/Adverse Reactions: Contraindicated in pregnancy. Asthenia, GI disturbances, headache, hot flashes, pain, dyspnea, rash, dry mouth, peripheral edema, depression, parenthesia, and vaginal bleeding may occur. Anastrozole may be associated with rash, including very rare cases of mucocutaneous disorders such as erythema multiforme and Stevens-Johnson Syndrome.

Administration: Oral

Preparations: Tablets, 1 mg.

ANCEF®, see Cefazolin Sodium

ANCOBON®, see Flucytosine

ANDRODERM®, see Testosterone

ANDROGEL®, see Testosterone Gel

AndroGel® 1% PUMP, see Testosterone Gel

ANECTINE®, see Succinylcholine Chloride

ANGIOMAX™, see Bivalirudin

ANISINDIONE—Miradon®

Description/Actions: Anticoagulant (indandione) indicated for the prophylaxis and treatment of conditions such as venous thrombosis and pulmonary embolism.

Preparations: Tablets, 50 mg.

ANISOTROPINE METHYLBROMIDE

Description/Actions: Anticholinergic agent indicated as adjunctive therapy in the management of peptic ulcer.

Preparations: Tablets, 50 mg.

ANISTREPLASE—Eminase®

Description/Actions: Thrombolytic agent also known as anisoylated plasminogen streptokinase activator complex (APSAC). Promotes the conversion of plasminogen to plasmin, which is fibrinolytic. Indicated for acute management of coronary thrombosis (myocardial infarction). Treatment should be initiated as soon as possible after the onset of AMI symptoms.

Precautions/Adverse Reactions: Contraindicated in patients who are hypersensitive to the drug or to streptokinase. Is also contraindicated in patients with active internal bleeding, history of cerebrovascular accident, recent intracranial or intraspinal surgery or trauma, intracranial neoplasm, arteriovenous malformation or aneurysm, known bleeding diathesis, or severe, uncontrolled hypertension. Serious bleeding reactions (e.g., internal bleeding and/or superficial or surface bleeding) may occur and appropriate precautions must be taken. Concurrent use of heparin anticoagulation may contribute to the bleeding. Warfarin, aspirin, and dipyridamole may increase the risk of bleeding if administered prior to anistreplase therapy. Intramuscular injections should be avoided during treatment with anistreplase. Other adverse reactions include hypotension and allergic-type reactions.

Administration: Intravenous.

Preparations: Vials, 30 units.

ANSAID®, see Flurbiprofen

ANSPOR®, see Cephradine

ANTABUSE®, see Disulfiram

ANTAGON®, see Ganirelix

ANTEPAR®, see Piperazine Citrate

ANTHRA-DERM®, see Anthralin

ANTHRALIN—Anthra-Derm®, Dithranol

Description/Actions: Used in the topical management of psoriasis and certain other dermatologic disorders.

Preparations: Cream and ointment, 0.1%, 0.2%, 0.25%, 0.4%, 0.5%, and 1%.

ANTILIRIUM®, see Physostigmine

ANTIMINTH®, see Pyrantel Pamoate

ANTISPAS®, see Dicyclomine Hydrochoride

ANTITHROMBIN III (HUMAN)—ATnativ®

Description/Actions: Is identical with heparin cofactor I, a factor that is necessary for heparin to exert its anticoagulant effect. Inactivates thrombin and the activated forms of Factors IX, X, XI, and XII. Indicated for the treatment of patients with hereditary antithrombin III deficiency in connection with surgical or obstetrical procedures or when they suffer from thromboembolism.

Precautions/Adverse Reactions: The anticoagulant effect of heparin is increased by concurrent treatment with antithrombin III, so the dosage of heparin should be reduced.

Administration. Intravenous. Plasma antithrombin III levels should be measured preceding and 30 minutes after the dose until the patient is stabilized, and thereafter measured once a day immediately before the next infusion.

Preparations: Infusion bottles, 500 international units.

ANTIVERT®, see Meclizine Hydrochloride

ANTURANE®, see Sulfinpyrazone

ANZEMET®, see Dolasetron Mesylate

APHTHASOL®, see Amlexanox 5%

A.P.L.®, see Chorionic Gonadotropin

APRACLONIDINE HYDROCHLORIDE—Lopidine®

Description/Actions: An alpha adrenergic agonist which, when instilled into the eye, reduces intraocular pressure. Indicated (1% solution) to control or prevent postsurgical elevations in intraocular pressure that occur in patients after argon laser trabeculoplasty or argon laser iridotomy. Also indicated (0.5% solution) for short-term adjunctive therapy in patients on maximally tolerated medical therapy who require additional intraocular pressure reduction.

Precautions/Adverse Reactions: Adverse reactions include upper lid elevation, conjunctival blanching, and mydriasis.

Administration: Ophthalmic.

Preparations: Ophthalmic solution, containing the equivalent of 0.5% and 1% apraclonidine base.

APREPITANT—Emend®

Description/Actions: Aprepitant is a selective high-affinity antagonist of human substance P/neurokinin 1(NK1) receptors. It crosses the blood-brain barrier and occupies brain NK1 receptors. Aprepitant augments the antiemetic activity of the $5-HT_3$ receptor antagonist ondansetron and the corticoid dexamethasone, and inhibits both the acute and delayed phases of cisplatin-induced emesis. Aprepitant is for the prevention of acute and delayed nausea and vomiting associated with highly emetogenic chemotherapy in combination with a corticosteroid and a $5-HT_3$ receptor antagonist. Aprepitant is NOT intended for the treatment of nausea and vomiting or for chronic continuous therapy.

Precautions/Adverse Reactions: Aprepitant is contraindicated in persons hypersensitive to aprepitant or any component of the formulation. Aprepitant is a moderate CYP3A4 inhibitor; it should not be used concurrently with pimozide, terfenadine, astemizole, or cisapride. Inhibition of cytochrome P450 isoenzyme 3A4(CYP3A4) by aprepitant could result in elevated plasma concentrations of these drugs, potentially causing serious or life-threatening reactions. Aprepitant should be used with caution in patients receiving concomitant medicinal products, including chemotherapy agents that are primarily metabolized through CYP3A4 (docetaxel, paclitaxel, etoposide, irinotecan, ifosfamide, imatinib, vinorelbine, vinblastine, and vincristine). Coadministration with warfarin may result in a clinically significant decrease in International Normalized Ration (INR) or prothrombin time. Patients on chronic warfarin therapy should have INR monitored in the 2-week period, especially at 7 to 10 days following initiation of the 3-day regimen. CYP3A4 inducers may decrease the levels/effects of aprepitant (i.e. carbamazepine, nafcillin, nevirapine, phenobarbital, phenytoins, and rifamycins). CYP3A4 inhibitors may increase the levels/effects of aprepitant (i.e., azole antifungals, ciprofloxacin, clarithromycin, diclofenac, erythromycin, imatinib, nicardipine, protease inhibitors, quinidine, and verapamil). Bioavailability of corticosteroids may be increased. Dexamethasone doses should be decreased by 50% (oral). Methylprednisolone doses should be decreased by 25% (IV) or 50% (oral). Oral contraceptive efficacy may be reduced; alternative or back-up methods of contraception recommended. Pregnancy Category B. Excretion in breast milk unknown/not recommended. Most common adverse reactions were asthenia, fatigue, weakness, nausea, hiccups, constipation, diarrhea, dizziness, dehydration, and headaches.

Administration: Oral.

Patient Care Implications: May take with or without food. Give 1 hour prior to chemotherapy; subsequent doses should be given in the morning. Avoid grapefruit juice and St. John's wort. Report unusual fatigue, weakness, dizziness, disorientation, abdominal discomfort, chest pain, respiratory distress, or other persistent side effects to physician.

Preparations: Capsule: 80 mg, 125 mg.

APRESOLINE®, see Hydralazine

APROBARBITAL—Alurate®

Description/Actions: Barbiturate sedative-hypnotic indicated for the treatment of anxiety and insomnia.

Preparations: Elixir, 40 mg/5 ml.

APROTININ—Trasylol®

Description/Actions: Is a natural protease inhibitor that inhibits fibrinolysis and decreases bleeding, and reduces the need for donor blood or blood products. Indicated for prophylactic use to reduce perioperative blood loss and the need for blood transfusion in patients undergoing cardiopulmonary bypass in the course of repeat coronary artery bypass graft (CABG) surgery. Is also indicated in selected cases of primary CABG surgery where the risk of bleeding is especially high or where transfusion is unavailable or unacceptable.

Precautions/Adverse Reactions: Adverse reactions include anaphylactic reactions, renal dysfunction, and abnormal liver function tests. All patients should first receive a test dose to assess the potential for allergic reactions. Patients who experience any allergic reaction to the test dose should not receive further administration of the drug. Particular caution is necessary when administering aprotinin (even test doses) to patients who have received the drug in the past. In reexposure cases, an antihistamine should be administered intravenously shortly before the loading dose. May inhibit the effects of fibrinolytic agents. May be administered concurrently with heparin; however, aprotinin prolongs the activated clotting time (ACT) and some patients may require additional heparin, even in the presence of ACT levels that appear to represent adequate anticoagulation.

Administration: Intravenous. Is administered through a central line and other drugs should not be administered using the same line. A 1 ml (10,000 Kallikrein Inhibitor Units [KIU]) test dose should be administered at least 10 minutes before the loading dose. The loading dose is given slowly over 20–30 minutes after induction of anesthesia but prior to sternotomy. When the loading dose is complete, it is followed by the constant infusion dose, which is continued until surgery is complete and the patient leaves the operating room. A "pump prime" dose is added to the priming fluid of the cardiopulmonary bypass circuit, by replacement of an aliquot of the priming fluid, prior to the institution of the cardiopulmonary bypass.

Preparations: Vials 1,000,000 and 2,000,000 Kallikrein Inhibitor Units (KIU). One million units represents 140 mg of the drug.

AQUA MEPHYTON®, see Phytonadione

AQUACARE®, see Urea

AQUASOL A®, see Vitamin A

AQUASOL E®, see Vitamin E

ARA-C, see Cytarabine

ARALEN®, see Chloroquine

ARAMINE®, see Metaraminol

ARANESP™, see Darbepoetin Alfa

ARDEPARIN—Normiflo®

Description/Actions: Antithrombolic indicated in the prevention of postop deep vein thrombosis in patients undergoing elective knee replacement.

Precautions/Adverse Reactions: Contraindicated in severe hemorrhagic diathesis, active major bleeding; type II thrombocytopenia associated with a positive in vitro test for antiplatelet antibody associated with ardeparin sodium, heparin, or pork allergy. Use cautiously in neuraxial anesthesia and postop indwelling epidural catheter or spinal puncture (risk of epidural or spinal hematoma), asthma, heparin-induced thrombocytopenia, bleeding disorders, severe renal dysfunction (monitor carefully if serum $Cr \geq 2$ mg/dl), severe uncontrolled hypertension, acute bacterial endocarditis, acute ulceration and angiodysplastic GI disease, bleeding diathesis, nonhemorrhagic stroke, invasive procedures, recent brain, spinal, or eye surgery. Adverse reactions include hemorrhage, hematoma, thrombocytopenia, local reactions (e.g., hematoma, pain), fever, allergic reaction, GI upset, constipation, rash, pruritus, edema, dizziness, insomnia, and anemia.

Administration: SQ injection.

Preparations: 5,000 anti-Xa units in 0.5 ml; 10,000 anti-Xa units in 0.5 ml.

ARDUAN®, see Pipecuronium Bromide

AREDIA®, see Pamidronate Disodium

ARGATROBAN

Description/Actions: Argatroban is an anticoagulant used in the prophylaxis or the treatment of thrombosis in adults with heparin-induced thrombocytopenia (HIT). Argatroban is also indicated for use during percutaneous coronary intervention (PTCI) in patients who have HIT or those who are at risk for HIT.

Precautions/Adverse Reactions: Argatroban is contraindicated in patients with active major bleeding, or in patients hypersensitive to this product or any of its product formulations. Because hemorrhage can occur with Argatroban, it should be used with extreme caution in patients with disease states or circumstances associated with increased risk of bleeding. Use caution in patients with hepatic impairment; initiate with a lower dose and titrate to desired effect. Concurrent use with warfarin will cause increased prolongation of the PT and INR greater than that of warfarin alone. Safety and efficacy for use with other thrombolytic agents have not been established. All parental anticoagulants should be discontinued before administration of Argatroban. Pregnancy Category B. No adequate and well-controlled studies have been done in pregnant women. Argatroban should be used in pregnant women only if clearly needed. It is not known if this drug is excreted in human milk; not recommended for nursing women. Safety and efficacy have not been established in children <18 years of age. Some adverse effects are gastrointestinal bleed, genitourinary bleeding and hematuria, hypotension, decrease in hemoglobin and hematocrit, fever, pain, diarrhea, nausea, and vomiting.

Administration: Intravenous.

Conversion to oral anticoagulant: Because there may be a combined effect on the INR when Argatroban is combined with warfarin, loading doses of warfarin should not be used. Warfarin therapy should be started at the expected daily dose.

Patient Care Implications: This medication can only be administered by intravenous infusion; vials must be diluted to 1 mg/ml prior to infusion and must not be mixed with other medications. Monitor aPTT, hemoglobin, and hematocrit. Inform patients to report any unusual bleeding or bruising while receiving Argatroban.

Preparations: Solution for injection: 100 mg/ml (2.5 ml) vials. Each vial contains 250 mg Argatroban.

ARGININE HYDROCHLORIDE—R-Gene®

Description/Actions: Diagnostic agent administered intravenously in the evaluation of pituitary function.

Preparations: Solution, 10%.

ARICEPT®, see Donepezil Hydrochloride

ARICEPT® ODT, see Donepezil

ARISTOCORT®, see Triamcinolone

ARIMIDEX, see Anastrozole

ARIPIPRAZOLE—Abilify®

Description/Actions: Aripiprazole is an atypical antipsychotic agent that exhibits high affinity for dopamine D_2 and D_3, serotonin 5-HT_{1A}, and 5-HT_{2A} receptors; moderate affinity for dopamine D_4, serotonin 5-HT_{2C} and 5-HT_7, alpha$_1$-adrenergic and histamine H_1 receptors, and moderate affinity for the serotonin reuptake site. Aripiprazole functions as a partial agonist at the dopamine D_2 and the serotonin 5-HT_{1A} receptors and as an agonist at the serotonin 5-HT_{2A} receptor. It is indicated for the treatment of schizophrenia and for the treatment of acute manic and mixed episodes associated with Bipolar Disorder.

Precautions/Adverse Reactions: Aripiprazole is contraindicated in patients with a known hypersensitivity to it or to any component of the formulation. There is an increased risk of mortality in elderly patients with dementia-related psychosis treated with atypical antipsychotic agents. Most deaths appeared to be either cardiovascular (e.g., heart failure, sudden death) or infectious (e.g., pneumonia). Aripiprazole is not approved for the treatment of patients with dementia-related psychosis. Cases of neuroleptic malignant syndrome (NMS) and tardive dyskinesia have been reported. Hyperglycemia associated with ketoacidosis or hyperosmolar coma or death has been reported in patients treated with atypical antipsychotics. Aripiprazole has been associated with orthostatic hypotension. Aripiprazole should be used with caution in patients with known cardiovascular disease (history of myocardial infarction or ischemic heart disease, heart failure, or conduction abnormalities), cerebrovascular disease or conditions that would predispose patients to hypotension (dehydration, hypovolemia, and treatment with antihypertensive medications). Seizures have been reported in patients treated with aripiprazole. Use with caution in patients with a history of seizures or with conditions that lower the seizure threshold. Aripiprazole has the potential to impair judgment, thinking, and motor skills. Use caution when operating hazardous machinery including automobiles. Aripiprazole may cause disruption of the body's ability to reduce core body temperature. Esophageal dysmotility and aspiration have been associated with aripiprazole. The possibility of a suicide attempt is inherent in psychotic illness. Close supervision of high-risk patients should accompany drug therapy. Coadministration of aripiprazole and cytochrome P450$_3$A4 (CYP$_3$A4) inducers such as carbamazepine can cause an increase in the clearance of aripiprazole and result in a decrease in aripiprazole plasma concentrations. Coadministration of aripiprazole and CYP$_3$A4 inhibitors (e.g., ketoconazole) and CYP$_2$D6 (quinidine, fluoxetine, or paroxetine) can inhibit aripiprazole elimination and lead to increased blood levels. No clinically significant effect of famotidine, valproate, or lithium was seen when aripiprazole was coadministered with these drugs. No significant pharmacokinetic interactions were observed when aripiprazole was coadministered with warfarin, dextromethorphan, or omeprazole. Pregnancy Category C. In animal studies, aripiprazole demonstrated developmental toxicity including possible teratogenic effects in rats and rabbits. No adequate and well-controlled studies in pregnant women. Use during pregnancy only if the potential benefit outweighs the potential risk to the fetus. Excretion in human breast milk is unknown. Breast feeding is not recommended. Safety and efficacy in pediatric and adolescent patients have not been established. Major adverse effects observed during therapy with aripiprazole include: headache, agitation, anxiety, insomnia, nausea, dyspepsia, somnolence, akathesia, lightheadedness, vomiting, constipation, asthenia, extrapyramidal syndrome, accidental injury, tremor, myalgia, pharyngitis, rhinitis, coughing, increased salivation, blurred vision, hypertension, and peripheral edema. Other adverse events observed during clinical trials include: weight gain, weight loss, gastroenteritis, flatulence, tooth caries, gastritis, gingivitis, gastrointestinal hemorrhage, hemorrhoids, colitis, gastroesophageal reflux, fecal incontinence, rectal hemorrhage, stomatitis, tongue edema, cholecystitis, mouth ulcer, oral moniliasis, fecal impaction, esophagitis, hematemesis, intestinal obstruction, gum hemorrhage, hepatitis, peptic ulcer, glossitis, melena, duodenal ulcer, cheilitis, hepatomegaly, pancreatitis, hyperthyroidism, hypothyroidism, ecchymosis, anemia, leukocytosis, leukopenia, lymphadenopathy, eosinophilia, macrocytic anemia, thrombocythemia, thrombocytopenia, increased creatinine phosphokinase, dehydration, hypercholesterolemia, hypokalemia, hyperkalemia, hypoglycemia, hyperlipidemia, hyponatremia, hypernatremia, cyanosis, increased alkaline phosphatase, increased blood urea nitrogen, increased SGPT, increased SGOT, increased creatinine, hyperuricemia, increased lactic dehydrogenase, gout, muscle cramps, arthralgias, myasthenia, bone pain, arthritis, myopathy, depression, nervousness, schizophrenic reaction, hallucinations, hostility, confusion, paranoid reaction, suicidal thought, abnormal gait, manic reaction, delusions, abnormal dreams, emotional lability, twitch, cogwheel rigidity, impaired concentration, dystonia, vasodilation, paresthesia, photosensitivity, migraine, fever, chest pain, heat stroke, flu syndrome, tachycardia, hypotension, bradycardia, palpitation, heart failure, myocardial infarction, cardiac arrest, atrial fibrillation, atrial flutter, AV block, prolonged QT interval, bundle branch block, deep vein thrombosis, angina, pallor, cardiomegaly, impotence, vertigo, stupor, bradykinesia, apathy, panic attack, decreased libido, increased libido, hypersomnia, dyskinesia, manic depressive reaction, ataxia, depersonalization, delirium, tardive dyskinesia, myoclonus, neuropathy, dysphoria, hyperkinesias, cerebral ischemia, increased reflexes, blunted affect, euphoria, intracranial hemorrhage, sinusitis, dyspnea, pneumonia, aspiration pneumonia, asthma, dry skin, rash, skin discoloration, alopecia, seborrhea, psoriasis, maculopapular rash, exfoliative dermatitis, pruritis, urticaria, conjunctivitis, ear pain, dry eye, eye pain, tinnitus, diplopia, urinary incontinence, urinary retention, cystitis, hematuria, dysuria, amenorrhea, vaginal hemorrhage, abnormal ejaculation, kidney failure, gynecomastia, albuminuria, breast pain, nocturia, polyuria, menorrhagia, anorgasmy, glycosuria, cervicitis, uterus hemorrhage, female lactation, priapism, and urolithiasis. Anaphylactic reactions, angioedema, and laryngospasm have been reported during post marketing surveillance.

Administration: Oral. No dosage adjustment in renal and/or hepatic impairment.

Patient Care Implications: Monitor patient for the development of neuroleptic malignant syndrome (NMS), and tardive dyskinesia. Patients should be monitored for symptoms of hyperglycemia including polydipsia, polyuria, polyphagia, and weakness. Patients should be instructed to avoid alcohol. Prescriptions should be written for the smallest quantity consistent with good patient management in order to reduce the risk of overdose.

Preparations: Tablets, 5mg, 10mg, 15mg, 20mg, and 30 mg. Oral solution, 1 mg/mL.

ARISTOSPAN®, see Triamcinolone Hexacetonide

ARIXTRA®, see Fondaparinux

AROMASIN®, see Exemestane

AROMATIC SPIRIT OF AMMONIA, see Ammonia, Aromatic Spirit

ARSENIC TRIOXIDE—Trisenox®

Description/Actions: Indicated for induction of remission and consolidation in patients with acute promyelocytic leukemia who are refractory to or have relapsed from retinoid and anthracycline chemotherapy and whose acute promyelocytic leukemia is characterized by the presence of the t(15;17) translocation or PML-RAR-alpha gene expression.

Precautions/Adverse Reactions: Arsenic trioxide is contraindicated in anyone with a known hypersensitivity to arsenic or to any component of the product. Arsenic trioxide should be administered only under the supervision of a physician who is experienced in the management of acute leukemia. May cause a syndrome known as retinoic acid acute promyelocytic leukemia (RA-APL) or APL differentiation syndrome. This syndrome can be fatal and requires prompt therapy with high dose dexamethasone. Arsenic trioxide may cause prolongation of the QT interval and complete atrioventricular block. It may lead to torsade de pointes, which can be fatal. The extent of the QT interval prolongation, coadministration of drugs known to prolong the QT interval, a history of torsade de pointes, preexisting QT interval prolongation, congestive heart failure, administration of potassium wasting diuretics, or other conditions that result in hypokalemia or hypomagnesemia are risk factors for the development of torsade de pointes. Baseline EKG (12 lead), serum potassium, magnesium, calcium, and creatinine values should be obtained prior to the initiation of therapy with arsenic trioxide. Electrolyte abnormalities should be corrected prior to the start of therapy. Potassium and magnesium levels should be kept at 4 mEq/dL and 1.8 mEq/dL respectively during treatment with arsenic trioxide. A QTc interval >500 msec should be corrected prior to the start of therapy with arsenic. If during therapy the QTc interval exceeds 500 msec, the patient should be reassessed and corrective action taken. If at any point syncope or rapid or irregular heartbeat develops, the patient should be hospitalized for monitoring. Hyperleukocytosis is possible during therapy with arsenic. Use cautiously in patients with renal insufficiency. Use caution when coadministering with other drugs known to prolong the QT interval or to cause electrolyte disturbances. Pregnancy category D. No adequate or well-controlled studies in pregnant women. May cause fetal harm. Excreted in human breast milk; not recommended in nursing women. Limited data in 5–16 year olds. No efficacy or safety data in children <5 years of age. Most serious adverse effects seen in patients treated with arsenic trioxide include: APL differentiation syndrome (22.5%), QTc interval prolongation (38%), hyperleukocytosis (50%), and EKG abnormalities. Adverse reactions occurring in ≥10% of patients include fatigue, fever, edema, rigors, chest pain, injection site, weakness, weight gain, nausea, anorexia, diarrhea, vomiting, abdominal pain, sore throat, constipation, loose stools, dyspepsia, hypokalemia, hypomagnesemia, headache, insomnia, paresthesia, dizziness, tremors, cough, dyspnea, epistaxis, hypoxia, pleural effusion, postnasal drip, wheezing, decreased breath sounds, crepitations, rales, dermatitis, pruritis, ecchymosis, dry skin, erythema, increased sweating, tachycardia, palpitations, sinusitis, herpes simplex, upper respiratory tract infections, arthralgias, myalgias, pain, anemia, thrombocytopenia, neutropenia, hypotension, hypertension, flushing, pallor, anxiety, depression, eye irritation, blurred vision, and vaginal hemorrhage.

Administration: Intravenous.

Patient Care Implications: Chemotherapeutic agent—handle and dispose of properly. Baseline, then twice weekly serum electrolytes, coagulation, and hematologic parameters. Baseline and weekly EKG (12 lead).

Preparations: Solution for injection: 10 mg/10 ml, 10 ml glass single-use ampules.

ARTANE®, see Trihexyphenidyl

ARTHROPAN®, see Choline Salicylate

ARTHROTEC®—Combination Agent Diclofenac Sodium and Misoprostol

ARTICAINE HYDROCHLORIDE AND EPINEPHRINE— Septocaine™

Description/Actions: Used as an anesthesia agent for infiltration and nerve block anesthesia in clinical dentistry. The onset of anesthesia occurs within 1 to 6 minutes after injection and the duration of complete anesthesia is approximately 1 to 2.5 hours.

Precautions/Adverse Reactions: This medication is contraindicated in patients with a hypersensitivity to Septocaine™/local anesthetics of the amide type or to sodium metabisulfite. Intravascular injections should be avoided; accidental intravascular injection may be associated with convulsions, followed by CNS or cardiorespiratory depression and respiratory arrest. Product contains epinephrine, which may cause local tissue necrosis or systemic toxicities. To avoid serious adverse effects and high plasma levels, use the lowest effective dose. Pregnancy Category C. Articaine should only be used during pregnancy if the potential benefit justifies a potential risk to the fetus. Some adverse effects are headache, dizziness, anxiety, agitations, paresthesia, pain (body as a whole), and hypersensitivity reactions.

Administration: Injection.

Patient Care Implications: Dental practitioners and/or clinicians using local anesthetics should be trained in diagnosis and management of emergencies that may arise from the utilization of these agents. Systemic absorption of local anesthetics may produce CNS and cardiovascular effects; careful monitoring of cardiovascular and respiratory status of the patient should be performed.

Preparations: Injection: Articaine hydrochloride 4% with epinephrine (as bitartrate), 1:100,000 (1.7 ml cartridges).

ASA, see Aspirin

ASACOL®, see Mesalamine

ASCORBIC ACID, see Vitamin C

ASENDIN®, see Amoxapine

A-SPAS®, see Dicyclomine

ASPARAGINASE—Elspar®

Description/Actions: Antineoplastic agent indicated in the treatment of acute lymphocytic leukemia.

Preparations: Vials, 10,000 IU.

ASPERCREME®, see Trolamine Salicylate

ASPIRIN—Acetylsalicylic acid, ASA, Bayer Aspirin®, Easprin®, Ecotrin®, Empirin®, ZORprin®

Description/Actions: A salicylate analgesic/antipyretic and anti-inflammatory agent used in the treatment of mild to moderate pain, fever, and arthritic and other disorders associated with inflammation. Also indicated for reducing the risk of stroke in male patients with recurrent ischemic attacks, and to reduce the risk of death and/or nonfatal myocardial infarction in patients with a previous infarction or unstable angina pectoris.

Precautions/Adverse Reactions: Contraindicated in patients known to be hypersensitive to salicylates or in individuals with the syndrome of nasal polyps, angioedema, and bronchospastic reactivity to aspirin. May cause GI effects, so use should be avoided in patients with active GI tract disease and closely supervised in patients with a previous history of such disorders. Other adverse reactions include rash, tinnitus, interference with hemostasis, aspirin intolerance, and salicylism. May interact with and increase the effect of anticoagulants, hypoglycemic agents, and methotrexate. May reduce the effect of probenecid and sulfinpyrazone. Discontinue the drug 7–10 days before elective surgical procedures. Use in children or teenagers with influenza or chicken pox may be associated with the development of Reye's syndrome. Use during pregnancy is best avoided, especially in the third trimester.

Administration: Oral and rectal. Enteric- coated and controlled-release formulations should be swallowed intact.

Preparations: Tablets, 81, 325, and 500 mg. Enteric-coated tablets/capsules, 325, 500, 650, and 975 mg. Controlled-release tablets, 650 and 800 mg. Suppositories, 60, 130, 200, 325, and 650 mg.

ASTELIN®, see Azelastine Hydrochloride

ASTRAMORPH PF®, see Morphine

ATACAND HCT™, Combination of Candesartan and Hydrochlorothiazide

ATARAX®, see Hydroxyzine

ATAZANAVIR—Reyataz™

Description/Actions: Atazanavir is an azapeptide HIV-1 protease inhibitor. It selectively inhibits the virus-specific processing of viral Gag and Gag-Pol polyproteins in HIV-1 infected cells, thus preventing formation of mature virions. It is indicated in combination with other antiretroviral agents for the treatment of HIV-1 infection.

Precautions/Adverse Reactions: Atazanavir is contraindicated in patients with a known hypersensitivity to it or to any component of the formulation. Atazanavir is contraindicated with drugs that are highly dependent on CYP3A for clearance and for which elevated plasma concentrations are associated with serious and/or life-threatening events. Atazanavir is an inhibitor of CYP3A and UGT1A1. Coadministration of atazanavir and sildenafil is expected to substantially increase sildenafil concentrations and may result in an increase in sildenafil-associated adverse events, including hypotension, visual changes, and priapism. Caution should be used if atazanavir is used concomitantly with atorvastatin. The risk of myopathy, including rhabdomyolysis, may be increased. Atazanavir has been shown to prolong the PR interval. Use with caution in patients with preexisting conduction system diseases such as marked first degree AV block or second or third degree AV block.

Dosage adjustments may be required when atazanavir is coadministered with drugs that prolong the PR interval. Exercise caution when coadministering atazanavir with didanosine buffered formulations, efavirenz, saquinavir, ritonavir, antacids, amiodarone, lidocaine, quinidine, warfarin, tricyclic antidepressants, rifabutin, diltiazem, felodipine, nifedipine, nicardipine, verapamil, histamine2 receptor antagonists, cyclosporine, sirolimus, tacrolimus, clarithromycin, and oral contraceptives containing ethinyl estradiol and norethindrone. Monitoring and dosage adjustments may be warranted. Hyperglycemia, exacerbations of preexisting diabetes mellitus, new onset diabetes mellitus, and diabetic ketoacidosis have been reported during therapy with protease inhibitors. Reyataz™ is primarily metabolized by the liver. Use caution when administering to patients with hepatic impairment because atazanavir concentrations may be increased. Patients with underlying hepatitis B or C viral infections or marked elevations in transaminases prior to treatment may be at an increased risk for developing further transaminase elevations or hepatic decompensation. Most patients on Reyataz™ experience asymptomatic elevations in unconjugated bilirubin (indirect). Increased bleeding, including spontaneous skin hematomas, has been reported in patients with hemophilia type A and B treated with protease inhibitors. Use caution when administering to these patients. Lactic acidosis, sometimes fatal, has been reported in patients receiving Reyataz™ and nucleoside analogues. Redistribution and accumulation of body fat, including central obesity, buffalo hump, peripheral wasting, facial wasting, breast enlargement, and "cushingoid appearance" have been observed in patients receiving antiretroviral therapy. Pregnancy Category B. No adequate and well-controlled studies in pregnant women. Atazanavir should be used during pregnancy only if the potential benefit justifies the potential risk to the fetus. Excretion in human breast milk is unknown. Breast-feeding is not recommended when receiving therapy with atazanavir. Optimal dosing regimen for use of Reyataz™ in pediatrics has not been established. Reyataz™ should not be administered to pediatric patients less than 3 months of age due to the risk of kernicterus. Most common adverse effects observed during therapy with atazanavir include nausea, headache, diarrhea, fever, pain, fatigue, back pain, jaundice, scleral icterus, abdominal pain, vomiting, lipodystrophy, arthralgia, depression, insomnia, dizziness, peripheral neurologic symptoms, increased cough, and rash. Allergic reactions, angioedema, and increases in amylase and lipase levels have also been reported.

Administration: Oral.

Patient Care Implications: Patients should be instructed to take Reyataz™ with food and take other concomitant antiretroviral therapy as prescribed. Patients should be informed that Reyataz™ is not a cure for HIV infection. Reyataz™ has many drug interactions. Therefore, patients should report the use of any other prescription, nonprescription, or herbal products to their doctors.

Preparations: Capsules, 100 mg, 150 mg, and 200 mg.

ATENOLOL—Tenormin®

Description/Actions: A cardioselective beta-adrenergic blocking agent indicated in the management of hypertension, angina pectoris, and myocardial infarction.

Precautions/Adverse Reactions: Contraindicated in patients with sinus bradycardia, heart block greater than first degree, cardiogenic shock, and overt cardiac failure. Adverse reactions include dizziness, fatigue, bradycardia, postural hypotension, and nausea. Avoid use in patients with bronchospastic diseases. Monitor diabetic patients closely.

Administration: Oral and intravenous. Patients should be cautioned about the interruption or discontinuation of therapy; exacerbation of angina pectoris has occurred following the abrupt cessation of therapy and, when therapy is to be discontinued, the dosage should be gradually reduced over a period of 1 to 2 weeks.

Preparations: Tablets, 25, 50, and 100 mg. Ampules, 5 mg/10 ml.

ATIVAN®, see Lorazepam

ATnativ®, see Antithrombin III (Human)

ATOMOXETINE HYDROCHLORIDE—Strattera™

Description/Actions: Atomoxetine is the first nonstimulant medication approved for the treatment of attention deficit/hyperactivity disorder (ADHD) in children, adolescents, and adults.

Precautions/Adverse Reactions: Atomoxetine is contraindicated in individuals hypersensitive to atomoxetine or any of its components, those with narrow angle glaucoma, or those who have used MAO inhibitors in the past 14 days. There have been reports of serious and fatal reactions when taken in combination with an MAOI. Use caution in patients with hypertension, tachycardia, or cardiovascular or cerebrovascular disease because blood pressure and heart rate can be increased. Metabolism is primarily through the CYP2D6-enzymatic pathway. Atomoxetine given with albuterol and sympathomimetics may increase heart rate and blood pressure. Use caution with pressor agents. Most common adverse effects were headache, abdominal pain, insomnia, xerostomia, decreased appetite, dyspepsia, nausea, vomiting, dizziness, and mood swings. Pregnancy Category C.

Administration: Oral, with or without food.

Preparations: Capsules, 10, 18, 25, 40, 60, 80, and 100 mg.

ATORVASTATIN—Lipitor®

Description/Actions: An HMG-CoA reductase inhibitor indicated as an adjunct to diet for the reduction of elevated total and LDL-cholesterol levels in patients with primary hypercholesterolemia and mixed dyslipidemia. Atorvastatin is also indicated for the treatment of heterozygous familial hypercholesterolemia in adolescent boys and post-menarchal girls aged 10–17 and as an adjunct to diet to reduce total cholesterol, low density lipoprotein cholesterol, and apolipoprotein B levels if after an adequate trial of diet, LDL-C levels are ≥190 mg/dL or LDLC levels are ≥160 mg/dL and there is a positive family history of premature cardiovascular disease or two or more other cardiovascular risk factors are present in the patient. Atorvastatin is indicated for the prevention of cardiovascular disease in adult patients without clinically evident coronary heart disease, but with multiple risk factors for coronary heart disease such as age ≥55 years, smoking, hypertension, low HDL-C, or a family history of early coronary heart disease. Lipitor® is indicated to reduce the risk of myocardial infarction and reduce the risk for revascularization procedures and angina.

Precautions/Adverse Reactions: Contraindicated in active liver disease, unexplained peristent elevated serum transaminases, and pregnancy. Monitor liver function before and during therapy. Reduce or discontinue dose if serum transaminase levels >3 times the upper limit of normal persist. Use cautiously in patients with chronic alcohol ingestion. Discontinue if myopathy or elevated CPK levels occur. Suspend therapy if predisposition to development of renal failure secondary to rhabdomyolysis develops. Adverse reactions include constipation, flatulence, dyspepsia, abdominal pain, headache, myalgia, arthralgia, rash, asthenia, and elevated serum transaminases.

Administration: Oral.

Preparations: Tablets, 10, 20, 40, and 80 mg.

ATOVAQUONE—Mepron®

Description/Actions: Antiprotozoal agent indicated for the treatment of mild to moderate *pneumocystis carinii* pneumonia (PCP) and prevention of PCP in patients who are intolerant to trimethoprim-sulfamethoxazole.

Precautions/Adverse Reactions: Adverse reactions include rash, nausea, vomiting, diarrhea, headache, fever, insomnia, and elevation of liver enzymes.

Administration: Oral. Should be taken with meals.

Preparations: Suspension, 750 mg/5 ml.

ATOVAQUONE AND PROGUANIL HYDROCHLORIDE—
Malarone™

Description/Actions: Fixed combination antimalarial agent, indicated for the prevention or treatment of acute, uncomplicated *P. falciparum* malaria, including in areas where chloroquine resistance has been reported.

Precautions/Adverse Reactions: Usage is contraindicated in patients with hypersensitivity to atovaquone, proguanil, or any formulation components and for the prophylaxis of *P. falciparum* malaria in patients with severe renal impairment (creatinine clearance <30 ml/min). Malarone™ is not indicated for severe or complicated manifestations of malaria. Absorption of atovaquone may be diminished in patients who have diarrhea or vomiting. Parasitemia should be closely monitored in these patients and treatment with an antiemetic should be considered. Recrudescent infections or infections following chemoprophylaxis with this medication should be treated with an alternative agent(s). Not for use in patients <11 kg. Delayed cases of *P. falciparum* may occur after stopping prophylaxis with Malarone™. Therefore, travelers returning from endemic areas who experience febrile illnesses should be investigated for malaria. Do not administer with other proguanil-containing products; concomitant treatment with tetracycline, metoclopramide, rifampin, or rifabutin with atovaquone has been associated with decreased bioavailability or plasma levels of atovaquone. Pregnancy Category C. Use in pregnant women only if the potential benefit outweighs the possible risk to the fetus. Excretion of atovaquone in breast milk is unknown; proguanil is excreted in small quantities. Exercise caution when administering to nursing women. Some adverse effects are abdominal pain, nausea, vomiting, diarrhea, headache, dizziness, and myalgia.

Administration: Oral.

Patient Care Implications: The daily dose should be given at the same time each day with food or a milky drink. If vomiting occurs within 1 hour of administration, repeat the dose.

Preparations: Tablet: atovaquone 250 mg and proguanil hydrochloride 100 mg. Tablet pediatric: atovaquone 62.5 mg and proguanil hydrochloride 25 mg.

ATRACURIUM BESYLATE—Tracrium®

Description/Actions: Nondepolarizing skeletal muscle relaxant administered intravenously as an adjunct to general anesthesia, to facilitate endotracheal intubation, and to provide skeletal muscle relaxation during surgery or mechanical ventilation.

Preparations: Ampules and vials, 10 mg/ml.

ATROMID-S®, see Clofibrate

ATROPINE SULFATE

Description/Actions: Anticholinergic, mydriatic, and cycloplegic agent used parenterally in a number of conditions including peptic ulcer, biliary and ureteral colic, bronchial spasm, and parkinsonism, to lessen the degree of AV heart block, to restore cardiac rate and arterial pressure during anesthesia in certain situations, and as preanesthetic medication. Used via ophthalmic administration for cycloplegic refraction, or for pupil dilation in certain acute ocular inflammatory conditions.

Preparations: Ampules, vials, and syringes, 0.05, 0.1, 0.3, 0.4, 0.5, 0.8, 1, and 1.2 mg/ml. Tablets, 0.4 mg. Hypodermic tablets, 0.3, 0.4, and 0.6 mg. Ophthalmic solution, 0.5%, 1%, 2%, and 3%. Ophthalmic ointment, 0.5% and 1%.

ATROVENT®, see Ipratropium

AUGMENTIN®, see Amoxicillin/Clavulanate Potassium

AURANOFIN—Ridaura®

Description/Actions: An orally administered gold-containing formulation indicated in the management of rheumatoid arthritis in adult patients who have had an insufficient therapeutic response to one or more nonsteroidal anti-inflammatory drugs or who are intolerant of such drugs.

Precautions/Adverse Reactions: Adverse reactions include loose stools or diarrhea, abdominal pain, nausea, vomiting, rash, pruritus, stomatitis, and proteinuria. A complete blood count (CBC) with differential and platelet count, urinalysis, and physical examination of the mouth and skin should be done at least monthly during therapy.

Administration: Oral.

Preparations: Capsules, 3 mg.

AUREOMYCIN®, see Chlortetracycline

AUROTHIOGLUCOSE—Solganal®

Description/Actions: Gold formulation administered intramuscularly in the treatment of rheumatoid arthritis.

Preparations: Vials, 50 mg/ml.

AVANDAMET™, see Rosiglitazone and Metformin

AVAPRO®, see Irbesartan

AVC®, see Sulfanilamide

AVELOX®, see Moxifloxacin Hydrochloride

AVENTYL®, see Nortriptyline

AVITA®, see Tretinoin

AVLOSULFON®, see Dapsone

AVODART™, see Dutasteride

AVONEX®, see Interferon beta-1A

AXERT™, see Almotriptan Maleate

AXID®, see Nizatidine

AZACTAM®, see Aztreonam

AZATADINE MALEATE—Optimine®

Description/Actions: Antihistamine indicated for the treatment of perennial and seasonal allergic rhinitis and chronic urticaria.

Preparations: Tablets, 1 mg.

AZATHIOPRINE—Imuran®

Description/Actions: Immunosuppressant indicated as an adjunct for the prevention of rejection in renal homotransplantation, and in the management of severe rheumatoid arthritis that has not responded satisfactorily to other agents.

Preparations: Tablets, 50 mg. Vials (sodium salt), 100 mg.

AZELAIC ACID—Azelex®

Description/Actions: Exerts antibacterial and keratolytic activity when applied topically. Indicated for treatment of mild to moderate inflammatory acne vulgaris.

Precaution/Adverse Reactions: Not recommended for use in children. Monitor patients with dark complexion for hypopigmentation. Discontinue if sensitivity or severe irritation develops. Pruritis, burning, stinging, tingling, exacerbation of acne, hypopigmentation, contact dermatitis, vitiligo, depigmentation, and hypertrichosis may occur.

Administration: Massage thin film on clean, dry affected areas twice daily. Wash hands after application. If persistent irritation occurs, may decrease to once daily.

Preparations: 20% topical cream.

AZELASTINE HYDROCHLORIDE—Astelin®, Optivar™

Description/Actions: Antihistamine indicated in the treatment of seasonal allergic rhinitis symptoms including rhinorrhea. A nasal spray formulation of an H_1 antagonist. Ophthalmic preparation used for the treatment of itching of the eye associated with seasonal allergic conjunctivitis in adults and children 3 years of age and older.

Precautions/Adverse Reactions: May potentiate CNS depression of other drugs or alcohol. Adverse reactions include bitter taste, somnolence, headache, weight increase, myalgia, nasal burning, sneezing, and nausea.

Administration: Two sprays in each nostril twice daily. Ophthalmic: Instill 1 drop into affected eye(s) twice daily.

Preparations: Aqueous nasal spray 137 mg/actuation, ophthalmic solution, 0.05%.

AZELEX®, see Azelaic Acid

AZITHROMYCIN—Zithromax®, ZPak ®, Zitromax® Tri-Pak

Description/Actions: Inhibits protein synthesis and usually exhibits a bacteriostatic action against gram-positive and gram-negative bacteria. Azithromycin is indicated for the treatment of patients with mild to moderate infections caused by susceptible strains of the designated microorganisms in the following conditions: acute bacterial exacerbations of chronic obstructive pulmonary disease and acute bacterial sinusitis due to *Haemophilus influenzae, Moraxella catarrhalis,* or *Streptococcus pneumoniae;* community acquired pneumonia due to *Chlamydia pneumoniae, Haemophilus influenzae, Mycoplasma pneumoniae,* or *Streptococcus pneumoniae;* pharyngitis/tonsillitis caused by *Streptococcus pyogenes* as an alternative to first-line therapy in individuals who cannot use first-line therapy. It is also indicated for use in the treatment of uncomplicated skin and skin-structure infections due to *Staphylococcus aureus, Streptococcus pyogenes,* or *Streptococcus agalactiae.* For the treatment of urethritis and cervicitis due to *Chlamydia trachomatis* or *Neisseria gonorrhoeae,* genital ulcer disease in men due to *Haemophilus Ducreyi* and for the treatment of acute otitis media in pediatric patients.

Precautions/Adverse Reactions: Contraindicated in patients with a known hypersensitivity to any of the macrolide antibiotics. Adverse reactions include diarrhea/loose stools, nausea, vomiting, abdominal pain, and vaginitis. Aluminum- and magnesium-containing antacids may reduce the rate of absorption, so the two agents should not be administered at the same time.

Administration: Oral (should be administered at least one hour before or 2 hours after a meal) and intravenous.

Preparations: Tablets 250 (scored), 500, and 600 mg. Oral suspension 100 mg/5 ml, and 200 mg/5 ml. Single-dose packets for oral suspension, 1 g. Vials for IV infusion after reconstitution, 500 mg/vial. Tablet (3 × 500mg).

AZMACORT®, see Triamcinolone Acetonide

AZO-STANDARD®, see Phenazopyridine Hydrochloride

AZT, see Zidovudine

AZTREONAM—Azactam®

Description/Actions: Monobactam antibiotic indicated for urinary tract infections, lower respiratory tract infections, septicemia, skin and skin-structure infections, intra-abdominal infections, and gynecologic infections caused by susceptible gram-negative bacteria. Among the organisms that are susceptible to the drug are *Pseudomonas aeruginosa, Haemophilus influenzae, Escherichia coli, Klebsiella pneumoniae, Proteus mirabilis, Serratia* species, *Enterobacter* species, and *Citrobacter* species. It is also indicated as adjunctive therapy to surgery in the management of infections caused by susceptible organisms.

Precautions/Adverse Reactions: It has only a weak potential to cause hypersensitivity reactions or to demonstrate cross-reactivity with the penicillins and cephalosporins. Adverse reactions include diarrhea, nausea and/or vomiting, rash, phlebitis/thrombophlebitis following intravenous administration, discomfort at the injection site following intramuscular administration, and superinfection with gram-positive bacteria such as enterococci.

Administration: Intravenous and intramuscular.

Preparations: Vials, 500 mg, 1 and 2 g. Intravenous infusion bottles, 500 mg, 1 and 2 g.

B

BACAMPICILLIN HYDROCHLORIDE—Spectrobid®

Description/Actions: Penicillin antibiotic. Is a prodrug that is hydrolyzed to ampicillin following administration. Indicated in the treatment of respiratory tract, urinary tract, and dermatologic infections caused by susceptible bacteria, and in the management of gonorrhea. Tablets may be given without regard to meals, but the suspension should be administered apart from meals.

Preparations: Tablets, 400 mg. Powder for oral suspension, 125 mg/5 ml when reconstituted.

BACITRACIN

Description/Actions: Anti-infective agent that is primarily active against gram-positive bacteria such as staphylococci. Most often used topically.

Preparations: Ointment and ophthalmic ointment, 500 units/g. Vials (for parenteral administration), 10,000 and 50,000 units.

BACLOFEN—Lioresal®

Description/Actions: Muscle relaxant and antispastic agent indicated for the alleviation of signs and symptoms of spasticity resulting from multiple sclerosis, as well as the management of certain spinal cord injuries and diseases. Intrathecal baclofen is indicated for use in the management of severe spasticity of cerebral and spinal origin.

Precautions/Adverse Reactions: Abrupt discontinuation of intrathecal baclofen, regardless of the cause, has resulted in sequelae that include high fever, altered mental status, exaggerated rebound spasticity, and muscle rigidity, which in rare cases has advanced to rhabdomyolysis, multiple organ-system failure, and death.

Preparations: Tablets, 10 and 20 mg. Ampules (for intrathecal use), 10 mg/5 ml and 10 mg/20 ml.

BACTRIM®, see Trimethoprim-sulfamethoxazole

BACTROBAN®, see Mupirocin

BAKING SODA, see Sodium Bicarbonate

BAL, see Dimercaprol

BALSALAZIDE—Colazal™

Description/Actions: Balsalazide is an anti-inflammatory agent used in the treatment of mild to moderate active ulcerative colitis.

Precautions/Adverse Reactions: Balsalazide is contraindicated in patients with hypersensitivity to salicylates or to any of the components of balsalazide or its metabolites. Patients with pyloric stenosis may have prolonged gastric retention of balsalazide capsules. Reports during clinical trials indicate that balsalazide may exacerbate symptoms of colitis. Because other mesalamine products have shown renal toxicity, balsalazide should be used with caution, and with careful monitoring, by persons with a history of or with current renal disease. The safety and efficacy have not been established beyond 12 weeks of therapy and in children. Pregnancy Category B. No adequate and well-controlled studies have been done in pregnant women. Balsalazide should be used in pregnant women only if clearly needed. It is not known whether balsalazide is excreted in breast milk. Caution should be used in administering to nursing women. Some adverse effects are headache, abdominal pain, nausea, diarrhea, vomiting, arthralgia, respiratory infections, and hepatotoxicity.

Administration: Oral.

Patient Care Implications: Do not chew or open capsules. Report abdominal pain, unresolved diarrhea, or severe headache to prescriber.

Preparations: Capsule: 750 mg.

BARIUM SULFATE

Description/Actions: Diagnostic agent used in the X-ray examination of the gastrointestinal tract.

BASALJEL®, see Aluminum Carbonate Gel, Basic

BASILIXIMAB—Simulect®

Description/Actions: Basiliximab is an immunosuppressive agent. It is indicated for the prophylaxis of acute organ rejection in patients receiving renal transplantation when used as part of an immunosuppressive regimen that includes cyclosporine and corticosteroids.

Precautions/Adverse Reactions: It is not known whether basiliximab will have a long-term effect on the ability of the immune system to respond to antigens first encountered during basiliximab-induced immunosuppression. Readministration after an initial course of therapy has not been studied in humans. Adverse effects include GI symptoms such as diarrhea, constipation, vomiting, abdominal pain, and dyspepsia.

Administration: Intravenous.

Patient Care Implications: Immunosuppressive therapy places patients at greater risk of developing an infection. Instruct patients in the measures to reduce the risk of infection as well as in signs and symptoms that should be reported promptly to the prescriber. Basiliximab is used as a part of an immunosuppressive regimen of corticosteroids and cyclosporine.

Preparations: Single-use vial containing 20 mg.

BAYER ASPIRIN®, see Aspirin

BECAPLERMIN—Regranex®

Description/Actions: Indicated as an adjunct to good ulcer care in the treatment of lower extremity diabetic neuropathic ulcers that extend into the subcutaneous tissue or beyond and have an adequate blood supply.

Precautions/Adverse Reactions: Contraindicated in neoplasia at the application site. Not for use in wounds that close by primary intention, in pregnancy (Category C), and in nursing mothers. Adverse reactions include erythematous rash.

Administration: Topical.

Preparations: 0.01% gel in 15 g tubes.

BECLOMETHASONE DIPROPIONATE—Beclovent®, Vanceril®, Beconase®, Beconase AQ®, Qvar™, Vancenase®, Vancenase AQ®, Double Strength®, Vanceril®, Double Strength

Description/Actions: Corticosteroid administered by oral inhalation (Beclovent®, Vanceril®) or nasal spray in patients who require chronic treatment with corticosteroids to control the symptoms of bronchial asthma. Also administered by nasal inhalation for the relief of symptoms of seasonal or perennial rhinitis.

Preparations: Aerosol, 42 and 84 mcg per actuation. Nasal spray (Beconase AQ®, Vancenase AQ®), 84 mcg/spray. Oral inhaler (Qvar™), 40 mcg and 80 mcg/inhalation.

BECLOVENT®, see Beclomethasone Dipropionate

BECONASE®, see Beclomethasone Dipropionate

BECONASE AQ®, see Beclomethasone Dipropionate

BEEPEN VK®, see Penicillin V Potassium

BELLADONNA

Description/Actions: Anticholinergic. Contains atropine, hyoscyamine, and scopolamine alkaloids and has been used in the treatment of gastrointestinal disorders and parkinsonism.

Preparations: Tincture of belladonna.

BENADRYL®, see Diphenhydramine

BENAZEPRIL HYDROCHLORIDE—Lotensin®

Description/Actions: An angiotensin-converting enzyme (ACE) inhibitor that is a prodrug. Following oral administration, is converted to its active metabolite, benazeprilat. Indicated for the treatment of hypertension and may be used alone or in combination with a thiazide diuretic.

Precautions/Adverse Reactions: Adverse reactions include headache, dizziness, fatigue, cough, and nausea. May cause an elevation in serum potassium levels; the risk of hyperkalemia is increased in patients also taking a potassium-sparing diuretic, a potassium supplement, and/or a potassium-containing salt substitute. May cause symptomatic postural hypotension. There have been infrequent reports of angioedema of the face, extremities, lips, tongue, glottis, and larynx, especially following the first dose. Patients should be told to report immediately any symptoms suggesting angioedema and to stop taking the drug. When drug is used during the second and third trimesters of pregnancy, ACE inhibitors have been reported to be associated with the development of neonatal hypertension, renal failure, and skull hypoplasia; use during pregnancy should be avoided. May increase serum lithium levels and concurrent therapy should be closely monitored. Monitor renal function, especially in the elderly.

Administration: Oral.

Preparations: Tablets, 5, 10, 20, and 40 mg.

BENDROFLUMETHIAZIDE—Naturetin®

Description/Actions: Thiazide diuretic indicated as adjunctive therapy in the treatment of edema and in the management of hypertension.

Preparations: Tablets, 2.5, 5, and 10 mg.

BENEMID®, see Probenecid

BENICAR™, see Olmesartan Medoxomil

BENOQUIN®, see Monobenzone

BENOXINATE HYDROCHLORIDE

Description/Actions: Local anesthetic sometimes employed to provide anesthesia in certain ophthalmic procedures.

BENTYL®, see Dicyclomine

BENYLIN COUGH®, see Diphenhydramine Hydrochloride

BENYLIN DM®, see Dextromethorphan

BENZALKONIUM CHLORIDE—Zephiran®

Description/Actions: Anti-infective agent used topically as an antiseptic, in the irrigation of certain tissues, and in the preoperative preparation of the skin. Also used as a preservative (e.g., in ophthalmic solutions) and in the sterile storage of instruments.

Preparations: Solution and tincture, 1:750. Concentrate (to be diluted), 17%.

BENZATHINE PENICILLIN G—Bicillin®, Permapen®

Description/Actions: Penicillin antibiotic that has a long duration of action following intramuscular administration. Indicated in infections caused by highly susceptible organisms such as streptococci. Also used in the prevention of recurrent rheumatic fever and in the treatment of syphilis.

Preparations: Vials, 300,000 units/ml. Syringes, 600,000, 1,200,000, and 2,400,000 units.

BENZEDREX®, see Propylhexedrine

BENZOCAINE—Ethyl Aminobenzoate, Zilabrace®, Ziladent®

Description/Actions: Local anesthetic administered topically in dermatologic disorders, locally to provide oral and mucosal anesthesia, and orally as an adjunct in a weight-reduction regimen.

Preparations: Cream, ointment, solution, and lotion, 0.5% to 20%. Gel, 6% and 10%. Candy and gum (in weight-reduction regimen), 6 mg.

BENZOIC ACID

Description/Actions: Anti-infective agent used topically in the treatment of fungal infections, usually in combination with salicylic acid in an ointment formulation known as Whitfield's ointment (6% benzoic acid and 3% salicylic acid).

BENZOIN

Description/Actions: Protectant used topically to protect the skin against irritants and to coat sores. Tincture and compound benzoin tincture have sometimes been placed in boiling water as steam inhalants to provide an expectorant and soothing action in certain respiratory conditions.

Preparations: Tincture.

BENZONATATE—Tessalon®

Description/Actions: Antitussive indicated for the symptomatic relief of cough.

Preparations: Capsules, 100 mg.

BENZPHETAMINE HYDROCHLORIDE—Didrex®

Description/Actions: Anorexiant indicated in the management of exogenous obesity as a short-term adjunct in a regimen of weight reduction based on caloric restriction.

Preparations: Tablets, 25 and 50 mg.

BENZTHIAZIDE—Exna®

Description/Actions: Thiazide diuretic indicated in the treatment of edema in the management of hypertension.

Preparations: Tablets, 50 mg.

BENZTROPINE MESYLATE—Cogentin®

Description/Actions: Exhibits anticholinergic activity, and is indicated for the treatment of parkinsonism and the control of drug-induced extrapyramidal reactions.

Precautions/Adverse Reactions: Adverse reactions include dry mouth, nausea, vomiting, blurred vision, tachycardia, confusion, nervousness, and urinary retention.

Administration: Oral, intravenous, and intramuscular.

Preparations: Tablets, 0.5, 1, and 2 mg. Ampules, 1 mg/ml.

BEPRIDIL HYDROCHLORIDE—Vascor®

Description/Actions: A calcium channel-blocking agent that is indicated for the treatment of chronic stable angina (classic effort-associated angina) in patients who have failed to respond optimally to, or are intolerant of, other antianginal medications. May be used alone or in combination with beta-blockers and/or nitrates.

Precautions/Adverse Reactions: Contraindicated in patients with a history of serious ventricular arrhythmias, sick sinus syndrome, or second- or third-degree AV block except in the presence of a functioning ventricular pacemaker, hypotension, uncompensated cardiac insufficiency, congenital QT interval prolongation, and in patients taking other drugs that prolong QT interval. May cause proarrhythmic effects including serious ventricular arrhythmias. May prolong the QT interval and the QTc interval, which has been associated with the development of torsade de pointes–type ventricular tachycardia. The risk of this reaction is increased by the presence of antecedent bradycardia, hypokalemia, and the use of potassium-depleting diuretics. If the concurrent use of a diuretic is needed, a potassium-sparing diuretic should be used if possible. Any potassium deficiency should be corrected before bepridil therapy is initiated, and serum potassium levels should be monitored periodically. Other adverse reactions include nausea, diarrhea, dyspepsia, GI distress, dizziness, asthenia, and nervousness. Agranulocytosis has been reported rarely. Other agents that may prolong the QT interval (e.g., quinidine, procainamide, tricyclic antidepressants) should not be used concurrently because of a greater potential for ventricular arrhythmias. Concurrent use with digoxin may result in an increase in serum digoxin levels and therapy should be closely monitored.

Administration. Oral.

Preparations: Tablets, 200, 300, and 400 mg.

BERACTANT—Survanta®

Description/Actions: A pulmonary surfactant of bovine origin that contains phospholipids, neutral lipids, fatty acids, and surfactant-associated proteins, to which colfosceril palmitate, palmitic acid, and tripalmitin are added to standardize the composition and to mimic the surface tension lowering properties of natural lung surfactant. Replenishes surfactant and restores surface activity to the lungs. Indicated for the prevention and treatment of respiratory distress syndrome in premature infants.

Precautions/Adverse Reactions: Adverse reactions include bradycardia and oxygen desaturation. May rapidly affect oxygenation and lung compliance.

Administration: Intratracheal. If settling has occurred during storage, swirl the vial gently (do not shake) to redisperse. Is stored refrigerated and, before administration, should be warmed by standing at room temperature for at least 20 minutes or warmed in the hand for at least 8 minutes. Is administered intratracheally by instillation through a 5 French end-hole catheter inserted into the infant's endotracheal tube. Each dose is divided into 4 quarter-doses, and each quarter-dose is administered with the infant in a different position.

Preparations: Vials, 200 mg phospholipids/8 ml.

BETADINE®, see Povidone-Iodine

BETAGAN®, see Levobunolol

BETAMETHASONE, BETAMETHASONE SODIUM PHOSPHATE, BETAMETHASONE ACETATE—Celestone®

Description/Actions: Corticosteroid indicated in a wide range of endocrine, rheumatic, allergic, dermatologic, respiratory, hematologic, neoplastic, and other disorders.

Preparations: Tablets, 0.6 mg. Syrup, 0.6 mg/5 ml. Vials (solution), 4 mg as the sodium phosphate per ml. Vials (suspension), 6 mg as the sodium phosphate and acetate per ml.

BETAMETHASONE BENZOATE—Uticort®

Description/Actions: Topical corticosteroid.

Preparations: Cream, lotion, and gel, 0.025%.

BETAMETHASONE DIPROPIONATE—Diprosone®, Maxivate®

Description/Actions: Topical corticosteroid.

Preparations: Cream, ointment, and lotion, 0.05%.

Administration: Topical aerosol, 0.1%.

BETAMETHASONE DIPROPIONATE AUGMENTED— Diprolene®, Diprolene AF®

Description/Actions: Specially formulated vehicle increases penetration and potency. Topical corticosteroid indicated for the short-term treatment of the inflammatory and pruritic manifestations of moderate to severe corticosteroid-responsive dermatoses.

Precautions/Adverse Reactions: Is highly potent and is more likely than less potent analogs to cause systemic effects including suppression of the hypothalamic-pituitary-adrenal (HPA) axis. Treatment period should be limited to 2 weeks and the total dosage should not exceed 45 g per week. Occlusive dressings should not be used.

Administration: Topical.

Preparations: Cream, ointment, and lotion, 0.05%.

BETAMETHASONE VALERATE—Luxig®, Valisone®

Description/Actions: Topical corticosteroid indicated for relief of the inflammatory and pruritic manifestations of corticosteroid-responsive dermatoses.

Precautions/Adverse Reactions: Adverse reactions include burning, itching, irritation, dryness, and a potential for systemic effect.

Administration: Topical.

Preparations: Cream, ointment, and lotion, 0.1%. Foam (Luxig®) 0.12%. Reduced-strength cream 0.01%.

BETAPACE®, see Sotalol Hydrochloride

BETAPACE AF™, see Sotalol Hydrochloride

BETAPEN VK®, see Penicillin V Potassium

BETASERON®, see Interferon Beta-1b

BETAXOLOL HYDROCHLORIDE—Betoptic®, Betoptic S®, Kerlone®

Description/Actions: A cardioselective beta-adrenergic blocking agent indicated in the treatment of hypertension, and for ophthalmic administration in the treatment of chronic open-angle glaucoma and ocular hypertension.

Precautions/Adverse Reactions: Contraindicated in patients with sinus bradycardia, second- and third-degree AV block in the absence of a functioning artificial pacemaker, overt cardiac failure, or cardiogenic shock. Adverse reactions include fatigue, dizziness, and bradycardia, and, when administered in the ophthalmic dosage forms, transient stinging during instillation. Use is best avoided in patients with bronchospastic diseases, and therapy in diabetic patients must be closely monitored.

Administration: Oral and ophthalmic. Patients should be cautioned about the interruption or discontinuation of oral therapy; exacerbation of angina pectoris has occurred following the abrupt cessation of therapy, and when therapy is to be discontinued, the dosage should be gradually reduced over a period of 2 weeks.

Preparations: Tablets (Kerlone), 10 and 20 mg. Ophthalmic suspension (Betoptic S), 0.25%. Ophthalmic solution (Betoptic), 0.5%.

BETAXON®, See Levobetaxolol HCl Ophthalmic Suspension 0.5%

BETHANECHOL CHLORIDE—Urecholine®

Description/Actions: Cholinergic agent indicated for the treatment of acute postoperative and postpartum nonobstructive urinary retention, and for neurogenic atony of the urinary bladder with retention.

Preparations: Tablets, 5, 10, 25, and 50 mg. Vials, 5 mg/ml.

BETIMOL®, see Timolol

BETOPTIC®, see Betaxolol

BEXAROTENE—Targretin®

Description/Actions: Indicated for the treatment of cutaneous manifestations of cutaneous T-cell lymphoma in patients who are refractory to at least one prior systemic therapy.

Precautions/Adverse Reactions: Targretin capsules are contraindicated in patients with a known hypersensitivity to bexaxrotene or other components of the product. Targretin should not be given to a pregnant woman or a woman who intends to become pregnant. Targretin can induce major lipid abnormalities, biochemical evidence of or clinical hypothyroidism, and leukopenia, so laboratory values should be followed and dosages adjusted as needed. Caution should be used in patients with a known hypersensitivity to retinoids, hepatic insufficiency, or diabetes mellitus. Retinoids have been associated with photosensitivity, and patients should be advised to minimize exposure to sunlight and artificial UV light while receiving Targretin capsules. Other adverse effects include headache, asthenia, infections, abdominal pain, rash, dry skin, nausea, diarrhea, vomiting, anorexia, peripheral edema, and insomnia.

Administration: Oral with meal.

Preparations: Capsules, 75 mg.

BIAXIN®, see Clarithromycin

BIAXIN XL®, see Clarithromycin Extended-Release Tablets

BICALUTAMIDE—Casodex®

Description/Actions: Antiandrogenic antineoplastic agent that antagonizes the effects of androgen (action is usually against a more potent androgen) at the cellular level. Indicated in the treatment of metastatic prostate carcinoma in conjunction with luteinizing hormone releasing hormone (LHRH) analogs (goserelin, leuprolide).

Precautions/Adverse Reactions: May cause moderate to severe hepatic impairment. Monitor hepatic function and prostate specific antigen (PSA). Adverse reactions include weakness, constipation, nausea, diarrhea, back pain, pelvic pain, hot flashes, and generalized pain.

Administration: Oral (must be given concurrently with LHRH analog).

Preparations: Tablets, 50 mg.

BICILLIN®, see Benzathine Penicillin G

BICITRA®, see Sodium Citrate and Citric Acid

BiCNU®, see Carmustine

BILTRICIDE®, see Praziquantel

BIMATOPROST—Lumigan®

Description/Actions: Bimatoprost is indicated for the reduction of elevated intraocular pressure in patients with open-angle glaucoma or ocular hypertension who are intolerant of other intraocular pressure–lowering medications or failed treatment with another intraocular pressure–lowering drug.

Precautions/Adverse Reactions: Pregnancy Category C. No adequate and well-controlled studies in pregnant women. Excretion in human breast milk is unknown. Safety and efficacy in children have not been established. The most common side effects observed in patients treated with bimatoprost include conjunctival hyperemia, growth of eyelashes, and ocular pruritus. Other side effects occurring less frequently include ocular dryness, visual disturbances, ocular burning, eye pain, eye discharge, tearing, photophobia, allergic conjunctivitis, and intraocular inflammation. Systemic side effects have been reported and include infections, headaches, abnormal liver function tests, asthenia, and hirsutism.

Administration: Ophthalmic.

Patient Care Implications: Remove contact lenses prior to using, and wait 15 minutes before reinserting. Contains benzalkonium chloride as a preservative. If more than one ophthalmic drug is being used, the drugs should be administered at least 5 minutes apart. Patients should be advised to avoid contamination of the solution. Patients should be informed that if only one eye is treated, cosmetic differences between the eyes may occur.

Preparations: Ophthalmic solution, 0.03% in 2.5 ml, 5 ml, and 7.5 ml.

BIPERIDEN—Akineton®

Description/Actions: Antiparkinson agent indicated for the treatment of parkinsonism and the control of extrapyramidal disorders secondary to neuroleptic drug therapy.

Preparations: Tablets (as the hydrochloride), 2 mg. Ampules (as the lactate), 5 mg.

BISACODYL—Dulcolax®

Description/Actions: Laxative indicated for acute constipation, chronic constipation, preparation for x-rays, preoperative preparation, and other situations.

Preparations: Tablets, 5 mg. Suppositories, 5 and 10 mg.

BISMUTH SUBCARBONATE

Description/Actions: Antacid included in some combination formulations.

BISMUTH SUBSALICYLATE—PeptoBismol®

Description/Actions: Antidiarrheal/antacid and analgesic used in the management of nausea, gas pains, abdominal cramps, and diarrhea. Has been used in the prevention and treatment of traveler's diarrhea. Also indicated in regimens for the treatment of gastrointestinal disorders caused by *Helicobacter pylori.*

Preparations: Chewable tablets, 262 mg. Suspension, 262 mg/15 ml and 524 mg/15 ml.

BISOPROLOL FUMARATE—Zebeta®

Description/Actions: Is a cardioselective beta-adrenergic-blocking agent that is indicated for the treatment of hypertension.

Precautions/Adverse Reactions: Contraindicated in patients in cardiogenic shock, or with overt cardiac failure, second- and third-degree heart block, or marked sinus bradycardia. Adverse reactions include headache, fatigue, dizziness, diarrhea, and cold extremities. Use is best avoided in patients with bronchospastic diseases, and therapy in diabetic patients must be closely monitored.

Administration: Oral. When therapy is to be discontinued, the dosage should be gradually reduced over a period of one week.

Preparations: Tablets, 5 and 10 mg. Also available in combination formulations (Ziac) with hydrochlorothiazide that contain 2.5, 5, and 10 mg of bisoprolol fumarate with 6.25 mg of the diuretic.

BITOLTEROL MESYLATE—Tornalate®

Description/Actions: Bronchodilator delivered by oral inhalation for prophylactic and therapeutic use for bronchial asthma and for reversible bronchospasm.

Preparations: Metered dose inhaler, 0.37 mg per actuation. Inhalation solution, 0.2%.

BIVALIRUDIN—Angiomax™

Description/Actions: Angiomax™ is used in conjunction with aspirin as an anticoagulant in patients with unstable angina undergoing percutaneous transluminal coronary angioplasty (PTCA).

Precautions/Adverse Reactions: Bivalirudin is contraindicated in patients with active major bleeding and hypersensitivity to bivalirudin or any of its formulation components. Safety and effectiveness have not been established when used in conjunction with platelet inhibitors other than aspirin (i.e., glycoprotein IIb/IIIa inhibitors) in patients with unstable angina who are not undergoing PTCA, in patients with other acute coronary syndromes, and in pediatrics. Because hemorrhage can occur with bivalirudin, exercise caution when utilizing in patients with disease states associated with increased risk of bleeding. Pregnancy Category B. Safety and efficacy for use in pregnant women have not been established. Use during pregnancy only if clearly needed. It is not known if bivalirudin is excreted in human milk; use with caution in nursing women. Some adverse effects are bleeding, hypotension, back pain, headache, nausea, and vomiting.

Administration: Intravenous.

Patient Care Implications: For IV administration only. Do not mix with other medications. In patients with renal impairment, monitor the ACT. Inform patient to report any unusual bleeding or bruising while on Angiomax™.

Preparations: Powder for injection. Each vial delivers 250 mg of Angiomax™.

BLENOXANE®, see Bleomycin

BLEOMYCIN SULFATE—Blenoxane®

Description/Actions: Antineoplastic agent indicated for parenteral use as a palliative treatment in the management of squamous cell carcinomas, lymphomas, and testicular carcinoma.

Preparations: Vials, 15 and 30 units.

BLOCADREN®, see Timolol

BONINE®, see Meclizine

BONTRIL®, see Phendimetrazine

BORIC ACID

Description/Actions: Antiseptic used topically for conditions associated with irritation of the skin, and for the treatment of irritated and inflamed eyelids.

Preparations: Ointment and ophthalmic ointment, 5% and 10%.

BORTEZOMIB—Velcade™

Description/Actions: Bortezomib is a protease inhibitor used for the treatment of multiple myeloma in patients who have had 2 prior therapies and have demonstrated disease progression on the last therapy. Bortezomib inhibits proteasomes, enzyme complexes that regulate protein homeostasis within the cell. It reversibly inhibits chymotrypsin-like activity at the 26S proteasome, leading to activation of signaling cascades, cell-cycle arrest and apoptosis.

Precautions/Adverse Reactions: Bortezomib is contraindicated in patients with a hypersensitivity to bortezomib, boron, mannitol, or any component of the formulation. Peripheral neuropathy may occur; risk may be increased with previous use of neurotoxic agents or preexisting peripheral neuropathy. Patients experiencing new or worsening peripheral neuropathy may require a change in the dose and schedule of bortezomib. May cause orthostatic/postural hypotension; caution should be used when treating patients with a history of syncope, patients receiving medications known to be associated with hypotension, and patients who are dehydrated. Bortezomib can cause nausea, diarrhea, constipation, and vomiting; fluid and electrolyte replacement should be administered to prevent dehydration. Thrombocytopenia occurs frequently; complete blood counts should be monitored throughout treatment. Use caution with hepatic or renal impairment; closely monitor for toxicities. Pregnancy Category D. Adverse effects observed in animal studies. Excretion in breast milk unkown; breastfeeding should be avoided. Most common side effects were asthenic conditions, peripheral neuropathy, pyrexia, headache, insomnia, edema, anxiety, rash, dehydration, dizziness, nausea, diarrhea, constipation, vomiting, arthralgia, limb pain, dyspnea, and upper respiratory tract infection. Bortezomib may increase levels/effects of CYP2C19 substrates (i.e., diazepam, phenytoin, propranolol, and sertraline). CYP3A4 inducers may decrease the levels/effects of bortezomib (i.e., carbamazepine, nafcillin, phenobarbital, nevirapine, and rifamycins). CYP3A4 inhibitors may increase the levels/effects of bortezomib (i.e., azole antifungals, ciprofloxacin, clarithromycin, diclofenac, isoniazid, nicardipine, protease inhibitors, and verapamil).

Administration: Intravenous.

Patient Care Implications: Inform patient he/she may experience fatigue, dizziness, syncope, orthostatic/postural hypotension, diplopia, or blurred vision; caution patients when driving or engaging in hazardous tasks until response to drug is known. Pregnancy Category D; use effective contraceptive measures to prevent pregnancy. Patients should inform physician if they experience new or worsening symptoms of peripheral neuropathy. Maintain adequate hydration. Small frequent meals, frequent mouth care, chewing gum, or sucking lozenges may help with nausea, vomiting, or abnormal taste. Report persistent headaches, cramping, loss of sensation, changes in vision, or other persistent adverse reactions.

Preparations: Injection, 3.5 mg single dose vial.

BOSENTAN—Tracleer™

Description/Actions: Bosentan is indicated for the treatment of pulmonary artery hypertension in patients with WHO class III or IV symptoms to improve exercise ability and to decrease the rate of clinical worsening.

Precautions/Adverse Reactions: Because of a high potential for liver injury effects and the risk associated with use in pregnancy, bosentan is available only through a distribution program directly from the manufacturer (866-228-3546). It is not available through wholesalers or individual pharmacies. Bosentan is contraindicated in persons hypersensitive to bosentan or any component of the medication. It is associated with significant transaminase elevations, indicating a potential for serious hepatic injury. Avoid use in moderate to severe hepatic impairment; caution should be exercised in patients with mild liver function impairment. Pregnancy category X. Based on animal studies, bosentan is likely to produce major birth defects. CYP3A3/4 inhibitors and cyclosporine may increase bosentan concentration. An increased risk of elevated liver aminotransferases was observed when given with glyburide. Most common adverse reactions include headache, flushing, increased serum transaminases (reversible), lower limb edema, nasopharyngitis, dyspepsia, hypotension, pruritis, and fatigue. Safety and efficacy in pediatric patients not established.

Administration: Oral.

Patient Care Implications: Pregnancy must be excluded before starting treatment and prevented thereafter by use of reliable contraception. Hormonal contraceptives (oral, injectable, and implanted) may not be reliable in the presence of bosentan and should not be used as the sole contraceptive method. Liver aminotransferase levels must be measured prior to initiation of treatment and then monthly. In patients developing elevated levels, dosage adjustment and monitoring of ALT/AST levels should be followed as per manufacturer's recommendations. If liver aminotransferase elevations are accompanied by clinical symptoms of liver injury (such as nausea, vomiting, fever, abdominal pain, jaundice, unusual lethargy, or fatigue) or increases in bilirubin ≥2 × ULN, treatment should be stopped. Hemoglobin levels should be monitored after 1 and 3 months of treatment, then every 3 months. Tablets should be administered morning and evening with or without food.

Preparations: Film-coated tablets: 62.5 and 125 mg.

BOTOX®, see Botulinum Toxin Type A

BOTULINUM TOXIN TYPE A—Botox®

Description/Actions: Is produced from a culture of *Clostridium botulinum* and, following injection into eye muscles, inhibits the release of acetylcholine, resulting in a localized reversible muscle paralysis. Indicated for the treatment of strabismus and blepharospasm associated with dystonia, including benign essential blepharospasm or seventh cranial nerve disorders. Botox® is indicated for the treatment of severe primary axillary hyperhidrosis that is inadequately managed with topical agents. Is also being evaluated in a number of other muscle disorders.

Precautions/Adverse Reactions: Adverse reactions when used in the treatment of strabismus include spatial disorientation, double vision, ptosis, vertical deviation, and retrobulbar hemorrhages resulting from needle penetrations into the orbit. Adverse reactions when used in the treatment of blepharospasm include ptosis, irritation/tearing, ecchymosis, rash, and local swelling of the eyelid skin.

Administration: Ocular injection. In the treatment of strabismus, the drug is injected using electromyographic guidance to facilitate placement within the target muscle. Paralysis of the injected muscles lasts for 2 to 6 weeks. In the treatment of blepharospasm, the drug is injected into the orbicularis oculi without electromygraphic guidance. Each treatment lasts approximately 3 months.

Preparations: Vials, 100 units.

BRETHAIRE®, see Terbutaline

BRETHINE®, see Terbutaline

BRETYLIUM TOSYLATE—Bretylol®

Description/Actions: Antiarrhythmic agent indicated for parenteral use in the prophylaxis and treatment of ventricular fibrillation and in the treatment of life-threatening ventricular arrhythmias that have not responded to other agents.

Preparations: Ampules, vials, and syringes, 500 mg.

BRETYLOL®, see Bretylium

BREVIBLOC®, see Esmolol

BREVITAL®, see Methohexital

BRICANYL®, see Terbutaline

BRIMONIDINE TARTRATE—Alphagan®, Alphagan®P

Description/Actions: Antiglaucoma agent used to lower intraocular pressure in patients with open-angle glaucoma or ocular hypertension.

Precautions/Adverse Reactions: Use cautiously in severe cardiovascular diseases, hepatic or renal impairment, depression, cerebral disease, Raynaud's phenomenon, orthostatic hypertension, and thromboangiitis obliterans. Contraindicated with concomitant MAOI use. Adverse reactions include xerostomia, ocular hyperemia, burning/stinging, headache, blurred vision, foreign body sensation, fatigue/drowsiness, conjunctival follicles, ocular allergic reactions, ocular pruritis, corneal staining/erosion, photophobia, eyelid erythema, ocular ache/pain/

dryness, tearing, upper respiratory symptoms, eyelid edema, conjunctival blanching, abnormal vision, and muscular pain.

Administration: Ophthalmic. Remove soft contact lenses before instillation and for 15 minutes after dose administration.

Preparations: 0.15% and 0.2% ophthalmic solution.

BRINZOLAMIDE—Azopt®

Description/Actions: Indicated for the treatment of elevated intraocular pressure in patients with ocular hypertension or open angle glaucoma.

Precautions/Adverse Reactions: Use not recommended in severe renal or hepatic impairment. Discontinue if serious systemic, ocular (e.g., conjunctivitis, lid edema), or hypersensitivity reactions occur. Brinzolamide is a sulfonamide and although administered topically, it is absorbed systemically. Therefore, the same types of reactions attributable to sulfonamides may occur with topical application. Advise patients that if serious or unusual ocular or systemic reactions occur they should discontinue the use of the medication and call the prescriber. Pregnancy Category C. Adverse reactions include blurred vision, bitter/sour taste, blepharitis, dermatitis, dry eye, foreign body sensation, headache, hyperemia, ocular discharge, pain, discomfort, or itching; keratitis, rhinitis, and possible systemic-like sulfa reactions.

Administration: Ophthalmic.

Patient Care Implications: Instruct patients to remove contact lenses prior to administration and to leave out for 15 minutes after application of the medication. Tell patients to shake the medication well prior to use. Separate use of this agent from other topical ocular medications by a minimum of 10 minutes.

Preparations: 1% ophthalmic suspension (contains benzalkonium chloride) in a dropper vial with a controlled dispensing tip. 5, 10, and 15 mL.

BROMOCRIPTINE MESYLATE—Parlodel®

Description/Actions: Dopamine receptor agonist indicated for the treatment of dysfunctions associated with hyperprolactinemia (e.g., amenorrhea, infertility), acromegaly, and parkinsonism. Is an ergot derivative.

Preparations: Tablets, 2.5 mg. Capsules, 5 mg.

BROMODIPHENHYDRAMINE HYDROCHLORIDE

Description/Actions: Antihistamine included in some combination formulations.

BROMPHENIRAMINE MALEATE—Dimetane®

Description/Actions: Antihistamine indicated for the management of allergic disorders.

Preparations: Tablets, 4 mg. Controlled-release tablets, 8 and 12 mg. Elixir, 2 mg/5 ml. Vials, 10 mg/ml.

BRONKAID MIST, see Epinephrine

BRONKEPHRINE®, see Isoetharine

BRONKOMETER®, see Isoetharine

BRONKOSOL®, see Isoetharine

BUCLADIN-S®, see Buclizine

BUCLIZINE HYDROCHLORIDE—Bucladin-S®

Description/Actions: Antiemetic indicated in the management of nausea, vomiting, and dizziness associated with motion sickness.

Preparations: Tablets, 50 mg.

BUDESONIDE—Entocort™ EC, Pulmicort Respules™, Pulmicort Turbuhaler®, Rhinocort®

Description/Actions: Pulmicort is a potent adrenocortical steroid with locally acting anti-inflammatory and immune modifer properties. Use of aerosolized steroids may decrease the requirement for or avoid use of systemic glucocorticoids and delay pulmonary damage that occurs from chronic asthma. Pulmicort is indicated in the maintenance and prophylactic treatment of asthma including patients who require systemic corticosteroids and those who may benefit from systemic dose reduction/elimination.

Precautions/Adverse Reactions: Contraindicated in acute asthma/status asthmaticus. Use cautiously in active untreated infections, patients with diabetes, glaucoma, underlying immunosuppression, systemic glucocorticoid therapy, pregnancy, nursing mothers, and children <6. Adverse reactions include headache, dysphonia, hoarseness, oropharyngeal fungal infections, bronchospasm, cough, wheezing, dry mouth, esophageal candidiasis, dyspepsia, gastroenteritis, back pain, and flulike symptoms.

Administration: Oral and oral inhalation.

Preparations: 160 mcg/actuation powder in a 200 dose turbohaler, inhalation solution, 0.25 mg/2 ml and 0.5 mg/2 ml. Capsules, 3 mg.

BUMETANIDE—Bumex®

Description/Actions: A loop diuretic indicated for the treatment of edema associated with congestive heart failure, hepatic disease, and renal disease, including the nephrotic syndrome.

Precautions/Adverse Reactions: Is contraindicated in anuria, and in patients in hepatic coma or in states of severe electrolyte depletion until the condition is improved or corrected. May cause volume and electrolyte depletion. Potential for hypokalemia warrants periodic measurement of serum potassium levels. Concurrent use with lithium is best avoided because of an increased risk of lithium toxicity. Parenteral administration is best avoided in patients receiving aminoglycoside antibiotics because of an increased risk of ototoxicity.

Administration: Oral, intravenous, and intramuscular.

Preparations: Tablets, 0.5, 1, and 2 mg. Ampules and vials, 0.25 mg/ml.

BUMEX®, see Bumetanide

BUMINATE®, see Albumin

BUPIVACAINE HYDROCHLORIDE—Marcaine®

Description/Actions: Local anesthetic administered by injection for the production of local or regional anesthesia or analgesia for surgery, dental and oral surgery procedures, diagnostic and therapeutic procedures, and obstetrical procedures. A formulation is also available for the production of subarachnoid block (spinal anesthesia).

Preparations: Ampules and vials, 0.25%, 0.5%, and 0.75%, and in combination with epinephrine. Ampules for spinal anesthesia, 15 mg.

BUPRENEX®, see Buprenorphine

BUPRENORPHINE—Subutex®

Description/Actions: Buprenorphine is a partial agonist at the mu-opioid receptor. It is one of the first medications approved for office-based induction treatment of opioid dependence. It is part of a complete addiction treatment program that includes counseling or behavior therapy.

Precautions/Adverse Reactions: Buprenorphine is contraindicated in individuals with a hypersensitivity to the product or any component of the formulation. May cause respiratory depression: use caution in patients with compromised respiratory function or preexisting respiratory depression. Chronic administration produces dependence of the opioid type, marked by withdrawal upon abrupt discontinuation or rapid taper. Buprenorphine may elevate cerebrospinal fluid pressure and should be used with caution in patients with head injury, intracranial lesions, and other circumstances where cerebrospinal pressure may be increased. In general, buprenorphine should be administered with caution in elderly or debilitated patients and those with severe impairment of hepatic, pulmonary, or renal function; myxedema or hyperthyroidism; adrenal cortical insufficiency; CNS depression or coma; toxic psychoses; prostatic hypertrophy or urethral stricture; acute alcoholism; delirium tremens; or kyphoscoliosis. Most common adverse reactions are headache, pain, insomnia, depression, nausea, back pain, abdominal pain, and constipation. Pregnancy category C. Withdrawal has been reported in infants of women receiving buprenorphine during pregnancy. Enters breast milk; not recommended while nursing.

Administration: Sublingual—The first dose should be given at least 4 hours after the patient last used opioids or preferably when early signs of opioid withdrawal appear.

Preparations: Sublingual tablets: 2 and 8 mg.

BUPRENORPHINE HYDROCHLORIDE—Buprenex®

Description/Actions: Demonstrates both opiate agonist and antagonist actions, and is indicated for the relief of moderate to severe pain.

Precautions/Adverse Reactions: Adverse reactions include sedation, dizziness, and vertigo. Caution should be exercised in patients also receiving other CNS depressants. Is less likely than many other potent analgesics to cause dependence and is included in Schedule V. May precipitate withdrawal symptoms in patients who are physically dependent on other opiates. Respiratory depression produced by buprenorphine is only partially reversed by naloxone, and doxapram may be used. Excreted in human breast milk. Nursing is not recommended.

Administration: Intravenous and intramuscular.

Preparations: Ampules, 0.3 mg.

BUPRENORPHINE AND NALOXONE—Suboxone®

Description/Actions: Suboxone® is one of two drugs first approved for office-based treatment of opioid dependence (e.g., morphine, heroin, or methadone). Suboxone® is indicated for maintenance treatment due to naloxone in the formulation. Naloxone is an antagonist at the mu-opioid receptor; it is intended to deter intravenous abuse by individuals dependent on other opiates.

Precautions/Adverse Reactions: Suboxone® is contraindicated in patients with a hypersensitivity to buprenorphine, naloxone, or any component of the formulation. Because Suboxone® may cause respiratory depression, use caution in patients with compromised respiratory function or preexisting respiratory depression. Buprenorphine is a partial agonist at the mu-opioid receptor, and chronic administration produced dependence of the opioid type, characterized by withdrawal upon abrupt discontinuation or rapid taper. Suboxone®, like other opioids, may elevate cerebrospinal fluid pressure and should be used with caution in patients with head injury, intracranial lesions, and other circumstances where cerebrospinal pressure may be increased. In general, it should be administered with caution in elderly or debilitated patients and those with severe impairment of hepatic, pulmonary, or renal function; CNS depression or coma; toxic psychoses; prostatic hypertrophy or urethral stricture; acute alcoholism; delirium tremens; or kyphoscoliosis. Most common adverse reactions are headache, pain, nausea, constipation, abdominal pain, vasodilation, and vomiting. Pregnancy Category C. Withdrawal has been reported in infants of women receiving buprenorphine during pregnancy. Buprenorphine enters breast milk; breast feeding not recommended.

Administration: Sublingual.

Preparations: Sublingual tablet, 2 mg buprenorphine with 0.5 mg naloxone, 8 mg buprenorphine with 2 mg naloxone.

BUPROPION HYDROCHLORIDE—Wellbutrin®, 2 g bar®, Wellbutrin® SR, Wellbutrin® XL, Zyban™

Description/Actions: Indicated for the treatment of depression and as an aid to smoking cessation treatment.

Precautions/Adverse Reactions: Contraindicated in patients undergoing abrupt discontinuation of alcohol or sedatives, including benzodiazepines. Contraindicated in patients with seizure disorders, and in patients with a current or prior diagnosis of bulimia or anorexia nervosa because of a higher incidence of seizures noted in such patients when treated with bupropion. Antidepressants increased the risk of suicidal thinking and behavior (suicidality) in short-term studies in children and adolescents with major depressive disorder (MDD) and other psychiatric disorders. Anyone considering the use of bupropion or any other antidepressant in a child or adolescent must balance this risk with the clinical need. Patients who are started on therapy should be observed closely for clinical worsening, suicidality, or unusual changes in behavior. Wellbutrin® is not approved for use in pediatric patients. Concurrent use with a monoamine oxidase inhibitor is contraindicated, and at least 14 days should elapse between discontinuation of an MAOI and initiation of treatment with bupropion. Adverse reactions most commonly encountered include nausea, vomiting, hallucinations, constipation, dry mouth, agitation, insomnia, headache, migraine, and tremor. Some patients experience weight loss. Patients should be cautioned regarding activities such as driving and operating machinery, as well as interactions with other CNS-acting drugs including alcohol. Extreme caution should be exercised in patients with a history of seizures or other predisposition toward seizure, and in patients treated with other medications (e.g., antipsychotics) that may lower seizure threshold. Is extensively metabolized and its activity may be changed by other medications known to affect hepatic enzyme systems (e.g., phenobarbital, cimetidine).

Administration: Oral. Because of a greater risk of seizures, no single dose should exceed 150 mg, and the total daily dosage should not exceed 450 mg. Consecutive 150 mg doses should be separated by an interval of at least 6 hours, and consecutive 100 mg doses by an interval of at least 4 hours. For smoking cessation, treat for 7–12 weeks; avoid bedtime dosing. Patients should aim to stop smoking within 1–2 weeks after starting bupropion. May be used with transdermal nicotine (quit smoking when starting nicotine).

Preparations: Tablets, 75 and 100 mg. Sustained release tabs, 100, 150, and 200 mg. Extended release tablets, 150 and 300 mg.

BUROW'S SOLUTION, see Aluminum Acetate

BuSpar®, see Buspirone

BUSPIRONE HYDROCHLORIDE—BuSpar®

Description/Actions: Indicated for the management of anxiety disorders or the short-term relief of the symptoms of anxiety.

Precautions/Adverse Reactions: Adverse reactions include dizziness, headache, nervousness, lightheadedness, excitement, and nausea. Buspirone is less likely than other antianxiety agents to cause effects such as sedation; however, because its CNS effects in any individual patient are usually not predictable, patients should be cautioned about engaging in activities such as operating an automobile or machinery. The concurrent use with other CNS-active drugs should be closely monitored, and the consumption of alcoholic beverages is best avoided. The drug should not be used concomitantly with a monoamine oxidase inhibitor because of the possibility of blood pressure elevations.

Administration: Oral.

Preparations: Tablets, 5, 10, and 15 mg.

BUSULFAN—Myleran®

Description/Actions: Antineoplastic agent indicated for the palliative treatment of chronic myelogenous leukemia.

Preparations: Tablets, 2 mg.

BUTABARBITAL SODIUM—Butisol Sodium®

Description/Actions: Barbiturate sedative-hypnotic indicated for the treatment of anxiety and insomnia.

Preparations: Tablets, 15, 30, 50, and 100 mg. Elixir, 30 mg/5 ml.

BUTALBITAL

Description/Actions: Barbiturate sedative used in combination with analgesics in the management of muscle-contraction headaches.

BUTAMBEN PICRATE—Butesin Picrate®

Description/Actions: Local anesthetic indicated for the temporary relief of pain due to minor burns.

Preparations: Ointment, 1%.

BUTENAFINE HYDROCHLORIDE—Mentax®

Description/Actions: Antifungal agent indicated in the treatment of tinea corporis, tinea cruris, interdigital tinea pedis, and tinea (pityriasis) versicolor due to *Malassezia furfur* (formerly *Pityrosporum orbiculare*).

Precautions/Adverse Reactions: Avoid eyes, nose, mouth, and mucous membranes. Do not occlude area of application. Discontinue if irritation develops and confirm diagnosis. Use cautiously in patients with hypersensitivity to allylamines. Adverse reactions include burning/stinging, worsening of condition, and other local irritation.

Administration: Apply to affected area and immediately surrounding area according to the following guidelines: Tinea pedis: once daily for 4 weeks. Tinea corporis, cruris: once daily for 2 weeks. If no improvement within 4 weeks, reconfirm diagnosis.

Preparations: 1% cream.

BUTESIN PICRATE®, see Butamben Picrate

BUTISOL®, see Butabarbital

BUTOCONAZOLE NITRATE—Femstat®

Description/Actions: Antifungal agent indicated for the treatment of vulvovaginal mycotic infections caused by *Candida* species.

Precautions/Adverse Reactions: Use during the first trimester of pregnancy should be avoided. Adverse reactions include vulvar/vaginal burning and/or vulvar itching.

Administration: Vaginal.

Preparations: Vaginal cream, 2%.

BUTORPHANOL TARTRATE—Stadol®, Stadol NS®

Description/Actions: Analgesic also possessing narcotic antagonist activity. Indicated for parenteral use in the relief of moderate to severe pain, for preoperative or preanesthetic medication, as a supplement to balanced anesthesia, and for the relief of prepartum pain. Also indicated for nasal use in the management of pain (including postoperative analgesia).

Preparations: Vials and syringes, 1 mg/ml and 2 mg/ml. Nasal spray, 10 mg/ml.

BUTYL METHOXYDIBENZOYLMETHANE/PADIMATE 0—
   Photoplex®

Description/Actions: A combination of padimate O, which is highly protective against shortwave ultraviolet radiation [UVB (290–320 nm)], and butyl methoxydibenzoylmethane, which protects against long-wave ultraviolet radiation [UVA (320–400 nm)]. The combination of the two agents has been designated as a "broad" or "full" spectrum sunscreen. Indicated to provide protection against the acute (e.g., sunburn) and long-term (e.g., photoaging, skin cancer) risks associated with UVA and UVB light exposure.

Precautions/Adverse Reactions: Contraindicated in patients with a history of allergy to para-aminobenzoic acid, sulfonamides, benzocaine, or aniline dyes. The formulation may stain some fabrics.

Administration: Topical.

Preparations: Lotion containing butyl methoxydibenzoylmethane in a 3% concentration and padimate O in a 7% concentration.

C

CABERGOLINE—Dostinex®

Description/Actions: Dopamine agonist indicated in treatment of hyperprolactinemic disorders, either idiopathic or due to pituitary tumors.

Precautions/Adverse Reactions: Not for pregnancy-induced hypertension or postpartum lactation inhibition or suppression. Use cautiously in hepatic dysfunction. Contraindicated in uncontrolled hypertension and previous sensitivity to ergot alkaloids. Monitor prolactin levels monthly, until normalized.

Administration: Oral.

Preparations: Scored tablets, 0.5 mg.

CAFERGOT®, Combination of Ergotamine Tartrate and Caffeine

CAFFEINE—NoDoz®

Description/Actions: Central nervous system stimulant used as an aid in staying awake and as an adjunct to analgesics in the management of pain.

Preparations: Tablets, 100 and 200 mg. Controlled-release capsules, 200 and 250 mg.

CAFFEINE AND SODIUM BENZOATE

Description/Actions: Central nervous system stimulant that has been administered parenterally as a diuretic, as a stimulant in acute circulatory failure, in the treatment of poisoning, and to alleviate headaches following spinal puncture.

Preparations: Ampules, 250 mg/ml (equal parts caffeine and sodium benzoate).

CALAMINE

Description/Actions: Protectant applied topically in the treatment of dermatologic conditions associated with itching, pain, and irritation.

Preparations: Lotion, 8% with 8% zinc oxide.

CALAN®, see Verapamil

CALAN SR®, see Verapamil

CALCIFEDIOL—Calderol®

Description/Actions: Vitamin D derivative indicated in the management of metabolic bone disease or hypocalcemia associated with chronic renal failure in patients undergoing renal dialysis. *Preparations:* Capsules, 20 and 50 mcg.

CALCIBIND®, see Sodium Cellulose Phosphate

CALCIJEX®, see Calcitriol

CALCIMAR®, see Calcitonin—Salmon

CALCIPOTRIENE—Dovonex®

Description/Actions: Is a synthetic analogue of vitamin D3 that is indicated for the topical treatment of moderate plaque psoriasis.

Precautions/Adverse Reactions: Contraindicated in patients with demonstrated hypercalcemia or evidence of vitamin D toxicity. Is also contraindicated for use on the face. Adverse reactions include burning, itching, skin irritation, and hypercalcemia. If an elevation in serum calcium outside the normal range should occur, treatment should be discontinued until normal calcium levels are restored.

Administration: Topical.

Preparations: Cream, ointment, scalp solution, 0.005%.

CALCITONIN—SALMON—Calcimar®, Miacalcin©

Description/Actions: Hormone indicated for the parenteral treatment of symptomatic Paget's disease of bone, hypercalcemia, and postmenopausal osteoporosis.

Preparations: Vials, 200 IU/ml. Nasal spray, 200 units/spray.

CALCITRIOL—Calcijex®, Rocaltrol®

Description/Actions: Vitamin D derivative indicated in the management of hypocalcemia and the resultant metabolic bone disease in patients undergoing chronic renal dialysis. Is also indicated in the management of hypocalcemia in patients with hypoparathyroidism.

Preparations: Capsules, 0.25 and 0.5 mcg. Ampules, 1 g/ml and 2 g/ml.

CALCIUM ACETATE—PhosLo®

Description/Actions: Phosphate binding agent indicated for the control of hyperphosphatemia in end stage renal failure.

Preparations: Tablets, 667 mg.

CALCIUM CARBONATE—Caltrate®, Os-Cal®, Tums®, Viactiv®

Description/Actions: Antacid and source of calcium used in the treatment of gastrointestinal conditions, in the treatment of hypocalcemic disorders and in situations in which calcium intake is inadequate.

Preparations: Chewable tablets, 350, 500, 750, and 850 mg. Tablets, 1.25 and 1.5 g. Calcium carbonate 500 mg in combination with vitamin D 100 units, vitamin K 400 mcg in soft chewable tablets (Viactiv®).

CALCIUM CHLORIDE

Description/Actions: Source of calcium and is administered intravenously in the treatment of hypocalcemic disorders. Also used IV in the treatment of magnesium intoxication, certain hyperkalemic conditions, and cardiac resuscitation.

Preparations: Ampules, vials, and syringes, 10%.

CALCIUM DISODIUM VERSENATE®, see Edetate
Calcium Disodium

CALCIUM GLUCEPTATE

Description/Actions: Source of calcium and is administered parenterally in the treatment of hypocalcemic disorders and certain other conditions.

Preparations: Ampules and vials, 1.1 g/5 ml.

CALCIUM GLUCONATE

Description/Actions: Source of calcium and is administered orally and intravenously in the treatment of hypocalcemic disorders and in situations in which calcium intake is inadequate.

Preparations: Tablets, 500 and 650 mg, 1 g. Ampules and vials, 10%.

CALCIUM LACTATE

Description/Actions: Source of calcium used in the treatment of hypocalcemic disorders and in situations in which calcium intake is inadequate.

Preparations: Tablets, 325 and 650 mg.

CALCIUM PHOSPHATE, TRIBASIC—Tricalcium Phosphate, Posture®

Description/Actions: Source of calcium used in the treatment of hypocalcemic disorders and in situations in which calcium intake is inadequate.

Preparations: Tablets, 300 and 600 mg.

CALCIUM UNDECYLENATE—Caldesene®

Description/Actions: Antifungal agent applied topically in the management of dermatologic fungal infections.

Preparations: Powder, 10%.

CALDEROL®, see Calcifediol

CALDESENE®, see Calcium Undecylenate

CALFACTANT—Infasurf®

Description/Actions: Indicated for the prevention of respiratory distress syndrome (RDS) in premature infants <29 weeks of gestational age at high risk for RDS and for treatment ("rescue") of premature infants 72 hours of age who develop RDS and require endotracheal intubation. Calfactant prophylaxis should be administered as soon as possible, preferably 30 minutes after birth.

Precautions/Adverse Reactions: Calfactant is for intratracheal use only. Reflux of the calfactant into the endotracheal tube, cyanosis, bradycardia, or airway obstruction has occurred during the dosing procedures. These events require stopping the calfactant administration and taking appropriate measures to relieve the condition. After the patient is stable, dosing can proceed with proper monitoring. The administration of lung surfactants often rapidly improves oxygenation and lung compliance. Following administration of calfactant, monitor patients carefully so that oxygen therapy and ventilatory support can be modified in response to changes in respiratory status. The most common adverse reactions associated with calfactant therapy are cyanosis, airway obstruction, bradycardia, reflux of surfactant into the endotracheal tube, requiring manual ventilation and reintubation. These events were generally transient and not associated with serious complication or death.

Administration: Administer through an endotracheal tube.

Preparations: Single-dose vials, 6 mL

CALTRATE®, see Calcium Carbonate

CAMPHOR

Description/Actions: Analgesic and antipruritic. Is used in topically applied formulations in the management of various dermatologic conditions.

CAMPHORATED OPIUM TINCTURE, see Paregoric

CANASA®, see Mesalamine

CANCIDAS®, see Caspofungin Acetate

CANDESARTAN—Atacand®

Description/Actions: Candesartan is an angiotensin II antagonist that is selective for the AT1 receptor subtype. It is indicated in the treatment of hypertension as monotherapy or in combination with other antihypertensive agents. Atacand® is also indicated for the treatment of heart failure (NYHA class II-IV) in patients with left ventricular systolic dysfunction (ejection fraction ≤40%) to reduce cardiovascular death and to reduce heart failure hospitalizations.

Precautions/Adverse Reactions: Correct hypovolemia before starting therapy or monitor patients closely. Use cautiously in patients with renal impairment, severe CHF, renal artery stenosis, and the elderly. Pregnancy Category C in the first trimester, Category D in second and third trimesters. Use not recommended in nursing mothers. Post marketing experience has identified reports of fetal and neonatal toxicity in babies born to women treated with candesartan during pregnancy. When pregnancy is detected candesartan should be discontinued as soon as possible. Adverse reactions include back pain, dizziness, upper respiratory tract infection, pharyngitis, and rhinitis.

Administration: Oral.

Patient Care Implications: Instruct patients that following recommended measures for control of hypertension (e.g., exercise, smoking cessation, weight control, dietary measures) will facilitate the action of the medication and does not eliminate the need for these measures. Warn patients that dehydration may enhance the effects of the drugs and to avoid prolonged sun and heat exposure. Caution patients to make position changes slowly to decrease the risk of orthostatic hypotension. Remind patients to continue taking the medication even if feeling well as medication controls but does not cure hypertension. This agent may not be as effective in Black patients and use of monotherapy in this population needs to be carefully assessed for effectiveness.

Preparations: Tablets, 4, 8, 16, and 32 mg.

CANTIL®, see Mepenzolate

CAPASTAT®, see Capreomycin

CAPECITABINE—Xeloda®

Description/Actions: Antineoplastic agent indicated in the treatment of patients with metastatic breast cancer resistant to both pacitaxel and an anthracycline-containing chemotherapy regimen or resistant to pacitaxel and for whom further anthracycline therapy is not indicated.

Capecitabine is also indicated as first-line treatment for patients with metastatic colorectal carcinoma when treatment with fluoropyrimidine therapy alone is preferred. Approved for use in combination with docetaxel for the treatment of metastatic breast cancer.

Precautions/Adverse Reactions: Capecitabine is contraindicated in patients with known hypersensitivity to it or to any component of the formulation. Capecitabine is contraindicated in patients who have a known hypersensitivity to 5–fluorouracil. Capecitabine is contraindicated in patients with known dihydropyrimidine dehydrogenase (DPD) deficiency. Capecitabine is also contraindicated in patients with severe renal impairment (creatinine clearance below 30 ml/min). The concomitant administration of capecitabine and warfarin has resulted in altered coagulation parameters (INR or prothrombin time) and/or bleeding, including death. These events occurred in patients with and without liver metastasis. Patients receiving capecitabine and warfarin should have their anticoagulant response monitored closely and the anticoagulant dose adjusted accordingly. Adverse effects include diarrhea, which can be severe. Provide supportive treatment to minimize dehydration and electrolyte imbalance. Other adverse effects are hand and foot syndrome (plantar erythrodyesthesia or chemotherapy-induced acral erythema), cardiotoxicity (MI, angina, dysrhythmias, cardiogenic shock, sudden death, ECG changes), hyperbilirubinemia, anemia, neutropenia, thrombocytopenia, nausea, vomiting, stomatitis, and others.

Administration: Oral.

Preparations: Tablets, 150 and 500 mg.

CAPOTEN®, see Captopril

CAPOZIDE®, Combination of Captopril and Hydrochlorothiazide

CAPREOMYCIN SULFATE—Capastat®

Description/Actions: Antitubercular agent used for the intramuscular treatment of tuberculosis, in conjunction with other antitubercular agents.

Preparations: Vials, 1 g.

CAPSAICIN—Zostrix®, Zostrix-HP®

Description/Actions: Topical analgesic indicated for the relief of neuralgias that may accompany herpes zoster infections, diabetic neuropathy, or follow surgery.

Preparations: Cream, 0.025% and 0.075%.

CAPTOPRIL—Capoten®

Description/Actions: Is an angiotensin-converting enzyme (ACE) inhibitor. Indicated for the treatment of hypertension, and in patients with congestive heart failure who have not responded adequately to treatment with diuretics and digitalis. Also indicated to improve survival following myocardial infarction in clinically stable patients with left ventricular dysfunction. Also indicated for the treatment of diabetic nephropathy.

Precautions/Adverse Reactions: Adverse reactions include cough, rash, pruritus, dysgeusia, hypotension, hyperkalemia, proteinuria, and nephrotic syndrome. Neutropenia and agranulocytosis have occurred, and patients should be advised to report promptly any indication of infection (e.g., sore throat, fever) that may be a sign of neutropenia. Use during pregnancy should be avoided.

Administration: Oral. Food reduces absorption and the drug should be given one hour before meals.

Preparations: Tablets, 12.5, 25, 50, and 100 mg.

CARAC™, see Fluorouracil

CARAFATE®, see Sucralfate

CARBACHOL—Isopto Carbachol®, Miostat®

Description/Actions: Cholinergic and miotic agent indicated for ophthalmic administration (Isopto Carbachol®) to lower intraocular pressure in the treatment of glaucoma, and for intraocular administration (Miostat®) to provide miosis during surgery.

Preparations: Ophthalmic solution (Isopto-Carbachol®, 0.75%, 1.5%, 2.25%, and 3%. Solution for intraocular administration (Miostat®), 0.01%.

CARBAMAZEPINE—Carbatrol®, Tegretol®, Equetro™

Description/Actions: Indicated in the following conditions in patients who have not responded satisfactorily to treatment with other agents such as phenytoin, phenobarbital, or primidone: (a) partial seizures with complex symptomatology, (b) generalized tonic-clonic seizures (grand mal), and (c) mixed seizure patterns that include the above, or other partial or generalized seizures. Also indicated in the treatment of pain associated with trigeminal neuralgia and glossopharyngeal neuralgia.

Precautions/Adverse Reactions: Is structurally related to the tricyclic antidepressants and should not be used in patients with a history of hypersensitivity to any of these agents. May cause serious hematologic reactions and should not be used in patients with a history of serious bone marrow depression. Patients should be advised to report immediately signs and symptoms of a potential hematologic problem, such as sore throat, fever, ulcers in the mouth, and easy brusing. Other adverse reactions include: dizziness, drowsiness, nausea, vomiting, and dermatologic effects. Concurrent use with a monoamine oxidase inhibitor is not recommended.

Administration: Oral.

Preparations: Tablets, 200 mg. Extended release, 100, 200, 300, and 400 mg. Chewable tablets, 100 mg. Suspension, 100 mg/5 ml. Extended release capsules, 100 mg, 200 mg, and 300 mg (Equetro).

CARBAMIDE PEROXIDE—Urea Peroxide, Debrox®, Gly-Oxide®

Description/Actions: Antiseptic and cleansing agent administered in the mouth for the treatment and prevention of minor oral inflammation such as canker sores, and in the ear to soften and remove earwax.

Preparations: Solution, 6.5% (otic use) and 10% (oral use).

CARBATROL®, see Carbamazepine

CARBENICILLIN INDANYL SODIUM—Geocillin®

Description/Actions: Penicillin antibiotic indicated in the oral treatment of urinary tract and prostatic infections caused by susceptible bacteria.

Preparations: Tablets, equivalent to 382 mg of carbenicillin.

CARBIDOPA—Lodosyn®, Parcopa™

Description/Actions: Inhibits the peripheral decarboxylation of levodopa and is used in combination with that agent in the treatment of parkinsonism.

Preparations: Tablets, 25 mg. Orally disintegrating tablets (carbidopa-levodopa), 10 mg/100 mg, 25 mg/100 mg, and 25 mg/250 mg.

CARBINOXAMINE MALEATE

Description/Actions: Antihistamine used in combination with other medications.

CARBOCAINE®, see Mepivacaine

CARBOL-FUCHSIN SOLUTION—Castellani Paint

Description/Actions: Antifungal formulation used topically in the management of dermatologic fungal infections. Fuchsin is a dye and causes staining.

Preparations: Solution containing phenol and resorcinol in addition to fuchsin.

CARBOLIC ACID, see Phenol

CARBON DIOXIDE

Description/Actions: Respiratory stimulant used by inhalation in conjunction with oxygen.

Preparations: Gas, available in mixtures with oxygen.

CARBOPLATIN—Paraplatin®

Description/Actions: A platinum compound related to cisplatin. Indicated for the palliative treatment of patients with ovarian carcinoma recurrent after prior chemotherapy, including patients who have been previously treated with cisplatin. Also indicated for the initial treatment of advanced ovarian carcinoma.

Precautions/Adverse Reactions: Should not be used in patients with severe bone marrow depression or significant bleeding. Thrombocytopenia, neutropenia, leukopenia, and anemia are often experienced and therapy must be closely monitored. Serious allergic reactions may occur. Other adverse reactions include nausea, vomiting, abdominal pain, diarrhea, constipation, peripheral neuropathies, abnormal hepatic and renal function tests, electrolyte changes, alopecia, and cardiovascular, respiratory, genitourinary, and mucosal effects. Concomitant treatment with aminoglycosides has resulted in increased renal and/or audiologic toxicity. The drug may cause fetal harm when administered during pregnancy.

Administration: Intravenous infusion (lasting 15 minutes or longer). Carboplatin reacts with aluminum, causing precipitate formation and loss of potency; therefore, needles or intravenous sets containing aluminum parts that may come in contact with the drug must not be used for the preparation or administration of carboplatin.

Preparations: Vials, 50, 150, and 450 mg.

CARBOPROST TROMETHAMINE—Hemabate®

Description/Actions: Abortifacient administered intramuscularly for the termination of pregnancy during the period from 13 to 20 gestational weeks. Also indicated for the treatment of postpartum hemorrhage due to uterine atony that has not responded to conventional management.

Preparations: Ampules, 250 μg carboprost and 83 μg tromethamine per ml.

CARBOWAX®, see Polyethylene Glycol

CARDENE®, see Nicardipine

CARDENE IV®, see Nicardipine

CARDILATE®, see Erythrityl Tetranitrate

CARDIOQUIN®, see Quinidine Polygalacturonate

CARDIZEM®, see Diltiazem

CARDIZEM CD®, see Diltiazem

CARDIZEM LA®, see Diltiazem

CARDIZEM SR®, see Diltiazem

CARDURA®, see Doxazosin Mesylate

CARISOPRODOL—Rela®, Soma®

Description/Actions: Skeletal muscle relaxant indicated as an adjunct to rest, physical therapy, and other measures for the relief of discomfort associated with acute, painful musculoskeletal conditions.

Preparations: Tablets, 350 mg.

CARMUSTINE—BiCNU®

Description/Actions: Antineoplastic agent administered intravenously as palliative therapy for brain tumors, multiple myeloma, Hodgkin's disease, and non-Hodgkin's lymphomas.

Preparations: Vials, 100 mg.

CARNITOR®, see L-Carnitine

CARTEOLOL HYDROCHLORIDE—Cartrol®, Ocupress®

Description/Actions: A nonselective beta-adrenergic blocking agent with intrinsic sympathomimetic activity. Indicated in the treatment of hypertension, and for ophthalmic administration in the treatment of chronic open-angle glaucoma and intraocular hypertension.

Precautions/Adverse Reactions: Contraindicated in patients with bronchial asthma, cardiogenic shock, severe bradycardia, and second and third degree atrioventricular conduction block in the absence of a functioning artificial pacemaker. Adverse reactions include weakness, tiredness, fatigue, and muscle cramps. Use is best avoided in patients with bronchospastic diseases, and therapy in diabetic patients must be closely monitored.

Administration: Oral and ophthalmic. Patients should be cautioned about the interruption or discontinuation of therapy; exacerbation of angina pectoris has occurred following the abrupt cessation of therapy and, when therapy is to be discontinued, the dosage should be gradually reduced over a period of 1 to 2 weeks.

Preparations: Tablets (Cartrol), 2.5 and 5 mg. Ophthalmic solution (Ocupress), 1%.

CARTROL®, see Carteolol

CARVEDILOL—Coreg®

Description/Actions: A noncardioselective beta-blocker/alpha-blocker. Carvedilol is indicated for the treatment of mild to severe heart failure of ischemic or cardiomyopathic origin, usually in addition to diuretics, ACE inhibitor, and digitalis, to increase survival, and also to reduce the risk of hospitalization. Carvedilol is indicated to reduce cardiovascular mortality in clinically stable patients who have survived the acute phase of a myocardial infarction and have a left ventricular ejection fraction ≤40% (with or without symptomatic heart failure). Carvedilol is also indicated for the management of essential hypertension. It can be used alone or in combination with other antihypertensive agents, especially thiazide-type diuretics.

Precautions/Adverse Reactions: Contraindicated in patients with bronchial asthma or related bronchospastic conditions, second- or third-degree AV block, sick sinus syndrome, severe bradycardia (unless paced), cardiogenic shock, and a history of carvedilol associated hepatic injury. Use cautiously in peripheral vascular disease, nonallergic bronchospasm, diabetes, hyperthyroidism, hepatic dysfunction, prinzemetal's angina, pheochromocytoma, and anesthesia. Monitor renal function in ischemic heart disease, diffuse vascular disease, underlying renal insufficiency, and/or if systolic BP <100 mm Hg. Avoid abrupt cessation. Pregnancy category C. Use not recommended in nursing mothers. Adverse reactions include bradycardia, orthostatic hypotension, edema, AV block, GI upset, hyperglycemia, increased weight, dizziness, and others.

Administration: Oral.

Preparations: Tablets, 3.125, 6.25, 12.5, and 25 mg.

CASANTHRANOL

Description/Actions: Laxative included in combination formulations indicated for constipation.

CASCARA SAGRADA

Description/Actions: Laxative used in the treatment of constipation.

Preparations: Tablets, 325 mg. Aromatic fluid extract.

CASODEX®, see Bicalutamide

CASPOFUNGIN ACETATE—Cancidas®

Description/Actions: Antifungal agent indicated for empirical therapy for presumed fungal infections in febrile, neutropenic patients. For the treatment of candidemia and the following candida infections: intra-abdominal abscesses, peritonitis, and pleural space infections. For the treatment of esophageal candidiasis and in the treatment of aspergillosis in patients who are refractory or intolerant to amphotericin B, lipid formulations of amphotericin B, or intraconazole. Cancidas® has not been studied as initial therapy for invasive aspergillosis.

Precautions/Adverse Reactions: Contraindicated in patients with hypersensitivity to caspofungin or to any component of the product. Concomitant use of caspofungin acetate with cyclosporine is not recommended. Concurrent use has resulted in elevations of hepatic transaminases. Use only if the potential benefit outweighs the potential risk to the patient. Safety on duration of therapy exceeding 2 weeks is limited; however, treatment appears to be well tolerated. Monitoring of tacrolimus blood concentrations is recommended when used concurrently with caspofungin acetate. Dosage adjustments may be necessary. Dosage of caspofungin acetate may need to be increased when administered concurrently with the enzyme inducers/mixed and inducer/inhibitors such as efavirenz, nelfinavir, nevirapine, phenytoin, rifampin, dexamethasone, or carbamazepine. The exact mechanism of the interaction is unknown. Pregnancy Category C. Caspofungin acetate has been shown to be embryotoxic in rats and rabbits. There are no adequate and well-controlled studies in pregnant women. Use in pregnancy only if the potential benefit justifies the potential risk to the fetus. Excretion in human breast milk is unknown. Safety and efficacy in pediatric patients have not been established. Adverse reactions noted in >10% of patients treated include headache, fever, increased hepatic transaminases, increased alkaline phosphatase, and phlebitis/thrombophlebitis. Less frequently observed adverse reactions include rash, pruritis, flushing, chills, edema, nausea, vomiting, diarrhea, pain, myalgias, decreased serum potassium, decreased total serum protein, decreased hemoglobin, hematocrit, platelets, white blood cell count, and decreased serum albumin levels. Possible histamine mediated symptoms have been reported during clinical trials.

Administration: Intravenous.

Patient Care Implications: Infuse slowly over at least 1 hour. Monitor patient during infusion. Do not use diluents containing dextrose. Do not mix or coinfuse with other medications. Reconstituted vials may be stored at room temperature for up to 1 hour prior to the preparation of the patient infusion solution. Diluted product is stable for 24 hours at room temperature. Vials should be stored in the refrigerator.

Preparations: Powder for injection: 50 mg and 70 mg single-use vials.

CASTELLANI PAINT, see Carbol-fuchsin Solution

CASTOR OIL

Description/Actions: Laxative indicated for the treatment of constipation and preparation of the colon for X-ray and endoscopic examination.

Preparations: Liquid. Emulsions, 36%, 60%, 67%, and 95%.

CATAPRES®, see Clonidine

CATAPRES-TTS®, see Clonidine

CATHFLO™, see Alteplase Recombinant

CAVERJECT®, see Alprostadil

CCNU®, see Lomustine

CECLOR®, see Cefaclor

CEDAX®, see Ceftibuten

CeeNU®, see Lomustine

CEFACLOR—Ceclor®, Raniclor™

Description/Actions: Spectrum of action includes many gram-positive and gram-negative bacteria. Indicated in upper and lower respiratory infections, otitis media, urinary tract infections, and skin and skin-structure infections caused by susceptible organisms.

Precautions/Adverse Reactions: Must be used cautiously in penicillin-sensitive patients, and use should be avoided in patients with a history of immediate and/or severe reactions to penicillin.

Administration: Oral. May be administered without regard to meals.

Preparations: Capsules, 250 and 500 mg. Extended release tablets, 375 and 500 mg. Powder for oral suspension, 125, 187, 250, and 375 mg/5 ml when reconstituted. Chewable tablets, 125 mg, 187 mg, 250 mg, and 375 mg.

CEFADROXIL—Duricef®, Ultracef®

Description/Actions: Spectrum of action includes many gram-positive and gram-negative bacteria. Indicated in pharyngitis and tonsillitis, urinary tract infections, and skin and skin-structure infections caused by susceptible organisms.

Precautions/Adverse Reactions: Must be used cautiously in penicillin-sensitive patients, and use should be avoided in patients with a history of immediate and/or severe reactions to penicillin.

Administration: Oral. May be administered without regard to meals.

Preparations: Capsules, 500 mg. Tablets, 1 g. Powder for oral suspension, 125, 250, and 500 mg/5 ml when reconstituted.

CEFADYL®, see Cephapirin

CEFAMANDOLE NAFTATE—Mandol®

Description/Actions: Active against many gram-positive and gram-negative bacteria. Indicated for lower respiratory infections, urinary tract infections, peritonitis, septicemia, skin and skin-structure infections, and bone and joint infections caused by susceptible organisms. May also be used for surgical prophylaxis.

Precautions/Adverse Reactions: Must be used cautiously, if at all, in penicillin-sensitive patients, and use should be avoided in patients with a history of immediate and/or severe reactions to penicillin. Therapy in patients at risk of bleeding reactions must be closely monitored. Disulfiram-like reactions may occur following the consumption of alcoholic beverages.

Administration: Intravenous and intramuscular.

Preparations: Vials, 500 mg, 1, 2, and 10 g of cefamandole activity.

CEFANEX®, see Cephalexin

CEFAZOLIN SODIUM—Ancef®, Kefzol®, Zolicef®

Description/Actions: Active against many gram-positive and gram-negative bacteria. Indicated for respiratory tract infections, genitourinary tract infections, skin and skin-structure infections, biliary tract infections, bone and joint infections, septicemia, and endocarditis caused by susceptible organisms. Is often used for surgical prophylaxis.

Precautions/Adverse Reactions: Must be used cautiously, if at all, in penicillin-sensitive patients, and use should be avoided in patients with a history of immediate and/or severe reactions to penicillin.

Administration: Intravenous and intramuscular.

Preparations: Vials, 250 and 500 mg, 1, 5, and 10 g of cefazolin.

CEFDINIR—Omnicef®

Description/Actions: Third-generation cephalosporin indicated in the treatment of susceptible community acquired pneumonia, acute exacerbations of chronic bronchitis, acute maxillary sinusitis, pharyngitis, tonsillitis, and uncomplicated infections of the skin and skin structures.

Precautions/Adverse Reactions: Use cautiously in patients with compromised renal or hepatic function, poor nutritional state, elderly or debilitated, and history of GI disease (especially colitis). Monitor prothrombin time. Contraindicated in patients with known allergy to cephalosporins. Adverse reactions include rash, pseudomembranous Colitis, and superinfection. Serious adverse events have been reported, including life-threatening or fatal occurrences of the following: encephalopathy (disturbance of consciousness including confusion, hallucinations, stupor, and coma), myoclonus, and seizures.

Administration: Oral.

Preparations: Capsules, 300 mg; suspension, 125 mg/5 ml. Oral suspension 250 mg/5 ml.

CEFDITOREN PIVOXIL—SPECTRACEF™

Description/Actions: Cefditoren pivoxil is indicated for the treatment of mild to moderate infections in adults and adolescents (12 years of age or older) that are caused by susceptible strains of the designated microorganisms in the following conditions: acute bacterial exacerbations of chronic bronchitis, pharyngitis/tonsillitis, and uncomplicated skin and skin-structure infections.

Precautions/Adverse Reactions: Cefditoren causes renal excretion of carnitine; therefore, it is contraindicated in patients with carnitine deficiency or inborn errors of metabolism that may result in clinically significant carnitine deficiency. Cefditoren tablets contain sodium caseinate, a milk protein, and should not be administered to patients with milk protein hypersensitivity. Use caution when using in patients with a history of hypersensitivity reactions to penicillins or to other beta-lactam antibiotics. Pseudomembranous colitis may occur and may range in severity from mild to life-threatening. Cefditoren is not recommended when prolonged antibiotic treatment is necessary. Cefditoren may be associated with a fall in prothrombin time. Coadministration with aluminum/magnesium-containing antacids is not recommended. Coadministraion of cefditoren and famotidine is not recommended. The coadministration of cefditoren and probenecid has resulted in increased plasma concentrations of cefditoren. Pregnancy Category B. No adequate and well-controlled studies in pregnant women. Use during pregnancy only if the potential benefit justifies the potential risk to the fetus. Excretion in human breast milk is unknown. Safety and efficacy in pediatric patients <12 years have not been established. Most common adverse effects noted in patients receiving cefditoren include diarrhea, nausea, headache, abdominal pain, vaginal moniliasis, dyspepsia, vomiting, decreased hematocrit, hematuria, increased urine white blood cells, and increased glucose. In addition, adverse reactions seen with cephalosporin antibiotics including allergic reactions, anaphylaxis, drug fever, Stevens-Johnson syndrome, serum sickness-like reactions, erythema multiforme, toxic epidermal necrolysis, colitis, renal dysfunction including cholestasis, aplastic anemia, hemolytic anemia, hemorrhage, superinfection, and seizures have been observed with cefditoren. Prolonged prothrombin time, positive direct Coombs' test, false-positive test for urinary glucose, elevated alkaline phosphatase, elevated bilirubin, elevated LDH, increased creatinine, pancytopenia, neutropenia, and agranulocytosis may also occur.

Administration: Oral.

Patient Care Implications: Take with meals. Avoid concomitant use of antacids or histamine$_2$ receptor antagonists. Not recommended when prolonged antibiotic therapy is needed.

Preparations: Tablets, 200 mg.

CEFEPIME—Maxipime®

Description/Actions: Fourth-generation cephalosporin indicated in treatment of susceptible uncomplicated or complicated urinary tract infections including pyelonephritis, uncomplicated skin and skin-structure infections, moderate to severe pneumonia, complicated intra-abdominal infection in adults (in conjunction with metronidazole), and empiric therapy in febrile neutropenia.

Precautions/Adverse Reactions: Use cautiously in patients with compromised renal or hepatic function, poor nutritional state, elderly, or debilitated, and history of GI disease (especially colitis). Monitor prothrombin time. Contraindicated in patients allergic to cephalosporins. Adverse reactions include local reactions to IV infusion (e.g., pain, phlebitis, inflammation), rash, pseudomembranous colitis, and superinfection. Serious adverse events have been reported, including life-threatening or fatal occurrences of the following: encephalopathy (disturbance of consciousness including confusion, hallucinations, stupor, and coma), myoclonus, and seizures.

Administration: Intravenous and intramuscular.

Preparations: Powder for reconstitution, 500 mg, 1 and 2 g.

CEFIXIME—Suprax®

Description/Actions: An orally administered, third-generation cephalosporin antibiotic that is especially active against gram-negative bacteria. Indicated in the treatment of otitis media, pharyngitis and tonsillitis, acute bronchitis and acute exacerbations of chronic bronchitis, uncomplicated gonorrhea, and uncomplicated urinary tract infections caused by susceptible bacteria. Among the bacteria that are susceptible are *Branhamella (Moraxella) catarrhalis, Escherichia coli, Haemophilus influenzae, Neisseria gonorrhoeae, Proteus mirabilis, Streptococcus pneumoniae, and Streptococcus pyogenes.*

Precautions/Adverse Reactions: Must be used cautiously in penicillin-sensitive patients, and use should be avoided in patients with a history of immediate and/or severe reactions to penicillin. Adverse reactions include diarrhea, loose or frequent stools, abdominal pain, nausea, dyspepsia, flatulence, headache, dizziness, pruritus, and rash.

Administration: Oral.

Preparations: Tablets, 400 mg. Powder for oral suspension, 100 mg/5 ml.

CEFIZOX®, see Ceftizoxime

CEFMETAZOLE SODIUM—Zefazone®

Description/Actions: Active against many aerobic and anaerobic gram-positive and gram-negative bacteria; spectrum of action includes *Bacteroides fragilis.* Indicated in the treatment of urinary tract, lower respiratory tract, skin and skin-structure, and intra-abdominal infections caused by susceptible bacteria. Is also indicated for surgical prophylaxis.

Precautions/Adverse Reactions: Must be used cautiously, if at all, in penicillin-sensitive patients, and use should be avoided in patients with a history of immediate and/or severe reactions to penicillin. Adverse reactions include diarrhea, nausea, epigastric pain, bleeding, allergic reactions, rash, pruritus, superinfection, pain and/or swelling at the injection site, thrombophlebitis, and prolonged prothrombin time. Prothrombin time should be monitored for patients at risk. Disulfiram-like reactions may occur when alcohol is ingested within 24 hours of cefmetazole administration.

Administration: Intravenous.

Preparations: Vials, 1 and 2 g.

CEFOBID®, see Cefoperazone

CEFONICID SODIUM—Monocid®

Description/Actions: Active against many gram-positive and gram-negative bacteria. Indicated for lower respiratory tract infections, urinary tract infections, septicemia, and bone and joint infections caused by susceptible organisms. May also be used for surgical prophylaxis.

Precautions/Adverse Reactions: Must be used cautiously, if at all, in penicillin-sensitive patients and use should be avoided in patients with a history of immediate and/or severe reactions to penicillin.

Administration: Intravenous and intramuscular.

Preparations: Vials, 500 mg, 1 and 10 g of cefonicid.

CEFOPERAZONE SODIUM—Cefobid®

Description/Actions: Highly active against many gram-negative bacteria and also effective against some gram-positive bacteria; spectrum of action includes *Pseudomonas aeruginosa.* Indicated for respiratory tract infections, peritonitis, and other intra-abdominal infections, septicemia, skin and skin-structure infections, urinary tract infections, and pelvic inflammatory disease and other female genital tract infections caused by susceptible organisms.

Precautions/Adverse Reactions: Must be used cautiously, if at all, in penicillin-sensitive patients, and use should be avoided in patients with a history of immediate and/or severe reactions to penicillin. Therapy in patients at risk of bleeding reactions must be closely monitored. Is excreted via biliary mechanisms to a greater extent than are other cephalosporins, and use is associated with a higher incidence of diarrhea. Disulfiram-like reactions may occur following the consumption of alcoholic beverages.

Administration: Intravenous and intramuscular.

Preparations: Vials, 1, 2, and 10 g of cefoperazone.

CEFOTAN®, see Cefotetan Disodium

CEFOTAXIME SODIUM—Claforan®

Description/Actions: Highly active against many gram-negative bacteria and also effective against some gram-positive bacteria. Indicated for lower respiratory tract infections, bacteremia/septicemia, skin and skin-structure infections, intra-abdominal infections, bone and/or joint infections, and central nervous system infections caused by susceptible organisms. May also be used for surgical prophylaxis.

Precautions/Adverse Reactions: Must be used cautiously, if at all, in penicillin-sensitive patients, and use should be avoided in patients with a history of immediate and/or severe reactions to penicillin.

Administration: Intravenous and intramuscular.

Preparations: Vials, 1, 2, and 20 g of cefotaxime.

CEFOTETAN DISODIUM—Cefotan®

Description/Actions: Active against many gram-positive and gram-negative bacteria; spectrum of action includes *Bacteroides fragilis*. Indicated for urinary tract infections, lower respiratory tract infections, skin and skin-structure infections, gynecologic infections, intra-abdominal infections, and bone and joint infections caused by susceptible organisms. May also be used for surgical prophylaxis.

Precautions/Adverse Reactions: Must be used cautiously, if at all, in penicillin-sensitive patients, and use should be avoided in patients with a history of immediate and/or severe reactions to penicillin. Disulfiram-like reactions may occur when alcohol is ingested within 72 hours of cefotetan administration. Prothrombin times should be monitored in patients at risk of bleeding reactions.

Administration: Intravenous and intramuscular.

Preparations: Vials, 1, 2, and 10 g of cefotetan activity.

CEFOXITIN SODIUM—Mefoxin®

Description/Actions: Second-generation cephalosporin antibiotic active against many gram-positive and gram-negative bacteria; spectrum of action includes *Bacteroides fragilis.* Indicated for lower respiratory tract infections, genitourinary infections, intra-abdominal infections, gynecological infections, septicemia, bone and joint infections, and skin and skin-structure infections caused by susceptible organisms. May also be used for surgical prophylaxis.

Precautions/Adverse Reactions: Must be used cautiously, if at all, in penicillin-sensitive patients, and use should be avoided in patients with a history of immediate and/or severe reactions to penicillins.

Administration: Intravenous and intramuscular.

Preparations: Vials, 1, 2, and 10 g of cefoxitin.

CEFPODOXIME PROXETIL—Vantin®

Description/Actions: Third-generation cephalosporin antibiotic. Is a prodrug that is converted to its active metabolite, cefpodoxime. Inhibits bacterial cell wall synthesis and exhibits a bactericidal action against many gram-positive and gram-negative bacteria. Indicated for upper respiratory tract infections, lower respiratory tract infections, uncomplicated skin and skin-structure infections, and uncomplicated urinary tract infections (cystitis) caused by susceptible organisms. Also indicated for acute, uncomplicated urethral and cervical gonorrhea, and acute, uncomplicated anorectal infections in women due to *Neisseria gonorrhoeae.*

Precautions/Adverse Reactions: Must be used cautiously in penicillin-sensitive patients, and use should be avoided in patients with a history of immediate and/or severe reactions to penicillin. Adverse reactions include diarrhea, nausea, abdominal pain, vomiting, vaginal fungal infections, rash, and headache. Absorption may be reduced by the concomitant administration of an antacid or histamine H_2-receptor antagonist.

Administration: Oral. Tablet formulation should be administered with food.

Preparations: Tablets, 100 and 200 mg. Powder for oral suspension, 50 mg/5 ml and 100 mg/5 ml.

CEFPROZIL—Cefzil®

Description/Actions: Second-generation cephalosporin antibiotic. Inhibits bacterial cell wall synthesis and exhibits a bactericidal action against many gram-positive and gram-negative bacteria. Indicated for upper respiratory tract infections (including pharyngitis and tonsilitis), lower respiratory tract infections, and uncomplicated skin and skin-structure infections caused by susceptible organisms.

Precautions/Adverse Reactions: Must be used cautiously in penicillin-sensitive patients, and use should be avoided in patients with a history of immediate and/or severe reactions to penicillins. Adverse reactions include diarrhea, nausea, vomiting, abdominal pain, rash, eosinophilia, vaginitis, and superinfection.

Administration: Oral.

Preparations: Tablets, 250 and 500 mg. Powder for oral suspension, 125 mg/5 ml and 250 mg/5 ml.

CEFTAZIDIME—Ceptaz®, Fortaz®, Tazicef®, Tazidime®

Description/Actions: Third-generation cephalosporin antibiotic. Highly active against many gram-negative bacteria and also effective against some gram-positive bacteria; spectrum of action includes *Pseudomonas aeruginosa.* Indicated for lower respiratory tract infections, skin and skin-structure infections, urinary tract infections, bacterial septicemia, bone and joint infections, gynecological infections, intra-abdominal infections, and central nervous system infections caused by susceptible organisms.

Precautions/Adverse Reactions: Must be used cautiously, if at all, in penicillin-sensitive patients, and use should be avoided in patients with a history of immediate and/or severe reactions to penicillin. Adverse reactions include hyperbilirubinemia, jaundice, renal impairment, urticaria, pain at injection site, anaphylaxis, and rare severe allergic reactions such as cardiopulmonary arrest. Myoclonia and coma have been reported in patients with renal insufficiency.

Administration: Intravenous and intramuscular.

Preparations: Vials, 500 mg, 1, 2, and 6 g.

CEFTIBUTEN—Cedax®

Description/Actions: Third-generation cephalosporin antibiotic. Indicated in susceptible mild to moderate acute bacterial exacerbations of chronic bronchitis, acute bacterial otitis media, and pharyngitis/tonsillitis.

Precautions/Adverse Reactions: May cause GI upset, headache, dizziness. Adjust dosing in renal impairment. Must be used cautiously in penicillin-sensitive patients, and use should be avoided in patients with a history of immediate and/or severe reactions to penicillin.

Administration: Oral. Suspension should be taken on an empty stomach. Capsules may be taken regardless of food intake.

Preparations: Capsules, 400 mg. Suspension, 90 mg/5 ml.

CEFTIN®, see Cefuroxime Axetil

CEFTIZOXIME SODIUM—Cefizox®

Description/Actions: Third-generation cephalosporin antibiotic. Highly active against many gram-negative bacteria and also effective against some gram-positive bacteria. Indicated for lower respiratory tract infections, urinary tract infections, gonorrhea, pelvic inflammatory disease, intra-abdominal infections, septicemia, skin and skin-structure infections, bone and joint infections, and meningitis caused by susceptible organisms.

Precautions/Adverse Reactions: Must be used cautiously, if at all, in penicillin-sensitive patients, and use should be avoided in patients with a history of immediate and/or severe reactions to penicillins.

Administration: Intravenous and intramuscular.

Preparations: Vials, 1, 2, and 10 g of ceftizoxime.

CEFTRIAXONE SODIUM—Rocephin®

Description/Actions: Third-generation cephalosporin antibiotic. Highly active against many gram-negative bacteria and also effective against some gram-positive bacteria. Indicated for lower respiratory tract infections, skin and skin-structure infections, urinary tract infections, gonorrhea, including pharyngeal gonorrhea, pelvic inflammatory disease, septicemia, bone and joint infections, intra-abdominal infections, and meningitis caused by susceptible organisms. May also be used for surgical prophylaxis.

Precautions/Adverse Reactions: Must be used cautiously, if at all, in penicillin-sensitive patients, and use should be avoided in patients with a history of immediate and/or severe reactions to penicillins.

Administration: Intravenous and intramuscular.

Preparations: Vials, 250 and 500 mg, 1, 2, and 10 g of ceftriaxone.

CEFUROXIME AXETIL—Ceftin®

Description/Actions: Second-generation cephalosporin antibiotic. Spectrum of action includes many gram-positive and gram-negative bacteria. Indicated in pharyngitis and tonsillitis, otitis media, lower respiratory tract infections, urinary tract infections, gonorrhea, and skin and skin-structure infections caused by susceptible organisms.

Precautions/Adverse Reactions: Must be used cautiously in penicillin-sensitive patients, and use should be avoided in patients with a history of immediate and/or severe reactions to penicillin.

Administration: Oral. Tablets may be administered without regard to meals, but the suspension should be administered with food.

Preparations: Tablets, 125, 250, and 500 mg. Powder for oral suspension, 125 mg/5 ml and 250 mg/5 ml.

CEFUROXIME SODIUM—Kefurox®, Zinacef®

Description/Actions: Second-generation cephalosporin antibiotic. Active against many gram-positive and gram-negative bacteria. Indicated for lower respiratory tract infections, urinary tract infections, skin and skin-structure infections, septicemia, bone and joint infections, meningitis, and gonorrhea caused by susceptible organisms. May also be used for surgical prophylaxis.

Precautions/Adverse Reactions: Must be used cautiously, if at all, in penicillin-sensitive patients, and use should be avoided in patients with a history of immediate and/or severe reactions to penicillins.

Administration: Intravenous and intramuscular.

Preparations: Vials, 750 mg, 1.5 and 7.5 g of cefuroxime.

CEFZIL®, see Cefprozil

CELECOXIB—Celebrex®

Description/Actions: An NSAID Cox-2 inhibitor indicated in the treatment of rheumatoid arthritis, osteoarthritis, management of acute pain, and treatment of primary dysmenorrhea.

Precautions/Adverse Reactions: Celecoxib is contraindicated in aspirin or sulfa allergy and the third trimester of pregnancy. Celebrex® may cause an increased risk of serious cardiovascular thrombotic events, myocardial infarction, and stroke, which can be fatal. All NSAIDs may have a similar risk. The risk may increase with duration of use. Patients with cardiovascular disease or risk factors for cardiovascular disease may be at greater risk. Celebrex® is contraindicated for the treatment of peri-operative pain in the setting of coronary artery bypass graft (CABG) surgery. NSAIDs, including Celebrex®, cause an increased risk of serious gastrointestinal adverse events including bleeding, ulceration, and perforation of the stomach or intestines, which can be fatal. These events can occur at any time during use and without warning symptoms. Elderly patients are at greater risk for serious gastrointestinal events. Use is not recommended in severe renal or hepatic impairment. Discontinue if liver impairment develops after initiation. Use cautiously in patients with the fluid retention, heart failure, hypertension, asthma, dehydration, debilitated, and the elderly. Monitor for GI ulcer/bleed. The risk of ulcer is increased if patient is otherwise at high risk, with extended drug treatment, high doses, history of GI bleed, or ulcer. Adverse reactions include GI upset, edema, pharyngitis, increase in liver tests (ALT/AST), and GI ulcer/bleed.

Administration: Oral.

Patient Care Implications: Instruct patients not to exceed dosing guidelines and not to independently increase the dose as this will increase the risk of serious adverse events. If pain relief is not achieved, call the doctor for other treatment options. If stomach discomfort is experienced, promptly call the doctor.

Preparations: Capsules, 100, 200, and 400 mg.

CELESTONE®, see Betamethasone

CELEXA®, see Citalopram Hydrobromide

CELLCEPT®, see Mycophenolate Mofetil.

CELONTIN®, see Methsuximide

CENESTIN®, see Estrogens, Conjugated

CENTRAX®, see Prazepam

CEPACOL®, see Cetylpyridinium

CEPHALEXIN—Cefanex®, Keflex®, Panixine DisperDose®

CEPHALEXIN HYDROCHLORIDE—Keftab®

Description/Actions: First-generation cephalosporin antibiotic. Spectrum of action includes many gram-positive and gram-negative bacteria. Indicated in respiratory tract infections, otitis media, skin and skin-structure infections, bone infections, and genitourinary tract infections caused by susceptible organisms.

Precautions/Adverse Reactions: Must be used cautiously in penicillin-sensitive patients and use should be avoided in patients with a history of immediate and/or severe reactions to penicillin.

Administration: Oral. May be administered without regard to meals.

Preparations: Capsules and tablets, 250 and 500 mg, 1 g. Powder for oral suspension, 125 and 250 mg/5 ml when reconstituted, and formulation for pediatric use, 100 mg/ml when reconstituted. Tablets for oral suspension, 125 and 250 mg.

CEPHALOTHIN SODIUM—Keflin®

Description/Actions: First-generation cephalosporin antibiotic indicated for the parenteral treatment of infections caused by susceptible organisms.

Preparations: Vials, 1, 2, 4, and 20 g.

CEPHAPIRIN SODIUM—Cefadyl®

Description/Actions: First-generation cephalosporin antibiotic indicated for the parenteral treatment of infections caused by susceptible organisms.

Preparations: Vials, 500 mg, 1, 2, 4, and 20 g.

CEPHRADINE—Anspor®, Velosef®

Description/Actions: First-generation cephalosporin antibiotic. Active against many gram-positive and gram-negative bacteria. Indicated for the oral treatment of respiratory tract infections, otitis media, skin and skin-structure infections, and urinary tract infections caused by susceptible organisms. May also be administered parenterally for these infections as well as for bone infections and septicemia caused by susceptible organisms. May be used parenterally for surgical prophylaxis.

Precautions/Adverse Reactions: Must be used cautiously, if at all, in penicillin-sensitive patients and use should be avoided in patients with a history of immediate and/or severe reactions to penicillins.

Administration: Oral, intravenous, and intramuscular. May be administered orally without regard to meals.

Preparations: Capsules, 250 and 500 mg. Powder for oral suspension, 125 and 250 mg/5 ml when reconstituted. Vials, 250 and 500 mg, 1, 2, and 4 g.

CEPHULAC®, see Lactulose

CEPTAZ®, see Ceftazidime

CEREBYX®, see Fosphenytoin

CEREDASE®, see Alglucerase

CEREZYME®, see Imiglucerase

CERUBIDINE®, see Daunorubicin

CETIRIZINE AND PSEUDOEPHEDRINE—Zyrtec-D 12 Hour™

Description/Actions: Zyrtec-D 12 Hour™ is indicated for the relief of nasal and nonnasal symptoms associated with seasonal or perennial allergic rhinitis in adults and children 12 years of age and older.

Precautions/Adverse Reactions: Zyrtec-D 12 Hour™ is contraindicated in patients with narrow-angle glaucoma or urinary retention, and in patients receiving monoamine oxidase inhibitor (MAOI) therapy or within 14 days of stopping therapy. Also contraindicated in patients with severe hypertension or severe coronary artery disease and in those who have shown hypersensitivity or idiosyncrasy to its components, to adrenergic agents, or to other drugs of similar chemical structure. Manifestations of patient idiosyncrasy to adrenergic agents include insomnia, dizziness, weakness, tremor, and arrhythmias. Pseudoephedrine produces peripheral effects similar to those of ephedrine and central effects similar to, but less intense than, amphetamines. It has the potential for excitatory side effects. Sympathomimetic amines should be used judiciously and sparingly in patients with hypertension, diabetes mellitus, ischemic heart disease, increased intraocular pressure, hyperthyroidism, renal impairment, or prostatic hypertrophy. Use with caution in patients older than 60 years of age; there is a decrease in cetirizine clearance that may be related to decreased renal function. The elderly are more likely to experience side effects. In general, dosing in the elderly should be cautious, because of the greater frequency of decreased hepatic, renal, or cardiac function, and of concomitant disease or other drug therapy. Zyrtec-D 12 Hour™ is not recommended in patients <12 years. Most common adverse reactions were somnolence, headache, fatigue, and dry mouth. Pregnancy Category C. No adequate, well-controlled studies in pregnant women. Use only if benefit justifies potential risk to fetus. Both cetirizine and pseudoephedrine are excreted in milk; use in nursing mothers is not recommended.

Administration: Oral.

Patient Care Implications: May be taken with or without food. Because of somnolence, caution should be exercised when driving a car or operating potentially dangerous machinery. Concurrent use with alcohol or other CNS depressants should be avoided because of additional decrease in alertness and additional impairment of CNS performance that may occur. Tablet should be swallowed whole; do not break, crush, or chew.

Preparations: Tablet, extended release: cetirizine hydrochloride, 5 mg, and pseudoephedrine hydrochloride, 120 mg.

CETIRIZINE HYDROCHLORIDE—Zyrtec®

Description/Actions: Antihistamine indicated for the treatment of seasonal rhinitis, for the relief of symptoms associated with perennial allergic rhinitis in adults and children 6 months of age and older, and for the treatment of the uncomplicated skin manifestations of chronic idiopathic urticaria in adults and children 6 months of age or older.

Precautions/Adverse Reactions: Contraindicated in hydroxyzine sensitivity. Use cautiously in hepatic or renal dysfunction. Use by nursing mothers is not recommended. Potentiates CNS depression with alcohol and other CNS depressants. Adverse reactions include somnolence, fatigue, dry mouth, and dizziness.

Administration: Oral.

Preparations: Tablets, 5 and 10 mg, syrup 1 mg/ml. Chewable tablets, 5 mg and 10 mg.

CETRORELIX ACETATE—Cetrotide®

Description/Actions: Indicated for the inhibition of premature LH surges in women undergoing controlled ovarian stimulation. The extent and duration of LH inhibition is dose dependent. Effects are reversible upon discontinuation of cetrorelix.

Precautions/Adverse Reactions: Contraindicated in patients with a known hypersensitivity to cetrorelix acetate, extrinsic peptide hormone, or mannitol. Known hypersensitivity to Gn-RH or any other Gn-RH analogs. Contraindicated in pregnancy and lactation. Caution is advised when administered to patients with a hypersensitivity to Gn-RH. Carefully monitor patients after the first injection. A severe anaphylactic reaction was observed in one patient after 7 months of treatment with cetrorelix for an indication other than infertility. Should only be prescribed by fertility specialists. No formal drug interaction studies have been performed. Pregnancy Category X. Cetrorelix is contraindicated in pregnant women. Animal studies have shown fetal resorption and loss of implantation. These results would also be expected in pregnant women. Excretion in human breast milk is unknown; therefore, cetrorelix should not be used by nursing mothers. Adverse reactions occurring in ≥1% of patients include ovarian hyperstimulation syndrome (3.5%), nausea, headache, increased alkaline phosphatase, and increased liver enzymes. Local site reactions such as redness, erythema, bruising, itching, swelling, and pruritis have been reported; however, they were usually mild and transient. Congenital anomalies and stillbirths have been reported.

Administration: SQ injection.

Patient Care Implications: Instruct patient and or caregiver on the proper administration of cetrorelix. Store drug in refrigerator.

Preparations: Injection: 0.25 mg vial and 3 mg vial each with one prefilled glass syringe, sterile water for injection, one 20 gauge needle, one 27 gauge needle, and two alcohol pads.

CETYLPYRIDINIUM CHLORIDE—Cepacol®

Description/Actions: Antiseptic included in formulations used in minor sore throat and in conditions in which there is minor irritation of the mouth or throat.

Preparations: Lozenges, 0.07%. Mouthwash, 0.05%.

CEVIMELINE HYDROCHLORIDE—Evoxac®

Description/Actions: Cholinergic agonist indicated in the treatment of symptoms of dry mouth in patients with Sjogren's syndrome.

Precautions/Adverse Reactions: Cevimeline is contraindicated in patients with uncontrolled asthma, known hypersensitivity to cevimeline, and when miosis is undesirable (e.g., in acute iritis and in narrow-angle glaucoma). Cevimeline should be used with caution in patients with cardiovascular disease, controlled asthma, chronic bronchitis, chronic obstructive pulmonary disease, or a history of nephrolithiasis or cholelithiasis. Caution should be advised while driving at night or performing hazardous activities in reduced lighting. Adverse effects include excessive sweating, nausea, rhinitis, diarrhea, excessive salivation, urinary tract infection, asthenia, flushing, and polyuria.

Administration: Oral.

Preparations: Capsules, 30 mg.

CHARCOAL, ACTIVATED

Description/Actions: Adsorbent used for relief of intestinal gas, diarrhea, and GI distress. Also used as an antidote in the treatment of poisoning by many drugs and chemicals.

Preparations: Capsules, 260 mg. Liquid. Powder.

CHEMET®, see Succimer

CHIBROXIN®, see Norfloxacin

CHILDREN'S ADVIL®—see Ibuprofen

CHILDREN'S MOTRIN®—see Ibuprofen

CHLORAL HYDRATE

Description/Actions: Sedative-hypnotic used in the treatment of insomnia and as an anesthetic adjunct for reduction of anxiety preoperatively.

Preparations: Capsules, 250 and 500 mg. Syrup, 500 mg/5 ml. Suppositories, 324, 500, and 648 mg.

CHLORAMBUCIL—Leukeran®

Description/Actions: Antineoplastic agent indicated in the treatment of chronic lymphocytic leukemia, malignant lymphomas, including lymphosarcoma, giant follicular lymphoma, and Hodgkin's disease.

Preparations: Tablets, 2 mg.

CHLORAMPHENICOL—Chloromycetin®

Description/Actions: Antibiotic with a broad spectrum of activity that has been used in the treatment of systemic, dermatologic, ophthalmic, and otic infections. Is of greatest value in systemic infections caused by *Salmonella typhi, Haemophilus influenzae* (e.g., meningitis), and rickettsial organisms.

Preparations: Vials (as the sodium succinate), 1 g. Ophthalmic solution (0.5%), and ointment (1%). Otic solution, 0.5%.

CHLORDIAZEPOXIDE—Librium®, Libritabs®

Description/Actions: Benzodiazepine indicated for the management of anxiety disorders or for the short-term relief of symptoms of anxiety, withdrawal symptoms of acute alcoholism, and preoperative apprehension and anxiety.

Precautions/Adverse Reactions: Adverse reactions include drowsiness and other CNS effects; patients should be cautioned regarding activities such as driving and operating machinery, as well as interactions with other CNS-acting drugs including alcohol. Can cause dependence and is included in Schedule IV.

Administration: Oral, intravenous, and intramuscular.

Preparations: Capsules (as the hydrochloride) and tablets, 5, 10, and 25 mg. Ampules (as the hydrochloride), 100 mg.

CHLORESIUM®, see Chlorophyll

CHLORHEXIDINE GLUCONATE—Hibiclens®, Hibistat®, Peridex®

Description/Actions: Antiseptic and cleanser indicated for topical use as a skin wound cleanser and general skin cleanser, as a surgical scrub, for patient preoperative showering and bathing, as a patient preoperative skin preparation, and as a health care personnel handwash or germicidal hand rinse. Also used as an oral rinse (Peridex®) for the treatment of gingivitis.

Preparations: Skin cleanser, 4%. Germicidal hand rinse, 0.5%. Oral rinse, 0.12%.

CHLORMEZANONE—Trancopal®

Description/Actions: Antianxiety agent indicated for the treatment of mild anxiety and tension states.

Preparations: Tablets, 100 and 200 mg.

CHLOROMYCETIN®, see Chloramphenicol

CHLOROPHYLL—Chloresium®, Derifil®

Description/Actions: Deodorizing agent used topically to reduce malodors in wounds, burns, and other dermatologic conditions, and orally for the control of fecal and urinary odor associated with incontinence and ostomy conditions, body odors, and odor of surface lesions.

Preparations: Solution, 0.2%. Ointment, 0.5%. Tablets, 100 mg.

CHLOROPROCAINE HYDROCHLORIDE—Nesacaine®, Nesacaine-CE®

Description/Actions: Local anesthetic indicated for the production of local anesthesia by infiltration and peripheral nerve block. Formulation without preservatives (Nesacaine-CE®) may also be used by central nerve block, including lumbar and caudal epidural blocks.

Preparations: Vials, 1% and 2%. Vials (Nesacaine-CE), 2% and 3%.

CHLOROQUINE—Aralen®

Description/Actions: Antimalarial agent and amebicide. Indicated for acute attacks of malaria and prophylaxis against malaria. Also indicated for the treatment of extraintestinal amebiasis.

Preparations: Tablets (as the phosphate), 500 mg. Vials (as the dihydrochloride), 50 mg/ml.

CHLOROTHIAZIDE—Diuril®

Description/Actions: Thiazide diuretic indicated as adjunctive therapy in edema and in the management of hypertension.

Preparations: Tablets, 250 and 500 mg. Suspension, 250 mg/5 ml.

CHLOROTRIANISENE—Tace®

Description/Actions: Estrogen indicated for the treatment of postpartum breast engorgement, moderate to severe vasomotor symptoms associated with the menopause, atrophic vaginitis, kraurosis vulvae, and female hypogonadism. Also used as palliative therapy of advanced prostatic carcinoma.

Preparations: Capsules, 12, 25, and 72 mg.

CHLORPHENESIN CARBAMATE—Maolate®

Description/Actions: Skeletal muscle relaxant indicated as an adjunct to rest, physical therapy, and other measures for relief of discomfort associated with acute, painful musculoskeletal conditions.

Preparations: Tablets, 400 mg.

CHLORPHENIRAMINE MALEATE—Chlor-Trimeton®, Teldrin®

Description/Actions: Antihistamine indicated in the treatment of various allergic disorders.

Precautions/Adverse Reactions: Adverse effects include drowsiness and other CNS effects; patients should be cautioned regarding activities such as driving and operating machinery, as well as interactions with other CNS-acting drugs including alcohol.

Administration: Oral, intravenous, intramuscular, and subcutaneous.

Preparations: Tablets, 2 and 4 mg. Controlled-release tablets and capsules, 8 and 12 mg. Syrup, 2 mg/5 ml. Vials, 10 mg/ml.

CHLORPROMAZINE—Thorazine®

Description/Actions: Phenothiazine antipsychotic and antiemetic agent. Indicated in the management of psychotic disorders, to control nausea and vomiting, as a preoperative medication, as an adjunct in the treatment of tetanus, for relief of intractable hiccups, to control the manifestations of the manic type of manic-depressive illness, and for acute intermittent porphyria. Also indicated for the treatment of certain severe behavioral problems in children, and in the short-term treatment of certain hyperactive children.

Preparations: Tablets, 10, 25, 50, 100, and 200 mg. Controlled-release capsules, 30, 75, 150, 200, and 300 mg. Syrup (as the hydrochloride), 10 mg/5 ml. Oral concentrate (as the hydrochloride), 30 and 100 mg/ml. Suppositories, 25 and 100 mg. Ampules and vials (as the hydrochloride), 25 mg/ml.

CHLORPROPAMIDE—Diabinese®

Description/Actions: Sulfonylurea hypoglycemic agent indicated as an adjunct to diet to lower the blood glucose in patients with noninsulin-dependent diabetes mellitus whose hyperglycemia cannot be controlled by diet alone.

Precautions/Adverse Reactions: May cause hypoglycemia and patients should be advised to contact their physician if symptoms of hypoglycemia develop.

Adverse reactions include nausea, vomiting, diarrhea, pruritus, and rash. Oral hypoglycemic agents have been suggested to be associated with increased cardiovascular mortality as compared with treatment by diet alone or diet plus insulin. May cause disulfiram-like reactions following the consumption of alcoholic beverages. Therapy in patients also receiving a beta-adrenergic-blocking agent should be monitored closely.

Administration: Oral.

Preparations: Tablets, 100 and 250 mg.

CHLORPROTHIXENE

Description/Actions: Antipsychotic agent indicated for the management of manifestations of psychotic disorders.

Preparations: Tablets, 10, 25, 50, and 100 mg. Oral concentrate (as the lactate and hydrochloride), 100 mg chlorprothixene/5 ml. Ampules (as the hydrochloride), 25 mg chlorprothixene/2 ml.

CHLORTETRACYCLINE—Aureomycin®

Description/Actions: Tetracycline antibiotic used in the treatment of dermatologic and ocular infections.

Preparations: Ointment, 3%.

CHLORTHALIDONE—Hygroton®

Description/Actions: Action is similar to that of the thiazide diuretics. Indicated in the management of hypertension, and as adjunctive therapy in edema associated with congestive heart failure, hepatic cirrhosis, and corticosteroid and estrogen therapy. Is also useful in edema due to various forms of renal dysfunction such as nephrotic syndrome.

Precautions/Adverse Reactions: May cause hypokalemia, and serum potassium levels should be determined periodically. Concurrent use with lithium is best avoided because of an increased risk of lithium toxicity. May cause hyperglycemia and hyperuricemia, and therapy in patients having diabetes or gout should be closely monitored.

Administration: Oral.

Preparations: Tablets, 25, 50, and 100 mg.

CHLOR-TRIMETON®, see Chlorpheniramine

CHLORZOXAZONE—Paraflex®, Parafon Forte DSC®

Description/Actions: Skeletal muscle relaxant indicated as an adjunct to rest, physical therapy, and other measures for the relief of discomfort associated with acute, painful skeletal muscle conditions.

Preparations: Tablets, 250 mg.

CHOLECALCIFEROL—Vitamin D3

Description/Actions: A form of vitamin D used as a supplement to treat or prevent vitamin D deficiency.

Preparations: Tablets 400 and 1000 IU.

CHOLEDYL®, see Oxtriphylline

CHOLESTYRAMINE—Questran®, Questran Light®

Description/Actions: Antihyperlipidemic agent indicated as adjunctive therapy to diet for the reduction of elevated serum cholesterol in patients with primary hypercholesterolemia. Also indicated for the relief of pruritus associated with partial biliary obstruction.

Preparations: Powder and packets, 4 g/9 g of powder. (Questran). Powder and packets, 4 g/5 g of powder (Questran Light with aspartame). Chewable bar, 4 g.

CHOLINE MAGNESIUM TRISALICYLATE—Trilisate®

Description/Actions: Salicylate analgesic/anti-inflammatory agent indicated in the treatment of rheumatoid arthritis, osteoarthritis, and acute painful shoulder.

Preparations: Tablets, 500 and 750 mg, 1 g of salicylate. Liquid, 500 mg salicylate/5 ml.

CHOLINE SALICYLATE—Arthropan®

Description/Actions: Salicylate analgesic/anti-inflammatory agent used in the treatment of conditions associated with mild to moderate pain and/or inflammation.

Preparations: Liquid, 870 mg/5 ml.

CHOLINE THEOPHYLLINATE, see Oxtriphylline

CHOLOXIN®, see Dextrothyroxine

CHORIONIC GONADOTROPIN—A.P.L.®, Follutein®

Description/Actions: Hormone indicated for intramuscular use for cryptorchidism not due to anatomic obstruction, selected cases of male hypogonadism secondary to pituitary failure, and induction of ovulation and pregnancy in the anovulatory, infertile woman in selected situations.

Preparations: Vials, 5000, 10,000, and 20,000 units.

CHYMODIACTIN®, see Chymopapain

CHYMOPAPAIN—Chymodiactin®

Description/Actions: Proteolytic enzyme indicated for intradiscal injection for the treatment of documented herniated lumbar intervertebral discs in patients whose symptoms and signs have not responded to adequate periods of conservative therapy.

Preparations: Vials, 4000 units.

CICLOPIROX—Penlac Nail Lacquer®

Description/Actions: Synthetic antifungal agent intended for topical use on fingernails, toenails, and immediately adjacent skin.

Precautions/Adverse Reactions: Penlac nail lacquer is contraindicated in individuals who have shown hypersensitivity to any of its components. Adverse reactions include periungual erythema of the proximal nail fold, nail shape change, nail irritation, ingrown toenail, and nail discoloration.

Administration: Topical.

Patient Care Implications: If reactions suggesting sensitivity or chemical irritation should occur with the use of Penlac Nail Lacquer, treatment should be discontinued and appropriate therapy instituted.

Preparations: Topical solution, 8%, 6.6 ml.

CICLOPIROX OLAMINE—Loprox®

Description/Actions: Antifungal agent indicated for the topical treatment of tinea pedis, tinea cruris, tinea corporis, candidiasis, and tinea versicolor.

Preparations: Cream, lotion, and shampoo, 1%.

CIDOFOVIR—Vistide®

Description/Actions: Nucleoside analogue indicated in the treatment of cytomegalovirus (CMV) retinitis in patients with AIDS.

Precautions/Adverse Reactions: Not recommended for use in patients with CrCl of <55 ml/min. Contraindicated in severe sulfa or probenecid allergy and within 7 days of discontinuing other nephrotoxic agents (e.g., aminoglycosides, foscarnet, IV pentamidine, NSAIDs, vancomycin). Do not exceed recommended dose as this may increase the risk of nephrotoxicity. Women should use effective contraception during and

1 month after therapy. Men should use barrier contraception during and 3 months after therapy. Monitor serum creatinine, urine protein, WBC, with differential before each dose; monitor intraocular pressure, visual acuity, and ocular symptoms periodically. Use cautiously in the elderly. Adverse reactions include elevated serum creatinine, proteinuria, neutropenia, ocular hypotony, metabolic acidosis, GI disturbances, fever, asthenia, rash, headache, alopecia, infection, chills, and dyspnea. Contraindicated in severe probenecid or other sulfa allergy. Not for intraocular injection.

Administration: Intravenous. Pretreat with oral probenecid and hydrate with normal saline as per manufacturer's guidelines.

Preparations: Solution for IV infusion after dilution, 75 mg/5 ml.

CILOSTAZOL—Pletal®

Description/Actions: Cilostazol is a quinolone derivative that is indicated in treatment of intermittent claudication. The medication preferentially enhances blood flow to the femoral arteries with a subsequent improvement in the patient's ability to walk distances.

Precautions/Adverse Reactions: In clinical trials, other PDE III inhibitors have caused a decreased survival compared to placebo in patients with class III-IV heart failure, so this product is contraindicated in CHF of any severity. Use cautiously in patients with severe underlying heart disease and moderate to severe hepatic dysfunction. Pregnancy Category C. Use not recommended in nursing mothers. Adverse reactions include headache, diarrhea, abnormal stools, palpitations, peripheral edema, dizziness, and tachycardia.

Administration: Oral. Take ½ hour before or 2 hours after breakfast and dinner.

Patient Care Implications: Instruct patients to avoid grapefruit juice. Take on an empty stomach. Instruct patients in the signs and symptoms of heart failure and to promptly report these symptoms to the prescriber. Patients should use this medication in combination with an exercise regimen of walking as prescribed by their health care provider.

Preparations: Tablets, 50 and 100 mg.

CILOXAN®, see Ciprofloxacin

CIMETIDINE—Tagamet®, Tagamet HB®

Description/Actions: A histamine H_2 receptor antagonist that inhibits gastric acid secretion. Indicated in (a) short-term treatment of active duodenal ulcer, (b) maintenance therapy for duodenal ulcer patients at reduced dosage after healing of active ulcer, (c) short-term treatment of active benign gastric ulcer, (d) the treatment of erosive gastroesophageal reflux disease, (e) the treatment of pathological hypersecretory conditions (e.g., Zollinger-Ellison syndrome), and (f) the prevention of upper gastrointestiinal bleeding in critically ill patients. Available without a prescription (Tagamet HB®) to relieve heartburn and acid indigestion.

Precautions/Adverse Reactions: Adverse reactions include diarrhea, rash, dizziness, somnolence, and confusional states. Has a weak antiandrogenic effect and has caused gynecomastia and impotence, particularly when used in high doses and/or for long periods.

Administration: Oral, intravenous, and intramuscular.

Preparations: Tablets, 100 (Tagamet HB®) 200, 300, 400, and 800 mg. Liquid (as the hydrochloride), 300 mg/5 ml. Vials and syringes (as the hydrochloride), 300 mg/2 ml. Plastic containers, 300 mg/50 ml.

CIPRO®, see Ciprofloxacin

CIPRO HC OTIC®—Combination Agent Ciprofloxacin and Hydrocortisone (Quinolone Antibiotic and Steroid)

CIPRO IV®, see Ciprofloxacin

CIPRO XR®, see Ciprofloxacin

CIPROFLOXACIN HYDROCHLORIDE—Ciloxan®, Cipro®, Cipro IV®, Cipro XR®

Description/Actions: A fluoroquinolone antibacterial agent with a broad spectrum of action. Indicated for lower respiratory tract, urinary tract, skin and skin-structure, and bone and joint infections, urethral/cervical gonococcal infections, typhoid fever, infectious diarrhea, complicated intra-abdominal infections (used with metranidazole), and ocular infections caused by susceptible bacteria. IV form is indicated in empicic therapy of febrile neutropenia and nosocomial pneumonia.

Precautions/Adverse Reactions: Contraindicated in patients with a known hypersensitivity to the drug and is also best avoided in patients with a history of hypersensitivity to other fluoroquinolone/quinolone derivatives. It should not be used in children or pregnant women because it and related drugs have been shown to cause arthropathy and damage to the weight-bearing joints in immature animals. Adverse reactions include nausea, vomiting, diarrhea, abdominal discomfort, headache, dizziness, restlessness, and rash. Because the drug may cause CNS effects, patients should be cautioned about engaging in activities that require mental alertness and coordination, and the drug should be used cautiously in patients with epilepsy or other CNS disorders. Concurrent use of ciprofloxacin and theophylline has resulted in elevated plasma concentrations of theophylline and a corresponding increase in the risk of adverse effects with this agent.

Administration: Oral, intravenous, and ophthalmic.

Preparations: Tablets, 250, 500, and 750 mg. Extended release tablets, 500 and 1000 mg. Oral suspension, 5% (250 mg/5 ml) and 10% (500 mg/5 ml) microcapsules for suspension after reconstitution in strawberry flavor. Vials, 200 and 400 mg. Ophthalmic solution, 0.3% (Ciloxan).

CISPLATIN—Platinol®

Description/Actions: Antineoplastic agent indicated for intravenous use as palliative therapy for metastatic testicular tumors, metastatic ovarian tumors, and advanced bladder cancer.

Preparations: Vials, 10 and 50 mg.

CITALOPRAM HYDROBROMIDE—Celexa®

Description/Actions: An antidepressant in the SSRI category. Indicated in the treatment of depression, obsessive-compulsive disorder, panic disorder, chronic schizophrenia (adjuvant treatment), and dementia.

Precautions/Adverse Reactions: Use is contraindicated within 14 days of use of MAOIs. Risk of serotonin syndrome when used in combination with linezolid. Increased risk of bleeding when used in combination with NSAIDs, aspirin, or other drugs that affect coagulation. Use cautiously in patients with a history of seizures or mania/hypomania, hepatic, or severe renal impairment, recent MI, or unstable heart disease. Antidepressants increased the risk of suicidal thinking and behavior (suicidality) in short-term studies in children and adolescents with Major Depressive Disorder (MDD) and other psychiatric disorders. Anyone considering the use of citalopram or any other antidepressant in a child or adolescent must balance this risk with the clinical need. Patients who are started on therapy should be observed closely for clinical worsening, suicidality, or unusual changes in behavior. Celexa® is not approved for use in pediatric patients. Reevaluate use frequently for patients with suicidal tendencies or undergoing ECT. Pregnancy Category C. Use in children and nursing mothers not recommended. Adverse reactions include GI upset, dry mouth, somnolence, insomnia, increased sweating, anorexia, rhinitis, sexual dysfunction, agitation, fatigue, arthralgia, myalgia, hyponatremia, and SIADH.

Administration: Oral.

Patient Care Implications: Monitor mood changes and notify therapist if patient demonstrates signifcant increase in anxiety, nervousness, or insomnia. Assess for suicidal tendencies, especially during early therapy. Restrict the amount of drug available to patient.

Preparations: Scored tablets, 10, 20, and 40 mg. Oral solution, 10 mg/5 mL.

CITANEST®, see Prilocaine

CITRATE OF MAGNESIA, see Magnesium Citrate

CITROVORUM FACTOR, see Leucovorin Calcium

CITRUCEL®, see Methylcellulose

CLADRIBINE—Leustatin®

Description/Actions: Antineoplastic agent. Also known as 2-chlorode-oxyadenosine or 2-CdA, it crosses lymphocyte cell membranes and is metabolized to a triphosphate derivative that disrupts cell metabolism and is cytotoxic to both actively dividing and resting cells. Indicated for the treatment of active hairy cell leukemia.

Precautions/Adverse Reactions: May cause myelosuppression (neutropenia, thrombocytopenia, anemia), and peripheral blood counts should be performed, particularly during the first 4–8 weeks following initiation of therapy. Caution should be exercised if cladribine is to be administered in conjunction with or following other drugs known to cause myelosuppression. Fever is often experienced (most often in neutropenic patients), and infection may develop; empiric antibiotic therapy should be initiated as necessary. Other adverse reactions include nausea, decreased appetite, vomiting, diarrhea, abnormal breath sounds, cough, fatigue, headache, injection site reactions, purpura, and rash. Women of childbearing age should be advised to avoid becoming pregnant.

Administration: Intravenous.

Preparations: Vials, 10 mg (1 mg/ml).

CLAFORAN®, see Cefotaxime Sodium

CLARINEX®, see Desloratadine

CLARINEX-D® 24-HOUR, extended release, see Desloratadine and Pseudoephedrine

CLARITHROMYCIN—Biaxin®

Description/Actions: Macrolide antibiotic. Is converted, in part, to an active metabolite, 14-hydroxyclarithromycin. Inhibits protein synthesis, and its spectrum of action includes many gram-positive and gram-negative bacteria, as well as organisms such as *Mycoplasma pneumoniae.* Indicated for upper respiratory tract infections, lower respiratory tract infections, and uncomplicated skin and skin structure infections caused by susceptible organisms. Is also used in combination with other agents for the treatment of disseminated infection due to *Mycobacterium avium* complex and in treatment of active duodenal ulcer associated with *H. pylori* infection in combination with omeprazole.

Precautions/Adverse Reactions: Contraindicated in patients with a known hypersensitivity to any of the macrolide antibiotics. Prescribers should review drug profiles to avoid interaction with contraindicated drugs. Adverse reactions include diarrhea, nausea, abnormal taste, dyspepsia, abdominal pain or discomfort, and headache. Should not be used in pregnant women unless no alternative therapy is appropriate. Concurrent use with terfenadine should be avoided. May increase serum concentrations of theophylline, carbamazepine, and other drugs that are metabolized via liver enzyme systems; concurrent therapy should be closely monitored.

Administration: Oral.

Preparations: Tablets, 250 and 500 mg. Granules for oral suspension, 125 mg/5 ml and 250 mg/5 ml when reconstituted.

CLARITHROMYCIN EXTENDED RELEASE—Biaxin XL®

Description/Actions: Macrolide antibiotic in an extended release formulation.

Precautions/Adverse Reactions: Contraindicated in patients with a known hypersensitivity to any of the macrolide antibiotics. Adverse reactions include diarrhea, nausea, abnormal taste, dyspepsia, abdominal pain or discomfort, and headache. Should not be used in pregnant women unless no alternative therapy is appropriate. Concurrent use with terfenadine should be avoided. May increase serum concentrations of theophylline, carbamazepine, and other drugs that are metabolized via liver enzyme systems; concurrent therapy should be closely monitored. Concurrent use with terfenadine, pimozide, cisapride, and astemizole should be avoided.

Administration: Oral.

Preparations: Extended-release tablet, 500 mg.

CLARITIN®, see Loratadine

CLARITIN-D®, Combination of Loratidine and Pseudoephedrine

CLEMASTINE FUMARATE—Tavist®

Description/Actions: Antihistamine indicated for the relief of symptoms associated with allergic rhinitis, and for the relief of mild, uncomplicated allergic skin manifestations of urticaria and angioedema.

Precautions/Adverse Reactions: Contraindicated in nursing mothers and in patients being treated with a monoamine oxidase inhibitor. Should not be used to treat lower respiratory tract symptoms including asthma. Adverse reactions include drowsiness and other CNS effects; patients should be cautioned regarding activities such as driving and operating machinery, as well as interactions with other CNS-acting drugs including alcohol. Exhibits anticholinergic activity and must be used with caution in patients with conditions such as narrow- angle glaucoma.

Administration: Oral.

Preparations: Tablets, 1.34 and 2.68 mg. Syrup, 0.67 mg/5 ml.

CLEOCIN®, see Clindamycin

CLIDINIUM BROMIDE—Quarzan®

Description/Actions: Anticholinergic agent indicated as adjunctive therapy in peptic ulcer disease.

Preparations: Capsules, 2.5 and 5 mg.

CLIMARA®, see Estradiol

CLIMARA PRO®, see Estradiol/Levonorgestrel

CLINDAMYCIN—Cleocin®, Cleocin T®, Evoclin®

Description/Actions: Antibiotic indicated for the treatment of infections caused by susceptible anaerobic bacteria including *Bacteroides fragilis,* and for the treatment of infections caused by susceptible gram-positive cocci. Topical solution, gel, and lotion formulations are indicated in the treatment of acne. Vaginal cream is indicated in the treatment of bacterial vaginosis.

Preparations: Capsules (as the hydrochloride), 75, 150, and 300 mg. For oral solution (as the palmitate), 75 mg clindamycin/5 ml. Ampules and vials (as the phosphate), 150 mg clindamycin/ml. Topical solution, gel, and lotion (as the phosphate), 1%. Vaginal cream, 2%. Foam, 50 g and 100 g cans (as the phosphate), 1%.

CLINDAMYCIN AND BENZOYL PEROXIDE—Duac™

Description/Actions: Duac™ is a topical skin product used for the treatment of acne vulgaris.

Precautions/Adverse Reactions: Duac™ topical gel is contraindicated in individuals who have shown hypersensitivity to benzoyl peroxide, lincomycin, clindamycin, or any component of the formulation. Also contraindicated in individuals with a history of regional enteritis, ulcerative colitis, pseudomembranous colitis, or antibiotic-associated colitis; or with concurrent use of erythromycin and clindamycin. Most common adverse reactions were erythema, peeling, and dry skin. Pregnancy Category C.

Administration: Topically.

Patient Care Implications: Skin should be clean and dry before applying. Avoid applying to inside of nose, mouth, eyes, and mucous membrane. Duac™ may bleach hair or colored fabrics. Protect skin from sun.

Preparations: Gel, topical: clindamycin 1% and benzoyl peroxide 5%.

CLINORIL®, see Sulindac

CLIOQUINOL—Lodochlorhydroxyquin, Vioform®

Description/Actions: Anti-infective agent used in the topical management of inflamed conditions of the skin (e.g., eczema, athlete's foot).

Preparations: Cream and ointment, 3%.

CLOBETASOL PROPIONATE—Olux™, Temovate®

Description/Actions: Topical corticosteroid indicated for the short-term treatment of inflammatory and pruritic manifestations of moderate to severe corticosteroid-responsive dermatoses.

Precautions/Adverse Reactions: Is highly potent and is more likely than less potent analogs to cause systemic effects, including suppression of the hypothalamic-pituitary-adrenal (HPA) axis. Treatment period should be limited to 2 weeks, and not more than 50 g of the cream or ointment should be used per week. Occlusive dressings should not be used.

Administration: Topical.

Preparations: Cream and ointment, 0.05% topical (scalp) foam.

CLOFAZIMINE—Lamprene®

Description/Actions: Antileprosy agent that exerts a slow bactericidal effect on *Mycobacterium leprae*. Indicated in the treatment of lepromatous leprosy, including dapsone-resistant lepromatous leprosy and lepromatous leprosy complicated by erythema nodosum leprosum.

Precautions/Adverse Reactions: The drug is a dye and will cause pink to brownish-black pigmentation of the skin within a few weeks of treatment. It will also cause discoloration of the conjunctivae, lacrimal fluid, sweat, sputum, urine, and feces. Other dermatologic reactions include ichthyosis, dryness, rash, and pruritus; the application of oil to the skin may help alleviate some of these effects. Many patients experience adverse gastrointestinal effects, such as abdominal and epigastric pain, diarrhea, nausea, vomiting, and gastrointestinal intolerance. Taking the medication with meals may reduce the occurrence of these effects. There have been rare reports of bowel obstruction, gastrointestinal bleeding, and splenic infarction.

Administration: Oral.

Preparations: Capsules, 50 and 100 mg.

CLOFIBRATE—Atromid-S®

Description/Actions: Antihyperlipidemic agent indicated for primary dysbetalipoproteinemia (type III hyperlipidemia) that does not respond adequately to diet. May be considered for the treatment of selected patients with very high serum triglyceride levels (types IV and V).

Preparations: Capsules, 500 mg.

CLOMID®, see Clomiphene

CLOMIPHENE CITRATE—Clomid®, Milophene®, Serophene®

Description/Actions: Ovulation stimulant indicated for the treatment of ovulatory dysfunction in patients desiring pregnancy, and whose partners are fertile and potent. Unlabeled uses include male infertility, menstrual abnormalities, gynecomastia, fibrocystic breast disease, regulation of cycles in patients using rhythm methods of contraception, endometrial hyperplasia, and persistent lactation.

Preparations: Tablets, 50 mg.

CLOMIPRAMINE HYDROCHLORIDE—Anafranil®

Description/Actions: A tricyclic antidepressant that acts primarily by inhibiting the reuptake of serotonin. Indicated for the treatment of obsessions and compulsions in patients with obsessive compulsive disorder.

Precautions/Adverse Reactions: Should not be given in combination, or within 14 days of treatment with a monoamine oxidase inhibitor. Is also contraindicated during the acute recovery period after a myocardial infarction. Adverse reactions include CNS effects, and patients should be cautioned regarding activities such as driving and operating machinery, as well as interactions with other CNS-acting drugs including alcohol. Other adverse reactions include dry mouth, blurred vision, nausea, dyspepsia, increased appetite, weight gain, sweating, orthostatic hypotension, and sexual dysfunction.

Administration: Oral. During the initial titration, clomipramine should be given in divided doses with meals to reduce gastrointestinal side effects. After titration, the total daily dose may be given once daily at bedtime to minimize daytime sedation.

Preparations: Capsules, 25, 50, and 75 mg.

CLONAZEPAM—Klonopin®

Description/Actions: Benzodiazepine anticonvulsant indicated in the treatment of the Lennox-Gastaut syndrome (petit mal variant), akinetic and myoclonic seizures, and panic disorder. May also be useful in absence seizures (petit mal).

Preparations: Tablets, 0.5, 1, and 2 mg.

CLONIDINE HYDROCHLORIDE—Catapres®, Catapres-TTS®

Description/Actions: Is a centrally acting alpha-adrenergic receptor agonist indicated in the treatment of hypertension.

Precautions/Adverse Reactions: Adverse reactions include drowsiness and other CNS effects. Patients should be cautioned regarding activities such as driving and operating machinery, as well as interactions with other CNS-acting drugs including alcohol. Other adverse reactions include dry mouth, headache, dizziness, and dermatological effects (primarily with the use of the transdermal formulation). Effect may be reduced by the concurrent administration of a tricyclic antidepressant. The abrupt discontinuation of therapy may be followed by a rapid rise in blood pressure. Patients should be advised of the importance of complying with the instructions for using the medication and, if therapy is to be discontinued, it should be done so gradually.

Administration: Oral and transdermal.

Preparations: Tablets, 0.1, 0.2, and 0.3 mg. Transdermal system, programmed delivery of 0.1, 0.2, and 0.3 mg clonidine base per day, for 1 week.

CLONOPIN®, former name for Klonopin®—see Clonazepam

CLOPIDOGREL—Plavix®

Description/Actions: An inhibitor of platelet aggregation indicated in the reduction of atherosclerotic events (MI, stroke, and vascular death) in patients with atherosclerosis documented by recent stroke or MI or established peripheral arterial disease. Clopidogrel is also indicated for the treatment of acute coronary syndrome (unstable angina and nonQ-wave MI) including patients who are to be managed medically and those who are to be managed with percutaneous coronary intervention (with or without stent) or CABG.

Precautions/Adverse Reactions: Contraindicated in active pathologic bleeding (e.g., peptic ulcer, intracranial hemorrhage). Use cautiously in the presence of the risk of bleeding (e.g., surgery, ulcers, trauma, concomitant NSAIDS), and severe hepatic disease. Consider discontinuing 7 days prior to surgery. Not recommended for use in children. Pregnancy Category C. Adverse reactions include diarrhea, rash, pruritus, purpura, other GI disturbances, GI ulcers, hemorrhage, neutropenia/agranulocytosis (rare). Instruct patients to report unusual or prolonged bleeding or fever.

Administration: Oral.

Preparations: Tablets, 75 mg.

CLORAZEPATE DIPOTASSIUM—Tranxene®

Description/Actions: Benzodiazepine indicated (a) for the management of anxiety disorders or for the short-term relief of the symptoms of anxiety, (b) for the symptomatic relief of acute alcohol withdrawal, and (c) as adjunctive therapy in the management of partial seizures.

Precautions/Adverse Reactions: Contraindicated in patients with acute narrow-angle glaucoma. Adverse reactions include drowsiness and other CNS effects. Patients should be cautioned regarding activities such as driving and operating machinery, as well as interactions with other CNS-acting drugs including alcohol. Can cause dependence and is included in Schedule IV.

Administration: Oral.

Preparations: Tablets, 3.75, 7.5, 11.25, 15, and 22.5 mg. Capsules, 3.75, 7.5, and 15 mg.

CLORPACTIN®, see Oxychlorosene

CLOTRIMAZOLE—Gyne-Lotrimin®, Lotrimin®, Lotrimin AF®, Mycelex®, Mycelex-G®, Trivagizole 3™

Description/Actions: Antifungal agent indicated for (a) dermal infections—tinea pedis, tinea cruris, tinea corporis, candidiasis, tinea versicolor, (b) vulvovaginal candidiasis, and (c) oropharyngeal candidiasis.

Precautions/Adverse Reactions: Adverse reactions include pruritus, stinging, erythema, vulval irritation.

Administration: Topical and vaginal.

Preparations: Cream, lotion, and solution, 1%. Vaginal cream, 1% and 2%. Vaginal tablets, 100 and 500 mg. Troches, 10 mg.

CLOVE OIL

Description/Actions: Local anesthetic included in some formulations used for the relief of toothache.

Preparations: Drops.

CLOXACILLIN SODIUM—Tegopen®

Description/Actions: Penicillin antibiotic indicated for the treatment of staphylococcal infections.

Preparations: Capsules, 250 and 500 mg. Powder for oral solution, 125 mg/5 ml when reconstituted.

CLOZAPINE—Clozaril®, Fazaclo™

Description/Actions: An atypical antipsychotic drug with effects on dopamine mediated behaviors that differ from those exhibited by the standard antipsychotic agents. Is much less likely than the standard antipsychotic drugs to cause extrapyramidal effects. Indicated for the management of severely ill schizophrenic patients who fail to respond adequately to standard antipsychotic drug treatment, either because of insufficient effectiveness or the inability to achieve an effective dose due to intolerable adverse effects from those drugs. Also indicated in the treatment of patients with schizophrenia or schizoaffective disorder to reduce the risk of recurrent suicidal behavior.

Precautions/Adverse Reactions: Contraindicated in patients with myeloproliferative disorders, or a history of clozapine-induced agranulocytosis or severe granulocytopenia. Should not be used simultaneously with other agents having a well-known potential to suppress bone marrow function. May cause agranulocytosis, and prior to initiating treatment, a white blood cell (WBC) count should be performed and subsequent WBC counts should be done at least weekly for the duration of therapy, as well as for 4 weeks past discontinuation. If the total WBC count falls below 2000/mm3 or granulocyte count below 1000/mm3 during clozapine therapy, the drug should be discontinued and not resumed because of an even higher risk of agranulocytosis upon rechallenge.

Patients should be advised to immediately report the appearance of lethargy, fever, sore throat, flu-like symptoms, or any other signs of infection. Use has also been associated with occurrence of seizures as well as other CNS effects (e.g., drowsiness/sedation, dizziness/vertigo). Patients should be cautioned regarding activities such as driving and operating machinery, as well as interactions with other CNS-acting drugs including alcohol. Other adverse reactions include tachycardia, hypotension, constipation, nausea, hypersalivation, sweating, dry mouth, visual disturbances, and fever.

Administration: Oral.

Preparations: Tablets, 25 and 100 mg. Orally disintegrating tablets, 25 mg and 100 mg.

CLOZARIL®, see Clozapine

COAL TAR

Description/Actions: Antipruritic and irritant used in the topical treatment of dermatologic disorders including scalp conditions.

Preparations: Solution, gel, cream, ointment, lotion, soap, and shampoo.

COCAINE

Description/Actions: Local anesthetic applied topically to provide anesthesia for mucous membranes.

Preparations: Powder. Topical solution, 40 mg/ml and 100 mg/ml. Soluble tablets, 135 mg.

CODEINE PHOSPHATE AND SULFATE

Description/Actions: Is a centrally acting analgesic indicated for the relief of pain and the management of cough.

Precautions/Adverse Reactions: Adverse reactions include sedation and other CNS effects. Patients should be cautioned regarding activities such as driving and operating machinery, as well as interactions with other CNS-acting drugs including alcohol. Other adverse reactions include constipation, nausea, vomiting, rash, and, in higher doses, respiratory depression. Can cause dependence, and formulations are covered under the provisions of the Controlled Substances Act.

Administration: Oral and parenteral.

Preparations: Tablets, 15, 30, and 60 mg. Vials, 30 and 60 mg/ml. Is often used in combination with other agents (e.g., acetaminophen, aspirin) in capsule, tablet, and liquid formulations.

COD LIVER OIL

Description/Actions: Vitamins A and D used to prevent and treat deficiences of these vitamins.

Preparations: Oil, emulsion, capsules.

COGENTIN®, see Benztropine

COGNEX®, see Tacrine Hydrochloride

COLACE®, see Docusate Sodium

COLAZAL®, see Balsalazide

COLCHICINE

Description/Actions: Agent for gout indicated for the relief of pain associated with acute attacks of gout. Has also been used in chronic gouty conditions for the prevention of acute attacks of gout.

Preparations: Tablets, 0.5 and 0.6 mg. Ampules, 1 mg.

COLESEVELAM—Welchol™

Description/Actions: Colesevelam is a nonabsorbable polymer that acts as a bile acid sequestering agent. It is indicated as adjunctive therapy to diet and exercise and used alone or in combination with an HMG-CoA reductase inhibitor for the management of elevated LDL in primary hypercholesterolemia (Fredrickson type IIa).

Precautions/Adverse Reactions: Usage is contraindicated in patients with hypersensitivity to colesevelam or any component of the formulation and in individuals with bowel obstructions. Because it has not been studied in persons having a triglyceride level greater than 300 mg/dl, caution should be used in treating such patients. Safety and efficacy have not been established in patients with dysphagia, swallowing disorders, severe gastrointestinal motility disorders, or major gastrointestinal tract surgery, and patients susceptible to fat-soluble vitamin deficiencies. Therefore, use in such patients should be with caution. Safety and efficacy have not been established in children. Prior to initiation, secondary causes of hypercholesterolemia should be excluded. Pregnancy Category B. Use only in pregnancy if clearly needed. Some adverse effects are constipation, dyspepsia, weakness, myalgia, and pharyngitis.

Administration: Oral.

Patient Care Implications: Inform patients to take with a liquid and a meal and to follow dietary guidelines.

Preparations: Tablet: 625 mg.

COLESTID®, see Colestipol

COLESTIPOL HYDROCHLORIDE—Colestid®

Description/Actions: Antihyperlipidemic agent indicated as adjunctive therapy to diet for the reduction of elevated serum cholesterol in patients with primary hypercholesterolemia.

Preparations: Tablets, 1 g. Granules, packets, 5 g.

COLFOSCERIL PALMITATE, CETYL ALCOHOL, AND TYLOXAPOL—Exosurf Neonatal®

Description/Actions: A synthetic pulmonary surfactant that contains colfosceril palmitate (also known as dipalmitoylphosphatidylcholine [DPPC]), cetyl alcohol, and tyloxapol. Replenishes surfactant and restores surface activity to the lungs. Indicated for the prophylactic treatment of infants with birth weights of less than 1350 g who are at risk of developing RDS, the prophylactic treatment of infants with birth weights greater than 1350 g who have evidence of pulmonary immaturity, and the rescue treatment of infants who have developed RDS.

Precautions/Adverse Reactions: Adverse reactions include pulmonary bleeding, apnea, and mucous plugging. Suctioning of infant before dosing may lessen the possibility of mucous plugs obstructing the endotracheal tube. May rapidly affect oxygenation and lung compliance.

Administration: Intratracheal. Before administration, the infant should be suctioned. Is administered in the form of a suspension by instillation into the trachea via the side port on a special endotracheal tube adapter without interrupting mechanical ventilation. Each dose is administered in two half doses. The infant is turned from the midline position to the right after the first half-dose, and from the midline position to the left after the second half-dose. If the suspension appears to separate, the vial should be gently shaken or swirled to resuspend the preparation.

Preparations: Vials, 108 mg colfosceril palmitate, 12 mg cetyl alcohol, 8 mg tyloxapol, and 47 mg sodium chloride.

COLISTIMETHATE SODIUM—Coly-Mycin M®,
see Colistin Sulfate

COLISTIN SULFATE—Coly-Mycin S®, Polymixin E®

Description/Actions: Antibiotic indicated for the treatment of infections caused by gram-negative bacteria including *Pseudomonas aeruginosa*. Colistimethate is used in the formulation administered parenterally, and colistin is used in the formulations administered orally (for gastrointestinal infections) and as otic drops.

Preparations: Vials, 150 mg. Oral suspension, 25 mg/5 ml when reconstituted. Otic drops (in combination with other agents), 3 mg/ml.

COLLAGENASE—Santyl®

Description/Actions: Enzyme indicated for debriding chronic dermal ulcers and severely burned areas.

Preparations: Ointment, 250 units/g.

COLLYRIUM®, see Sodium Borate

COLY-MYCIN®, see Colistimethate

COLYTE®, see Polyethylene Glycol 3350

COMBIVIR®—Combination Agent Lamivudine and Zidovudine

COMBIVENT®—Combination Agent Ipratopium Bromide and Albuterol

COMPAZINE®, see Prochlorperazine

COMTAN®, see Entacapone

CONCERTA™, see Methylphenidate Hydrochloride

CONDYLOX®, see Podofilox

CONJUGATED ESTROGENS, see Estrogens, Conjugated

CORDARONE®, see Amiodarone

CORDRAN®, see Flurandrenolide

COREG®, see Carvedilol

CORGARD®, see Nadolol

CORTEF®, see Hydrocortisone

CORTICOTROPIN—Adrenocorticotropic Hormone, ACTH, Acthar®

Description/Actions: Hormone indicated for parenteral use in the diagnostic testing of adrenocortical function. Is of limited value in conditions responsive to corticosteroid therapy.

Preparations: Vials, 25 and 40 units. Vials (gel for repository effect), 40 and 80 units/ml.

CORTISOL, see Hydrocortisone

CORTISONE ACETATE—Cortone Acetate®

Description/Actions: Corticosteroid indicated for oral or intramuscular use in a wide range of endocrine, rheumatic, allergic, dermatologic, respiratory, hematologic, neoplastic, and other disorders.

Preparations: Tablets, 5, 10, and 25 mg. Vials, 25 and 50 mg/ml.

CORTISPORIN OTIC®, Combination of Hydrocortisone, Neomycin, and Polymyxin B

CORTONE®, see Cortisone Acetate

CORTROSYN®, see Cosyntropin

CORVERT®, see Ibutilide Fumarate

COSMEGEN®, see Dactinomycin

COSOPT®—Combination Agent Dorzolamide Hcl 2% and Timolol Maleate 0.5%

COSYNTROPIN—Cortrosyn®

Description/Actions: Synthetic ACTH analogue indicated for parenteral use in the diagnostic testing of adrenocortical function.

Preparations: Vials, 0.25 mg.

COTRIMOXAZOLE, see Trimethoprim-Sulfamethoxazole

COUMADIN®, see Warfarin

COVERA-HS®, see Verapamil

COZAAR®, see Losartan Potassium

CRIXIVAN®, see Indinavir

CROFAB®, see Crotalidae Polyvalent, Immune Fab (Ovine)

CROMOLYN SODIUM—Crolom®, Gastrocrom®, Intal®, Nasalcrom®

Description/Actions: Antiasthmatic agent used by oral inhalation in the prophylactic management of bronchial asthma, and shortly before exposure to factors (e.g., exercise) that precipitate bronchoconstriction. Instruct patients that this agent is not for treatment of acute bronchial asthmatic attacks. Ophthalmic solution is indicated for the treatment of vernal keratoconjunctivitis, vernal conjunctivitis, and vernal keratitis. Nasal solution is indicated for the prevention and treatment of symptoms of allergic rhinitis. Capsules for oral administration are used in the treatment of mastocytosis.

Preparations: Capsules, 100 mg. Oral solution, 100 mg/5 ml. Nebulizer solution (20 mg/2 ml). Metered dose inhalation unit. Nasal solution, 40 mg/ml. Ophthalmic solution, 4%.

CROTALIDAE POLYVALENT IMMUNE FAB (OVINE)— Crofab®

Description/Actions: Indicated for the management of patients with minimal or moderate North American envenomation. Use within 6 hours of a snakebite to prevent coagulation abnormalities.

Precautions/Adverse Reactions: Crotalidae should not be administered to patients with a known history of hypersensitivity to papaya or papain unless the benefits outweigh the risks and appropriate management for anaphylactic reactions is available. Should be used within 6 hours of a snakebite in order to prevent coagulation abnormalities. Recurrent coagulopathy may persist for 1–2 weeks or more. Retreatment may be necessary; monitor patient. Patients with allergies to papain, chymopapain, other papaya extracts, or the pineapple enzyme bromelain may also experience a hypersensitivity reaction to crotalidae. Cross sensitivity with dust mites and latex allergens is a possibility due to similar antigenic structures with papain. Contains thimeresal. Anaphylactic reactions are possible due to foreign proteins in the antivenom. Patients should be monitored for the development of delayed hypersensitivity reactions or serum sickness. Caution should be exercised when administering a repeat course of treatment for a second envenomation episode as patients may become sensitized to the foreign protein. Drug interaction studies have not been conducted. Pregnancy Category C. Reproductive studies have not been conducted. Crotalidae contains thimeresal, which has been associated with neurologic and renal toxicities. Developing fetuses and very young children are most at risk. Excretion in human breast milk is unknown. No specific studies have been conducted in children. The absolute venom dose following a snakebite is expected to be the same in children and adults; therefore, no dosage adjustment for age should be made. Adverse reactions observed during therapy with crotalidae include urticaria, rash, pruritis, nausea, coagulation disorders, back pain, chest pain, cellulitis, wound infection, chills, allergic reactions, hypotension, asthma, cough, increased sputum, anorexia, myalgia, ecchymosis, nervousness, and paresthesias.

Administration: Intravenous.

Patient Care Implications: Infusion should proceed slowly during the first 10 minutes. Patient should be monitored for signs and symptoms of an allergic reaction.

Preparations: Injection, 2 vials per box.

CROTAMITON—Eurax®

Description/Actions: Scabicide indicated for the treatment of scabies and for the symptomatic treatment of pruritic skin.

Preparations: Cream and lotion, 10%.

CRYSTICILLIN®, see Procaine Penicillin G

CUPRIMINE®, see Penicillamine

CURARE, see Tubocurarine

CUROSURF®, see Poractant Alfa

CUTIVATE®, see Fluticasone Propionate

CYANOCOBALAMIN—Vitamin B$_{12}$, Nascobal®

Description/Actions: Vitamin indicated in the treatment of pernicious anemia, dietary deficiency of vitamin B$_{12}$, malabsorption of vitamin B$_{12}$, and other situations in which there is inadequate utilization of vitamin B$_{12}$. Also used for the Schilling test. Nascobal® is indicated to maintain therapeutic levels of cyanocobalamin in patients in remission following intramuscular vitamin B$_{12}$ administration and for the maintenance of therapeutic levels of vitamin B_{12} in patients with HIV, AIDS, multiple sclerosis, or Crohn's disease.

Preparations: Tablets, 25, 50, 100, 250, 500, and 1000 mcg. Vials, 100 and 1000 mcg/ml. Intranasal gel, 500 mcg/0.1 ml. Nasal spray scent-free, 500 mcg/0.1 ml.

CYCLANDELATE—Cyclospasmol®

Description/Actions: Vasodilator indicated for adjunctive therapy in intermittent claudication, Raynaud's phenomenon, nocturnal leg cramps, and other peripheral vascular disorders. Has also been used in selected cases in ischemic cerebral vascular disease.

Preparations: Tablets, 400 mg. Capsules, 200 and 400 mg.

CYCLESSA™, see Desogestrel/Ethinyl Estradiol

CYCLIZINE—Marezine®

Description/Actions: Antiemetic indicated in the management of nausea and vomiting of motion sickness.

Preparations: Tablets (as the hydrochloride), 50 mg. Ampules (as the lactate), 50 mg.

CYCLOBENZAPRINE HYDROCHLORIDE—Flexeril®

Description/Actions: Skeletal muscle relaxant indicated as an adjunct to rest and physical therapy for relief of muscle spasm associated with acute, painful musculoskeletal conditions.

Precautions/Adverse Reactions: Contraindicated during the acute recovery phase of myocardial infarction, in patients with arrhythmias, heart block or conduction disturbances, congestive heart failure, or hyperthyroidism, and in patients being treated with a monoamine oxidase inhibitor. Adverse reactions include drowsiness and other CNS effects. Patients should be cautioned regarding activities such as driving and operating machinery, as well as interactions with other CNS-acting drugs including alcohol. Has an anticholinergic effect and adverse reactions such as dry mouth are common; caution should be exercised in patients with conditions such as angle-closure glaucoma, and in those taking other anticholinergic medications.

Administration: Oral.

Preparations: Tablets, 5 and 10 mg.

CYCLOCORT®, see Amcinonide

CYCLOGYL®, see Cyclopentolate

CYCLOMEN®, see Danazol

CYCLOPENTOLATE HYDROCHLORIDE—Cyclogyl®

Description/Actions: Anticholinergic agent used to produce mydriasis and cycloplegia in diagnostic procedures.

Preparations: Ophthalmic solution, 0.5% and 1%.

CYCLOPHOSPHAMIDE—Cytoxan®, Neosar®

Description/Actions: Antineoplastic agent indicated in the oral and parenteral treatment of malignant lymphomas, leukemias, multiple myeloma, carcinoma of the breast, neuroblastoma, adenocarcinoma of the ovary, retinoblastoma, and mycosis fungoides.

Preparations: Tablets, 25 and 50 mg. Vials, 100, 200, and 500 mg, 1 and 2 g.

CYCLOSERINE—Seromycin®

Description/Actions: Antibiotic indicated in the treatment of tuberculosis when therapy with the primary medications has not been successful. Has also been used for urinary tract infections in which conventional therapy has failed.

Preparations: Capsules, 250 mg.

CYCLOSPASMOL®, see Cyclandelate

CYCLOSPORINE—Sandimmune®, Neoral®

Description/Actions: Immunosuppressant used orally and intravenously, in conjunction with a corticosteroid, for the prophylaxis of organ rejection in kidney, liver, and heart transplants and severe, active rheumatoid arthritis unresponsive to methotrexate alone.

Preparations: Capsules, 25 and 100 mg. Oral solution, 100 mg/ml. Ampules, 50 mg.

CYCRIN®, see Medroxyprogesterone

CYKLOKAPRON®, see Tranexamic Acid

CYLERT®, see Pemoline

CYPROHEPTADINE HYDROCHLORIDE—Periactin®

Description/Actions: Antihistamine indicated for allergic disorders. Also possesses antiserotonin and appetite-stimulating properties.

Preparations: Tablets, 4 mg. Syrup, 2 mg/5 ml.

CYSTAGON®, see Cysteamine Bitartrate

CYSTEAMINE BITARTRATE—Cystagon®

Description/Actions: Cystine-depleting agent indicated in the management of nephropathic cystinosis in children and adults.

Precautions/Adverse Reactions: Contraindicated in patients with known hypersensitivity to this agent or penicillamine. Adverse reactions include vomiting, anorexia, fever, diarrhea, lethargy, and rash. If rash develops, the drug should be withheld until the rash clears. If a severe skin rash (e.g., erythema multiforme) develops, should not be readministered. Has occasionally been associated with reversible leukopenia and abnormal liver function studies. Therefore, blood counts and liver function studies should be monitored.

Administration: Oral.

Preparations: Capsules, 50 and 150 mg.

CYTARABINE—Cytosine Arabinoside, ARA-C, Cytosar-U®

Description/Actions: Antineoplastic agent indicated for the parenteral treatment of leukemias (primarily acute myelocytic leukemia) and as part of a combination regimen in children with non-Hodgkin's lymphoma.

Preparations: Vials, 100 and 500 mg.

CYTOMEL®, see Liothyronine

CYTOSAR-U®, see Cytarabine

CYTOSINE ARABINOSIDE, see Cytarabine

CYSTOSPAZ®, see Hyoscyamine Sulfate

CYTOTEC®, see Misoprostol

CYTOVENE®, see Ganciclovir

CYTOXAN®, see Cyclophosphamide

D

DACARBAZINE—DTIC®

Description/Actions: Antineoplastic agent indicated for the parenteral treatment of metastatic malignant melanoma, refractory Hodgkin's disease, various sarcomas, and neuroblastoma.

Preparations: Vials, 100 and 200 mg.

DACTINOMYCIN—Cosmegen®

Description/Actions: Antineoplastic agent indicated for the parenteral treatment of Wilms' tumor, testicular carcinoma, choriocarcinoma, rhabdomyosarcoma, and other neoplasms.

Precautions/Adverse Reactions: This drug is highly toxic and both powder and solution must be handled and administered with care. Inhalation of dust vapors and contact with skin or mucous membranes, especially those of the eyes, must be avoided. Avoid exposure during pregnancy. Due to the toxic properties of dactinomycin, special handling procedures should be reviewed prior to handling and followed diligently. Dactinomycin is extremely corrosive to soft tissue. If extravasation occurs during intravenous use, severe damage to soft tissue will occur.

Preparations: Vials, 0.5 mg.

DALFOPRISTIN/QUINUPRISTIN—Synercid®

Description/Actions: Synercid has been approved for vancomycin-resistant *Enterococcus faecium bacteremia* and *Staphylococcus aureus* skin infections.

Precautions/Adverse Reactions: Patients who are known to have a hypersensitivity reaction to dalfopristin, quinupristin, or any other streptogramin should not take Synercid. Synercid has also not been proven to be safe in children under 16, in pregnant women, and/or in women who breast-feed. Also Synercid should be used carefully in patients with hepatic disease. Synercid in general has few side effects in patients. The most common reasons for discontinuing this drug are nausea, vomiting, pruritus, and a rash. Other possible side effects are arthralgia, myalgia, hepatotoxicity, hyperbilirubinemia, and pseudomembranous colitis.

Administration: Intravenous.

Patient Care Implications: Patients with hepatic impairment may need a reduction in dosage. Monitor liver function enzymes while patient on medicine. Not proven to be safe in pregnant women, women who breast-feed, and children under 16.

Preparations: Vials, 500 mg.

DALGAN®, see Dezocine

DALMANE®, see Flurazepam

DALTEPARIN—Fragmin®

Description/Actions: Dalteparin is indicated for the prophylaxis of ischemic complications in unstable angina and non-Q-wave myocardial infarction, when concurrently administered with aspirin therapy. Dalteparin is also indicated for the prophylaxis of deep vein thrombosis (DVT), which may lead to pulmonary embolism (PE) in patients undergoing hip replacement surgery, in patients undergoing abdominal surgery who are at risk for thromboembolic complications, and in medical patients who are at risk for thromboembolic complications due to severely restricted mobility during acute illness.

Precautions/Adverse Reactions: Contraindicated in active major bleeding and thrombocytopenia associated with positive in vitro tests for antiplatelet antibody in the presence of dalteporin, heparin, or pork allergy. Adverse effects include local hematoma, anaphylaxis, and thrombocytopenia.

Administration: SQ injection.

Preparations: 2500 and 5000 IU/0.2 ml single-dose, prefilled syringe.

DANAPAROID SODIUM—Orgaran®

Description/Actions: Antithrombolic indicated in prevention of post-op DVT.

Precautions/Adverse Reactions: Contraindicated in severe hemorrhagic diathesis, active major bleeding, type II thrombocytopenia associated with a positive in vitro test for anitiplatelet antibody associated with danaparoid sodium, heparin, or pork allergy. May cause bleeding or hematomas within the spinal column if used concurrently with spinal or epidural anesthesia analgesia. Use cautiously in asthma, heparin-induced thrombocytopenia, bleeding disorders, severe renal dysfunction (monitor carefully if serum $Cr \geq 2$ mg/dl), severe uncontrolled hypertension, acute bacterial endocarditis, acute ulceration, and angiodysplastic GI disease, bleeding diathesis, nonhemorrhagic stroke, invasive procedures, recent brain, spinal, or eye surgery. Not interchangeable (unit for unit) with heparin or other low molecular weight heparin products. Pregnancy Category C. Adverse reactions include hemorrhage, thrombocytopenia, local reactions (e.g., hematoma, pain), fever, GI upset, constipation, rash, pruritus, edema, dizziness, insomnia, and anemia.

Administration: SQ injection.

Preparations: 750 units/0.6 ml solution for SC injection; contains sulfites.

DANAZOL—Cyclomen®, Danocrine®

Description/Actions: Androgen indicated for the treatment of endometriosis unresponsive to more conventional treatment, fibrocystic breast disease, and hereditary angioedema.

Preparations: Capsules, 50, 100, and 200 mg.

DANOCRINE®, see Danazol

DANTRIUM®, see Dantrolene

DANTROLENE SODIUM—Dantrium®

Description/Actions: Muscle relaxant and antispastic agent used in controlling the manifestations of spasticity resulting from upper motor neuron disorders (e.g., stroke, cerebral palsy, multiple sclerosis). Also used intravenously in the management of malignant hyperthermia crisis, and orally to prevent or reduce the development of signs of malignant hyperthermia in susceptible patients.

Preparations: Capsules, 25, 50, and 100 mg. Vials, 20 mg.

DAPIPRAZOLE HYDROCHLORIDE—Rev-Eyes™

Description/Actions: An alpha-adrenergic blocking agent that reverses the mydriasis caused by agents used in ocular examinations. Indicated in the treatment of iatrogenically induced mydriasis produced by adrenergic (phenylephrine) and parasympatholytic (tropicamide) agents.

Precautions/Adverse Reactions: Contraindicated in patients in whom constriction is undesirable (e.g., acute iritis). Adverse reactions include conjunctival injection, burning on instillation, ptosis, lid erythema, lid edema, chemosis, itching, punctate keratitis, corneal edema, browache, photophobia, and headaches.

Administration: Ophthalmic.

Preparations: Ophthalmic solution, 0.5%.

DAPSONE, Avlosulfan®, DDS®

Description/Actions: Antileprosy agent indicated for the management of all forms of leprosy. Also indicated in the treatment of dermatitis herpetiformis.

Preparations: Tablets, 25 and 100 mg.

DAPTOMYCIN—Cubicin™

Description/Actions: Daptomycin is a cyclic lipopeptide natural product that has clinical utility in the treatment of infections caused by aerobic gram-positive bacteria. Daptomycin retains potency against antibiotic-resistant gram-positive bacteria including isolates resistant to methicillin, vancomycin, and linezolid. Daptomycin exhibits rapid concentration dependent bactericidal activity against gram-positive organisms in vitro. Daptomycin binds to bacterial membranes and causes a rapid depolarization of membrane, potentially leading to inhibition of protein, DNA and RNA synthesis, which results in bacterial cell death. Daptomycin is indicated for the treatment of complicated skin and skin structure infections caused by susceptible strains of the following gram-positive microorganisms: *Staphylococcus aureus* (including methicillin-resistant strains), *Streptococcus pyogenes, Streptococcus agalactiae, Streptococcus dysgalactiae* subsp. *equismillis,* and *Enterococcus faecalis* (vancomycin susceptible strains only). Daptomycin is not indicated for the treatment of pneumonia.

Precautions/Adverse Reactions: Daptomycin is contraindicated in patients with a known hypersensitivity to it or to any component of the formulation. Pseudomembranous colitis has been reported with the use of daptomycin, ranging in severity from mild to life threatening. Elevations in creatinine phosphokinase (CPK) have been reported during therapy with daptomycin. Daptomycin should be discontinued in patients with unexplained signs and symptoms of myopathy in conjunction with CPK elevations greater than 5x the upper limit of normal or in patients without symptoms who have marked elevations in CPK greater than 10x the upper limit of normal. Consideration should be given to temporarily suspending agents associated with rhabdomyolysis, such as HMG-CoA reductase inhibitors, in patients receiving daptomycin. No clinically significant drug interactions have been found. Pregnancy Category B. No adequate and well-controlled studies in pregnant women. Use during pregnancy only if clearly needed. Excretion in human breast milk is unknown. Exercise caution when administering daptomycin to women who are nursing. Safety and efficacy of daptomycin in patients under the age of 18 have not been established. Most common adverse effects observed during treatment with daptomycin include: constipation, nausea, diarrhea, vomiting, dyspepsia, injection site reactions, fever, headache, insomnia, dizziness, rash, pruritis, abnormal liver function tests, elevated CPK, fungal infections, urinary tract infections, hypotension, hypertension, renal failure, anemia, dyspnea, limb pain, and arthralgia. Less common side effects include: edema, cellulitis, hypoglycemia, cough, back pain, hypokalemia, hypomagnesemia, increased serum bicarbonate, electrolyte disturbances, myalgia, muscle cramps, muscle weakness, osteomyelitis, vertigo, mental status changes, paresthesia, taste disturbance, leukocytosis, thrombocytopenia, thrombocytosis, eosinophilia, increased INR, hypersensitivity, and candida infections.

Administration: Intravenous.

Patient Care Implications: Monitor patient for the development of muscle pain or weakness. CPK levels should be monitored weekly during therapy with daptomycin.

Preparations: Lyophilized powder for injection, 250 mg and 500 mg single-use vials.

DARANIDE®, see Dichlorphenamide

DARAPRIM®, see Pyrimethamine

DARBEPOETIN ALFA—Aranesp™

Description/Actions: Darbepoetin alfa is indicated for the treatment of anemia associated with chronic renal failure, including patients on dialysis and patients not on dialysis. It is also indicated in the treatment of anemia in patients with nonyeloid malignancies where anemia is due to the effect of concomitantly administered chemotherapy.

Precautions/Adverse Reactions: Treatment with darbepoetin has been associated with cardiovascular and neurologic events (including seizures, stroke, and death) in patients with chronic renal failure. Monitor blood pressure and neurologic status during treatment. Supplemental iron therapy is recommended for all patients whose serum ferritin is below 100 mg/l or whose serum transferrin saturation is below 20%. Folic acid and/or vitamin B_{12} deficiencies should be corrected or excluded prior to initiation of therapy with darbepoetin. Infections, inflammatory or malignant processes, osteofibrosis cystica, occult blood loss, hemolysis, severe aluminum toxicity, and bone marrow fibrosis may compromise an erythropoietic response. Pregnancy Category C. There are no adequate and well-controlled studies in pregnant women. Use during pregnancy only if the potential benefit justifies the potential risk to the fetus. Excretion in human breast milk is unknown. Use with caution in nursing women. Safety and efficacy have not been established in pediatric patients. Safety and efficacy have not been established in patients with underlying hematologic diseases such as hemolytic anemia, sickle cell anemia, thalassemia, and porphyria. Most commonly reported adverse reactions include hypertension, hypotension, infection, headache, myalgia, and diarrhea. The most commonly reported serious side effects associated with darbepoetin therapy are vascular access thrombosis, congestive heart failure, sepsis, and cardiac arrhythmia. Aranesp® and other erythropoietic therapies may increase the risk of cardiovascular events, including death. The higher risk may be associated with higher hemoglobin and or higher rates of rise of hemoglobin. Avoid exceeding a target hemoglobin level of 12 g/dL. An increased incidence of thrombotic events (pulmonary emboli, thrombophlebitis, and thrombosis) and increased mortality have been observed in patients treated with Aranesp®. The most commonly reported adverse reactions resulting in discontinuation of darbepoetin, dosage adjustment, or the need for concomitant medication to treat an adverse reaction symptom were hypotension, hypertension, fever, myalgia, nausea, and chest pain.

Administration: For intravenous or subcutaneous administration.

Patient Care Implications: Do not exceed a target hemoglobin concentration of 12 g/dl. Do not shake darbepoetin. Shaking will render it inactive. Do not dilute darbepoetin. Monitor blood pressure and neurologic status of patients treated with darbepoetin. Store in refrigerator.

Preparations: Available in 2 solutions for injection: Polysorbate 80 solution (contains 0.05 mg/ml polysorbate/ml) in 1 ml single-dose vials containing 25, 40, 60, 100, and 200 mg/ml. Albumin solution (contains 2.5 mg/ml human albumin) in 1 ml single-dose vials containing 25, 40, 60, 100, and 200 mg/ml.

DARICON®, see Oxphencyclimine

DARVOCET-N®, Combination of Propoxyphene Napsylate and Acetaminophen

DARVON®, see Propoxyphene Hydrochloride

DARVON-N®, see Propoxyphene Napsylate

DAUNORUBICIN HYDROCHLORIDE—Cerubidine®

Description/Actions: Antineoplastic agent indicated for the parenteral treatment of acute nonlymphocytic leukemia in adults and in acute lymphocytic leukemia in children.

Preparations: Vials, 20 mg (of the base).

DAYPRO®, see Oxaprozin

DDAVP®, see Desmopressin Acetate

DDC, see Zalcitabine

DDI, see Didanosine

DDS®, see Dapsone

DEBRISAN®, see Dextranomer

DEBROX®, see Carbamide Peroxide

DECADRON®, see Dexamethasone

DECA-DURABOLIN®, see Nandrolone Decanoate

DECHOLIN®, see Dehydrocholic Acid

DECLOMYCIN®, see Demeclocycline

DEFEROXAMINE MESYLATE—Desferal®

Description/Actions: Antidote that chelates iron. Indicated for parenteral use to facilitate the removal of iron in the treatment of acute iron intoxication and in chronic iron overload due to transfusion-dependent anemias.

Preparations: Vials, 500 mg.

DEHYDROCHOLIC ACID—Decholin®

Description/Actions: Hydrocholeretic indicated for the relief of constipation. Has also been used as an adjunct in the treatment of various biliary conditions.

Preparations: Tablets, 250 mg.

DELATESTRYL®, see Testosterone Enanthate

DELAVIRDINE MESYLATE—Rescriptor®

Description/Actions: Antiretroviral indicated in the treatment of HIV-1 infection in combination with other antiretroviral agents when therapy is warranted. When used as monotherapy viral resistance emerged rapidly.

Precautions/Adverse Reactions: Discontinue if serious rash (or rash with other symptoms) occurs. Use cautiously in patients with impaired liver function or achlorhydria (take with an acidic beverage). Adverse reactions include rash, GI upset.

Administration: Oral.

Preparations: Tablets, 100 mg.

DELESTROGEN®, see Estradiol Valerate

DELSYM®, see Dextromethorphan

DELTA-CORTEF®, see Prednisolone

DELTASONE®, see Prednisone

DEMADEX®, see Torsemide

DEMECARIUM BROMIDE—Humorsol®

Description/Actions: Cholinesterase inhibitor exhibiting miotic activity. Indicated for ophthalmic use in the treatment of open-angle glaucoma, conditions obstructing aqueous outflow, accommodative esotropia, and following iridectomy.

Preparations: Ophthalmic solution, 0.125% and 0.25%.

DEMEROL®, see Meperidine

DEMECLOCYCLINE HYDROCHLORIDE—Declomycin®

Description/Actions: Tetracycline antibiotic indicated for the treatment of infections caused by susceptible organisms.

Preparations: Tablets, 150 and 300 mg. Capsules, 150 mg.

DEMSER®, see Metyrosine

DENAVIR®, see Penciclovir

DENILEUKIN DIFTITOX—Ontak®

Description/Actions: Denileukin diftitox is used for the treatment of persistent or recurrent cutaneous T-cell lymphoma (CTCL) with CD25 expression of the IL-2 receptor.

Precautions/Adverse Reactions: The drug should be administered in a facility that is equipped for cardiopulmonary resuscitation and where the patient can be monitored for hypersensitivity reactions. Women should discontinue breast-feeding while receiving the drug. Most patients experience some kind of adverse reaction from the drug. The most common is a flu-like syndrome (91%), then hypersensitivity reaction (69%), infection (48%), vascular leak syndrome (27%), and nervous system disturbances.

Administration: Intravenous.

Patient Care Implications: Should be administered to patients in a facility equipped and staffed for cardiopulmonary resuscitation and where the patient can be closely monitored.

Preparations: Vials, 300 mcg/2 ml.

DEPAKENE®, see Valproic Acid

DEPAKOTE®, see Valproic Acid

DEPAKOTE® ER, see Valproic Acid

DEPEN®, see Penicillamine

DEPO-ESTRADIOL®, see Estradiol Cypionate

DEPO-MEDROL®, see Methylprednisolone Acetate

DEPONIT®, see Nitroglycerin

DEPO-PROVERA®, see Medroxyprogesterone Acetate

DEPO-TESTOSTERONE®, see Testosterone Cypionate

DERIFIL®, see Chlorophyll

DERMATOP®, see Prednicarbate

DES, see Diethylstilbestrol

DESENEX®, see Undecylenic Acid

DESFERAL®, see Deferoxamine Mesylate

DESFLURANE—Suprane®

Description/Actions: Is a halogenated volatile liquid that is administered via a vaporizer as a general inhalation anesthetic. Indicated as an inhalation agent for induction or maintenance of anesthesia for inpatient and outpatient surgery in adults. Also indicated for maintenance of anesthesia in infants and children after induction of anesthesia with other agents, and for tracheal intubation.

Precautions/Adverse Reactions: Contraindicated in patients with a known or suspected genetic susceptibility to malignant hyperthermia. Adverse reactions include coughing, breathholding, apnea, increased secretions, laryngospasm, pharyngitis, nausea, and vomiting. Because it may increase heart rate, it is recommended that it should not be used as the sole agent for anesthetic induction in patients with coronary artery disease or in any patients in whom increases in heart rate or blood pressure are undesirable. May trigger a skeletal muscle hypermetabolic state that results in malignant hyperthermia. Concurrent use of preanesthetic medications such as an opioid or benzodiazepine may decrease the amount of desflurane required to produce anesthesia. Use will probably reduce the dose of a neuromuscular blocking agent required during anesthesia; however, for endotracheal intubation, it is recommended that the dose of the neuromuscular blocking agent not be reduced.

Administration: Inhalation. Should be administered using a vaporizer (Tec 60) specifically designed for use with the drug.

Preparations: Bottles, 240 ml.

DESIPRAMINE HYDROCHLORIDE—Norpramin®, Pertofrane®

Description/Actions: Tricyclic antidepressant indicated for the relief of depression.

Precautions/Adverse Reactions: Should not be given concomitantly with a monoamine oxidase inhibitor, or following recent myocardial infarction. Adverse reactions include drowsiness and other CNS effects. Patients should be cautioned regarding activities such as driving and operating machinery, as well as interactions with other CNS-acting drugs including alcohol. Other adverse reactions include anticholinergic effects (e.g., dry mouth, blurred vision), GI effects (e.g., nausea), and cardiovascular effects (e.g., orthostatic hypotension). Caution should be exercised in patients with cardiovascular disorders.

Administration: Oral.

Preparations: Tablets, 10, 25, 50, 75, 100, and 150 mg. Capsules, 25 and 50 mg.

DESLORATADINE—Clarinex®, Clarinex® Reditabs,
Clarinex-D® 24-Hour (Combination of Desloratadine and Pseudephedrine) see Desloratadine and Pseudephedrine

Description/Actions: Desloratadine is indicated for the relief of nasal and nonnasal symptoms of allergic rhinitis (seasonal and perennial) and for symptomatic relief of chronic idiopathic urticaria.

Precautions/Adverse Reactions: Desloratadine is contraindicated in patients who are hypersensitive to desloratadine, loratadine, or any component of the formulation. There are no adequate and well-controlled studies in pregnant women. Pregnancy Category C. Excreted in breast milk/breast-feeding not recommended. Safety and efficacy have not been established for children <12.

Administration: Oral.

Patient Care Implications: May be taken with or without food. Patients should be warned of possible drowsiness and advised not to drive or operate machinery until they see how they react to medication. Dosage should not be increased, because no greater efficacy may be expected and drowsiness might result. No clinically significant changes in the safety profile of desloratadine were observed in clinical studies when combined with erythromycin and ketoconazole. Both of these agents have been associated with potentially dangerous interactions with some other antihistamines.

Preparations: Tablets, 5 mg. Rapidly disintegrating tables, 5 mg. Syrup, 2.5 mg/5 ml. Extended release tablets, desloratadine 5 mg and pseudephedrine 240 mg.

DESMOPRESSIN ACETATE—DDAVP®, Stimate®

Description/Actions: Antidiuretic hormone indicated for the intranasal or parenteral treatment of diabetes insipidus, intranasal treatment of primary nocturnal enuresis, and parenteral treatment of patients with hemophilia A and von Willebrand's disease.

Preparations: Nasal solution (DDAVP), 0.1 mg/ml. (available as a nasal tube delivery system and as a nasal spray pump). Nasal solution (Stimate), 1.5 mg/ml. Ampules and vials, 4 µg/ml. Tablets, 0.1 mg, 0.2 mg.

DESOGEN®, see Desogestrel/Ethinyl Estradiol

DESOGESTREL/ETHINYL ESTRADIOL—Cyclessa™, Desogen®, Ortho-Cept®

Description/Actions: Is a progestin/estrogen combination oral contraceptive that acts primarily by the suppression of gonadotropins and inhibition of ovulation. Desogestrel exhibits a highly selective progestational action and minimal androgenicity. Indicated for the prevention of pregnancy in women who elect to use oral contraceptives as a method of contraception.

Precautions/Adverse Reactions: Contraindicated in women who have thrombophlebitis or a thromboembolic disorder, a past history of such disorders, cerebral vascular or coronary artery disease, known or suspected carcinoma of the breast, carcinoma of the endometrium, or other known or suspected estrogen-dependent neoplasia, undiagnosed abnormal genital bleeding, cholestatic jaundice of pregnancy or jaundice with prior oral contraceptive use, hepatic adenomas or carcinomas, or known or suspected pregnancy. Adverse reactions include bleeding irregularities (e.g., breakthrough bleeding, spotting, changes in menstrual flow), gastrointestinal effects (e.g., nausea, vomiting, abdominal cramps), fluid retention, melasma, rash, reduced tolerance to carbohydrates, and vaginal candidiasis. Women should be strongly advised not to smoke because of the increased risk of cardiovascular effects.

Administration: Oral.

Preparations: Tablets, 0.15 mg of desogestrel and 30 mcg of ethinyl estradiol in 21-day and 28-day regimens.

DESONIDE—Tridesilon®

Description/Actions: Corticosteroid indicated for the topical treatment of corticosteroid-responsive dermatoses and, in combination with acetic acid in an otic solution, for the management of superficial infections of the external auditory canal.

Preparations: Cream and ointment, 0.05%. Otic solution, 0.05% with 2% acetic acid.

DESOXIMETASONE—Topicort®

Description/Actions: Corticosteroid indicated for the topical treatment of corticosteroid-responsive dermatoses.

Preparations: Cream, 0.05% and 0.25%. Ointment, 0.25%. Gel, 0.05%.

DESOXYN®, see Methamphetamine

DESYREL®, see Trazodone

DETROL®, see Tolterodine Tartrate

DETROL® LA, see Tolterodine Tartrate

DEXAMETHASONE—Decadron®, Hexadrol®

Description/Actions: Corticosteroid indicated in a wide range of endocrine, rheumatic, allergic, dermatologic, respiratory, hematologic, neoplastic, and other disorders.

Preparations: Tablets, 0.5, 0.75, 1, 1.5, 2, 3, and 6 mg. Liquid, 0.5 mg/5 ml. Oral concentrate, 0.5 mg/0.5 ml. Vials (as the acetate for intramuscular, intra-articular, and intralesional use), 8 mg/ml. Vials and ampules (as the sodium phosphate for parenteral use), 4, 10, 20, and 24 (for IV use only) mg/ml. Topical gel, 0.1%. Topical aerosol, 10 mg/25 g. Cream (as sodium phosphate), 0.1% Ophthalmic solution (as sodium phosphate), 0.1%. Ophthalmic ointment (as sodium phosphate), 0.05%. Aerosols (as sodium phosphate) for oral inhalation and intranasal administration.

DEXCHLORPHENIRAMINE MALEATE—Polaramine®

Description/Actions: Antihistamine indicated in the treatment of allergic disorders.

Preparations: Tablets, 2 mg. Controlled-release tablets, 4 and 6 mg. Syrup, 2 mg/5 ml.

DEXEDRINE®, see Dextroamphetamine

DEXMEDETOMIDINE HYDROCHLORIDE INJECTION— Precedex®

Description/Actions: Indicated for sedation of initially intubated and mechanically ventilated patients during treatment in an intensive care setting.

Precautions/Adverse Reactions: Precedex should be administered by continuous infusion not to exceed 24 hours. Hypotension and bradycardia have been associated with Precedex infusion. Caution should be used when administering this drug to patients with advanced heart block. Transient hypertension has also been observed, primarily during the loading dose, in association with the initial peripheral vasoconstrictive effects of Precedex. In these cases, reduction of the loading infusion rate may be desirable. Precedex should not be coadministered through the same IV catheter with blood or plasma as physical compatibility has not been established. Withdrawal symptoms, including nervousness, agitation, and headaches, may occur if Precedex is administered chronically and stopped abruptly. Adverse effects of the drug include hypotension, hypertension, nausea, bradycardia, fever, vomiting, hypoxia, tachycardia, and anemia.

Administration: Intravenous.

Patient Care Implications: Precedex should be administered only by persons skilled in the management of patients in the intensive care setting. Due to known pharmacologic effects of Precedex, patients should be continuously monitored while receiving the drug.

Preparations: Vials and ampules, 2 mL, 100 mcg/mL.

DEXMETHYLPHENIDATE HYDROCHLORIDE—Focalin™

Description/Actions: Dexmethylphenidate is indicated for the treatment of ADHD.

Precautions/Adverse Reactions: Contraindicated in patients with marked anxiety, tension, and agitation because the drug may aggravate these symptoms. Contraindicated in patients with motor tics or with a family history or diagnosis of Tourette's syndrome. Contraindicated during treatment with monoamine oxidase inhibitors (MAOIs) and also within a minimum of 14 days following discontinuation of an MAOI (hypertensive crisis may occur). Contraindicated in patients with glaucoma. Should not be used to treat severe depression or for the prevention or treatment of normal fatigue states. Suppression of growth (weight and/or height gain) has been reported with long-term use of stimulants in children. Patients requiring long-term therapy should be monitored carefully. Administration of methylphenidate may exacerbate symptoms of behavior disturbance and thought disorder in psychotic children. In the presence of seizures, this drug should be discontinued. Use cautiously in patients with hypertension and in patients whose underlying medical conditions might be compromised by increases in blood pressure or heart rate (preexisting hypertension, heart failure, recent myocardial infarction, or hyperthyroidism). Should be given cautiously to patients with a history of drug dependence or alcoholism. Chronic abusive use can lead to marked tolerance and psychological dependence, with varying degrees of abnormal behavior. Most common adverse reactions were abdominal pain, fever, nausea, and anorexia. Methylphenidate may decrease the effectiveness of drugs used to treat hypertension because of possible effects on blood pressure. Use cautiously with pressor agents. Severe toxic reactions reported when combined with clonidine. Avoid use with linezolid, due to MAO inhibition. Pregancy Category C. Safety and efficacy not established in pregnant women. Use during pregnancy only if the potential benefit to mother outweighs the possible risks to the fetus.

Administration: Oral.

Patient Care Implications: When this drug is used for extended periods, physicians should periodically reevaluate the long-term usefulness of the drug for the individual patient. If improvement is not observed after appropriate dosage adjustment over a 1-month period, the drug should be discontinued. Dexmethylphenidate is administered twice a day at least 4 hours apart. It may be given with or without food. Avoid alcohol, caffeine, and other stimulants. Use caution when driving or engaging in tasks requiring alertness until response to drug is known. Do not store medicine in hot, damp, or humid places.

Preparations: Tablets, 2.5, 5, and 10 mg.

DEXPANTHENOL—Ilopan®

Description/Actions: Pantothenic acid derivative used as a GI stimulant. Indicated for parenteral treatment of intestinal atony causing abdominal distention, postoperative and postpartum retention of flatus, or postoperative delay in resumption of intestinal motility, paralytic ileus, and for prophylactic use immediately after major abdominal surgery to minimize the possibility of paralytic ileus.

Preparations: Ampules, vials, and syringes, 250 mg/ml. Has been used orally in combination with choline bitartrate.

DEXRAZOXANE—Zinecard®

Description/Actions: Cardioprotective agent indicated for reducing the incidence and severity of cardiomyopathy associated with doxorubicin administration in women with metastatic breast cancer who have received a cumulative doxorubicin dose of 300 mg/m2 and who would benefit from continuing doxorubicin therapy. Not recommended for use with the initiation of doxorubicin therapy.

Precautions/Adverse Reactions: Contraindicated in chemotherapy regimens that do not contain an anthracycline. Additive myelosuppressive effect of this agent with antineoplastic agents requires careful blood count monitoring.

Administration: Intravenous.

Preparations: Vials, 250 and 500 mg.

DEXTRAN, LOW MOLECULAR WEIGHT—Dextran 40, Gentran 40®, Rheomacrodex®

DEXTRAN, HIGH MOLECULAR WEIGHT—Dextran 70, Dextran 75, Gentran 75®, Macrodex®

Description/Actions: Synthetic polysaccharide administered parenterally primarily as a plasma expander as adjunctive treatment of shock or impending shock due to hemorrhage, burns, surgery, or other trauma.

Preparations: Injection, 10% low molecular weight dextran and 6% high molecular weight dextran.

DEXTRANOMER—Debrisan®, Envisan®

Description/Actions: Applied topically for use in cleaning wet ulcers and wounds such as venous stasis ulcers, pressure ulcers, infected traumatic and surgical wounds, and infected burns.

Preparations: Beads. Paste.

DEXTROAMPHETAMINE SULFATE—Dexedrine®

Description/Actions: Central nervous system stimulant indicated in the treatment of narcolepsy, attention-deficit disorder with hyperactivity, and in exogenous obesity as a short-term adjunct in a regimen of weight reduction based on caloric restriction.

Preparations: Tablets, 5 mg. Controlled-release capsules, 15 mg.

DEXTROMETHORPHAN—Benylin DM®, Delsym®

Description/Actions: Antitussive indicated for the relief of cough.

Preparations: Syrup (as a hydrobromide) 5, 10, and 15 mg/5 ml.

DEXTROSE—Glucose, Glutose®, Instaglucose®

Description/Actions: Carbohydrate administered parenterally as a source of calories. Oral forms are used to correct hypoglycemia in conscious patients.

Preparations: Solutions, 2.5%, 5%, 10%, 20%, 25%, 30%, 40%, 50%, 60%, and 70%. Oral gel, 40% in 25 g and 30 g tubes and 80 g bottle. Chewable tablets, 5 g.

DEXTROTHYROXINE SODIUM—Choloxin®

Description/Actions: Antihyperlipidemic agent used as an adjunct to diet and other measures for the reduction of elevated serum cholesterol levels. May also reduce beta lipoprotein and triglyceride levels.

Preparations: Tablets, 1, 2, and 4 mg.

DEZOCINE—Dalgan®

Description/Actions: An opioid agonist/antagonist analgesic that exhibits analgesic efficacy, as well as an onset and duration of action that are comparable to those of morphine. Is most often used in the management of postoperative pain, and pain associated with surgery and orthopedic trauma.

Precautions/Adverse Reactions: Adverse reactions include sedation, dizziness/vertigo, and psychotomimetic effects. Patients should be cautioned regarding activities such as driving and operating machinery, as well as interactions with other CNS-acting drugs including alcohol. Other adverse reactions include nausea, vomiting, and injection site reactions. Should not be used in patients who are physically dependent on narcotics because its antagonist action may precipitate withdrawal symptoms.

Administration: Intramuscular and intravenous.

Preparations: Single-dose vials and syringes, 5, 10, and 15 mg. Multiple-dose vials, 10 mg/ml.

DHE 45®, see Dihydroergotamine

DHT®, see Dihydrotachysterol

DIABETA®, see Glyburide

DIABINESE®, see Chlorpropamide

DIACETYLMORPHINE, see Heroin

DIAMOX®, see Acetazolamide

DIASTAT®, see Diazepam

DIAZEPAM—Diastat®, Valium®, Valrelease®

Description/Actions: Benzodiazepine indicated (a) for the management of anxiety disorders or for the short-term relief of the symptoms of anxiety; (b) in acute alcohol withdrawal; (c) as an adjunct for the relief of skeletal muscle spasm due to reflex spasm to local pathology, athetosis, stiff-man syndrome, and tetanus; (d) as an adjunct in convulsive disorders; (e) as an adjunct in status epilepticus and severe recurrent convulsive seizures; (f) as an adjunct prior to endoscopic procedures; and (g) as a premedication in patients who are to undergo surgical procedures.

Precautions/Adverse Reactions: Contraindicated in patients with acute narrow-angle glaucoma. Adverse reactions include drowsiness and other CNS effects; patients should be cautioned regarding activities such as driving and operating machinery, as well as interactions with other CNS-acting drugs including alcohol. Can cause dependence and is included in Schedule IV. Intramuscular injections are painful and erratically absorbed. If IM route is essential for administration, inject deeply into a large muscle mass and rotate sites.

Administration: Oral, intravenous, and intramuscular.

Preparations: Tablets, 2, 5, and 10 mg. Controlled-release capsules, 15 mg. Oral solution, 5 mg/5 ml. Concentrated oral solution, 5 mg/ml. Ampules, vials, and syringes, 5 mg/ml. Rectal gel, 2.5, 5, 10, 15, and 20 mg. Sterile emulsion for injection, 5 mg/ml (contains egg phospholipids, and soybean oil).

DIAZOXIDE—Hyperstat®, Proglycem®

Description/Actions: Antihypertensive agent administered intravenously for short-term use in the emergency reduction of blood pressure in severe hypertension. Also used orally in the management of hypoglycemia due to hyperinsulinism associated with various conditions (e.g., inoperable islet cell carcinoma or adenoma).

Preparations: Ampules, 300 mg. Capsules, 50 mg. Oral suspension, 50 mg/ml.

DIBENT®, see Dicyclomine

DIBENZYLINE®, see Phenoxybenzamine

DIBUCAINE—Nupercainal®

Description/Actions: Local anesthetic used for painful skin conditions and hemorrhoids.

Preparations: Cream, 0.5%. Ointment, 1%.

DICHLORPHENAMIDE—Daranide®, Oratrol®

Description/Actions: Carbonic anhydrase inhibitor indicated for adjunctive treatment of open-angle glaucoma, secondary glaucoma, and preoperatively in acute angle-closure glaucoma.

Preparations: Tablets, 50 mg.

DICLOFENAC POTASSIUM—Cataflam®

DICLOFENAC SODIUM—Voltaren®

Description/Actions: A non-steroidal anti-inflammatory agent that inhibits prostaglandin synthesis. Diclofenac sodium is indicated for the treatment of rheumatoid arthritis, osteoarthritis, and ankylosing spondylitis. Also indicated for ophthalmic use for the treatment of postoperative inflammation following cataract extraction and in photophobia due to incisional refractive surgery. Diclofenac potassium is indicated for the management of pain and primary dysmenorrhea.

Precautions/Adverse Reactions: Should not be given to patients in whom aspirin or another NSAID causes asthma, rhinitis, urticaria, or other allergic-type reactions. May cause GI effects, and use should be avoided in patients with active GI tract disease and closely monitored in patients with a previous history of such disorders. Other adverse reactions include headache, dizziness, rash, pruritus, tinnitus, and fluid retention. Elevations in liver function tests have occurred, and it is recommended that hepatic function tests be performed no later than 8 weeks after starting therapy and periodically thereafter.

Administration: Oral and ophthalmic.

Preparations: Tablets (Cataflam), 25, 50, and 75 mg. Enteric-coated tablets (Voltaren), 25, 50, and 75 mg. Enteric- coated tablets (Cataflam), 75 mg and 100 mg. Ophthalmic solution, 0.1%. Suppositories, 50 and 100 mg, 100 mg extended-release tabs (Voltarum-XR).

DICLOXACILLIN SODIUM—Dycill®, Dynapen®, Pathocil®

Description/Actions: Penicillin antibiotic indicated for the treatment of staphylococcal infections.

Preparations: Capsules, 125, 250, and 500 mg. Powder for oral solution, 62.5 mg/5 ml when reconstituted.

DICUMAROL

Description/Actions: Coumarin anticoagulant indicated for conditions such as prophylaxis and treatment of venous thrombosis and its extension. During period of dosage adjustment, prothrombin activity should be measured daily and dose order obtained.

Preparations: Tablets, 25 and 50 mg.

DICYCLOMINE HYDROCHLORIDE—Antispas®, A-spas®, Bentyl®, Dibent®, Di-Spaz®, Spasmoject®

Description/Actions: Anticholinergic agent that relieves smooth muscle spasms of the GI tract and is indicated for the treatment of functional bowel/irritable bowel syndrome (irritable colon, spastic colon, and mucous colitis).

Precautions/Adverse Reactions: Contraindicated in patients with obstructive uropathy, obstructive disease of the GI tract, paralytic ileus, intestinal atony, unstable cardiovascular status in acute hemorrhage, severe ulcerative colitis, myasthenia gravis, and glaucoma. Adverse reactions include dry mouth, blurred vision, and nausea. Anticholinergic psychosis and heat prostration (in the presence of a high environmental temperature) have been reported in sensitive patients. May cause drowsiness and other CNS effects; patients should be cautioned regarding activities such as driving and operating machinery, as well as interactions with other CNS-acting drugs including alcohol.

Administration: Oral and intramuscular.

Preparations: Tablets, 10 and 20 mg. Extended-release tablets, 30 mg. Capsules, 10 and 20 mg. Syrup, 10 mg/5 ml. Solution for injection, 10 mg/ml.

DIDANOSINE—Videx®, Videx® EC

Description/Actions: Also known as dideoxyinosine or ddI. Antiviral agent that inhibits the replication of the human immunodeficiency virus (HIV). Is converted by cellular enzymes to the active antiviral metabolite that inhibits viral replication, in part, by interfering with reverse transcriptase. Indicated for adult and pediatric patients (>6 months of age) with advanced HIV infection who are intolerant of zidovudine therapy or who have demonstrated significant clinical or immunologic deterioration during zidovudine therapy. Also indicated for adult patients with advanced HIV infection who have received prolonged prior zidovudine therapy.

Precautions/Adverse Reactions: Fatal lactic acidosis has been reported in pregnant women who received the combination of didanosine and stavudine with other antiretroviral agents. The combination of didanosine and stavudine should be used with caution during pregnancy and is recommended only if the potential benefits clearly outweigh the potential risks. Redistribution of body fat including central obesity, dorsocervical fat enlargement, peripheral wasting, facial wasting, breast enlargement, and "cushingoid appearance" has been observed in patients receiving antiretroviral therapy. May cause pancreatitis and, if a patient develops abdominal pain and nausea, vomiting, or elevated amylase levels, use of the drug should be interrupted until the possibility of pancreatitis is excluded. Use of didanosine in patients with a history of pancreatitis or alcoholism is best avoided, as is the concurrent use with other agents known to be associated with pancreatic toxicity (e.g., intravenous pentamidine). May cause peripheral neuropathy, particularly in patients with a history of neuropathy or neurotoxic drug therapy. Patients should be advised to report symptoms such as tingling, burning, pain, or numbness in the hands or feet. Other adverse reactions include headache, diarrhea, insomnia, rash, pruritus, depression, pain, constipation, stomatitis, taste disturbance, myalgia, arthritis, hepatic enzyme elevations, leukopenia, granulocytopenia, and thrombocytopenia. Because two of the three formulations contain (or have added) magnesium and aluminum antacids (to reduce the degradation of the drug by gastric acid), tetracyclines, fluoroquinolones, or other drugs that interact with metals should not be administered within 2 hours of taking didanosine. Ketoconazole should be administered at least 2 hours before dosing with didanosine. Each tablet contains 15.7 mEq of magnesium, 264.5 mg of sodium, as well as a quantity of phenylalanine. Caution should be exercised in patients with significant renal impairment, on a sodium-restricted diet, and/or who are phenylketonuric.

Administration: Oral. Food reduces absorption by as much as 50%; therefore, the drug should be administered on an empty stomach (i.e., having nothing to eat or drink, except water, for 1 hour before and 1–2 hours after taking the drug). Each dose of the tablet formulation must consist of 2 tablets to achieve adequate acid-neutralizing capacity for maximal absorption. The tablets should be thoroughly chewed, manually crushed, or dispersed in water. The buffered powder for oral solution is provided in packets, the contents of which should be poured into a container with about 4 oz of water. The drug must not be mixed with fruit juice or other acid-containing liquid. The pediatric powder for oral solution is initially constituted with purified water, to which the pharmacist then adds an appropriate quantity of an antacid (Mylanta Double Strength Liquid or Maalox TC Suspension). Videx® EC capsules should be swallowed whole; the capsules should not be opened.

Preparations: Chewable/dispersible buffered tablets, 25, 50, 100, and 150 mg. Packets of powder for oral solution, 100, 167, 250, and 375 mg. Bottles of pediatric powder for oral solution, 2 and 4 g. Sustained-release capsules, 125, 200, 250, and 400 mg.

DIDREX®, see Benzphetamine

DIDRONEL®, see Etidronate

DIENESTROL

Description/Actions: Estrogen indicated for intravaginal use in the treatment of atrophic vaginitis and kraurosis vulvae.

Preparations: Vaginal cream, 0.01%.

DIETHYLPROPION HYDROCHLORIDE—Tenuate®, Tepanil®

Description/Actions: Anorexiant indicated in the management of exogenous obesity as a short-term adjunct in a regimen of weight reduction based on caloric restriction.

Preparations: Tablets, 25 mg. Controlled-release tablets, 75 mg.

DIETHYLSTILBESTROL—DES DIETHYLSTILBESTROL DIPHOSPHATE—Stilphostrol®

Description/Actions: Estrogen indicated in the treatment of moderate to severe vasomotor symptoms associated with menopause, atrophic vaginitis, kraurosis vulvae, female hypogonadism, female castration, primary ovarian failure, and breast cancer. Both oral and parenteral (diphosphate) dosage forms are indicated in the treatment of prostatic carcinoma.

Preparations: Tablets, 1 and 5 mg. Enteric-coated tablets, 0.1, 1, and 5 mg. Tablets (diphosphate), 50 mg. Ampules (diphosphate), 250 mg/5 ml.

DIFENOXIN HYDROCHLORIDE/ATROPINE SULFATE—Motofen®

Description/Actions: Difenoxin is the principal active metabolite of diphenoxylate. A subtherapeutic dose of atropine is included in the formulation to discourage abuse of difenoxin. Indicated as adjunctive therapy in the management of diarrhea.

Precautions/Adverse Reactions: Contraindicated in patients with diarrhea associated with pseudomembranous colitis. Is also contraindicated in children under 2 years of age because of an increased risk of adverse reactions. Adverse reactions include drowsiness and other CNS effects Patients should be cautioned regarding activities such as driving and operating machinery, as well as interactions with other CNS-acting drugs including alcohol. Should not be administered to patients being treated with a monoamine oxidase inhibitor. Is included in Schedule IV.

Administration: Oral.

Preparations: Tablets containing 1 mg difenoxin hydrochloride and 0.025 mg atropine sulfate.

DIFFERIN®, see Adapalene

DIFLORASONE DIACETATE—Florone®, Maxiflor®

Description/Actions: Corticosteroid used topically in the treatment of corticosteroid-responsive dermatoses.

Preparations: Cream and ointment, 0.05%.

DIFLUCAN®, see Fluconazole

DIFLUNISAL—Dolobid®

Description/Actions: A salicylate analogue that exhibits analgesic, anti-pyretic, and anti-inflammatory effects. Indicated for the treatment of mild to moderate pain, rheumatoid arthritis, and osteoarthritis.

Precautions/Adverse Reactions: Contraindicated in patients in whom acute asthmatic attacks, urticaria, or rhinitis are precipitated by aspirin or other nonsteroidal anti-inflammatory drugs. May cause GI effects, so use should be avoided in patients with active GI tract disease and closely supervised in patients with a previous history of such disorders. Other adverse reactions include headache and rash. Effect may be reduced by antacids.

Administration: Oral.

Preparations: Tablets, 250 and 500 mg.

DIGIBIND®, see Digoxin Immune FAB

DIGITALIS

Description/Actions: Cardiac glycosides primarily used in the treatment of congestive heart failure.

Preparations: Tablets, 100 mcg.

DIGITOXIN

Description/Actions: Cardiac glycoside indicated in the treatment of heart failure, atrial flutter, atrial fibrillation, and supraventricular tachycardia.

Preparations: Tablets, 0.1 and 0.2 mg.

DIGOXIN—Lanoxicaps®, Lanoxin®

Description/Actions: Cardiac (digitalis) glycoside that exhibits a positive inotropic action and also causes a slowing of heart rate and decreased conduction velocity through the AV node. Indicated in the management of heart failure, atrial fibrillation, atrial flutter, and paroxysmal atrial tachycardia.

Precautions/Adverse Reactions: Contraindicated in patients in ventricular fibrillation. May cause serious cardiac toxicity (e.g., arrhythmias), and therapy must be closely supervised. Other adverse reactions include anorexia, nausea, and vomiting, visual disturbances, headache, weakness, apathy, psychosis, and gynecomastia. Certain diuretics and corticosteroids may cause potassium depletion and increase the risk of digoxin toxicity. Simultaneous administration of antacids, cholestyramine, or colestipol may reduce absorption, and as long an interval as possible should separate the administration of digoxin and one of these agents.

Administration: Oral, intravenous, and intramuscular.

Preparations: Tablets, 0.125, 0.25, and 0.5 mg. Liquid in caps, 0.05, 0.1, and 0.2 mg. Elixir (pediatric), 0.05 mg/ml. Ampules, 0.1 mg/ml (pediatric) and 0.25 mg/ml. Elixir 0.05 mg/ml.

DIGOXIN IMMUNE FAB (OVINE)—Digibind®

Description/Actions: Antidote for digoxin toxicity. Indicated for the treatment of potentially life-threatening digoxin or digitoxin intoxication.

Precautions/Adverse Reactions: A potential for hypersensitivity reactions exists. Low cardiac output states and congestive heart failure may be exacerbated by the withdrawal of the inotropic effects of digoxin. Hypokalemia may result from the rapid reversal of the hyperkalemia associated with digoxin intoxication, and potassium concentrations should be monitored closely.

Administration: Intravenous.

Preparations: Vials, 40 mg.

DIHYDROCODEINE BITARTRATE

Description/Actions: Opioid analgesic indicated for the relief of moderate to moderately severe pain. Used in combination with other analgesics.

DIHYDROERGOTAMINE MESYLATE—DHE 45®

Description/Actions: Vasoconstrictor administered parenterally to abort or prevent vascular headaches (e.g., migraine). In conjunction with low-dose heparin to prevent postoperative deep vein thrombosis and pulmonary embolism.

Preparations: Ampules, 1 mg.

DIHYDROTACHYSTEROL—DHT®, Hytakerol®

Description/Actions: Vitamin D analogue indicated for the treatment of hypoparathyroidism, postoperative tetany, and idiopathic tetany.

Preparations: Capsules, 0.125 mg. Tablets, 0.125, 0.2, and 0.4 mg. Solution, 0.2 mg/5 ml. Concentrated solution, 0.2 mg/ml. Solution in oil, 0.25 mg/ml.

DILACOR XR®, see Diltiazem

DILANTIN®, see Phenytoin

DILAUDID®, see Hydromorphone

DILOR®, see Dyphylline

DILTIAZEM HYDROCHLORIDE—Cardizem®, Cardizem CD®, Cardizem LA®, Cardizem SR®, Dilacor XR®, Tiazac®

Description/Actions: Is a calcium channel-blocking agent that is indicated in the treatment of (a) angina pectoris due to coronary artery spasm; (b) chronic stable angina in patients who cannot tolerate therapy with beta-blockers and/or nitrates or who remain symptomatic despite adequate doses of these agents; (c) hypertension (Cardizem SR, Cardizem CD, Dilacor XR); (d) atrial fibrillation or flutter (intravenously); and (e) paroxysmal supraventricular tachycardia (intravenously).

Precautions/Adverse Reactions: Contraindicated in patients with sick sinus syndrome (except in the presence of a functioning ventricular pacemaker), second- or third-degree AV block, and hypotension. Adverse reactions include edema, headache, nausea, dizziness, and rash. Although usually well tolerated, concomitant therapy with a beta-adrenergic blocking agent or digitalis glycoside should be monitored closely because there may be additive effects in prolonging AV conduction.

Administration: Oral and intravenous.

Preparations: Tablets, 30, 60, 90, and 120 mg. Long-acting tablets, 120, 180, 240, and 300 mg (Cardizem LA). Sustained-release capsules, 60, 90, and 120 mg (Cardizem SR); 120, 180, 240, and 300 mg and 360 mg (Cardizem CD); 180 and 240 mg (Dilacor XR); 120, 180, 240, 300, 360, and 420 mg (Tiazac). Vials, 25 and 50 mg.

DIMENHYDRINATE—Dramamine®

Description/Actions: Antinauseant/antiemetic indicated for the prevention and treatment of the nausea, vomiting, or vertigo of motion sickness. When used for prophylaxis of motion sickness, administer at least 30 minutes and preferably 1–2 hr before exposure to conditions that may precipitate motion sickness.

Preparations: Tablets and capsules, 50 mg. Extended-release capsules, 25 mg. Chewable tablets, 50 mg. Liquid, 12.5 mg/4 ml. Elixir, 12.5 mg/5 ml and 15 mg/5 ml. Ampules and vials, 50 mg/ml. Suppositories, 50 mg.

DIMERCAPROL—BAL

Description/Actions: Antidote indicated in the parenteral treatment of arsenic, gold, and mercury poisoning. As an adjunct with edetate calcium disodium in the treatment of severe lead poisoning accompanied by encephalopathy.

Preparations: Ampules, 100 mg/ml.

DIMETANE®, see Brompheniramine

DIMETHYL SULFOXIDE—Rimso-50®, DMSO

Description/Actions: Agent for symptomatic relief of interstitial cystitis and is instilled directly into the bladder. Is being evaluated for the topical treatment of conditions such as scleroderma and a wide range of musculoskeletal disorders. Also used to protect living cells and tissues during cold storage (cryoprotection).

Preparations: Aqueous solution, 50%.

DINOPROST TROMETHAMINE—Prostaglandin F_2 alpha, Prostin F_2 alpha®

Description/Actions: Abortifacient injected into the amniotic sac for the termination of pregnancy during the period from 16–20 gestational weeks.

Preparations: Ampules, 5 mg/ml.

DINOPROSTONE—Prostaglandin E$_2$, Cervidil®, Prepidil®, Prostin E$_2$®

Description/Actions: Abortifacient (Prostin E$_2$) indicated for intravaginal use for the termination of pregnancy during the period from 12–20 gestational weeks. Used for the evacuation of the uterine content in the management of missed abortion or intrauterine fetal death up to 28 weeks gestational age. Indicated in the management of nonmetastatic gestational trophoblastic disease (benign hydatiform mole).

Agent for cervical ripening (Cervidil®, Prepidil®): used to ripen an unfavorable cervix in pregnant women at or near term with a medical or obstetrical need for labor induction.

Preparations: Vaginal suppositories (Prostin E$_2$), 20 mg. Gel (Prepidil), 0.5 mg. Vaginal insert (Cervidil®), 10 mg.

DIOVAN®, see Valsartan

DIOVAN HCT®—Combination Agent Valsartan and Hydrochlorothiazide (Angiotensin II Receptor Antagonist and Diuretic) see individual discussion on Valsartan and Hydrochlorothiazide

DIPENTUM®, see Olsalazine Sodium

DIPHENHYDRAMINE HYDROCHLORIDE—Benadryl®, Benylin Cough®, Nytol®, Sominex®

Description/Actions: Antihistamine, hypnotic, and antitussive used in the treatment of various allergic disorders, management of cough, treatment of insomnia, prevention of motion sickness, and drug-induced Parkinson's disease or dystonic reactions.

Preparations: Capsules and tablets, 25 and 50 mg. Chewable tablets, 25 mg. Liquid, 12.5 mg/5 ml. Ampules and vials, 10 and 50 mg/ml. Cream and gel, 1%, 2%. Spray, 1%.

DIPHENATOL, see Diphenoxylate Hydrochloride with Atropine Sulfate

DIPHENIDOL—Vontrol®

Description/Actions: Antiemetic indicated in the treatment of peripheral vertigo and associated nausea and vomiting, and in the control of nausea and vomiting as seen in conditions such as postoperative states, malignant neoplasms, and labyrinth disturbances.

Preparations: Tablets, 25 mg.

DIPHENOXYLATE HYDROCHLORIDE WITH ATROPINE SULFATE—Lomotil®, Diphenatol®, Lofene®, Lomanate®, Lonox®, Lo-Trol®, Low Qual®, Nor-Mil®

Description/Actions: Diphenoxylate is structurally related to meperidine. Indicated as adjunctive therapy in the management of diarrhea.

Precautions/Adverse Reactions: Contraindicated in patients with obstructive jaundice, and in diarrhea associated with pseudomembranous enterocolitis. Adverse reactions include drowsiness and other CNS effects. Patients should be cautioned regarding activities such as driving and operating machinery, as well as interactions with other CNS-acting drugs including alcohol. Effects attributed to the atropine include dry mouth. Use is not recommended for children under 2 years of age because of an increased risk of adverse reactions. Should not be administered to patients being treated with a monoamine oxidase inhibitor. Is included in Schedule V.

Administration: Oral.

Preparations: Tablets and liquid. Each tablet and 5 ml of liquid contains 2.5 mg and 0.025 mg atropine sulfate.

DIPHENYLHYDANTOIN—former name for Phenytoin

DIPIVEFRIN HYDROCHLORIDE—Propine®

Description/Actions: Sympathomimetic agent. A prodrug that is converted to epinephrine following administration. Indicated for ophthalmic use in the treatment of chronic open-angle glaucoma.

Preparations: Ophthalmic solution, 0.1%.

DIPRIVAN®, see Propofol

DIPROLENE®, see Betamethasone Dipropionate Augmented

DIPROLENE AF®, see Betamethasone Dipropionate Augmented

DIPROSONE®, see Betamethasone Dipropionate

DIPYRIDAMOLE—Persantine®, Persantine IV®

Description/Actions: Indicated as an adjunct to coumarin anticoagulants in the prevention of postoperative thromboembolic complications of cardiac valve replacement. Also indicated for intravenous use as an alternative to exercise in thallium myocardial perfusion imaging for the evaluation of coronary artery disease in patients who cannot exercise regularly.

Precautions/Adverse Reactions: Adverse reactions include dizziness, abdominal distress, headache, and rash.

Administration: Oral and intravenous.

Preparations: Tablets, 25, 50, and 75 mg. Ampules, 10 mg/2 ml.

DIRITHROMYCIN—Dynabac®

Description/Actions: Anti-infective agent. Macrolide antibiotic indicated in the treatment of mild to moderate susceptible infections including acute and chronic bronchitis, secondary bacterial infection of acute bronchitis, community acquired pneumonia, pharyngitis/tonsillitis, uncomplicated skin and skin structure infections. Should not be used in patients with bacteremia.

Precautions/Adverse Reactions: Adverse reactions include abdominal pain, headache, GI upset, dizziness, pain, asthenia, cough, rash, dyspnea, pruritus, insomnia, blood dyscrasias, electrolyte imbalance, and pseudomembranous colitis.

Administration: Oral. Take with food. Do not crush, chew, or cut.

Preparations: Enteric-coated tablets, 250 mg.

DISALCID®, see Salsalate

DISODIUM EDTA®, see Edetate

DISOPYRAMIDE PHOSPHATE—Norpace®, Norpace CR®

Description/Actions: Antiarrhythmic agent indicated for the prevention and suppression of premature ventricular contractions and episodes of ventricular tachycardia.

Preparations: Capsules and controlled-release capsules, 100 and 150 mg.

DISOTATE, see Edetate

DI-SPAZ®, see Dicyclomine Hydrochloride

DISPERMOX®, see Amoxiciilin

DISULFIRAM—Antabuse®

Description/Actions: Agent for alcoholism indicated as an aid in the management of selected chronic alcoholic patients who want to remain in a state of enforced sobriety.

Preparations: Tablets, 250 and 500 mg.

DITHRANOL, see Anthralin

DITROPAN® and **DITROPAN XL®**, see Oxybutynin

DIUCARDIN®, see Hydroflumethiazide

DIURIL®, see Chlorothiazide

DIVALPROEX SODIUM, see Valproic Acid

DMSO®, see Dimethyl Sulfoxide

DOAN'S PILLS®, see Magnesium Salicylate

DOBUTAMINE HYDROCHLORIDE—Dobutrex®

Description/Actions: Inotropic catecholamine indicated in the short-term intravenous treatment of adults with cardiac decompensation due to depressed contractility resulting either from organic heart disease or from cardiac surgical procedures.

Preparations: Vials, 250 mg.

DOBUTREX®, see Dobutamine Hydrochloride

DOCETAXEL—Taxotere®

Description/Actions: Antineoplastic agent used for the treatment of patients with locally advanced or metastatic breast cancer after failure of prior chemotherapy. Docetaxel, in combination with doxorubicin and cyclophosphamide, is indicated for the adjuvant treatment of patients with operable node-positive breast cancer. Taxotere® as a single agent is indicated for the treatment of patients with locally advanced or metastatic nonsmall-cell lung cancer after failure of prior platinum-based chemotherapy. Docetaxel in combination with cisplatin is indicated for the treatment of patients with unresectable, locally advanced, or metastatic nonsmall-cell lung cancer who have not previously received chemotherapy for this condition. It is also indicated in combination with prednisone for the treatment of patients with androgen independent (hormone refractory) metastatic prostate cancer.

Precautions/Adverse Reactions: Contraindicated in patients with history of severe hypersensitivity reactions to docetaxel or to other drugs formulated with polysorbate 80 or neutrophil counts <1500 cells/mm3. Toxic deaths have occurred when docetaxel was administered at doses of 100 mg/m2 in patients with and without impaired liver function. Sepsis accounted for the majority of these deaths. Fatal GI bleeds in patients with severe liver impairment have been associated with drug-induced thrombocytopenia. Fluid retention, neutropenia, and cutaneous reactions have also been reported with docetaxel. Careful monitoring of blood counts, liver, and renal functions is recommended.

Administration: Intravenous.

Preparations: Injection, 20 and 80 mg in single dose vials with diluent.

DOCOSANOL 10% CREAM—Abreva®

Description/Actions: Docosanol is indicated in the treatment of herpes labialis of the lips or face.

Precautions/Adverse Reactions: Docosanol is contraindicated in patients with a hypersensitivity to docosanol or to any component of the product. For external use only. Use on lips and face only. Docosanol is not indicated for the treatment of genital herpes. Pregnancy Category B. Excretion in human breast milk is unknown. Adverse effects observed with docosanol were similar to those observed with placebo. Headache and dermatological effects (rash, pruritis, and dry skin) occurred most often.

Administration: Topical.

Patient Care Implications: Use at the first sign of a cold sore or fever blister. Wash hands prior to applying cream. Apply a thin layer, cover entire area, and rub until cream completely disappears. Wash hands after applying cream to prevent the spread of the virus.

Preparations: Cream, topical 10% in 2 g tubes.

DOCUSATE CALCIUM—Dioctyl Calcium Sulfosuccinate, Surfak®

DOCUSATE POTASSIUM—Dioctyl Potassium Sulfosuccinate

DOCUSATE SODIUM—DSS, Dioctyl Sodium
Sulfosuccinate, Colace®

Description/Actions: Stool softener used in the treatment of constipation due to hard stools.

Preparations: Docusate calcium—Capsules, 50 and 240 mg. Docusate potassium—Capsules, 100 and 240 mg. Docusate sodium—Capsules, 50, 100, and 240 mg. Liquid, 50, 60, and 150 mg/ml and other potencies.

DOFETILIDE—Tikosyn®

Description/Actions: Dofetilide is used for patients in atrial fibrillation/flutter. Used to convert and maintain normal sinus rhythm.

Precautions/Adverse Reactions: Dofetilide can cause a variety of arrhythmias including torsade de pointes and ventricular tachycardia. The drug is contraindicated in patients who already have QT prolongation (QTc >440 msec), torsade de pointes, renal failure (increases plasma concentration of drug), hypokalemia, and hypomagnesemia because of the increased risk of arrhythmias. Other side effects that can occur are headache, chest pain, and dizziness. Patients taking dofetilide should discontinue breast feeding, and the drug is not proven to be safe in children <18. Concomitant administration with cimetidine, ketoconazole, megestrol, prochlorperazine, trimethoprim, or verapamil is contraindicated. The concomitant use of dofetilide with hydrochlorothiazide (alone or in combinations such as with triamterene) is contraindicated due to increased dofetilide plasma concentrations and QT interval prolongation. The use of dofetilide in conjunction with other drugs (e.g., phenothiazines, cisapride, bepridil, tricyclic antidepressants, certain oral macrolides, and certain fluoroquinolones) that prolong the QT interval has not been studied and is not recommended.

Administration: Oral.

Patient Care Implications: Patients starting dofetilide should be kept in a monitored facility where ECG and creatinine clearance can be monitored and cardiac resuscitation can be performed. The dose of dofetilide must be adjusted based on creatinine clearance levels to avoid arrhythmias. Women taking the drug should discontinue breast-feeding, and the drug should not be used in children under 18 years of age.

Preparations: Capsule, 125 mcg, 250 mcg, and 500 mcg.

DOLASETRON MESYLATE—Anzemet®

Description/Actions: Dolasetron mesylate is indicated in the prevention of nausea and vomiting associated with emetogenic cancer chemotherapy, including initial and repeat courses. Also indicated in the prevention and treatment of post-op nausea and vomiting.

Precautions/Adverse Reactions: Use cautiously in patients at risk of developing prolongation of cardiac conduction intervals, especially Qtc (e.g., congenital QT syndrome, hypokalemia, hypomagnesemia). Pregnancy Category B. Not recommended for use in nursing mothers. Adverse reactions include headache, dizziness, pain, fatigue, diarrhea, tachycardia, and ECG changes.

Administration: Oral and intravenous.

Preparations: Tablets, 50 and 100 mg. Injection, single use ampules 12.5 mg/0.625 mL. Single use vials 100 mg/5 mL.

DOLOBID®, see Diflunisal

DOLOPHINE®, see Methadone

DONEPEZIL HYDROCHLORIDE—Aricept®, Aricept® ODT

Description/Actions: Reversible acetylcholinesterase inhibitor. Indicated in mild to moderate dementia of the Alzheimer's type.

Precautions/Adverse Reactions: Adverse reactions include nausea, diarrhea, insomnia, vomiting, muscle cramps, fatigue, and anorexia. Donepezil may have vagotonic effects on the sinoatrial and atrioventricular nodes. This effect may be seen as bradycardia or heart block in patients both with and without known underlying cardiac conduction abnormalities. Syncope and neuroleptic malignant syndrome have also been reported. Monitor for GI bleeding, seizures, and asthma.

Administration: Oral.

Preparations: Tablets, 5 and 10 mg. Orally disintegrating tablets, 5 and 10 mg.

DONNATAL®, Combination of Belladonna Alkaloids and Phenobarbital. See individual discussion on Belladonna and Phenobarbital

DOPAMINE HYDROCHLORIDE—Intropin®

Description/Actions: Inotropic catecholamine indicated for intravenous use in the correction of hemodynamic imbalances present in the shock syndrome due to myocardial infarctions, trauma, endotoxic septicemia, open heart surgery, renal failure, and chronic cardiac decompensation as in congestive failure.

Preparations: Ampules, vials, and syringes, 40, 80, and 160 mg/ml. Bottles (in 5% dextrose), 80, 160, and 320 mg/100 ml.

DOPAR®, see Levodopa

DORIGLUTE®, see Glutethimide

DOPRAM®, see Doxapram

DORAL®, see Quazepam

DORNASE ALFA—Pulmozyme®

Description/Actions: Mucolytic agent for cystic fibrosis. Is a recombinant form of natural human deoxyribonuclease I (also known as DNase), and contains 260 amino acids in a sequence that is identical to that of the native human enzyme. Is administered by inhalation of an aerosol mist and selectively breaks down extracellular DNA, making the accumulated respiratory secretions less viscous and easier to clear. Indicated for daily use in conjunction with standard therapies in the management of cystic fibrosis patients to reduce the frequency of respiratory infections requiring parenteral antibiotics, and to improve pulmonary function.

Precautions/Adverse Reactions: Adverse reactions include sore throat, hoarseness, laryngitis, chest pain, rash, and conjunctivitis.

Administration: Inhalation, using a recommended nebulizer. The drug should not be diluted or mixed with other drugs in the nebulizer.

Preparations: Ampules, 2.5 mg in 2.5 ml of a sterile aqueous solution.

DORYX®, see Doxycycline

DORZOLAMIDE HYDROCHLORIDE—Trusopt®

Description/Actions: Carbonic anhydrase inhibitor indicated in the treatment of elevated intraocular pressure in patients with ocular hypertension or open-angle glaucoma.

Precautions/Adverse Reactions: Adverse reactions include ocular burning, stinging, or discomfort and bitter taste following administration. Superficial punctate keratitis, and signs and symptoms of ocular allergic reaction may also occur. Use is not recommended in patients with a creatinine clearance of less than 30 ml/min or concurrently with orally administered carbonic anhydrase inhibitor. Do not administer while wearing soft contact lenses, as the formulation contains benzalkonium chloride as a preservative, which may damage soft contact lenses.

Administration: Ophthalmic.

Preparations: Ophthalmic solution, 2%.

DOSTINEX®, see Cabergoline

DOVONEX®, see Calcipotriene

DOXACURIUM CHLORIDE—Nuromax®

Description/Actions: Nondepolarizing neuromuscular blocking agent that acts by competing for cholinergic receptors at the motor end-plate, resulting in a block of neuromuscular transmission. Has a long duration of action. Indicated as an adjunct to general anesthesia to provide skeletal muscle relaxation during surgery. Also used to provide skeletal muscle relaxation for endotracheal intubation.

Precautions/Adverse Reactions: May cause excessive skeletal muscle weakness resulting in respiratory insufficiency and apnea. Action may be antagonized by neostigmine. Must be used with caution in patients with myasthenia gravis or myasthenic syndrome, and in patients receiving other medications that may increase neuromuscular blockade (e.g., inhalation anesthetics, aminoglycosides, quinidine, magnesium salts).

Administration: Intravenous.

Preparations: Vials, 1 mg/ml.

DOXAPRAM HYDROCHLORIDE—Dopram®

Description/Actions: Respiratory stimulant indicated for intravenous use in the treatment of drug-induced central nervous system depression, chronic pulmonary disease associated with acute hypercapnia, postanesthesia respiratory depression, or apnea other than that due to muscle relaxant drugs.

Precautions/Adverse Reactions: Doxapram should not be used with mechanical ventilation. Pulse oximetry is recommended for assessing oxygenation. Monitor blood pressure, heart rate, and deep tendon reflexes. Doxapram contains the preservative benzyl alcohol, which has been associated with a fatal "gasping syndrome" in neonates. Therefore, doxapram is contraindicated in neonates. Anticonvulsants such as intravenous short-acting barbiturates along with oxygen resuscitative equipment should be readily available to manage overdosage.

Preparations: Vials, 20 mg/ml.

DOXAZOSIN MESYLATE—Cardura®

Description/Actions: An alpha$_1$-adrenergic blocking agent that acts on the peripheral vasculature to decrease systemic vascular resistance and lower blood pressure. Indicated for the treatment of hypertension and may be used alone or in combination with a diuretic or beta-adrenergic blocking agent. Also indicated for the treatment of benign prostatic hyperplasia.

Precautions/Adverse Reactions: May cause orthostatic hypotension, resulting in symptoms such as dizziness, lightheadedness, vertigo, and syncope. Orthostatic effects are more common with the first dose (i.e., the "first dose" effect). Treatment should be initiated at a dosage level of 1 mg daily. Patients should be advised of the need to sit or lie down when symptoms of lowered blood pressure occur, and to be careful when rising from a sitting or lying position. Other adverse reactions include edema, fatigue, and somnolence.

Administration: Oral.

Preparations: Tablets, 1, 2, 4, and 8 mg.

DOXEPIN HYDROCHLORIDE—Sinequan®, Zonalon®

Description/Actions: Tricyclic antidepressant indicated in patients with (a) depression and/or anxiety, (b) depression and/or anxiety associated with alcoholism, (c) depression and/or anxiety associated with organic disease, and (d) psychotic depressive disorders with associated anxiety including involutional depression and manic-depressive disorders. Also indicated for the short-term topical management of moderate pruritus in adults with atopic dermatitis and lichen simplex chronicus.

Precautions/Adverse Reactions: Contraindicated in patients with glaucoma or with a tendency to urinary retention. Should not be used in patients being treated with a monoamine oxidase inhibitor. Adverse reactions include CNS effects, and patients should be cautioned regarding activities such as driving and operating machinery, as well as interactions with other CNS-acting drugs including alcohol. Reportedly the most sedating of the tricyclic antidepressants. Other adverse reactions include anticholinergic effects (e.g., dry mouth, blurred vision), GI effects (e.g., nausea, vomiting), and cardiovascular effects (e.g., hypotension).

Administration: Oral and topical.

Preparations: Capsules, 10, 25, 50, 75, 100, and 150 mg. Oral concentrate, 10 mg/ml. Cream, 5%.

DOXERCALCIFEROL—Hectorol®

Description/Actions: Doxercalciferol is a synthetic vitamin D analogue that is used for the treatment of secondary hyperparathyroidism in patients receiving chronic renal dialysis.

Precautions/Adverse Reactions: Doxercalciferol should not be given to patients who are hypercalcemic, hyperphosphatemic, or hypervitaminosis D. Also doxercalciferol's safety has not been determined in children or in breast-feeding women. Patients with hepatic failure should be monitored closely. Some common side effects are edema, headache, malaise, nausea/vomiting, dizziness, dyspnea, confusion, constipation, increased thirst, and sinus bradycardia. Also, long-term use of the drug can lead to hypercalcemia, hyperphosphatemia, and ectopic calcifications.

Administration: Oral.

Patient Care Implications: Patients on the medication should be monitored weekly for PTH levels and calcium-phosphorus product. Also, patients should restrict intake of other vitamin D products while on the medication. Doxercalciferol should not be given to children, breast-feeding women, and pregnant women. Also, hepatic impairment patients should be monitored closely.

Preparations: Tablet, 2.5 mcg. Capsule, 0.5 mcg.

DOXORUBICIN HYDROCHLORIDE—Adriamycin PFS®, Adriamycin RDF®, Rubex®

Description/Actions: Antineoplastic agent indicated for intravenous use in the treatment of a number of neoplastic disorders such as acute lymphoblastic leukemia, acute myeloblastic leukemia, Wilms' tumor, neuroblastoma, soft tissue and bone sarcomas, breast carcinoma, ovarian carcinoma, transitional cell bladder carcinoma, thyroid carcinoma, lymphomas of both Hodgkin and non-Hodgkin types, and bronchogenic carcinoma. Serious, irreversible myocardial toxicity with delayed CHF, ventricular arrhythmias, and acute left ventricular failure may occur with use of this agent. Follow vesicant precautions for IV administration.

Precautions/Adverse Reactions: Myocardial damage may lead to congestive heart failure and may be encountered as the total cumulative dose of doxorubicin approaches 550 mg/m². Acute infusion related reactions including flushing, shortness of breath, facial swelling, headache, chills, back pain, tightness in the chest or throat, and/or hypotension have occurred in patients treated with doxorubicin. Serious and sometimes life-threatening or fatal allergic/anaphylactoid-like infusion reactions have been reported. Severe myelosuppression may occur. Dosage should be reduced in patients with impaired hepatic function.

Preparations: Vials, 10, 20, and 50 mg.

DOXYCYCLINE CALCIUM—Vibramycin®

Preparations: Syrup, 50 mg/5 ml.

DOXYCYCLINE HYCLATE—Doryx®, Vibramycin®, Vibra-Tabs®, Periostat®

Description/Actions: Tetracycline antibiotic active against many gram-positive and gram-negative bacteria, mycoplasmal, chlamydial, and rickettsial organisms, and certain spirochetes. Indicated in the treatment of respiratory tract infections, urinary tract infections, sexually transmitted infections, and a number of other types of infections. Effective in the treatment of infections caused by *Chlamydia trachomatis* and *Ureaplasma urealyticum*. Also indicated for prophylaxis of malaria due to *Plasmodium falciparum* in short-term travelers (less than 4 months) to areas with chloroquine or pyrimethaminesulfadoxine resistant strains.

Precautions/Adverse Reactions: Use is best avoided during the last half of pregnancy and in childhood to the age of 8 years because of the risk of discoloration of the teeth. Other adverse reactions include nausea, vomiting, diarrhea, rash, and fungal superinfections. May cause photosensitivity reactions, so patients should be cautioned to limit their exposure to sunlight and ultraviolet light. Absorption may be reduced by the simultaneous administration of antacids.

Administration: Oral and intravenous. May be administered orally without regard to meals.

Preparations: Tablets, 20 mg. Capsules and tablets, 50 and 100 mg. Delayed-release capsules, 100 mg. Oral suspension, 25 mg/5 ml. and 50 mg/5 ml. Vials, 100 and 200 mg.

DOXYCYCLINE MONOHYDRATE—Monodox®, Vibramycin®

Preparations: Capsules, 100 mg. Powder for oral suspension, 25 mg/5 ml when reconstituted.

DOXYLAMINE SUCCINATE—Unisom®

Description/Actions: Antihistamine and hypnotic. Primarily used for the treatment of insomnia.

Preparations: Tablets, 25 mg.

DRAMAMINE®, see Dimenhydrinate

DRISDOL®, see Ergocalciferol

DRONABINOL—Marinol®

Description/Actions: Antiemetic and appetite stimulant. Is the principal psychoactive substance in marijuana. Indicated for the treatment of nausea and vomiting associated with cancer chemotherapy in patients who have failed to respond adequately to conventional antiemetic treatments. Also indicated for the treatment of anorexia associated with weight loss in patients with AIDS.

Precautions/Adverse Reactions: Can produce physical and psychological dependence and is included in Schedule II of the Controlled Substances Act. CNS adverse reactions include drowsiness, dizziness, impairment of coordination, easy laughing, elation, hallucinations, and brief psychotic reactions.

Administration: Oral.

Preparations: Capsules, 2.5, 5, and 10 mg.

DROPERIDOL—Inapsine®

Description/Actions: Droperidol is indicated to reduce the incidence of nausea and vomiting associated with surgical and diagnostic procedures. It is not recommended for any other use other than for the treatment of perioperative nausea and vomiting in patients for whom other treatments are ineffective or inappropriate.

Precautions/Adverse Reactions: Droperidol is contraindicated in patients with a known hypersensitivity to any component of the formulation. It is contraindicated in patients with a known or suspected QT prolongation (QTc interval greater than 440 msec for males or 450 msec for females), including patients with congenital long QT syndrome. Cases of QT prolongation and serious arrhythmias (torsades de pointes, ventricular arrhythmias, cardiac arrest, and death) have been reported in patients receiving droperidol at doses at or below recommended doses. Some cases have occurred in patients with no known risk factors for QT prolongation. A dose-dependent prolongation of the QT interval has been observed in clinical trials. Droperidol should be administered with extreme caution to patients who may be at risk for development of prolonged QT syndrome, for example, congestive heart failure, bradycardia, use of a diuretic, cardiac hypertrophy, hypokalemia, hypomagnesemia, or administration of other drugs known to increase the QT interval. Other risk factors may include age >65, alcohol abuse, and use of agents such as benzodiazepines, volatile anesthetics, and IV opiates. Droperidol should be initiated at a low dose and adjusted upward with caution to achieve the desired effect. All patients should undergo a 12-lead ECG prior to administration of droperidol to determine if a prolonged QT interval is present. If there is a prolonged QT interval, droperidol should not be used. For patients in whom the potential benefit of droperidol treatment outweighs the potential risks of serious arrhythmias, ECG monitoring should be performed prior to treatment and continued for 2–3 hours after completing treatment to monitor for arrhythmias. Droperidol should not be administered with drugs known to prolong the QT interval, such as class I or class III antiarrhythmics, antihistamines that prolong the QT interval, antimalarials, calcium channel blockers, neuroleptics that prolong the QT interval, and antidepressants. Exercise caution when using droperidol with drugs known to induce hypokalemia or hypomagnesemia (diuretics, laxatives, supraphysiological use of steroid hormones with mineralocorticoid potential) as they may precipitate QT prolongation. Concomitant administration of droperidol and central nervous system depressant drugs, such as barbiturates, tranquilizers, opioids, and general anesthetics, requires a reduction in the dose of the CNS depressant drug.

Administration: IM or slow IV.

Patient Care Implications: ECG monitoring prior to treatment and continued for 2–3 hours after completing treatment to monitor for arrhythmias. Physicians should be alert to palpitations, syncope, or other symptoms suggestive of episodes of irregular cardiac rhythm and promptly evaluate these patients. Monitor vital signs. Fluids and other countermeasures to manage hypotension should be readily available.

Preparations: Ampules and vials 2.5 mg/ml.

DROTRECOGIN ALFA—Xigris™

Description/Actions: Drotrecogin alfa (activated) is indicated for the reduction of mortality in adult patients with severe sepsis (sepsis associated with acute organ dysfunction) who have a high risk of death (e.g., APACHE II score ≥25).

Precautions/Adverse Reactions: Drotrecogin alfa is contraindicated in anyone with a known hypersensitivity to it or to any component of the formulation. Drotrecogin alfa increases the risk of bleeding; therefore, it is contraindicated in patients with the following clinical situations in which bleeding could be associated with a high risk of death or significant morbidity: active internal bleeding, recent (within 3 months) hemorrhagic stroke, recent (within 2 months) intracranial or intraspinal surgery or severe head trauma, trauma with an increased risk of life-threatening bleeding, presence of an epidural catheter, intracranial neoplasm or mass lesion, or evidence of cerebral herniation. Clinical trials have shown an increased incidence of all-cause mortality in patients with single organ dysfunction and recent surgery treated with drotrecogin alfa. Patients with single organ dysfunction and recent surgery may not be at high risk of death irrespective of Apache II score and therefore, may not be among the indicated population. Xigris™ should be used in these patients only after careful consideration of the risks and benefits. Xigris™ may prolong the activated partial thromboplastin time (aPTT); therefore, its use to access the status of the coagulopathy during drotrecogin alfa infusion is not reliable. The most common adverse reaction associated with the use of drotrecogin alfa is bleeding. Bleeding may occur from any site. Some common sites include gastrointestinal, intra-abdominal, intrathoracic, retroperitoneal, intracranial, genitourinary, and skin/soft tissue (patients requiring the administration of ≥3 units of packed red blood cells per day for 2 consecutive days without an identified site of bleeding). There is no known antidote for drotrecogin alfa. In cases of overdose, stop the infusion and monitor closely for hemorrhagic complications.

Administration: Intravenous.

Patient Care Implications: Monitor patient for bleeding. Xigris should be administered via a dedicated line. The only solutions that can be administered through the same line are 0.9% sodium chloride injection, lactated Ringer's injection, dextrose, or dextrose and saline mixtures.

Preparations: Powder for injection (preservative free), 5 and 20 mg.

DTIC®, see Dacarbazine

DUAC™, see Clindamycin and Benzoyl Peroxide

DULCOLAX® see Bisacodyl

DURABOLIN®, see Nandrolone

DURAGESIC®, see Fentanyl

DURALUTIN®, see Hydroxyprogesterone

DURAMORPH®, see Morphine

DURANEST®, see Etidocaine

DURICEF®, see Cefadroxil

DUTASTERIDE—Avodart™

Description/Actions: Dutasteride is indicated for the treatment of symptomatic benign prostatic hyperplasia in men with enlarged prostates 18 years of age or older.

Precautions/Adverse Reactions: Dutasteride is contraindicated for use in women and children. Pregnancy Category X. Because it is absorbed through the skin, handling of the drug should be avoided by any pregnant woman. Preclinical data suggest that the suppression of circulating levels of DHT may inhibit the development of the external genital organs in a male fetus carried by a woman exposed to dutasteride.

Other urological diseases including cancer should be ruled out before starting therapy. Use caution in hepatic impairment and with the concurrent use of potent chronic CYP3A3/4 inhibitors. Dutasteride is not indicated for use in the pediatric population; safety and efficacy have not been established in this population. Most common adverse reaction was sexual dysfunction. This may include impotence, decreased libido, ejaculation disorders, and gynecomastia.

Administration: Oral.

Patient Care Implications: May be taken with or without food. Capsule should be swallowed whole. Dutasteride is a soft gelatin capsule that may become soft and leak or stick to other capsules if kept at high temperatures. Store at room temperature. If capsules are cracked or leaking, do not use them. Do not donate blood for at least 6 months after last dose to prevent administration of dutasteride to a pregnant transfusion recipient. A new baseline PSA concentration should be established after 3–6 months of treatment. Results may take several months.

Preparations: Capsules, soft gelatin, 0.5 mg.

DYAZIDE®, Combination of Triamterene and Hydrochlorothiazide

DYCILL®, see Dicloxacillin

DYCLONE®, see Dyclonine

DYCLONINE HYDROCHLORIDE—Dyclone®

Description/Actions: Local anesthetic used primarily for anesthetizing mucous membranes (e.g., mouth, pharynx) prior to endoscopic procedures. Also used to suppress gag reflex, to relieve pain of minor burns or trauma, and to alleviate itching of pruritis ani or vulvae.

Preparations: Topical solution, 0.5% and 1%.

DYFLEX®, see Dyphylline

DYLLINE®, see Dyphylline

DYMELOR®, see Acetohexamide

DYNABAC®, see Dirithromycin

DynaCirc®, see Isradipine

DYNAPEN®, see Dicloxacillin

DYPHYLLINE—Dilor®, Dyflex®, Dylline®, Lufyllin®, Neothylline, Thylline

Description/Actions: Bronchodilator related to theophylline. Indicated for relief of acute bronchial asthma and for reversible bronchospasm associated with chronic bronchitis and emphysema.

Preparations: Tablets, 200 and 400 mg. Elixir, 33.3 mg/5 ml, 53.3 mg/5 ml, and 100 mg/15 ml. Injection, 250 mg/ml.

DYRENIUM®, see Triamterene

E

EASPRIN®, see Aspirin

ECHOTHIOPHATE IODIDE—Phospholine iodide®

Description/Actions: Antiglaucoma agent, cholinesterase inhibitor indicated for ophthalmic use in the treatment of glaucoma and accommodative esotropia. Use is usually reserved for patients not satisfactorily controlled by less potent miotics.

Preparations: For ophthalmic solution, 1.5 mg (0.03%), 3 mg (0.06%), 6.25 mg (0.125%), and 12.5 mg (0.25%) when reconstituted.

EC-NAPROSYN®, see Naproxen

ECONAZOLE NITRATE—Spectazole®

Description/Actions: Imidazole antifungal agent indicated for topical use in the treatment of tinea pedis, tinea cruris, tinea corporis, cutaneous candidiasis, and tinea versicolor.

Preparations: Cream, 1%.

ECOTRIN®, see Aspirin

EDECRIN®, see Ethacrynic Acid

EDETATE CALCIUM DISODIUM—EDTA, Calcium EDTA, Calcium Disodium Versenate®

Description/Actions: Antidote indicated in the parenteral management of acute and chronic lead poisoning and lead encephalopathy.

Preparations: Ampules, 200 mg/ml.

EDETATE DISODIUM—Disotate®, Disodium EDTA®, Endrate®

Description/Actions: Indicated in selected patients for the emergency treatment of hypercalcemia and for the control of ventricular arrhythmias associated with digitalis toxicity.

Preparations: Ampules and vials, 150 mg/ml.

EDEX®, see Alprostadil

EDROPHONIUM CHLORIDE—Enlon®, Tensilon®, Reversol®

Description/Actions: Cholinesterase inhibitor administered parenterally for the differential diagnosis of myasthenia gravis and as an adjunct in the evaluation of treatment requirements in this disease. Also useful when a curare antagonist is needed to reverse the neuromuscular block produced by tubocurarine and related agents.

Preparations: Ampules and vials, 10 mg/ml.

EDTA, see Edetate Calcium Disodium

EES®, see Erythromycin Ethylsuccinate

EFALIZUMAB Raptiva™

Description/Actions: Efalizumab is a monoclonal antibody indicated for the treatment of adult patients (18 years or older) with moderate to severe plaque psoriasis who are candidates for systemic therapy or phototherapy. Efalizumab binds to CD11a, a subunit of leukocyte function antigen-1 (LFA-1) found on leukocytes. By binding to CD11a, efalizumab blocks multiple T-cell mediated responses involved in the pathogenesis of psoriatic plaques.

Precautions/Adverse Reactions: Efalizumab is contraindicated in patients hypersensitive to efalizumab or any of the formulation's components. Efalizumab is an immunosuppressant and has the potential to increase the risk of infection and reactivate latent, chronic infections. Use caution with chronic infections, history of recurrent infection, or the elderly. Discontinue if serious infection develops. Thrombocytopenia occurred in clinical trials; follow patients closely for signs and symptoms of thrombocytopenia. Platelet counts should be obtained upon initiation of treatment and monthly during treatment. Worsening of psoriasis can occur during or after discontinuation of efalizumab. First-dose reactions that include headache, chills, fever, nausea, and myalgia are associated with efalizumab; they are dose-level related.

Concomitant use with other immunosuppressant agents and vaccines is not recommended. Pregnancy Category C. Excretion in breast milk unknown; breast-feeding not recommended. Most common adverse reactions were first-dose reaction that occurred within 2 days of the first injection (e.g., lymphocytosis, pain, myalgia, and weakness).

Administration: Subcutaneous.

Patient Care Implications: Inform patient he/she may experience dizziness and sedation. Monitor for signs of infections, worsening of psoriasis, and signs of low platelet count and inform physician.

Preparations: Injection: Lyophilized, sterile powder for reconstitution: 150 mg (delivers 125 mg/1.25 mL).

EFAVIRENZ—Sustiva®

Description/Actions: Indicated for use in combination with other antiretroviral agents for the treatment of HIV-1 infection. Efavirenz should always be initiated in combination with one other antiretroviral agent to which the patient has not already been exposed.

Precautions/Adverse Reactions: Coadministration with astemizole, cisapride, midazolam, triazolam, ergot derivatives, or voriconazole is contraindicated. Concomitant use with St. John's Wort or St. John's Wort-containing products is not recommended. Use cautiously in patients with CNS disturbances and hepatic dysfunction. Monitor liver function and lipid levels in patients with hepatitis. Discontinue the medication if severe rash (with blistering, desquamation, mucosal involvement, or fever) occurs. Exclude pregnancy before starting. Adverse reactions include CNS/psychiatric effects (e.g. insomnia, drowsiness, dizziness, depression, abnormal thinking, impaired concentration, confusion, abnormal dreaming), rash (possibly severe, e.g., Stevens-Johnson, erythema multiforme), GI upset, fever, and cough.

Administration: Oral.

Patient Care Implications: Administer at bedtime for the first 2 weeks to minimize CNS effects. May be taken without regard to food, but avoid taking with a high fat meal. Instruct patients to use appropriate barrier precautions and contraceptives when engaging in sexual intercourse as this medication controls but does not cure HIV.

Preparations: Capsules, 50, 100, and 200 mg. Tablets, 600 mg.

EFEDRON®, see Ephedrine

EFFEXOR®, see Venlafaxine Hydrochloride

EFFEXOR® XR, see Venlafaxine Hydrochloride

EFIDAC/24®, see Pseudoephedrine Hydrochloride

EFLORNITHINE (Topical)—Vaniqa™

Description/Actions: Vaniqa™ is a topical skin product indicated for the reduction of unwanted facial hair and hair in or on adjacent areas under the chin in women.

Precautions/Adverse Reactions: Usage is contraindicated in patients with a hypersensitivity to eflornithine or any component of the formulation. Discontinue if hypersensitivity occurs. For external use only; not for ophthalmic, oral, or intravaginal use. Pregnancy Category C. There are no adequate and well-controlled studies of topical eflornithine cream in pregnant women. The potential risks to the fetus versus the benefit of the medication to the mother should be considered before use. Excretion into breast milk is unknown. Exercise caution when administering to nursing women. Safety and efficacy in children <12 years have not been established. Some adverse effects (topical): acne, pseudofolliculitis barbe, headache, dizziness, vertigo, pruritus, burning skin, tingling skin, dry skin, skin irritation, and dyspepsia.

Administration: Topical.

Patient Care Implications: Patients should be informed of the following: 1. This medication is not a depilatory, but appears to retard hair growth to improve appearance. Patients will likely need to continue using a hair removal method in conjunction with Vaniqa™. 2. Onset of improvement was seen after as little as 4–8 weeks of treatment; the condition may return to pretreatment levels 8 weeks after cessation of treatment. 3. If skin irritation develops, direct the patient to temporarily reduce the frequency of application (i.e., once daily); if irritation persists, discontinue therapy.

Preparations: Topical cream: 13.9% (30 g) tube.

EFUDEX®, see Fluorouracil

ELAVIL®, see Amitriptyline

ELASE®, see Fibrinolysin

ELDEPRYL®, see Selegiline

ELDOQUIN®, see Hydroquinone

ELESTAT™, see Epinastine

ELETRIPTAN HYDROBROMIDE—Relpax®

Description/Actions: Eletriptan is indicated for the acute treatment of migraines with or without aura in adults. It is not intended for the prophylactic therapy of migraine or for use in the management of hemiplegic or basilar migraine. Safety and effectiveness have not been established for cluster headaches, which occur in an older, predominantly male population.

Precautions/Adverse Reactions: Eletriptan is contraindicated in patients hypersensitive to eletriptan or any component of the formulation; patients with ischemic heart disease (e.g., angina pectoris, history of myocardial infarction, or documented silent ischemia) or patients who have symptoms or findings consistent with ischemic heart disease, coronary artery vasospasm, or other significant underlying cardiovascular disease. Eletriptan should not be given to patients with cerebrovascular syndromes, including (but not limited to) strokes of any type as well as transient ischemic attacks. It should not be given to patients with peripheral vascular disease, including (but not limited to) ischemic bowel disease. Eletriptan may elevate blood pressure. It should not be given to patients with uncontrolled hypertension. Do not give to patients with hemiplegic or basilar migraine. Do not use within 24 hours of treatment with another 5-HT1 agonist, ergotamine-containing or ergot-type medication such as dihydroergotamine (DHE) or methysergide. Eletriptan should not be used within at least 72 hours of treatment with the following potent CYP3A4 inhibitors: ketoconazole, itraconazole, nefazodone, troleandomycin, clarithromycin, ritonavir, and nelfinavir. CYP3A4 inhibitors increase serum concentration and half life of eletriptan. Most common adverse reactions are pain or pressure sensation in chest or throat, dizziness, somnolence, nausea, xerostomia, and weakness.

Administration: Oral.

Preparations: Tablet (film coated), 20 and 40 mg.

ELIDEL®, see Pimecrolimus

ELIGARD®, see Leuprolide Acetate

ELIMITE®, see Permethrin

ELITEK™, see Rasburicase

ELIXOPHYLLIN®, see Theophylline

ELLENCE®, see Epirubicin

ELMIRON®, see Pentosan Polysulfate Sodium

ELOCON®, see Mometasone Furoate

ELOXATIN™, see Oxaliplatin

ELSPAR®, see Asparaginase

ELTROXINE®, see Levothyroxine

EMCYT®, see Estramustine

EMINASE®, see Anistreplase

EMKO®, see Nonoxynol 9

EMLA®

Description/Actions: Eutectic mixture of local anesthetics (lidocaine and prilocaine) that is applied topically.

Precautions/Adverse Reactions: Use on normal intact skin. Contraindicated in methemoglobinemia. Not recommended for use in infants <37 weeks gestational age.

Administration: Apply thick layer of cream over selected site 1 hour prior to routine procedures and 2 hours prior to painful procedures. Cover with an occlusive dressing. Prior to procedure remove cream and cleanse area with antiseptic.

Preparations: Topical cream and disk.

EMLA CREAM®, see Lidocaine and Prilocaine Cream

EMTRICITABINE—Emtriva™

Description/Actions: Emtricitabine is a synthetic nucleoside analog of cytosine with activity against Human Immunodeficiency Virus type 1 (HIV-1) reverse transcriptase. It is indicated for the treatment of HIV-1 infection in adults in combination with other antiretroviral agents.

Precautions/Adverse Reactions: Emtricitabine is contraindicated in patients with a known hypersensitivity to it or to any component of the formulation. Lactic acidosis and severe hepatomegaly with steatosis, including fatal cases, have been reported with the use of nucleoside analogs alone or in combination with other antiretrovirals. Treatment with emtricitabine should be suspended in any patient who develops clinical or laboratory findings suggestive of lactic acidosis or pronounced hepatotoxicity. Exacerbations of hepatitis B have been reported in patients after the discontinuation of emtricitabine. No clinically significant drug interactions have been found when emtricitabine is coadministered with other drugs metabolized via the cytochrome P450 system. Redistribution/accumulation of body fat, including central obesity, buffalo hump, peripheral wasting, facial wasting, breast enlargement and "cushingoid appearance" have been reported in patients receiving antiretroviral therapy. Pregnancy Category B. No adequate and well-controlled studies in pregnant women. Use during pregnancy only if clearly needed. Secretion in human breast milk is unknown. Breast-feeding is not recommended while receiving emtricitabine. Safety and efficacy in pediatric patients have not been established. Most common adverse effects observed during treatment with emtricitabine include: headache, diarrhea, nausea, and rash. Skin discoloration manifested by hyperpigmentation on the palms and/or soles has also been reported during therapy with emtricitabine. Other reported adverse effects include: abdominal pain, asthenia, dyspepsia, vomiting, myalgia, arthralgia, abnormal dreams, depression, dizziness, insomnia, neuropathy, neuritis, paresthesia, increased cough, rhinitis, increased AST, ALT, bilirubin, creatinine kinase, amylase, lipase, glucose, and triglycerides.

Administration: Oral.

Patient Care Implications: Patients should be informed that emtricitabine is not a cure for HIV infection.

Preparations: Capsules, 200 mg.

EMTRIVA™, see Emtricitabine

E-MYCIN®, see Erythromycin Base

E-MYCIN 333®, see Erythromycin Base

ENALAPRIL/HYDROCHLOROTHIAZIDE—Vaseretic®

Description/Actions: Enalapril and hydrochlorothiazide are combined in an oral formulation for the treatment of hypertension. The extent of blood pressure reduction with the combination of these drugs is approximately additive.

Precautions/Adverse Reactions: Thiazide diuretics, such as hydrochlorothiazide, are contraindicated in patients with sulfonamide hypersensitivity or thiazide diuretic hypersensitivity because of the risk of cross-sensitivity. Enalapril is contraindicated in patients with a history of ACE inhibitor-induced, hereditary, or idiopathic angioedema. Enalapril/hydrochlorothiazide should be used with caution in patients with hypotension, hepatic disease, renal artery stenosis, gout, diabetes mellitus, pregnancy, pancreatitis, SLE, and potassium imbalances. Adverse effects include dizziness, headache, fatigue, cough, muscle cramps, nausea/vomiting, asthenia, impotence, and diarrhea.

Administration: Oral.

Preparations: Tablets, 5/12.5 mg and 10/25 mg.

ENALAPRIL MALEATE—Vasotec®

Description/Actions: Is a prodrug which, after oral administration, is hydrolyzed to enalaprilat, a potent angiotensin converting enzyme (ACE) inhibitor. Indicated for the treatment of hypertension, and as adjunctive therapy in the management of heart failure in patients who are not responding adequately to diuretics and digitalis. Also indicated for clinically stable asymptomatic patients with left ventricular dysfunction.

Precautions/Adverse Reactions: Angioedema has occurred infrequently, sometimes after the first dose. Adverse reactions include headache, dizziness, fatigue, cough, proteinuria, and hyperkalemia. Excessive hypotension may occur, particularly in patients with severe salt/volume depletion (e.g., those being treated vigorously with diuretics). Use during pregnancy should be avoided. Nonsteroidal anti-inflammatory drugs may diminish the antihypertensive effect of ACE inhibitors.

Administration: Oral.

Preparations: Tablets, 2.5, 5, 10, and 20 mg.

ENALAPRILAT—Vasotec IV®, see discussion on Enalapril

Administration: Intravenous.

Preparations: Vials, 1.25 mg/ml.

ENDRATE®, see Edetate Disodium

ENDURON®, see Methyclothiazide

ENFLURANE—Ethrane®

Description/Actions: General anesthetic administered by inhalation in the induction and maintenance of general anesthesia.

Preparations: Bottles, 125 and 250 ml.

ENFUVIRTIDE—Fuzeon™

Description/Actions: Enfuvirtide is an antiretroviral agent indicated for the treatment of HIV-1 infection in combination with other antiretroviral agents in treatment-experienced patients with evidence of HIV-1 replication despite ongoing antiretroviral therapy. Enfuvirtide interferes with the entry of HIV-1 into cells by inhibiting fusion of viral and cellular membranes. Enfuvirtide binds to the first heptad-repeat (HR1) in the gp41 subunit of the viral envelope lipoprotein and prevents the conformational changes required for the fusion of viral and cellular membranes.

Precautions/Adverse Reactions: Enfuvirtide is contraindicated in patients with known hypersensitivity to enfuvirtide or any of its components. The most common adverse events are local injection site reactions. Patients must be familiar with injection instructions and know how to monitor carefully for signs or symptoms of cellulitis or local infection. Bacterial pneumonia observed in clinical trials; patients with HIV infection should be carefully monitored for signs and symptoms of pneumonia, especially if they have underlying conditions that may predispose them to pneumonia. Risk factors include low initial CD4 cell count, high initial viral load, intravenous drug use, smoking, and a prior history of lung disease. Hypersensitivity reactions have been associated with enfuvirtide therapy and may recur on rechallenge. Patients developing signs and symptoms suggestive of a systemic hypersensitivity reaction should discontinue enfuvirtide and should seek medical evaluation immediately. Therapy should not be restarted. Pregnancy Category B. Excretion in breast milk unknown/breast-feeding not recommended. Most common adverse reactions were insomnia, injection site reactions, depression, decreased appetite, diarrhea, neuropathy, and cough.

Administration: Subcutaneous.

Patient Care Implications: Inject into the upper arm, abdomen, or anterior thigh. Do not inject in the same area as the time before and do not inject around the navel, into scar tissues, a bruise, a mole, or where there is an injection site reaction. There may be injection site reactions such as itching, swelling, redness, pain, hardened skin, or bumps. Monitor for signs or symptoms of cellulitis or local infection. Advise patients to seek medical attention if signs or symptoms of pneumonia develop. May experience dizziness. Do not operate heavy machinery or drive a car until effect of enfuvirtide in known. Insomnia is common; may cause depression and anxiety.

Preparations: Injection: 108 mg (90 mg/mL following reconstitution).

ENLON®, see Edrophonium

ENOXACIN—Penetrex®

Description/Actions: Fluoroquinolone anti-infective agent. Inhibits DNA gyrase, an essential bacterial enzyme, and exhibits a bactericidal action against many gram-positive and gram-negative bacteria. Indicated for urinary tract infections caused by susceptible organisms. Also indicated for uncomplicated urethral or cervical gonorrhea.

Precautions/Adverse Reactions: Contraindicated in patients with a known hypersensitivity to any of the fluoroquinolones or the related quinolone antibacterial agents (i.e., nalidixic acid, cinoxacin). Fluoroquinolones have caused erosion of cartilage in weight-bearing joints and other signs of arthropathy in juvenile animals, and use in children under 18, pregnant women, and women who are nursing is best avoided. Adverse reactions include nausea and/or vomiting, abdominal pain, diarrhea, dyspepsia, dizziness, and headache. Because of the possibility of photosensitivity reactions, patients should be advised to avoid excessive sunlight and artificial ultraviolet light during the period of treatment. May cause dizziness, lightheadedness, and other central nervous system effects, and patients should know how they tolerate the drug before they engage in activities that require mental alertness and coordination.

Administration: Oral. Should be administered at least 1 hour before or 2 hours after a meal.

Preparations: Tablets, 200 and 400 mg.

ENOXAPARIN—Lovenox®

Description/Actions: Is a low molecular weight heparin fraction that is prepared by the degradation of heparin benzyl ester derived from porcine intestinal mucosa. Does not significantly influence platelet aggregation or the plasma fibrinogen concentration, and does not affect global blood clotting tests (i.e., prothrombin time [PT] or activated partial thromboplastin time [APTT]). Enoxaparin is indicated for the prophylaxis of deep vein thrombosis, which may lead to pulmonary embolism in patients undergoing abdominal surgery, in patients undergoing hip replacement surgery, and for the prophylaxis of ischemic complications of unstable angina and non-Q-wave myocardial infarction when concurrently administered with aspirin. Enoxaparin is indicated for the inpatient treatment of acute deep vein thrombosis with or without pulmonary embolism when administered with warfarin and for the outpatient treatment of acute deep vein thrombosis without pulmonary embolism when administered with warfarin and, for the prevention of deep vein thrombosis in patients at risk due to severely restricted mobility during acute illness.

Precautions/Adverse Reactions: Contraindicated in patients who are hypersensitive to the drug heparin or to pork products. Also contraindicated in patients with active major bleeding and in patients with thrombocytopenia associated with a positive in vitro test for antiplatelet antibody in the presence of enoxaparin. May cause bleeding episodes, although the incidence of such reactions was similar to that with placebo in the clinical studies. Should be used with extreme caution in patients with conditions that are associated with an increased risk of hemorrhage (e.g., congenital or acquired bleeding disorders, active ulceration, or a history of recent gastrointestinal ulceration and hemorrhage, uncontrolled arterial hypertension, and hemorrhagic stroke). Cases of epidural or spinal hematomas have been reported with the use of enoxaparin injection and spinal/epidural anesthesia or spinal puncture resulting in long-term or permanent paralysis. The use of enoxaparin is not recommended for thromboprophylaxis in patients with prosthetic heart valves. Cases of prosthetic heart valve thrombosis have been reported in patients with prosthetic valves who have received enoxaparin for thromboprophylaxis. May cause thrombocytopenia. Periodic complete blood counts, including platelet count, and stool occult blood tests should be conducted during the course of treatment with enoxaparin.

Administration: Subcutaneous injection.

Preparations: Prefilled syringes, 30, 40, 60, 80, 100, 120, 150, and 300 mg.

ENTACAPONE—Comtan®

Description/Actions: Entacapone is used with levodopa/carbidopa in the treatment of Parkinson's disease.

Precautions/Adverse Reactions: Entacapone should be given with caution to patients with hepatic impairment, biliary obstruction, hypotension, and syncope. Also, the safety is questionable in pregnant women, breast-feeding women, and children. Some common adverse effects are dyskinesia, nausea/vomiting, hyperkinesia, diarrhea, brownish-orange urine, hypokinesia, rhabdomyolysis, orthostatic hypotension, and dizziness. Entacapone should not be discontinued abruptly because neuroleptic malignant syndrome could occur.

Administration: Oral.

Patient Care Implications: Patients with hepatic impairment or biliary obstruction may need dosage adjustments. The safety of the drug is not proven in pregnant women, children, or breast-feeding women. The drug should not be discontinued abruptly.

Preparations: Tablet, 200 mg.

ENTEX LA®, Combination of Phenylephrine and Guaifenesin

ENTOCORT™ EC, see Budesonide

ENVISAN®, see Dextranomer

EPHEDRINE HYDROCHLORIDE—Efedron®

Description/Actions: Nasal decongestant often used in combination with other agents. See also pseudoephedrine. Has also been used as a central nervous system stimulant to counteract the depressant effect of certain other agents with which it may be used in combination.

Preparations: Capsules, 25 and 50 mg.

EPHEDRINE SULFATE

Description/Actions: Pressor agent administered parenterally in the management of hypotensive states.

Preparations: Ampules, 25 and 50 mg/ml.

EPI E-Z PEN®, see Epinephrine

EPINEPHRINE—Adrenalin®, Bronkaid Mist®, Epinephrine Pediatric®, Epi E-Z Pen®, Epipen AutoInjector®, Primatene Mist Suspension®

Description/Actions: Sympathomimetic agent used to relieve respiratory distress due to bronchospasm, to provide rapid relief of hypersensitivity reactions to drugs and other allergens, to restore cardiac rhythm in cardiac arrest due to various causes, and to prolong the action of infiltration anesthetics. Also used in the treatment of mucosal congestion of hay fever and rhinitis, to relieve bronchial asthmatic paroxysms, for symptomatic relief of serum sickness, urticaria, and angioneurotic edema, for the management of glaucoma and other ocular conditions, and selected other disorders.

Preparations: Ampules and vials (as the hydrochloride), 1:1000, 1:10,000, and 1:100,000. Solution for nebulization (as the hydrochloride), 1.25% and 2.25%. Aerosol, 0.2 and 0.27 mg per spray. Aerosol (as the bitartrate), 0.16 mg per spray. Solution for nasal administration (as the hydrochloride), 0.1%. Ophthalmic solution (as the bitartrate, borate, and hydrochloride), 0.1%, 0.25%, 0.5%, 1%, and 2%. Autoinjector syringes, 0.3 mg and 0.15 mg.

EPINASTINE—Elestat™

Description/Actions: Epinastine is a selective H1-receptor antagonist and an inhibitor of histamine release from the mast cell. Epinastine is indicated for the prevention of itching associated with allergic conjunctivitis.

Precautions/Adverse Reactions: Epinastine is contraindicated in patients who have shown hypersensitivity to epinastine or any components of the formulation. Contact lenses should be removed prior to instillation and may be reinserted after 10 minutes following its administration. The most common adverse reactions were burning sensation in the eyes, infection (i.e., cold symptoms and upper respiratory infections), headache, rhinitis, sinusitis, increased cough, and pharyngitis. Pregnancy risk factor C. No adequate and well-controlled studies in pregnant women. Excretion in breast milk unknown; use caution when administered to nursing women.

Administration: Ophthalmic.

Patient Care Implications: Instruct to avoid allowing the tip of the dispensing container to contact the eye, surrounding structures, fingers, or any other surface in order to avoid contamination of the solution by common bacteria known to cause ocular infections.

Preparations: Solution, ophthalmic: 0.05%

EPIPEN AUTOINJECTOR®—see Epinephrine

EPIRUBICIN—Ellence®

Description/Actions: Epirubicin is used as adjuvant treatment in patients with node-positive breast cancer.

Precautions/Adverse Reactions: Epirubicin dosage has to be adjusted in patients with hepatic impairment and renal impairment. Epirubicin should not be administered to patients with neutropenia, thrombocytopenia, pregnant women, and breast-feeding women. The drug should be administered carefully in patients with cardiac disease. Some side effects are bone marrow suppression, cardiotoxicity, alopecia, nausea, vomiting, urine discoloration, skin ulcers, tissue necrosis, and anorexia.

Administration: Intravenous.

Patient Care Implications: Patients with hepatic disease and renal disease need dosage adjustment. CBC with differential, echocardiogram, LFTs, MUGA, bilirubin, and creatinine should be checked before initiation of drug and monitored during therapy.

Preparations: Vials, 50 mg/25 ml, 200 mg/100 ml.

EPIVIR®—see Lamivudine

EPLERENONE—Inspra™

Description/Actions: Eplerenone is a blocker of aldosterone binding at the mineralocorticoid receptor. Eplerenone is indicated for the treatment of hypertension either alone or in combination with other antihypertensives. It is also indicated to improve survival of stable patients with left ventricular systolic dysfunction (ejection fraction ≤40%) and clinical evidence of congestive heart failure after an acute myocardial infarction.

Precautions/Adverse Reactions: Eplerenone is contraindicated in patients with a known hypersensitivity to it or to any component of the formulation. It is contraindicated in patients with the following conditions: serum potassium >5.5 meq/L, type 2 diabetes with microalbuminuria, serum creatinine >2.0 mg/dL in males and 1.8 mg/dL in females, and in patients with creatinine clearances <50 mL/min. Eplerenone is also contraindicated in patients treated concomitantly with the following medications: potassium supplements or potassium-sparing diuretics (amiloride, spironolactone, or triamterene) and strong inhibitors of CYP450 3A4 (ketoconazole, itraconazole). The principal risk of eplerenone is hyperkalemia, which can cause serious, sometimes fatal arrhythmias. Monitor potassium levels every 2 weeks for the first 1–2 months and then monthly thereafter. Pregnancy Category B. Concomitant administration of eplerenone and St. John's Wort resulted in a 30% decrease in eplerenone's AUC. Most common adverse reactions observed during therapy with eplerenone include dizziness (3%), diarrhea (2%), coughing (2%), fatigue (2%), influenza-like symptoms (2%), and albuminuria (1%). Hypercholesterolemia occurred in approximately 0.3% of patients treated with eplerenone (dose-related effect). Gynecomastia occurred in 0.5%–1% of patients treated with eplerenone. Abnormal vaginal bleeding occurred in 0.6%–2.1% of female patients treated with eplerenone. Increases in AST, ALT, GGT, BUN, serum creatinine, and uric acid levels were observed during therapy with eplerenone. Hyperkalemia (dose-related) was observed in <1% of patients and increased with decreasing renal function. Hyponatremia was observed in approximately 2.3% of patients receiving eplerenone.

Administration: Oral.

Preparations: Tablets, 25, 50, and 100 mg.

EPO, see Epoetin Alfa

EPOETIN ALFA—EPO, Epogen®, Procrit®

Description/Actions: Agent for anemia. Also known as recombinant human erythropoietin or EPO. Stimulates red blood cell production in anemic patients, decreasing the need for transfusions in these patients. Indicated in the treatment for anemia associated with chronic renal failure, management of anemia secondary to zidovudine therapy (AZT) in HIV-infected patients, and the management of anemia from chemotherapy in patients with nonmyeloid malignancies.

Precautions/Adverse Reactions: Contraindicated in patients with uncontrolled hypertension. Adverse reactions include hypertension, headache, arthralgias, nausea, vomiting, diarrhea, and seizures. For patients who respond to epoetin alfa with a rapid increase in hematocrit (e.g., more than 4 points in any 2-week period), the dose should be decreased to reduce the risk of hypertension. Because of the risk of seizures, patients should be cautioned to avoid potentially hazardous activities such as driving or operating machinery. During hemodialysis, patients treated with epoetin alfa may require increased anticoagulation with heparin to prevent clotting of the artificial kidney.

Administration: Intravenous or subcutaneous. The vials should not be shaken as shaking may denature the glycoprotein, rendering it biologically inactive.

Preparations: Vials, 2000, 3000, 4000, 10,000, and 40,000 units.

EPOGEN®, see Epoetin Alfa

EPOPROSTENOL—Flolan®, Prostacyclin®, Prostaglandin 12 (PG 12)®, Prostaglandin X (PGX)®

Description/Actions: Prostaglandin, vasodilator. Directly dilates pulmonary and systemic arterial vasculature. Also inhibits platelet aggregation. Indicated in the management of primary pulmonary hypertension in selected patients.

Precautions/Adverse Reactions: Side effects include headache, anxiety, dizziness, tachycardia, nausea, vomiting, flushing, myalgia, hypesthesia, hyperesthesia/paresthesia, and flu-like symptoms. Dosage adjustments may be necessary in geriatric patients. Unless contraindicated, concurrent anticoagulant therapy is usually administered to decrease the risk of pulmonary or systemic embolism.

Administration: Intravenously via continuous infusion.

Preparations: Powder for injection, 0.5 mg and 1.5 mg vials.

EPTIFIBATIDE—Integrilin®

Description/Actions: Platelet aggregation inhibitor indicated in combination with heparin for treating acute coronary syndrome (unstable angina/non-Q-wave myocardial infarction), including patients who are to be managed medically and those undergoing percutaneous transluminal angioplasty or artherectomy.

Precautions/Adverse Reactions: Contraindicated in the following conditions within previous 30 days: active internal bleeding, bleeding diathesis, stroke, major surgery, or severe trauma. Contraindicated with a history of intracranial hemorrhage, intracranial neoplasm, arteriovenous malformation, aneurysm, hemorrhagic stroke, thrombocytopenia after previous Integrilin therapy, symptoms or findings suggestive of aortic dissection, severe hypertension, acute pericarditis, and concomitant parenteral GI 11b/111A inhibitor. Use cautiously in patients with renal failure, platelet count <150,000/mm3 or hemorrhagic retinopathy. Properly care for femoral artery access site to minimize bleeding. Minimize other arterial and venous punctures, IM injections, catheter use, and other invasive procedures to minimize bleeding risk. Avoid use of noncompressible IV access sites. Do baseline platelet counts, hemoglobin, hematocrit, and monitor during therapy. Discontinue Integrilin if confirmed thrombocytopenia occurs. Adjust heparin to maintain aPTT at 2 times control. Adverse reactions include bleeding, decreased hemoglobin and/or hematocrit, reduced platelet counts, edema, vasovagal reaction, and others.

Administration: Intravenous.

Preparations: Vials, 2 mg/ml (10 ml for bolus dose). Vials, 0.75 mg/ml (100 ml for infusion).

EQUALACTIN®, see Polycarbophil

EQUANIL®, see Meprobamate

EQUETRO™, see Carbamazepine

ERGAMISOL®, see Levamisole

ERGOCALCIFEROL—Vitamin D$_2$, Drisdol®

Description/Actions: A form of vitamin D indicated in the treatment of rickets, familial hypophosphatemia, hypoparathyroidism, osteomalacia, anticonvulsant-induced rickets, osteoporosis, and renal osteodystrophy.

Preparations: Capsules, 25,000 and 50,000 IU. Liquid, 8000 IU/ml. Ampules, 500,000 IU/ml and 500,000 IU/5 ml.

ERGOLOID MESYLATES—Hydergine®

Description/Actions: Ergot derivatives indicated in patients over 60 years of age who manifest signs and symptoms of an idiopathic decline in mental capacity (i.e., cognitive and interpersonal skills, mood).

Preparations: Sublingual tablets, 0.5 and 1 mg. Capsules (liquid) and tablets, 1 mg. Liquid, 1 mg/ml.

ERGOMETRINE, see Ergonovine

ERGONOVINE MALEATE—Ergometrine®, Ergotrate®

Description/Actions: Ergot derivative indicated for the prevention and treatment of postpartum and postabortal hemorrhage due to uterine atony.

Preparations: Tablets, 0.2 mg. Ampules, 0.2 mg/ml.

ERGOSTAT®, see Ergotamine

ERGOTAMINE TARTRATE—Ergostat®

Description/Actions: Ergot derivative indicated to abort or prevent vascular headache such as migraine and cluster.

Preparations: Sublingual tablets, 2 mg, tablets, 1 mg.

ERGOTRATE®, see Ergonovine

ERTAPENEM—Invanz™

Description/Actions: Ertapenem is indicated in adults for treatment of moderate to severe infections caused by susceptible strains of gram-positive and gram-negative aerobic and anaerobic organisms.

Precautions/Adverse Reactions: Contraindicated in patients with a known hypersensitivity to lidocaine or other amide-type anesthetics. Serious and fatal anaphylactic reactions noted in patients receiving therapy with betalactams. These reactions are more likely to occur in individuals with a history of sensitivity to multiple allergens. Seizures have occurred most commonly in patients with CNS disorders and/or compromised renal function. Prolonged use of ertapenem may result in pseudomembranous colitis that may range in severity from mild to life threatening. Pregnancy Category B. There are no well-controlled studies in pregnant women. Use only if clearly needed. Ertapenem is excreted in breast milk. Most common adverse reactions were diarrhea, infused vein complication, nausea, headache, constipation, increased platelet count, and elevated hepatic enzymes.

Administration: Intravenous, intramuscular.

Patient Care Implications: Avoid inadvertent injection of intramuscular preparation into intravenous line. The reconstituted solution, after immediately being diluted in NS, may be stored at room temperature (25° C) and used within 6 hours or stored for 24 hours under refrigeration (5° C) and used within 4 hours after removal from refrigeration. Solutions should not be frozen.

Preparations: Sterile lyophilized powder for injection, 1 g ertapenem.

ERYC®, see Erythromycin Base

ERYCETTE®, see Erythromycin Base (Topical)

ERYDERM®, see Erythromycin Base (Topical)

ERYGEL®, see Erythromycin Base (Topical)

ERYMAX®, see Erythromycin Base (Topical)

ERYPED®, see Erythromycin Ethylsuccinate

ERY-TAB®, see Erythromycin Base

ERYTHRITYL TETRANITRATE—Cardilate®

Description/Actions: Antianginal agent indicated for the prophylaxis and treatment of patients with frequent or recurrent anginal pain.

Preparations: Oral/sublingual tablets, 10 mg.

ERYTHROMYCIN BASE—EMycin ®, E-Mycin 333®, Ery-Tab®, Ilotycin®, Robimycin®, ERYC®, PCE®

Description/Actions: Macrolide antibiotic active against most gram-positive and a number of gram-negative bacteria, mycoplasmal, and chlamydial organisms, and certain spirochetes. Indicated in the treatment of respiratory tract and a number of other types of infections. Effective in the treatment of primary atypical pneumonia, Legionnaires' disease, infections caused by *Chlamydia trachomatis* and *Ureaplasma urealyticum*, and GI infections caused by *Campylobacter jejuni*. Used with neomycin for prophylaxis in colorectal surgery.

Precautions/Adverse Reactions: Adverse reactions include nausea, vomiting, abdominal cramps, and hepatic dysfunction (primarily associated with the use of the estolate). Should not be used concurrently with terfenadine or astemizole.

Administration: Oral. Some formulations may be administered without regard to meals whereas others should be administered apart from meals. Labeling for individual product should be consulted.

Preparations: Enteric-coated tablets, 250, 333, and 500 mg. Capsules with enteric-coated pellets (ERYC), 125 and 250 mg. Tablets with polymer-coated particles (PCE), 333 and 500 mg. Film-coated tablets, 250 and 500 mg.

ERYTHROMYCIN BASE (for topical use)—Akne-mycin®, Erycette®, EryDerm®, Erygel®, Erymax®, Staticin®

Description/Actions: Antibiotic for the topical treatment of acne.

Administration: Topical.

Preparations: Solution, 1.5% and 2%. Gel, 2%.

ERYTHROMYCIN ESTOLATE—Ilosone® (See discussion on Erythromycin Base.)

Administration: Oral. May be administered without regard to meals.

Preparations: Capsules, 250 mg. Tablets, 500 mg. Suspension, 125 and 250 mg/5 ml.

ERYTHROMYCIN ETHYLSUCCINATE—EES®, EryPed® (See discussion on Erythromycin Base.)

Administration: Oral. May be administered without regard to meals.

Preparations: Suspension, 200 and 400 mg/5 ml. Powder for oral suspension, 200 and 400 mg/5 ml when reconstituted. Tablets, 400 mg. Chewable tablets, 200 mg.

ERYTHROMYCIN GLUCEPTATE—Ilotycin Gluceptate® (See discussion on Erythromycin Base.)

Administration: Intravenous.

Preparations: Vials, 250 and 500 mg, 1 g.

ERYTHROMYCIN LACTOBIONATE (See discussion on Erythromycin Base.)

Administration: Intravenous.

Preparations: Vials, 500 mg, 1 g.

ERYTHROMYCIN STEARATE (See discussion on Erythromycin Base.)

Administration: Oral. Should be administered apart from meals.

Preparations: Tablets, 250 and 500 mg.

ERYTHROPOIETIN, see Epoetin Alfa

ESCITALOPRAM OXALATE—Lexapro™

Description/Actions: Escitalopram is the S-enantiomer of citalopram, which selectively inhibits the reuptake of serotonin with minimal effects on norepinephrine and dopamine reuptake. Escitalopram is indicated for the treatment of Major Depressive Disorder (MDD) and for the treatment of Generalized Anxiety Disorder (GAD).

Precautions/Adverse Reactions: Escitalopram is contraindicated in individuals with a hypersensitivity to escitalopram, citalopram, or any component of the formulation. It should not be administered with or within 2 weeks of use of monoamine oxidase inhibitors (MAOIs). There have been reports of serious, sometimes fatal reactions when serotonin reuptake inhibitors are given in combination with MAOIs. At least 14 days should be allowed to pass after stopping escitalopram before starting an MAOI. May precipitate a shift to mania/hypomania. Use cautiously in patients with a history of mania. Psychoactive drugs may impair judgment, thinking, or motor skills. Use caution in patients with a previous seizure disorder or condition predisposing to seizures such as brain damage, alcoholism, or concurrent therapy with other drugs that lower the seizure threshold. May cause hyponatremia/SIADH (syndrome of inappropriate antidiuretic hormone secretion). Use caution if suicidal risk may be present; the possibility of a suicide attempt is inherent in major depressive disorder. Pregnancy Category C. Enters breast milk; breast feeding not recommended. Most common adverse reactions were nausea, insomnia, somnolence, diarrhea, xerostomia, and ejaculation disorder. Escitalopram use with buspirone, linezolid, MAOI, meperidine, moclobemide, nefazodone, selegiline, SSRIs, sumatriptan, trazodone, and venlaflaxine may cause serotonin syndrome; avoid concurrent use. Antidepressants increased the risk of suicidal thinking and behavior (suicidality) in short-term studies in children and adolescents with Major Depressive Disorder (MDD) and other psychiatric disorders. Anyone considering the use of escitalopram or any other antidepressant in a child or adolescent must balance this risk with the clinical need. Patients who are started on therapy should be observed closely for clinical worsening, suicidality, or unusual changes in behavior. Lexapro™ is not approved for use in pediatric patients.

Administration: Oral, with or without food.

Preparations: Solution (oral), 1 mg/ml (240 ml). Tablet (film coated), 5, 10, and 20 mg.

ESERINE, see Physostigmine

ESGIC-PLUS—Combination Barbiturate and Analgesic.
Butalbital, Acetaminophen, and Caffeine. See individual discussion on butalbital, acetaminophen and caffeine.

ESIDRIX®, see Hydrochlorothiazide

ESKALITH®, see Lithium Carbonate

ESMOLOL HYDROCHLORIDE—Brevibloc®

Description/Actions: A beta-adrenergic blocking agent indicated for the rapid control of ventricular rate in patients with atrial fibrillation or atrial flutter in perioperative, postoperative, or other emergent circumstances where short-term control of ventricular rate with a short-acting agent is desirable. Also indicated in noncompensatory sinus tachycardia, where the rapid heart rate requires specific intervention.

Precautions/Adverse Reactions: Contraindicated in patients with sinus bradycardia, heart block greater than first degree, cardiogenic shock, or overt heart failure. Hypotension is the most important adverse reaction, and some patients experience manifestations such as dizziness and diaphoresis. Other adverse reactions include peripheral ischemia, sedation, agitation, nausea, and local reactions at the infusion site; to reduce the incidence of venous irritation and thrombophlebitis, infusion concentrations greater than 10 mg/ml should be avoided. Therapy must be closely monitored in patients with bronchospastic diseases. It must also be used with caution in diabetic patients.

Administration: Intravenous infusion.

Preparations: Ampules, 10 mg/ml, 250 mg/ml.

ESOMEPRAZOLE—Nexium™

Description/Actions: Esomeprazole is a proton pump inhibitor indicated for the short-term treatment (4–8 weeks) in the healing and symptomatic resolution of diagnostically confirmed erosive esophagitis, for the maintenance of healing of erosive esophagitis, for the treatment of heartburn and other symptoms of GERD, and for the reduction in the occurrence of gastric ulcers associated with continuous NSAID therapy in patients at risk for developing gastric ulcers. Esomeprazole, in combination with clarithromycin and amoxicillin, is indicated for the treatment of patients with *H-pylori* infection and duodenal ulcer disease to eradicate *H-pylori.*

Precautions/Adverse Reactions: Usage is contraindicated in patients with hypersensitivity to esomeprazole, any component of the formulation, or to substituted benzimidazoles. Symptomatic response to therapy does not preclude the presence of gastric malignancy. Atrophic gastritis has been noted by biopsy from patients treated long-term with omeprazole; this may occur with esomeprazole therapy. Safety and efficacy of esomeprazole have not been established in pediatric patients. Pregnancy Category B. This drug should be used during pregnancy only if clearly needed. Excretion in the breast milk is unknown; therefore, breast-feeding is not recommended. Some adverse effects are headache, diarrhea, nausea, flatulence, abdominal pain, constipation, and dry mouth.

Administration: Oral.

Patient Care Implications: Capsule should be swallowed whole and taken at least 1 hour before eating. In patients with swallowing difficulties, open capsule and mix contents with 1 tbsp of applesauce. The mixture should be swallowed immediately and should not be chewed; do not store the mixture for future use.

Preparations: Capsule, delayed release: 20 mg, 40 mg.

ESTAZOLAM—ProSom®

Description/Actions: Usually initiates sleep within 15–30 minutes following administration and action continues for an average of 6–8 hours. Classified as an intermediate-acting benzodiazepine hypnotic. Indicated for the short-term management of insomnia characterized by difficulty in falling asleep, frequent nocturnal awakenings, and/or early morning awakenings.

Precautions/Adverse Reactions: Contraindicated in pregnancy. Adverse reactions include daytime sedation, hypokinesia, dizziness, and abnormal coordination. Patients should be cautioned regarding activities such as driving and operating machinery, as well as interactions with other CNS-acting drugs including alcohol. Can cause dependence and is included in Schedule IV.

Administration: Oral.

Preparations: Tablets, 1 and 2 mg.

ESTINYL®, see Ethinyl Estradiol

ESTRACE®, see Estradiol

ESTRADERM®, see Estradiol

ESTRADIOL—Alora®, Climara®, Estrace®, Estraderm®, Estring®, Vivelle®, EstroGel®

Description/Actions: Estrogen indicated in the treatment of moderate to severe vasomotor symptoms associated with menopause, atrophic vaginitis, kraurosis vulvae, female hypogonadism, female castration, primary ovarian failure, breast cancer, and prostatic cancer. Transdermal system is also indicated for postmenopausal osteoporosis. Remove vaginal ring when treating vaginal infections and during treatment with other vaginally administered preparations.

Preparations: Tablets, 1 and 2 mg. Transdermal systems 0.025 mg, 0.0375 mg, 0.05 mg, 0.06 mg, 0.075 mg, 0.1 mg, 4 and 8 mg. Vaginal cream, 0.1 mg/g. Vaginal ring (Estring®) 2 mg Estradiol/90 days. Metered dose pump delivering 1.25 g of a gel containing 0.75mg of estradiol/depression (EstroGel®).

ESTRADIOL CYPIONATE—Depo-Estradiol Cypionate® (See discussion on Estradiol.)

Preparations: Vials (for intramuscular administration), 1 mg/ml and 5 mg/ml.

ESTRADIOL/ETHINYL ESTRADIOL—Vagifem®

Description/Actions: Estradiol/ethinyl estradiol is a vaginal tablet used to prevent osteoporosis and relieve symptoms associated with menopause.

Precautions/Adverse Reactions: Estradiol/ethinyl estradiol should not be administered in patients with breast, endometrial, or any estrogen-dependent carcinoma. The drug is also contraindicated in patients with abnormal vaginal bleeding, thromboembolic disorder, and thrombophlebitis. The drug should be avoided in pregnant women and children. Some side effects are gallbladder disease, thromboembolic disorders, spotting, rash, genital pruritis, and endometrial hyperplasia.

Administration: Vaginal tablets.

Patient Care Implication: Estradiol/ethinyl estradiol should not be given to pregnant women or children. Patients receiving the drug should be checked every 3–6 months to see if the drug is working. Patients on the drug should be monitored for LFTs, lipid profile, and cervical dysplasia.

Preparations: Vaginal tablets, 25 mcg.

ESTRADIOL/LEVONORGESTREL—Climara Proz® (See discussion on Estradiol.)

Preparations: Transdermal system, 0.015 mg/day of levonorgestrel and 0.045 mg/day of estradiol.

ESTRADIOL VALERATE—Delestrogen® (See discussion on Estradiol.)

Preparations: Vials (for intramuscular administration), 10 mg/ml, 20 mg/ml, and 40 mg/ml.

ESTRAMUSTINE PHOSPHATE SODIUM—Emcyt®

Description/Actions: Antineoplastic agent indicated in the treatment of metastatic and/or progressive carcinoma of the prostate.

Preparations: Capsules, 140 mg.

ESTROGEL®, see Estradiol

ESTROGEN—Cenestin®

Description/Actions: Cenestin is a conjugated estrogen product synthesized from soy and yam plants indicated in the treatment of moderate to severe vasomotor spasms associated with menopausal symptoms.

Precautions/Adverse Reactions: Estrogen replacement therapy is contraindicated in breast or estrogen-dependent carcinomas (unless palliative), undiagnosed abnormal vaginal bleeding, thromboembolic disorders, thrombophlebitis, and pregnancy. Use cautiously in women with increased risk of endometrial carcinoma or hyperplasia, in women with an intact uterus (consider adding progestin), hepatic or renal dysfunction, gallbladder disease, familial hyperlipoproteinemia, bone disease associated with hypercalcemia, diabetes, depression, uterine leiomyomas, and conditions aggravated by fluid retention (e.g., asthma, epilepsy, migraine, cardiac or renal dysfunction). Monitor patients for hypertension. Do an initial complete physical and repeat at 6–12 months. Discontinue if jaundice occurs and during immobilization or at least 4 weeks before surgery associated with thromboembolism. Adverse reactions include nausea, vomiting, abdominal pain, irregular bleeding, headache, insomnia, edema, weight changes, hypertonia, leg cramps, hypertension, mastodynia, intolerance to contact lenses, and increased size of uterine fibromyomata, chloasma. Long-term continuous use may increase the risk of estrogen-dependent cancers. Use of this medication may increase the incidence of gallbladder disease and thromboembolic disorders.

Administration: Oral.

Patient Care Implications: Instruct the patient in the signs and symptoms of fluid retention, thromboembolic disorders, gallbladder disease, and to report them promptly to the prescriber. Inform patients that exercise has been shown to be of benefit when taking estrogen because of bone loss.

Preparations: Tablet, 0.45 mg.

ESTROGENS, CONJUGATED—Premarin®, Cenestin®

Description/Actions: Estrogen indicated in the treatment of (a) moderate to severe vasomotor symptoms associated with menopause and

(b) osteoporosis in postmenopausal women. Intravenous dosage form is indicated in the treatment of abnormal uterine bleeding due to hormonal imbalance in the absence of organic pathology. Vaginal cream is indicated in the treatment of atrophic vaginitis and kraurosis vulvae.

Precautions/Adverse Reactions: Contraindicated (a) during pregnancy; (b) in patients with known or suspected cancer of the breast, except in appropriately selected patients being treated for metastatic disease; (c) in patients with known or suspected estrogen-dependent neoplasia; (d) in patients with undiagnosed abnormal genital bleeding; (e) in patients with thrombophlebitis or thromboembolic disorders; and (f) in patients with a past history of thrombophlebitis, thrombosis, or thromboembolic disorders associated with previous estrogen use (except when used in treatment of breast or prostatic malignancy). Estrogens have been reported to increase the risk of endometrial carcinoma. Premarin® alone or in combination with a progestin is not indicated and should not be used to prevent coronary heart disease. Adverse reactions include thromboembolic effects, increased incidence of gallbladder disease, edema, headache, nausea, vomiting, abdominal cramps, tenderness and enlargement of the breasts, and genitourinary effects.

Administration: Oral, intravenous, and vaginal.

Preparations: Tablets, 0.3, 0.45, 0.625, 0.9, 1.25, and 2.5 mg. Vials, 25 mg. Vaginal cream, 0.625 mg/g.

ESTROGENS, ESTERIFIED—Menest®

Description/Actions: Estrogen indicated for moderate to severe vasomotor symptoms of menopause, atrophic vaginitis, kraurosis vulvae, female hypogonadism, female castration, primary ovarian failure, prostatic carcinoma, and breast cancer.

Preparations: Tablets, 0.3, 0.45, 0.625, 1.25, and 2.5 mg.

ESTRONE—Theelin®

Description/Actions: Estrogen indicated for intramuscular use for moderate to severe vasomotor symptoms associated with menopause, atrophic vaginitis, kraurosis vulvae, female hypogonadism, female castration, primary ovarian failure, and prostatic carcinoma.

Preparations: Vials, 2 mg/ml and 5 mg/ml.

ESTROPIPATE—Piperazine Estrone Sulfate, Ogen®

Description/Actions: Estrogen indicated for moderate to severe vasomotor symptoms of menopause, atrophic vaginitis, kraurosis vulvae, female hypogonadism, female castration, primary ovarian failure, and postmenopausal osteoporosis.

Preparations: Tablets, 0.625, 1.25, 2.5, and 5 mg (equivalent, respectively, to 0.75, 1.5, 3, and 6 mg estropipate). Vaginal cream, 1.5 mg/g.

ESTROSTEP 21®—Oral Contraceptive with Progestin and Estrogen. Also, Estrostep®.

ESTROVIS®, see Quinestrol

ETANERCEPT—Enbrel®

Description/Actions: Indicated for reducing signs and symptoms, inducing major clinical response, inhibiting the progression of structural damage, and improving physical function in patients with moderately to severely active rheumatoid arthritis either in combination with methotrexate or used alone. It is also indicated for reducing signs and symptoms of moderately to severely active polyarticular course juvenile rheumatoid arthritis in patients who have had an inadequate response to one or more disease-modifying antirheumatic drugs (DMARDs), for reducing signs and symptoms, inhibiting the progression of structural damage of active arthritis, and improving physical function in patients with psoriatic arthritis. Etanercept can be used in combination with metotrexate in patients who do not respond adequately to methotrexate alone. Enbrel® is also indicated for reducing signs and symptoms in patients with active ankylosing spondylitis and for the treatment of adult patients (18 years of age or older) with chronic moderate to severe plaque psoriasis who are candidates for systemic therapy or phototherapy.

Precautions/Adverse Reactions: Etanercept is contraindicated in patients with active infection. The needle cover of the diluent syringe contains latex, which should not be handled by persons sensitive to this substance (e.g., nurses, caregivers, patients, etc.). Live vaccines should not be administered during therapy with etanercept. Use cautiously in patients with recurrent infections and diseases that may predispose to infections (diabetes, CHF). Monitor closely if a new infection does develop and discontinue if a serious infection or sepsis develops. Temporarily suspend therapy if a significant varicella exposure occurs. Attempt to complete childhood immunizations prior to initiating therapy. Pregnancy Category B. Use in nursing mothers not recommended. Adverse reactions include injection site reactions (may be serious, e.g., sepsis), development of autoantibodies, respiratory disorders, headache, rhinitis, and dyspepsia. In children, abdominal pain and vomiting have also been reported.

Administration: SQ injection. Inject into the thigh, upper arm, or abdomen.

Patient Care Implications: Instruct patients in correct self administration techniques to ensure safe administration and to reduce the incidence of infection at the injection site. Tell patients to keep vials in the refrigerator and to administer the medication promptly after reconstitution. Corticosteroids, salicylates and NSAIDs, and analgesics may be continued during etanercept therapy. Inform patients that response is generally seen within 1–2 weeks after starting therapy but may not be evident for up to 3 months.

Preparations: Vial, 25 mg powder for reconstitution (diluent contains benzyl alcohol), prefilled syringe, 50 mg/mL.

ETHACRYNIC ACID—Edecrin®

Description/Actions: Diuretic indicated for the treatment of edema associated with various conditions, including the nephrotic syndrome, the short-term management of ascites, the short-term management of hospitalized pediatric patients with congenital heart disease or the nephrotic syndrome, and, intravenously, when a rapid onset of diuresis is desired.

Preparations: Tablets, 25 and 50 mg. Vials (using ethacrynate sodium), 50 mg.

ETHAMBUTOL HYDROCHLORIDE—Myambutol®

Description/Actions: Antitubercular agent indicated in the treatment of tuberculosis or other mycobacterial diseases in conjunction with at least one other antitubercular drug.

Precautions/Adverse Reactions: Ethambutol is contraindicated in patients with a known hypersensitivity to it or to any component of the formulation. It is also contraindicated in patients with known optic neuritis unless clinical judgment determines that it can be used. Ethambutol may produce decreases in visual acuity that appear to be due to optic neuritis. This effect may be related to dose and duration of treatment. This effect is generally reversible when administration of the drug is discontinued promptly. However, irreversible blindness has been reported. Liver toxicities including fatalities have been reported. Baseline and periodic assessment of hepatic function should be performed.

Preparations: Tablets, 100 and 400 mg.

ETHAMOLIN®, see Ethanolamine Oleate

ETHANOLAMINE OLEATE—Ethamolin®

Description/Actions: Sclerosing agent that acts primarily by irritation of the intimal endothelium of the vein and produces a sterile inflammatory response that results in fibrosis and occlusion of the vein. Indicated for the treatment of patients with esophageal varices that have recently bled, to prevent rebleeding.

Precautions/Adverse Reactions: Adverse reactions include pleural effusion/infiltration, esophageal ulcer, pyrexia, retrosternal pain, esophageal stricture, and pneumonia. Anaphylactic reactions have occurred infrequently.

Administration: Intravenous (directly into the varix).

Preparations: Ampules, 5%.

ETHAQUIN®, see Ethaverine

ETHATAB®, see Ethaverine

ETHAVERINE HYDROCHLORIDE—Ethaquin®, Ethatab®, Ethavex-100®, Isovex®

Description/Actions: Peripheral vasodilator indicated in the management of peripheral and cerebral vascular insufficiency associated with arterial spasm. Also used as a smooth muscle spasmolytic in spastic conditions of the gastrointestinal and genitourinary tracts.

Preparations: Tablets, 100 mg.

ETHAVEX-100®, see Ethaverine

ETHCHLORVYNOL—Placidyl®

Description/Actions: Hypnotic indicated for short-term use in the management of insomnia for periods of up to 1 week.

Preparations: Capsules, 200, 500, and 750 mg.

ETHER

Description/Actions: General anesthetic administered by inhalation to produce anesthesia.

Preparations: Liquid.

ETHINYL ESTRADIOL—Estinyl®

Description/Actions: Estrogen indicated in the treatment of moderate to severe vasomotor symptoms associated with menopause, female hypogonadism, prostatic carcinoma, and breast cancer in appropriately selected women. Also used as the estrogen component of many oral contraceptive formulations.

Preparations: Tablets, 0.02, 0.05, and 0.5 mg.

ETHINYL ESTRADIOL AND DROSPIRENONE—Yasmin®

Description/Actions: Yasmin® is indicated for the prevention of pregnancy in women who elect to use an oral contraceptive.

Precautions/Adverse Reactions: Yasmin® is contraindicated in women with any of the following conditions: renal insufficiency, hepatic dysfunction, adrenal insufficiency, thrombophlebitis or thrombo-embolic disorders, a past history of deep vein thrombophlebitis or thromboembolic disorders, cerebrovascular or coronary artery disease, known or suspected carcinoma of the breast, carcinoma of the endometrium, or other known or suspected estrogen-dependent neoplasia, undiagnosed abnormal genital bleeding, cholestatic jaundice of pregnancy or jaundice with prior pill use, liver tumor (benign or malignant) or active liver disease, known or suspected pregnancy, heavy smoking (≥15 cigarettes per day), and over age 35. Cigarette smoking increases the risk of serious cardiovascular side effects from oral contraceptive use. Oral contraceptive use has been associated with an increased risk of myocardial infarction, thromboembolism, stroke, hepatic neoplasia, gallbladder disease, hypertension, ocular lesions, carbohydrate and lipid metabolic effects, headache, and bleeding irregularities. Women should be advised that this product does not protect against HIV infection and other sexually transmitted diseases. Concomitant administration of oral contraceptives and rifampin, phenobarbital, phenytoin, griseofulvin, Saint John's Wort, or phenylbutazone may decrease the effectiveness of the oral contraceptive and lead to menstrual irregularities. Coadministration of oral contraceptives and atorvastatin has resulted in increased plasma concentrations of norethindrone and ethinyl estradiol. Ascorbic acid and acetaminophen may increase plasma concentrations of some synthetic estrogens. Oral contraceptives may inhibit the metabolism of cyclosporine, prednisolone, and theophylline, resulting in increased plasma concentrations of these drugs. Increased clearance of temazepam, salicylic acid, morphine, and clofibric acid has resulted when these drugs were coadministered with oral contraceptives. Pregnancy Category X. Known or suspected pregnancy is a contraindication for the use of Yasmin®. Excreted in human breast milk. Nursing is not recommended. Most common adverse effects associated with Yasmin® therapy and occurring in >1% of women include headache, menstrual disorders, breast pain, abdominal pain, nausea, leukorrhea, flu syndrome, acne, vaginal moniliasis, depression, diarrhea, asthenia, dysmenorrhea, back pain, infection, sinusitis, cystitis, bronchitis, gastroenteritis, allergic reaction, urinary tract infection, pruritis, emotional lability, surgery, rash, and upper respiratory infection. Most common adverse reactions associated with other oral contraceptives include nausea, vomiting, abdominal cramps, bloating, breakthrough bleeding, spotting, change in menstrual flow, amenorrhea, temporary infertility after discontinuation of treatment, edema, melasma, breast changes (tenderness, enlargement, or secretion), weight changes, changes in cervical erosion and secretion, cholestatic jaundice, migraine, rash, depression, vaginal candidiasis, change in corneal curvature, intolerance to contact lenses, acne, Budd-Chiari syndrome, changes in libido, colitis, cystitis-like syndrome, dizziness, erythema multiforme, erythema nodosum, hemolytic uremic syndrome, hemorrhagic eruption, hirsutism, impaired renal function, loss of scalp hair, nervousness, porphyria, premenstrual syndrome, and vaginitis. Some noncontraceptive benefits of oral contraceptives include: increased menstrual cycle regularity, decreased blood loss and decreased incidence of iron-deficiency anemia, decreased incidence of dysmenorrhea, functional ovarian cysts, ectopic pregnancies, fibroadenomas, and fibrocystic disease of the breast, decreased incidence of acute pelvic inflammatory disease, and decreased incidence of endometrial and ovarian cancer.

Administration: Oral. Missed pills: see package insert.

Patient Care Implications: Instruct patient to take the pills exactly as prescribed. Instruct patient to take the pills at the same time each day either after the evening meal or at bedtime. Monitor serum potassium levels during the first treatment cycle and in high-risk patients. Monitor blood pressure. Advise patients not to smoke.

Preparations: Tablets, ethinyl estradiol, 0.03 mg, and drospirenone, 3 mg (21 active—yellow pills, 7 inactive—white pills).

ETHINYL ESTRADIOL AND ETONOGESTREL—NuvaRing®

Description/Actions: NuvaRing® is indicated for the prevention of pregnancy in women who elect to use this product as a method of contraception.

Precautions/Adverse Reactions: NuvaRing® is contraindicated in women with thrombophlebitis or thromboembolic disorders, a past history of deep vein thrombophlebitis or thromboembolic disorders, cerebral vascular or coronary artery disease, valvular heart disease with complications, severe hypertension, diabetes with vascular involvement, headache with focal neurologic symptoms, major surgery with prolonged immobilization, known or suspected carcinoma of the breast or history of breast cancer, carcinoma of the endometrium or other known or suspected estrogen-dependent neoplasia, undiagnosed abnormal genital bleeding, cholestatic jaundice of pregnancy or jaundice with prior hormonal contraceptive use, hepatic tumors, active liver disease, known or suspected pregnancy, heavy smoking (≥15 cigarettes/day), and over age 35. Cigarette smoking increases the risk of serious cardiovascular side effects. May lead to increased risk of myocardial infarction, thromboembolism, stroke, hepatic neoplasia, and gallbladder disease. Retinal thrombosis has also been seen in women using oral contraceptives. The risk of morbidity and mortality increases significantly in the presence of hypertension, hyperlipidemias, obesity, and diabetes. There are no data available to determine whether or not safety and efficacy with the vaginal route of administration of combination hormonal contraceptives would be different than the oral route. Hormonal contraceptives have been shown to cause a decrease in glucose tolerance and hypertriglyceridemia among users. Women with a history of hypertension, hypertension-related disease, or renal disease should be encouraged to use another method of birth control. Breakthrough bleeding and spotting have been reported with NuvaRing®. Fluid retention and depression have also been reported. Patients should be informed that this product does not protect against HIV or other sexually transmitted diseases. Coadministration of herbal products containing St. John's Wort may decrease the effectiveness of contraceptive steroids. Coadministration of atorvastatin and certain oral contraceptives containing ethinyl estradiol results in an increase in ethinyl estradiol area under the curve. Ascorbic acid and acetaminophen may increase blood levels of ethinyl estradiol. Coadministration with itraconazole or ketoconazole may increase blood hormone levels. Coadministration of oral contraceptives containing ethinyl estradiol and cyclosporine, prednisolone, and/or theophylline results in increased plasma concentrations of these drugs. Concomitant use of oral contraceptives and acetaminophen results in decreased plasma concentrations of acetaminophen. Coadministration of oral contraceptives and temazepam results in the increased clearance of temazepam. Increased clearance of salicylic acid, morphine, and clofibric acid has been observed when these drugs were administered with oral contraceptives. Pregnancy Category X. Pregnancy should be ruled out prior to starting NuvaRing®. Effects of NuvaRing® in nursing mothers have not been evaluated. Women who are breast-feeding should be advised not to use NuvaRing®. Safety and efficacy in pediatric patients have not been established. Use before menarche is not indicated. The most common adverse reactions noted in patients using NuvaRing® were vaginitis, headache, upper respiratory tract infection, leukorrhea, sinusitis, weight gain, and nausea. Most frequently reported adverse reactions leading to discontinuation of NuvaRing® include device-related problems (foreign body sensation, coital problems, device expulsion), vaginal symptoms (discomfort, vaginitis, leukorrhea), headache, emotional lability, and weight gain.

Administration: For vaginal use only—1 ring inserted into the vagina. The ring is to remain in place continuously for 3 weeks. It is then removed for 1 week, during which withdrawal bleeding usually occurs. A new ring is inserted 1 week after the last ring was removed even if menstrual bleeding has not stopped.

Patient Care Implications: Patient should be informed that this product does not protect against HIV or other sexually transmitted diseases. Patient should be advised not to smoke. Patient should be instructed to wash her hands prior to removing the ring from the pouch (save foil pouch for disposal of ring). Ring may be inserted lying down, squatting, or standing with one leg up. Patient should be instructed to hold NuvaRing® between her thumb and index finger and to press the opposite sides of the ring together. Ring should be pushed into the vagina. To remove the ring, hook the index finger under the forward rim or hold the rim between the index and middle finger and pull it out. The used ring should be placed in the foil pouch and disposed of in a waste receptacle out of reach of children and pets. It should not be thrown in the toilet. A new ring should be inseted on the same day of the week as it was inserted in the last cycle and at about the same time. Patient should be warned that the ring may fall out of the vagina due to incorrect insertion, bowel movements, straining due to severe constipation, or during tampon removal. If the ring accidentally falls out, it may be rinsed with cool or lukewarm water and reinserted as soon as possible within 3 hours of expulsion. Patient should be advised to have an annual health assessment, including blood pressure, laboratory tests, breast exam, Pap test, and abdominal pelvic organ and vaginal examination.

Preparations: Vaginal ring (delivers ethinyl estradiol 0.015 mg/day and etonogestrel 0.12 mcg/day).

ETHINYL ESTRADIOL AND NORELGESTROMIN—
Ortho Evra™

Description/Actions: Ortho Evra™ is a combination contraceptive patch for the prevention of pregnancy.

Precautions/Adverse Reactions: Ortho Evra™ is contraindicated in patients with a known hypersensitivity to ethinyl estradiol, norelgestromin, or any components of the formulation. It should not be used in women who currently have the following conditions: thrombophlebitis or thromboembolic disorders, past history of deep vein thrombophlebitis or thromboembolic disorders, cerebrovascular or coronary disease (past or current), valvular heart disease with complications, severe hypertension, diabetes with vascular involvement, headaches with focal neurologic symptoms, major surgery with prolonged immobilization, known or suspected carcinoma of the breast or personal history of breast cancer, carcinoma of the endometrium or other known or suspected estrogen-dependent neoplasia, undiagnosed abnormal genital bleeding, cholestatic jaundice of pregnancy or jaundice with prior hormonal contraceptive use, acute or chronic hepatocellular disease with abnormal liver function, hepatic adenomas or carcinomas, and known or suspected pregnancy. Cigarette smoking increases the risk of serious cardiovascular side effects from hormonal contraceptive use. Risk increases with age and with heavy smoking (15 or more cigarettes/day). It is quite marked in women over 35 years of age. Women using hormonal contraceptives should be strongly advised not to smoke. Smoking in combination with oral contraceptives has been shown to contribute substantially to the incidence of myocardial infarctions in women in their mid-30s or older. There is an increased risk of thromboembolic and thrombotic disease, myocardial infarction, and both relative and attributable risks of cerebrovascular events (thrombotic and hemorrhagic strokes). A positive association has been observed between the amount of estrogen and progestin in hormonal contraceptives and the risk of vascular disease. Benign hepatic adenomas are associated with hormonal contraceptive use; rupture of benign hepatic adenomas may cause death through intra-abdominal hemorrhage. Cases of retinal thrombosis have been reported. Combination hormonal contraceptives may worsen existing gallbladder disease and may accelerate the development of this disease in previously asymptomatic women. Oral contraceptives have been shown to cause a decrease in glucose tolerance in some users. Women being treated for hyperlipidemias should be followed closely; some progestins may elevate LDL levels and may render the control of hyperlipidemias more difficult. If jaundice develops, the medication should be discontinued; the hormones in Ortho Evra™ may be poorly metabolized in patients with impaired liver function. If there is onset or exacerbation of migraine headache or the development of headache with a new pattern that is recurrent, persistent, or severe, Ortho Evra should be discontinued. Common adverse reactions were abdominal pain, application site reaction, breast symptoms, headache, nausea, upper respiratory infections, and emotional lability. Contraceptive effectiveness may be reduced when coadministered with some antibiotics, antifungals, anticonvulsants, and other drugs that increase metabolism of contraceptive steroids. Pregnancy Category X. Enters breast milk; not recommended in nursing mothers.

Administration: Topical. This system uses a 28-day (4-week) cycle. Apply 1 patch each week for 3 weeks (21 days), followed by 1 week that is patch-free. There should be no more than a 7-day patch-free interval. Withdrawal bleeding is expected during this week.

Patient Care Implications: Patients should be counseled that this product does not protect against HIV infection and other sexually transmitted diseases. New patches should be applied on the same day each week. Apply to clean, dry, intact healthy skin on the buttock, abdomen, upper outer arm, or upper torso, or in a place where it will not be rubbed by tight clothing. Should not be placed on skin that is red, irritated, or cut, nor on the breasts. Do not apply makeup, creams, lotions, powders, or any topical products where the patch will be placed. If an uncomfortable irritation should occur, remove patch; a new patch may be applied to a different location until the next change day. Only one patch should be worn at a time. Store patches in their protective pouches. Do not store in refrigerator or freezer. Used patches still contain some active hormones; carefully fold old patch in half so that it sticks to itself before throwing out.

Preparations: Patch (transdermal); ethinyl estradiol, 20 mcg, and norelgestromin, 150 mcg/day.

ETHIONAMIDE—Trecator-SC®

Description/Actions: Antitubercular agent indicated in the treatment of tuberculosis in conjunction with other drugs after failure of treatment with the primary antitubercular agents.

Preparations: Tablets, 250 mg.

ETHMOZINE®, see Moricizine

ETHOPROPAZINE HYDROCHLORIDE—Parsidol®

Description/Actions: Antiparkinson agent indicated in the treatment of parkinsonism and to control extrapyramidal reactions due to drugs such as the phenothiazines.

Preparations: Tablets, 10 and 50 mg.

ETHOSUXIMIDE—Zarontin®

Description/Actions: Anticonvulsant indicated in the treatment of absence (petit mal) epilepsy, myoclonic seizures, and akinetic epilepsy.

Preparations: Capsules, 250 mg. Syrup, 250 mg/5 ml.

ETHOTOIN—Peganone®

Description/Actions: Anticonvulsant indicated for the control of tonic-clonic (grand mal) and complex partial (psychomotor) seizures.

Preparations: Tablets, 250 and 500 mg.

ETHRANE®, see Enflurane

ETHYL ALCOHOL, see Alcohol

ETHYL AMINOBENZOATE, see Benzocaine

ETHYL CHLORIDE

Description/Actions: Local anesthetic used to provide local anesthesia and analgesia when sprayed on the skin.

Preparations: Topical spray.

ETHYLENE

Description/Actions: General anesthetic administered by inhalation to produce anesthesia.

Preparations: Gas.

ETHYLNOREPINEPHRINE HYDROCHLORIDE—
Bronkephrine®

Description/Actions: Bronchodilator indicated for parenteral use in the treatment of bronchial asthma and for reversible bronchospasm that may occur in association with bronchitis and emphysema.

Preparations: Ampules, 2 mg/ml.

ETHYNODIOL DIACETATE

Description/Actions: Progestin included in certain oral contraceptive formulations.

ETHYOL®, see Amifostine

ETIDOCAINE HYDROCHLORIDE—Duranest®

Description/Actions: Local anesthetic indicated for infiltration anesthesia, peripheral nerve blocks, and central neural blocks (i.e., lumbar or caudal epidural blocks).

Preparations: Vials, 1% solution. Vials, 1% and 1.5% solutions, both with epinephrine bitartrate, 1:200,000.

ETIDRONATE DISODIUM—Didronel®

Description/Actions: Acts primarily on bone and is indicated for the treatment of symptomatic Paget's disease of bone, and for the prevention and treatment of heterotopic ossification following total hip replacement or due to spinal cord injury. Also used parenterally for the management of hypercalcemia of malignancy inadequately managed by dietary modification or oral hydration, and in the hypercalcemia of malignancy that persists after adequate hydration has been restored.

Preparations: Tablets, 200 and 400 mg. Ampules, 300 mg.

ETODOLAC—Lodine®

Description/Actions: Non-steroidal anti-inflammatory agent that inhibits prostaglandin synthesis and is indicated for the management of osteoarthritis and rheumatoid arthritis. Is also indicated for the management of pain.

Precautions/Adverse Reactions: Should not be given to patients in whom aspirin or another NSAID causes asthma, rhinitis, urticaria, or other allergic-type reactions. May cause GI effects and use should be avoided in patients with active GI tract disease and closely monitored in patients with a previous history of such disorders.

Administration: Oral.

Preparations: Capsules, 200 and 300 mg. Tablets, 400 and 500 mg. Extended-release tablets, 400, 500, and 600 mg.

ETOPOSIDE—VePesid®, VP-16®

Description/Actions: Antineoplastic agent used in treatment of refractory testicular neoplasms in patients who have already received appropriate surgical, chemotherapeutic, and radiation therapy. Indicated for the treatment of choriosarcoma in women and small cell carcinoma.

Administration: Oral, intravenous.

Preparations: Capsules, 50 mg. Injection, 50 mg/ml.

ETOMIDATE—Amidate®

Description/Actions: General anesthetic indicated for induction of general anesthesia and for supplementation of subpotent anesthetic agents (e.g., nitrous oxide in oxygen) during maintenance of anesthesia for short surgical procedures.

Preparations: Ampules, 2 mg/ml.

EUGENOL

Description/Actions: Local anesthetic used in some formulations used for the relief of toothache.

Preparations: Drops.

EULEXIN®, see Flutamide

EURAX®, see Crotamiton

EVISTA®, see Raloxifene HCl

EVOCLIN®, see Clindamycin

EVOXAC®, see Cevimeline Hydrochloride

EXCEDRIN®—Combination Agent Acetaminophen, Aspirin, and Caffeine (Analgesic and Salicylate)

EXELDERM®, see Sulconazole Nitrate

EXELON®, see Rivastigmine Tartrate

EXEMESTANE—Aromasin®

Description/Actions: Exemestane is used as a second-line agent for the treatment of breast cancer in postmenopausal women.

Precautions/Adverse Reactions: Exemestane should not be given to pregnant women, breast-feeding women, or children. Also, the drug should not be given to premenopausal women because exemestane will not be effective. Patients on exemestane should not take any exogenous estrogens. Some common side effects are hot flashes, fever, leg swelling, constipation, weight gain, fatigue, pain, depression, insomnia, anxiety, dyspnea, dizziness, headache, diaphoresis, nausea, and vomiting.

Administration: Oral.

Patient Care Implications: Patients should not take any exogenous estrogens while on the medication. Also, the drug should not be given to pregnant women, breast-feeding women, premenopausal women, and children.

Preparations: Tablets, 25 mg.

EXNA®, see Benzthiazide

EXOSURF NEONATAL®, see Colfosceril Palmitate

EZETIMIBE—Zetia™

Description/Actions: Ezetimibe belongs to a class of lipid-lowering compounds that selectively inhibit the intestinal absorption of cholesterol and related phytosterols. It may be used alone or in combination with an HMG-CoA reductase inhibitor (atorvastatin, fluvastatin, lovastatin, pravastatin, or simvastatin) or as adjunctive therapy to diet for the reduction of elevated total cholesterol, LDL-C, and APo B in patients with primary heterozygous familial and nonfamilial hypercholesterolemia and homozygous sitosterolemia.

Precautions/Adverse Reactions: Ezetimibe is contraindicated in patients with a known hypersensitivity to any component of the formulation. It is contraindicated in combination with an HMGCoA reductase inhibitor in patients with active liver disease or unexplained persistent elevations in serum transaminases. Hypersensitivity reactions, including rash and angioedema, have been reported during treatment with ezetimibe. Not recommended for use in patients with moderate or severe hepatic insufficiency. Pregnancy Category C. Most common adverse effects observed during treatment with ezetimibe (as monotherapy or in combination with an HMG-CoA reductase inhibitor) include headache, diarrhea, abdominal pain, fatigue, pharyngitis, sinusitis, arthralgias, back pain, coughing, chest pain, and dizziness. When ezetimibe is used in combination with an HMG-CoA reductase inhibitor, liver function tests should be performed at initiation of therapy and according to the package labeling for the HMG-CoA reductase inhibitor. Ezetimibe does not appear to be an inducer or inhibitor of the cytochrome P450 enzyme system.

Administration: Oral, with or without food.

Preparations: Tablets, 10 mg.

F

FACTREL®, see Gonadorelin

FAMCICLOVIR—Famvir®

Description/Actions: Is a prodrug that is rapidly converted following administration to the antiviral compound penciclovir. Antiviral agent indicated for the management of acute herpes zoster (shingles), treatment or suppression of recurrent episodes of genital herpes in immunocompetent patients, and treatment of recurrent mucocutaneous herpes simplex infections in HIV-infected patients.

Precautions/Adverse Reactions: Adverse reactions include headache, nausea, and fatigue.

Administration: Oral.

Preparations: Tablets, 125, 250, and 500 mg.

FAMOTIDINE—Mylanta AR®, Pepcid®, Pepcid AC®, Pepcid RDP®

Description/Actions: Indicated in (a) short-term treatment of active duodenal ulcer; (b) maintenance therapy for duodenal ulcer patients at reduced dosage after healing of an active ulcer; (c) short-term treatment of active, benign gastric ulcer; (d) treatment of gastroesophageal reflux disease including erosive esophagitis; and (e) treatment of pathological hypersecretory conditions (e.g., Zollinger-Ellison syndrome, multiple endocrine adenomas). Available without a prescription (Pepcid AC®) to relieve and prevent acid indigestion.

Precautions/Adverse Reactions: Adverse reactions include headache, dizziness, constipation, diarrhea, and transient irritation at the injection site when administered intravenously. Dosage adjustments are required for patients with moderate renal impairment (creatinine clearance <50 ml/min).

Administration: Oral and intravenous.

Preparations: Tablets, 10 (Pepcid AC®), 20, and 40 mg. Disintegrating tablets (Pepcid RDP®), 20 and 40 mg. Oral suspension containing 40 mg/5 ml when reconstituted. Vials, 10 mg/ml.

FAMVIR®, see Famciclovir

FANSIDAR®, Combination of Sulfadoxine and Pyrimethamine

FARESTON®, see Toremifene

FASLODEX®, see Fulvestrant

FASTIN®, see Phentermine

FAZACLO™, see Clozapine

FELBAMATE—Felbatol®

Description/Actions: Antiepileptic agent. Because of the risks of aplastic anemia and acute liver failure, should only be used in patients whose epilepsy is so severe that the risk is deemed acceptable in light of the benefits conferred by its use. Indicated as monotherapy and adjunctive therapy in the treatment of partial seizures with and without generalization in adults with epilepsy, and as adjunctive therapy in the treatment of partial and generalized seizures associated with Lennox-Gastaut syndrome in children.

Precautions/Adverse Reactions: Adverse reactions include aplastic anemia, acute liver failure, anorexia, nausea, vomiting, insomnia, somnolence, dizziness, and headache. Do full baseline hematologic evaluation and hepatic function tests before, during, and after therapy. Discontinue if hepatic tests are abnormal or bone marrow depression occurs. Consult hematologist if hematologic abnormalities occur.

Administration: Oral.

Preparations: Tablets, 400 and 600 mg. Oral suspension, 600 mg/5 ml.

FELBATOL®, see Felbamate

FELDENE®, see Piroxicam

FELODIPINE—Plendil®

Description/Actions: A calcium channel-blocking agent that is indicated in the management of hypertension. May be used alone or concurrently with other antihypertensive agents.

Precautions/Adverse Reactions: Adverse reactions include peripheral edema, headache, flushing, dizziness, asthenia, cough, paresthesia, dyspepsia, chest pain, nausea, muscle cramps, and palpitation. Mild gingival hyperplasia has been reported and may be reduced by good dental hygiene. Caution should be exercised in patients with congestive heart failure, particularly if a beta-blocker is used concurrently. Action may be increased by the concurrent use of cimetidine. Bioavailability of the drug has been reported to be significantly increased when taken with doubly concentrated grapefruit juice. Coadministration of felodipine and cimetidine results in an increase in felodipine plasma levels.

Administration: Oral.

Preparations: Extended-release tablets, 2.5, 5, and 10 mg.

FEMARA®, see Letrozole

FEMSTAT®, see Butoconazole

FENOFIBRATE—Tricor®

Description/Actions: Indicated as an adjunct to diet in treating adults with very high elevations of serum triglyerceride levels (types IV and V hyperlipidemias) who are at risk of pancreatitis and who do not adequately respond to a strict dietary measure of control. Fenofibrate reduces serum uric acid levels in both hyperuricemic and normal individuals by increasing urinary excretion of uric acid.

Precautions/Adverse Reactions: Contraindicated in hepatic dysfunction (including primary biliary cirrhosis and unexplained persistent liver function abnormality), severe renal dysfunction, and gallbladder disease. Fenofibrate can cause dose-related hepatoxicity. Liver function should be monitored at baseline and at regular intervals for the duration of treatment. Pancreatitis has been reported in patients taking fenofibrate, but it is a secondary phenomenon through biliary tract stone or sludge formation and obstruction of the bile duct. Use cautiously in patients with renal impairment. Monitor CBC for at least a year. Monitor liver function regularly and discontinue if ALT (SGPT) levels are >3 times upper limit of normal (ULN). Discontinue if myopathy or gallstones occur. Pregnancy Category C. Not recommended in nursing mothers. Adverse reactions include rash, flu-like symptoms, eye irritation, dizziness, eructation, myopathy, rhabdomyolysis, increased serum transaminases, hepatitis, cirrhosis, cholelithiasis, pancreatitis, increased BUN/Cr., transient moderate hematologic changes, thrombocytopenia, and agranulocytosis (rare).

Administration: Oral. Give with meals. Discontinue if significant improvement is not seen in 2 months.

Preparations: Tablets, 48, and 145 mg.

FENOPROFEN CALCIUM—Nalfon®

Description/Actions: Non-steroidal anti-inflammatory agent indicated for the relief of mild to moderate pain, rheumatoid arthritis, and osteoarthritis.

Precautions/Adverse Reactions: Should not be used in patients with a history of significantly impaired renal function. Should not be given to patients in whom aspirin or another NSAID causes asthma, rhinitis, urticaria, or other allergic-type reactions. May cause GI effects, so use should be avoided in patients with active GI tract disease and closely monitored in patients with a previous history of such disorders. Other adverse reactions include dizziness, pruritus, palpitations, and nervousness.

Administration: Oral.

Preparations: Capsules, 200 and 300 mg. Tablets, 600 mg.

FENTANYL—Duragesic®

Description/Actions: *Opioid analgesic* indicated for the management of chronic pain. Transdermal system provides analgesic activity for up to 72 hours.

Preparations: Transdermal system, 12 mcg/hr, 25 mcg/hour (2.5 mg), 50 mcg/hour (5 mg), 75 mcg/hour (7.5 mg), and 100 mcg/hour (10 mg).

FENTANYL CITRATE—Actiq®, Sublimaze®, Oralet®

Description/Actions: Opioid analgesic/anesthetic indicated for parenteral use for (a) analgesic action before, during, and following surgery; (b) as an analgesic supplement in general or as a regional anesthesia; (c) administration with a neuroleptic in conjunction with anesthesia; and (d) as an anesthetic agent with oxygen in selected high-risk patients. Also indicated for oral transmucosal use (as a lozenge) for anesthetic premedication in children and adults, and for use in anesthesia or monitored anesthesia care.

Preparations: Ampules, 50 mcg/ml. Lozenges, 200, 300, 400, 600, 800, and 1200 mcg.

FEOSOL®, see Ferrous Sulfate Exsiccated

FEOSTAT®, see Ferrous Fumarate

FERGON®, see Ferrous Gluconate

FER-IN-SOL®, see Ferrous Sulfate

FERO-GRADUMET®, see Ferrous Sulfate

FERRIC SODIUM GLUCONATE—Ferrlecit®

Description/Actions: Ferric sodium gluconate is used to treat iron deficiency in patients who receive chronic hemodialysis and epoetin alfa.

Precautions/Adverse Reactions: Ferric sodium gluconate should not be administered in neonates, in patients with benzyl alcohol hypersensitivity, and in patients who have an anemia not caused by iron deficiency. The drug may be given to pregnant women but should be administered with caution in breast-feeding patients. One adverse reaction is a hypersensitivity reaction that can cause cardiovascular collapse, cardiac arrest, bronchospasm, angioedema, urticaria, or pruritus. Other side effects are hemosiderosis, flu-like syndrome, dizziness, infection, insomnia, upper respiratory infection, hypertension, syncope, tachycardia, bradycardia, pulmonary edema, flatulence, electrolyte disturbance, leg edema, flushing, and hypotension.

Administration: Intravenous.

Patient Care Implications: The drug should not be administered in neonates, in patients with benzyl alcohol hypersensitivity, or in patients who have an anemia not caused by iron deficiency. Ferritin, hemoglobin, hematocrit, iron, and transferrin should be checked before and during therapy.

Preparations: Ampule, 62.5 mg/5 ml.

FERRLECIT®, see Ferric Sodium Gluconate

FERROUS FUMARATE—Feostat®

Description/Actions: Hematinic indicated for the prevention and treatment of iron deficiency anemias.

Preparations: Tablets, 100, 200, and 325 mg. Suspension, 100 mg/5 ml. Drops, 45 mg/0.6 ml.

FERROUS GLUCONATE—Fergon®

Description/Actions: Hematinic indicated for the prevention and treatment of iron deficiency anemias.

Preparations: Tablets, 325 mg. Capsules, 325 and 435 mg. Elixir, 300 mg/5 ml.

FERROUS SULFATE—Fero-Gradumet®, Fer-In-Sol®

Description/Actions: Hematinic indicated for the prevention and treatment of iron deficiency anemias.

Preparations: Controlled-release tablets, 525 mg. Syrup, 90 mg/5 ml. Drops, 75 mg/0.6 ml.

FERROUS SULFATE, EXSICCATED—Feosol®, Slow FE®

Description/Actions: Hematinic indicated for the prevention and treatment of iron deficiency anemias.

Preparations: Tablets, 200 mg. Controlled-release capsules and tablets, 160 mg.

FEXOFENADINE HYDROCHLORIDE—Allegra®

Description/Actions: A nonsedating antihistamine with selective peripheral H_1-receptor antagonist activity indicated in the treatment of seasonal allergic rhinitis.

Precautions/Adverse Reactions: Adverse reactions include viral infection, nausea, dysmenorrhea, drowsiness, dyspepsia, and fatigue. Use cautiously in patients with renal impairment. Rash, urticaria, pruritis, and hypersensitivity reactions, with manifestations such as angiocdcma, chest tightness, dyspnea, flushing, and anaphylaxis, have been reported.

Administration: Oral.

Preparations: Capsules, 60 mg. Tablets, 30, 60, and 180 mg.

FEXOFENADINE/PSEUDOEPHEDRINE—Allegra-D®, Allegra-D® 24 Hour

Description/Actions: Fexofenadine and pseudoephedrine are used together in an oral preparation to relieve symptoms of seasonal allergic rhinitis in adults and children 12 years of age and older.

Precautions/Adverse Reactions: Adverse reactions include headache, insomnia, nausea/vomiting, dry mouth, agitation, dizziness, nervousness, anxiety, palpitations, dyspepsia, throat irritation, upper respiratory infection, back pain, and abdominal pain. Central nervous system stimulation resulting in restlessness, tremor, seizures, and psychological disturbances can be seen. Use cautiously in patients with renal impairment, narrow-angle glaucoma, diabetes mellitus, urinary retention, hyperthyroidism, or prostatic hypertrophy. In addition, because pseudoephedrine is a vasoconstrictor, it should be used cautiously in patients with uncontrolled hypertension or severe coronary artery disease. Due to its pseudoephedrine component, Allegra-D is contraindicated in patients receiving MAOI therapy or within 14 days of stopping such treatment.

Administration: Oral.

Preparations: Extended release tablets, fexofenadine 180 mg/pseudoephedrine 240 mg.

FIBERCON® see Polycarbophil

FIBRINOLYSIN—in Elase®

Description/Actions: Fibrinolytic agent used in combination with deoxyribonuclease for topical use as debriding agents in a variety of inflammatory and infected lesions.

Preparations: Ointment and powder for solution.

FILGRASTIM—Neupogen®

Description/Actions: A human granulocyte colony stimulating factor (G-CSF) produced by recombinant DNA technology. It regulates the production of neutrophils within the bone marrow. It is indicated to decrease the incidence of infection, as manifested by febrile neutropenia in patients with nonmyeloid malignancies receiving myelosuppressive anticancer drugs associated with a significant incidence of severe neutropenia, with fever. May also be used to reduce the time of neutrophil recovery and fever duration after induction and consolidation chemotherapy treatment of adults with AML. Also indicated in patients with nonmyeloid malignancies undergoing chemotherapy followed by marrow transplantation. Also indicated to reduce the incidence and duration of sequelae of severe chronic neutropenia.

Precautions/Adverse Reactions: May cause bone pain and leukocytosis. Caution must be exercised in patients with any malignancy with myeloid characteristics because of the possibility that the drug may act as a growth factor for the tumor.

Administration: Intravenous and subcutaneous. Should be administered no earlier than 24 hours after the administration of cytotoxic chemotherapy, and should not be administered in the period 24 hours before the administration of chemotherapy. Vials should not be shaken.

Preparations: Vials, 300 and 480 mcg.

FINASTERIDE—Propecia®

Description/Actions: Indicated in the treatment of male pattern hair loss (androgenetic alopecia) in men only.

Precautions/Adverse Reactions: Contraindicated in women and children. Women of childbearing potential must not handle crushed or broken tablets. Pregnancy Category X. Use cautiously in hepatic dysfunction. Consider that the PSA may double in men ≥41 years of age without BPH who are undergoing PSA test. Instruct patients that the benefits may not be seen for 3 months. Must continue to sustain effect. Reversal of effects seen within 12 months of discontinuation. Adverse reactions include decreased libido, erectile dysfunction, and ejaculation disorder (all rare).

Administration: Oral.

Preparations: Tablets, 1 mg.

FINASTERIDE—Proscar®

Description/Actions: Inhibits steroid 5-alpha-reductase that converts testosterone into 5-alpha-dihydrotestosterone (DHT), a potent androgen. Indicated for the treatment of symptomatic benign prostatic hyperplasia to improve symptoms and reduce risks of acute urinary retention and the need for prostate surgery. Proscar® administered in combination with the alpha blocker doxazocin is indicated to reduce the risk of symptomatic progression of benign prostatic hyperplasia (BPH).

Precautions/Adverse Reactions: Contraindicated during pregnancy and in nursing mothers. Adverse reactions include impotence, decreased libido, and decreased volume of ejaculate. May cause harm to a male fetus, and women who are pregnant should avoid exposure to the drug—crushed tablets should not be handled by a woman who is pregnant, and, when the patient's sexual partner is or may become pregnant, the patient should avoid exposure of his partner to semen or discontinue the medication. May cause a decrease in serum prostate-specific antigen (PSA).

Administration: Oral. A minimum of 6 months of treatment may be necessary to determine whether an individual will respond to the drug.

Preparations: Tablets, 5 mg.

FIORICET®, Combination of Butalbital, Acetaminophen, and Caffeine. See individual discussion on Butalbital, Acetaminophen and Caffeine.

FIORINAL®, Combination of Butalbital, Aspirin, and Caffeine. See individual discussion on Butalbital, Aspirin and Caffeine.

5 FU®, see Fluorouracil

FLAGYL®, see Metronidazole

FLAVOXATE HYDROCHLORIDE—Urispas®

Description/Actions: Spasmolytic agent indicated for the symptomatic relief of urinary tract problems such as dysuria, urgency, nocturia, suprapubic pain, frequency, and incontinence.

Preparations: Tablets, 100 mg.

FLAXEDIL®, see Gallamine

FLECAINIDE ACETATE—Tambocor®

Description/Actions: A class IC antiarrhythmic agent. Indicated for the treatment of life-threatening ventricular arrhythmias such as sustained ventricular tachycardia. Also indicated for paroxysmal atrial fibrillation/flutter associated with disabling symptoms and paroxysmal supraventricular tachycardias associated with disabling symptoms in patients without structural heart disease.

Precautions/Adverse Reactions: Contraindicated in patients with second- or third-degree AV block, with right bundle branch block when associated with a left hemiblock (unless a pacemaker is present), or in the presence of cardiogenic shock. Adverse reactions include proarrhythmic events, worsening of congestive heart failure, dizziness, visual disturbances, dyspnea, headache, nausea, fatigue, and palpitation.

Administration: Oral.

Preparations: Tablets, 50, 100, and 150 mg.

FLEXERIL®, see Cyclobenzaprine

FLOLAN®, see Epoprostenol

FLOMAX®, see Tamsulosin Hydrochloride

FLONASE®, see Fluticasone Propionate

FLORINEF®, see Fludrocortisone

FLORONE®, see Diflorasone

FLOROPRYL®, see Isoflurophate

FLOVENT®, see Fluticasone Propionate

FLOVENT® DISKUS, see Fluticasone Propionate

FLOXIN®, see Ofloxacin

FLOXIN IV®, see Ofloxacin

FLOXIN® OTIC, see Ofloxacin

FLOXIN® OTIC SINGLES®, see Ofloxacin

FLOXURIDINE—FUDR®

Description/Actions: Antineoplastic agent administered by intra-arterial infusion in the management of gastrointestinal adenocarcinoma metastatic to the liver.

Preparations: Vials, 5 mg.

FLUCONAZOLE—Diflucan®

Description/Actions: Antifungal agent indicated for the treatment of cryptococcal meningitis, serious systemic candidal infections including urinary tract infection, peritonitis, and pneumonia, as well as oropharyngeal and esophageal candidiasis. Also indicated as a single-dose treatment for vaginal candidiasis.

Precautions/Adverse Reactions: Adverse reactions include nausea, vomiting, abdominal pain, diarrhea, headache, rash, and hepatic reactions. May increase the plasma concentrations and/or activity of warfarin, phenytoin, cyclosporine, and oral hypoglycemic agents. Rifampin may increase the rate of metabolism, and it may be necessary to increase the dosage of the antifungal agent during the period of concurrent therapy.

Administration: Oral and intravenous.

Preparations: Tablets, 50, 100, and 200 mg. Oral suspension, 10 mg/ml. Glass bottles and plastic containers, 200 mg/100 ml and 400 mg/200 ml.

FLUCYTOSINE—Ancobon®

Description/Actions: Antifungal agent indicated for systemic infections caused by *Candida* and *Cryptococcus*.

Precautions/Adverse Reactions: Bone marrow toxicity can be irreversible and may lead to death in immunosuppressed patients.

Preparations: Capsules, 250 and 500 mg.

FLUDARA®, see Fludarabine

FLUDARABINE PHOSPHATE—Fludara®

Description/Actions: Antineoplastic agent that is an analog of the antiviral agent vidarabine. Indicated for the treatment of patients with B-cell chronic lymphocytic leukemia who have not responded to or have progressed during treatment with at least one standard regimen containing an alkylating agent.

Precautions/Adverse Reactions: May cause fetal harm and should not be used during pregnancy unless safer alternatives are not available. Pulmonary toxicity (e.g., ARDS, respiratory distress, pulmonary hemorrhage, pulmonary fibrosis, and respiratory failure) has occurred in patients treated with fludarabine. Myelosuppression may be severe; several instances of trilineage bone marrow depression or aplastic aplasia resulting in pancytopenia, sometimes death, have been reported. These effects have occurred in both previously treated and untreated patients. Decrease dose of fludarabine by 20% in patients with moderate renal impairment (creatinine clearance 30–70 ml/min/1.73 m2). Fludarabine should not be administered to patients with severe renal impairment (creatinine clearance <30 ml/min/1.73 m2).

Administration: Intravenous.

Preparations: Vials, 50 mg.

FLUDROCORTISONE ACETATE—Florinef®

Description/Actions: Mineralocorticoid indicated for the treatment of Addison's disease and salt-losing adrenogenital syndrome.

Preparations: Tablets, 0.1 mg.

FLUMADINE®, see Rimantadine Hydrochloride

FLUMAZENIL—Romazicon®

Description/Actions: Benzodiazepine antagonist that reverses the sedating and psychomotor effects of benzodiazepines (e.g., diazepam, midazolam); however, amnesia is less completely and less consistently reversed. Indicated for the complete or partial reversal of the sedative effects of benzodiazepines in cases where general anesthesia has been induced and/or maintained with benzodiazepines, where sedation has been produced with benzodiazepines for diagnostic and therapeutic procedures, and for the management of benzodiazepine overdose.

Precautions/Adverse Reactions: Contraindicated in patients who may be relying on the effects of a benzodiazepine to control potentially life-threatening conditions (e.g., status epilepticus, increased intracranial pressure). Is also contraindicated in cases of serious cyclic antidepressant (e.g., amitriptyline) overdose. May cause seizures, including withdrawal seizures in patients who are physically dependent on benzodiazepines. Other adverse reactions include nausea, vomiting, dizziness, agitation, and injection site pain. In situations in which a patient has received a neuromuscular blocking agent, flumazenil should not be used until the effects of neuromuscular blockade have been fully reversed. Duration of action is shorter than that of the benzodiazepines, and a return of sedation (resedation) may occur following initial reversal. Patients should be monitored for resedation, as well as respiratory depression and other residual benzodiazepine effects. Patients should be advised not to engage in any activities requiring complete alertness until at least 18–24 hours after discharge and not to take any alcohol or nonprescription drugs for 18–24 hours after flumazenil administration or if the effects of the benzodiazepine persist. Because flumazenil does not consistently reverse amnesia, patients cannot be expected to remember information told to them in the postprocedure period, and instructions given to patients should be reinforced in writing or given to a responsible family member.

Administration: Intravenous. Should be administered through a freely running intravenous infusion into a large vein to minimize the likelihood of pain or inflammation at the injection site.

Preparations: Vials, 0.1 mg/ml.

FLUMETHIAZIDE

Description/Actions: Thiazide diuretic used in combination with other agents in the treatment of hypertension.

FLUNISOLIDE—Aerobid®, Aerobid-M® (menthol flavor), Nasalide®, Nasarel®

Description/Actions: Corticosteroid. Nasalide®: indicated for the topical treatment of the symptoms of seasonal or perennial rhinitis when effectiveness of or tolerance of conventional treatment is unsatisfactory. Nasarel®: for the treatment of seasonal or perennial rhinitis. Aerobid®: Maintenance treatment of asthma as prophylactic therapy or to reduce the need for systemic corticosteroids in individuals requiring systemic steroid therapy.

Precautions/Adverse Reactions: Adverse reactions include transient nasal burning and stinging and nasal congestion. Caution must be exercised when transferring a patient from systemic corticosteroid therapy to flunisolide therapy. Contraindicated as primary treatment of an acute attack, in varicella and vaccinia.

Administration: Oral and nasal.

Preparations: Nasal solution spray bottle, 6.25 mg, metered dose inhaler 250 µg/inh.

FLUOCINOLONE ACETONIDE—Synalar®

Description/Actions: Corticosteroid applied topically for relief of inflammatory and pruritic manifestations of corticosteroid-responsive dermatoses.

Preparations: Cream, 0.01%, 0.025%, and 0.2%. Ointment, 0.025%. Topical solution, 0.01%.

FLUOCINONIDE—Lidex®, Lidex-E®, Vanos®

Description/Actions: Topical corticosteroid indicated for the relief of the inflammatory and pruritic manifestations of corticosteroid-responsive dermatoses.

Precautions/Adverse Reactions: Adverse reactions include burning, itching, dryness, irritation, and a potential for systemic effects.

Administration: Topical.

Preparations: Cream, gel, ointment, and solution, 0.05%. Lidex-E cream utilizes water-washable aqueous base. Cream 0.1%.

FLUORESCEIN SODIUM

Description/Actions: Diagnostic aid used in various ocular conditions.

Preparations: Solution, 2%. Strips, 0.6 and 1 mg. Ampules, 10% and 25%.

FLUOROMETHOLONE—FML®

Description/Actions: Corticosteroid indicated for ophthalmic use in the treatment of inflammatory conditions of the eye.

Preparations: Ophthalmic suspension and ointment, 0.1%.

FLUOROPLEX®, see Fluorouracil

FLUOROURACIL—Adrucil®, Carac™, Efudex®, 5 FU®, Fluoroplex®

Description/Actions: Antineoplastic agent indicated for intravenous use in the management of carcinoma of the colon, rectum, breast, stomach, and pancreas, and for the topical treatment of active or solar keratoses and superficial basal cell carcinomas.

Preparations: Ampules, 500 mg. Cream, 05%, 1%, and 5%. Topical solution, 1%, 2%, and 5%.

FLUOTHANE®, see Halothane

FLUOXETINE HYDROCHLORIDE—Prozac®, Prozac® Weekly™, Sarafem™

Description/Actions: Fluoxetine is a selective serotonin reuptake inhibitor. It is indicated for the treatment of depression, obsessive-compulsive disorder (OCD), bulimia nervosa, and panic disorder, and for the treatment of premenstrual dysphoric disorder (PMDD). It is also indicated for the treatment of depression and OCD in pediatric patients.

Precautions/Adverse Reactions: Antidepressants increased the risk of suicidal thinking and behavior (suicidality) in short-term studies in children and adolescents with Major Depressive Disorder (MDD) and other psychiatric disorders. Anyone considering the use of fluoxetine or any other antidepressant in a child or adolescent must balance this risk with the clinical need. Patients who are started on therapy should be observed closely for clinical worsening, suicidality, or unusual changes in behavior. Prozac® is approved for use in pediatric patients with MDD and obsessive compulsive disorder (OCD). Adverse reactions include anxiety, nervousness, insomnia, nausea, diarrhea, and rash and/or urticaria. Dizziness and other CNS effects may develop, so patients should be cautioned regarding activities such as driving and operating machinery, as well as interactions with other CNS-acting drugs including alcohol. Concurrent use with tryptophan has resulted in the development of agitation and restlessness in some patients. Use in combination with a monoamine oxidase inhibitor should be avoided and at least 14 days should elapse between discontinuation of an MAO inhibitor and initiation of treatment with fluoxetine. At least 5 weeks should elapse between discontinuation of fluoxetine and initiation of therapy with an MAOI.

Administration: Oral.

Preparations: Tablets, 10 mg. Capsules, 10 and 20 mg. Liquid, 20 mg/ 5 ml. Sustained release capsules, 90 mg.

FLUOXYMESTERONE—Halotestin®

Description/Actions: Androgen indicated in male patients for replacement therapy in conditions associated with symptoms of deficiency or absence of endogenous testosterone (e.g., primary hypogonadism—testicular failure), and delayed puberty. Also indicated in the treatment of recurrent mammary cancer in selected female patients.

Preparations: Tablets, 2, 5, and 10 mg.

FLUPHENAZINE DECANOATE—Prolixin Decanoate®

FLUPHENAZINE ENANTHATE—Prolixin Enanthate®

Description/Actions: Phenothiazine antipsychotic agent indicated for the parenteral treatment of patients requiring prolonged parenteral neuroleptic therapy (e.g., chronic schizophrenics).

Preparations: Vials and syringes, 25 mg/ml.

FLUPHENAZINE HYDROCHLORIDE—Permitil®, Prolixin®

Description/Actions: Phenothiazine antipsychotic agent indicated for the management of manifestations of psychotic disorders.

Preparations: Tablets, 1, 2.5, 5, and 10 mg. Elixir, 2.5 mg/5 ml. Concentrate, 5 mg/ml. Vials, 2.5 mg/ml.

FLURANDRENOLIDE—Cordran®

Description/Actions: Corticosteroid applied topically for the relief of inflammatory and pruritic manifestations of corticosteroid-responsive dermatoses.

Preparations: Cream and ointment, 0.025% and 0.05%. Lotion, 0.05%. Tape, 4 mcg/sq. cm. Patch, 2 × 3 inches.

FLURAZEPAM HYDROCHLORIDE—Dalmane®

Description/Actions: A benzodiazepine hypnotic indicated for the management of insomnia.

Precautions/Adverse Reactions: Contraindicated during pregnancy. Adverse reactions include residual sedation and other CNS effects upon awakening; patients should be cautioned regarding activities such as driving and operating machinery, as well as interactions with other CNS-acting drugs, including alcohol. Can cause dependence and is included in Schedule IV.

Administration: Oral.

Preparations: Capsules, 15 and 30 mg.

FLURBIPROFEN—Ansaid®

Description/Actions: Nonsteroidal anti-inflammatory agent that inhibits prostaglandin synthesis and is indicated for the treatment of rheumatoid arthritis and osteoarthritis.

Precautions/Adverse Reactions: Should not be given to patients in whom aspirin or another NSAID causes asthma, rhinitis, urticaria, or other allergic-type reactions. May cause GI effects, so use should be avoided in patients with active GI tract disease and closely monitored in patients with a previous history of such disorders.

Administration: Oral.

Preparations: Tablets, 50 and 100 mg.

FLURBIPROFEN SODIUM—Ocufen®

Description/Actions: Nonsteroidal anti-inflammatory agent indicated for the inhibition of intraoperative miosis to reduce the risk of complications associated with procedures such as cataract surgery.

Precautions/Adverse Reactions: Contraindicated in epithelial herpes simplex keratitis. Adverse reactions include transient burning and stinging upon instillation; the drug may also delay wound healing. Caution should be exercised in the treatment of patients having a history of sensitivity to aspirin or another nonsteroidal anti-inflammatory drug.

Administration: Ophthalmic.

Preparations: Ophthalmic solution, 0.03%.

FLUTAMIDE—Eulexin®

Description/Actions: An antiandrogenic antineoplastic agent that inhibits the uptake and binding of androgen. Is rapidly converted to hydroxyflutamide, which is the major active metabolite. Indicated in the treatment of locally confined stage A2–C or metastatic prostatic carcinoma (stage D2) in combination with an analog of luteinizing hormone-releasing hormone (LH-RH) such as leuprolide.

Precautions/Adverse Reactions: Adverse reactions include diarrhea, nausea, vomiting, hot flashes, loss of libido, impotence, and gynecomastia. Has caused elevations of hepatic enzyme levels, as well as clinically evident hepatitis, and periodic liver function tests should be considered in patients on long-term therapy.

Administration: Oral. It is recommended that treatment be started simultaneously with both flutamide and leuprolide. Patients should be informed that the two drugs are to be administered concurrently and that they should not discontinue taking either medication without consulting their physician.

Preparations: Capsules, 125 mg.

FLUTICASONE PROPIONATE—Cutivate®, Flonase®, Flovent®, Flovent® Diskus™

Description/Actions: Corticosteroid indicated (Cutivate®) for the relief of the inflammatory and pruritic manifestations of corticosteroid-responsive dermatoses. Also administered (Flonase®) by nasal inhalation for the management of seasonal and perennial allergic rhinitis.

Precautions/Adverse Reactions: Adverse reactions include pruritus, dryness, burning, increased erythema, hypertrichosis, and numbness of fingers.

Administration: Topical, nasal, and inhalation.

Preparations: Cream, 0.05%; ointment, 0.005%. Nasal spray, 44 mcg, 50 mcg, 110 mcg, 220 mcg per actuation. Metered dose inhaler, 44, 110, and 220 mcg/inh. Rotadisk, 50, 100, and 250 mcg/inh. via dry powder.

FLUVASTATIN SODIUM—Lescol®, Lescol® XL

Description/Actions: Produces a significant reduction in total and low-density lipoprotein (LDL) cholesterol concentrations, a modest reduction in triglyceride concentrations, and an increase in high-density lipoprotein (HDL) cholesterol concentrations. Indicated as an adjunct to diet in the treatment of elevated total cholesterol and low-density lipoprotein cholesterol in patients with primary hypercholesterolemia whose response to dietary restriction of saturated fat and cholesterol and other nonpharmacological measures has not been adequate. Also indicated to slow the progression of coronary atherosclerosis in patients with coronary heart disease. In patients with coronary artery disease, Lescol® and Lescol® XL are indicated to reduce the risk of undergoing coronary revascularization procedures.

Precautions/Adverse Reactions: Contraindicated in patients with active liver disease or unexplained, persistent elevations of serum transaminases. Is also contraindicated in pregnant women and nursing mothers. Increases in serum transaminases may occur, so it is recommended that liver function tests be performed before the initiation of treatment, at 6 and 12 weeks after initiation of therapy or elevation in dose, and periodically thereafter (e.g., every 6 months). Should be used with caution in patients with a history of liver disease or heavy alcohol ingestion. Adverse reactions include dyspepsia, abdominal pain, arthropathy, and exercise-related muscle pain. Patients should be advised to promptly report unexplained muscle pain, tenderness, or weakness. The concurrent use of clofibrate or gemfibrozil is best avoided, and caution should be exercised if cyclosporine or erythromycin is used concurrently. When used concomitantly with a bile acid-binding resin, fluvastatin sodium should be administered at least 4 hours after the resin.

Administration: Oral. Should be administered at bedtime.

Preparations: Capsules, 20 and 40 mg, extended-release tablets, 80 mg.

FLUVOXAMINE MALEATE—Luvox®

Description/Actions: Selective serotonin reuptake inhibitor indicated for the treatment of obsessive compulsive disorder.

Precautions/Adverse Reactions: Antidepressants increased the risk of suicidal thinking and behavior (suicidality) in short-term studies in children and adolescents with Major Depressive Disorder (MDD) and other psychiatric disorders. Anyone considering the use of fluvoxamine or any other antidepressant in a child or adolescent must balance this risk with the clinical need. Patients who are started on therapy should be observed closely for clinical worsening, suicidality, or unusual changes in behavior. Luvox® is not approved for use in pediatric patients. Concurrent administration of terfenadine or astemizole is contraindicated. Adverse reactions include somnolence, insomnia, nervousness, dizziness, and tremor. Advise patients to avoid driving or operating machinery until response is ascertained. Alcohol should be avoided. It is recommended that fluvoxamine not be used in combination with MAOIs or within 14 days of discontinuing an MAOI.

Administration: Oral.

Preparations: Tablets, 50 and 100 mg.

FML®, see Fluorometholone

FOCALIN™, see Dexmethylphenidate Hydrochloride

FOLIC ACID—Folvite®

Description/Actions: Agent for anemias that is indicated in the prevention and treatment of megaloblastic anemias due to a deficiency of folic acid as may be seen in sprue, anemias of nutritional origin, pregnancy, infancy, or childhood.

Preparations: Tablets, 0.1, 0.4, 0.8, and 1 mg. Vials 5 mg/ml and 10 mg/ml.

FOLINIC ACID, see Leucovorin

FOLLUTEIN®, see Chorionic Gonadotropin

FOLVITE®, see Folic Acid

FOMIVIRSEN NA—Vitravene®

Description/Actions: Indicated for the local treatment of human cytomegalovirus (CMV) retinitis in patients with AIDS who are intolerant of or have a contraindication to other treatment for CMV retinitis or who are insufficiently responsive to previous treatment for CMV retinitis.

Precautions/Adverse Reactions: Fomivirsen is contraindicated in patients who have recently (within 2–4 weeks) been treated with either intravenous or intravitreal cidofovir because of the risk of exaggerated ocular inflammation. CMV retinitis may be associated with CMV disease elsewhere in the body. Fomivirsen provides localized therapy limited to the treated eye. The use of fomivirsen does not provide treatment for systemic CMV disease. Patients should be monitored for extraocular CMV disease or disease of the contralateral eye. Adverse reactions include ocular inflammation, uveitis, including iritis and vitreitis. Inflammation is more commonly reported during the induction dosing.

Administration: Intravitreal injection.

Patient Care Implications: If inflammatory reactions are severe, delaying additional treatment and using topical corticosteroids have been shown to be useful in medical management of these reactions. For patients whose disease progresses while on fomivirsen, an attempt at reinduction at the same dose may result in resumed disease control. Instruct patients that fomivirsen is not a cure for their opthalmic CMV and that adherence to consistent follow-up appointments is necessary. Warn patients that their disease may still progress despite treatment with fomivirsen.

Preparations: Single-use vial, 0.25 ml (6.6 mg/ml).

FONDAPARINUX—Arixtra®

Description/Actions: Fondaparinux is indicated for the prophylaxis of deep vein thrombosis, which may lead to a pulmonary embolism in patients undergoing hip fracture surgery, including extended prophylaxis, in patients undergoing knee replacement surgery, and in patients undergoing abdominal surgery who are at risk for thromboembolic complications. It is also indicated for the treatment of acute deep vein thrombosis when administered in conjunction with warfarin and for the treatment of acute pulmonary embolism when administered in conjunction with warfarin when initial therapy is administered in the hospital.

Precautions/Adverse Reactions: Fondaparinux is contraindicated in patients with severe renal impairment (creatinine clearance <30 mL/min). Prophylactic therapy with fondaparinux in patients weighing less than 50 Kg is contraindicated in patients undergoing hip fracture, hip replacement, or knee replacement surgery. The use of fondaparinux is contraindicated in patients with active major bleeding, bacterial endocarditis, in patients with thrombocytopenia associated with a positive in vitro test for anti-platelet antibody in the presence of fondaparinux, or in patients with a hypersensitivity to fondaparinux or any component of the formulation. Fondaparinux cannot be used interchangeably (unit for unit) with heparin, low molecular weight heparins (LMWHs), or heparinoids. Each of these medicines has its own instructions for use. Use with extreme caution in conditions with increased risk of hemorrhage, such as congenital or acquired bleeding disorders, active ulcerative and angiodysplastic disease, and hemorrhagic stroke, shortly after brain, spinal, or opthalmological surgery, or in patients treated concomitantly with platelet inhibitors. Discontinue agents that may increase the risk of hemorrhage before starting fondaparinux. Should be used with caution in elderly patients and in patients with a history of heparin-induced thrombocytopenia. When neuraxial anesthesia or spinal puncture is used, patients anticoagulated or scheduled to be anticoagulated with LMWH, heparinoids, or fondaparinux for prevention of thromboembolic complications are at risk of developing an epidural or spinal hematoma, which can result in long-term or permanent paralysis. Pregnancy Category B. Excretion in breast milk unknown; use caution. The most common adverse reactions were bleeding complications. Other adverse reactions were mild local irritation, edema, fever, nausea, constipation, vomiting, and insomnia. Antiplatelet agents (anagrelide, clopidogrel, dipyridamole, abciximab), NSAIDs, and salicylates may increase its anticoagulant effect.

Administration: SQ injection.

Patient Care Implications: Inform patients they may have tendency to bleed easily while on fondaparinux; brush teeth with soft brush, floss with waxed floss, use electric razor, and avoid potentially harmful activities.

Preparations: Injection: 2.5 mg in 0.5 ml single-dose prefilled syringe, affixed with a 27 gauge × ½ inch needle with an automatic needle protection system.

FORADIL®—see Formoterol Fumarate

FORMOTEROL FUMARATE—Foradil®

Description/Actions: Formoterol fumarate is indicated for long-term, twice daily (morning and evening) administration in the maintenance treatment of asthma and in the prevention of bronchospasm in adults and children >5 years of age with reversible obstructive airway disease, including patients with symptoms of nocturnal asthma who require regular treatment with inhaled, short-acting beta-2-agonists. Formoterol is also indicated for the acute prevention of exercise-induced bronchospasm in adults and children 12 years of age when administered on an occasional, as-needed basis. Formoterol is indicated for the long-term, twice daily (morning and evening) administration in the maintenance treatment of bronchoconstriction in patients with chronic obstructive pulmonary disease, including chronic bronchitis and emphysema.

Precautions/Adverse Reactions: Therapy with formoterol should not be initiated in patients with worsening or acutely deteriorating asthma that may be a life-threatening condition. Formoterol is not a substitute for inhaled or oral corticosteroids. Corticosteroid therapy should not be stopped or reduced at the time formoterol is initiated. When initiating therapy with formoterol in patients who have been taking inhaled, short-acting beta-2-agonists on a regular basis, patients should be instructed to discontinue the regular use of the short-acting beta-2-agonists and to use them only on an as-needed basis for symptomatic relief of acute asthma symptoms. Formoterol can produce paradoxical bronchospasms that may be life threatening. If one occurs, discontinue formoterol immediately. Formoterol should not be used more frequently than twice daily at the recommended dose. Worsening asthma may warrant a reevaluation of the patient and treatment regimen. Formoterol can produce clinically significant cardiovascular effects in some patients, such as increased heart rate, increased blood pressure, and/or symptoms. Use with caution in patients with cardiovascular disorders such as coronary insufficiency, cardiac arrhythmias, and hypertension. Use with caution in patients with seizure disorders and thyrotoxicosis and in patients who are unusually sensitive to sympathomimetic amines. Beta-2-agonists have been reported to produce ECG changes such as flattening of the T wave, prolongation of the QTc interval, and ST segment depression. Immediate hypersensitivity reactions (anaphylactic reactions, urticaria, angioedema, rash, and bronchospasm) may occur following the administration of formoterol. Concurrent use of formoterol with xanthine derivatives, steroids, or diuretics may potentiate the hypokalemic effects of adrenergic agonists. Concomitant administration of formoterol with monoamine oxidase inhibitors, tricyclic antidepressants, or drugs known to prolong the QTc interval may potentiate cardiovascular side effects. Coadministration of beta-blockers and formoterol may inhibit the effects of each other. Beta-blockers not only block the therapeutic effects of beta agonists, but may produce severe bronchospasms in asthmatic patients. Use a cardioselective beta-blocker if therapy with a beta-blocker is necessary. Concurrent administration of formoterol and adrenergic drugs may potentiate the sympathetic effects of formoterol. Pregnancy Category C. Excretion in human breast milk is unknown. Beta-2-agonists may potentially interfere with uterine contractility. Use during labor only if the potential benefit justifies the potential risk. Safety and efficacy in children <5 years of age have not been established. Most common adverse effects noted in patients treated with formoterol include angina, hypertension or hypotension, tachycardia, arrhythmias, nervousness, headache, tremor, dry mouth, palpitation, muscle cramps, nausea, dizziness, fatigue, malaise, dysphonia, hypokalemia, hyperglycemia, metabolic acidosis, and insomnia. Most common adverse events seen in children include viral infection, inflammation, abdominal pain, nausea, and dyspepsia.

Administration: Foradil® capsules should be administered by the oral inhalation route and only using the Aerolizer inhaler.

Patient Care Implications: Patients should be advised not to increase the dose or frequency of formoterol without consulting their physician. Patients should be informed that formoterol is not intended to relieve acute asthma symptoms. When formoterol is used for the prevention of exercise-induced bronchospasms, the contents of 1 capsule should be taken at least 15 minutes prior to exercise. Formoterol should not be used as a substitute for oral or inhaled corticosteroids. The dosage of these medications should not be changed, and they should not be stopped without consulting a physician. Patients should be informed that treatment with beta-2-agonists may cause palpitations, chest pain, rapid heart rate, tremor, or nervousness. Patients should be advised never to use formoterol with a spacer and never to exhale into the device. Patients should be instructed to avoid exposing formoterol capsules to moisture and should be instructed to handle the capsule with dry hands. The Aerolizer inhaler should never be washed and should be kept dry. Patients should be informed that in rare cases the gelatin capsule may break into small pieces. These pieces should be retained by the screen built into the Aerolizer inhaler. However, tiny pieces of gelatin may reach the mouth or throat after inhalation. Patients should be informed that formoterol capsules should always be stored in the blister and only removed immediately before use. Formoterol capsules should only be administered by oral inhalation. Formoterol capsules should not be ingested.

Preparations: Gelatin capsules containing 12 mg of formoterol fumarate for oral inhalation, and one Aerolizer inhaler.

FORTAZ®, see Ceftazidime

FORTEO™, see Teriparatide

FORTOVASE®, see Saquinavir

FOSAMAX®, see Alendronate

FOSAMPRENAVIR—Lexiva®

Description/Actions: Fosamprenavir is a prodrug of amprenavir, an inhibitor of human immunodeficiency virus (HIV-1) protease. Fosamprenavir is rapidly converted to amprenavir by cellular phosphatases in vivo. Amprenavir binds to the active site of HIV-1 protease and thereby prevents the processing of viral Gag and Gag-Pol polyprotein precursors, resulting in the formation of immature, noninfectious viral particles. Fosamprenavir is indicated for use in combination with other antiretroviral agents for the treatment of HIV-1 infection in adults.

Precautions/Adverse Reactions: Fosamprenavir is contraindicated in patients with a known hypersensitivity to it or to any component of the formulation or to amprenavir. Fosamprenavir should be used with caution in patients with a known sulfonamide allergy. Coadministration of fosamprenavir with drugs that are highly dependent on CYP4503A4 for clearance and for which elevated plasma concentrations are associated with serious and/or life-threatening events is contraindicated. These include dihydroergotamine, ergonovine, ergotamine, methylergonovine, cisapride, pimozide, midazolam, and triazolam. If fosamprenavir is coadministered with ritonavir, the antiarrhythmic agents flecainide and propafenone are also contraindicated. Serious and/or life-threatening drug interactions could occur between fosamprenavir and amiodarone, lidocaine, tricyclic antidepressants, and quinidine. Monitoring drug levels is recommended if these drugs are coadministered. Severe and life-threatening skin reactions, including Stevens-Johnson syndrome, have occurred in patients receiving fosamprenavir. Acute hemolytic anemia has also been reported. Coadministration of fosamprenavir and delavirdine is not recommended. Concomitant administration of fosamprenavir and rifampin and/or St. John's Wort is not recommended due to decreased protease inhibitor concentrations. The risk of myopathy including rhabdomyolysis may be increased when HIV protease inhibitors are used in combination with lovastatin or simvastatin or other HMG-CoA reductase inhibitors metabolized by the CYP3A4 enzyme system. Coadministration of fosamprenavir and sildenafil or vardenafil is expected to substantially increase sildenafil and or vardenafil concentrations and may result in an increase in sildenafil- or vardenafil-associated adverse events including hypotension, visual changes, and priapism. New onset diabetes mellitus, exacerbation of preexisting diabetes mellitus, hyperglycemia, and diabetic ketoacidosis have been reported during therapy with fosamprenavir. Primarily metabolized by the liver. Exercise caution when administering to patients with hepatic impairment. There have been reports of spontaneous bleeding in patients with hemophilia A and B treated with fosamprenavir. Accumulation of body fat, including central obesity, buffalo hump, peripheral wasting, facial wasting, breast enlargement, and "cushingoid appearance" have been observed in patients receiving antiretroviral therapy. Treatment with fosamprenavir plus ritonavir has resulted in increases in triglycerides. Alterations in dose or regimen may be warranted when fosamprenavir is included in combination with efavirenz, nevirapine, indinavir, nelfinavir, lopinavir/ritonavir, and saquinavir. Dosage adjustments may be required when fosamprenavir is coadministered with bepridil, warfarin, carbamazepine, phenobarbital, phenytoin, ketoconazole, itraconazole, rifabutin, alprazolam, clorazepate, diazepam, flurazepam, diltiazem, felodipine, nifedipine, nicardipine, nimodipine, verapamil, amlodipine, nisolpidine, isradipine, dexamethasone, histamine2 receptor antagonists, cyclosporine, tacrolimus, rapamycin, and methadone. Pregnancy Category C. No adequate and well-controlled studies in pregnant women. Fosamprenavir should be used during pregnancy only if the potential benefit justifies the potential risk to the fetus. Excretion in human breast milk is unknown. Mothers should be instructed not to breast-feed if they are receiving fosamprenavir. Safety and efficacy in pediatric patients have not been established. Most common adverse effects observed during treatment with fosamprenavir include diarrhea, nausea, vomiting, headache, and rash. Severe or life-threatening skin reactions were reported in <1% of patients treated with fosamprenavir. Other reported adverse effects include: abdominal pain, pruritis, fatigue, depression, paresthesia, increased AST, ALT, lipase, increased triglycerides, neutropenia, and hyperglycemia.

Administration: Oral.

Patient Care Implications: Patients should be informed that Lexiva® is not a cure for HIV infection. Patients should inform their health care provider if they have a sulfa allergy. Lexiva® may interact with many drugs; therefore, patients should report to their health care provider the use of any other prescription, nonprescription medication, or herbal products. Patients receiving hormonal contraceptives should be instructed to use alternative measures of contraception during therapy with Lexiva® because hormonal levels may be altered.

Preparations: Tablets, 700 mg.

FOSCARNET SODIUM—Foscavir®

Description/Actions: Antiviral agent that inhibits replication of herpes viruses including cytomegalovirus (CMV). Indicated for the treatment of cytomegalovirus retinitis in patients with AIDS. Also indicated for the treatment of acyclovir-resistant mucocutaneous herpes simplex virus infections in immunocompromised patients.

Precautions/Adverse Reactions: May cause renal impairment, and creatinine clearance should be determined at baseline, 2–3 times per week during induction therapy, and at least once every 1 or 2 weeks during maintenance therapy. Concurrent use with other potentially nephrotoxic drugs (e.g., aminoglycosides) should be avoided when possible. Has the potential to chelate divalent metal ions such as calcium and has been associated with changes in serum electrolytes, including hypocalcemia and hypomagnesemia, as well as hypokalemia, hypophosphatemia, and hyperphosphatemia. Serum calcium, magnesium, potassium, and phosphorus should be monitored on a schedule similar to that recommended for serum creatinine. Patients should be advised to report symptoms such as perioral tingling, numbness in the extremities, and paresthesias, which may be associated with electrolyte abnormalities. The concomitant use with intravenous pentamidine may increase the risk of severe hypocalcemia. Other adverse reactions include seizures, anemia, granulocytopenia, fever, nausea, vomiting, diarrhea, and headache.

Administration: Intravenous infusion. Must not be administered by rapid or bolus injection because of the increased risk of toxicity.

Preparations: Bottles, 250 and 500 ml containing the drug in a concentration of 24 mg/ml.

FOSCAVIR®, see Foscarnet

FOSFOMYCIN—Monurol®

Description/Actions: Synthetic, broad spectrum antibiotic that has bactericidal activity in the urine at therapeutic doses. Indicated in the treatment of uncomplicated susceptible UTIs in women.

Precautions/Adverse Reactions: Adverse reactions include diarrhea, vaginitis, nausea, headache, dizziness, asthenia, and dyspepsia.

Administration: Oral.

Preparations: Single-dose sachet packets of 3 g.

FOSINOPRIL SODIUM—Monopril®

Description/Actions: An angiotensin converting enzyme (ACE) inhibitor that is a prodrug. Following oral administration, it is converted to its active metabolite, fosinoprilat. Indicated for the treatment of hypertension and may be used alone or in combination with a thiazide diuretic. Also indicated in the management of congestive heart failure.

Precautions/Adverse Reactions: Adverse reactions include headache, dizziness, fatigue, cough, diarrhea, and nausea/vomiting. May cause an elevation in serum potassium levels; the risk of hyperkalemia is increased in patients also taking a potassium-sparing diuretic, a potassium supplement, and/or a potassium-containing salt substitute. May cause symptomatic postural hypotension. There have been infrequent reports of angioedema of the face, extremities, lips, tongue, glottis, and larynx, especially following the first dose. Patients should be told to report immediately any symptoms suggesting angioedema and to stop taking the drug. When used during the second and third trimesters of pregnancy, ACE inhibitors have been reported to be associated with the development of neonatal hypertension, renal failure, and skull hypoplasia; use during pregnancy should be avoided. May increase serum lithium levels, and concurrent therapy should be closely monitored.

Administration: Oral.

Preparations: Tablets, 10 and 20 mg.

FOSPHENYTOIN SODIUM—Cerebyx®

Description/Actions: For short-term (up to 5 days) IV/IM administration when other forms of phenytoin administration are unavailable or deemed less advantageous. See phenytoin.

FRAGMIN®, see Dalteparin

FROVA™, see Frovatriptan

FROVATRIPTAN—Frova™

Description/Actions: Frovatriptan is indicated for acute treatment of migraine with or without aura in adult patients.

Precautions/Adverse Reactions: Because of the potential of this class of compound (5-HT1 agonists) to cause coronary vasospasm, frovatriptan should not be given to patients with documented ischemic or vasospastic coronary artery disease (CAD). Not intended for the prophylactic therapy of migraine or for use in the management of hemiplegic or basilar migraine. Frovatriptan is contraindicated in the following conditions: cerebrovascular syndromes, peripheral vascular disease, and uncontrolled hypertension. It is strongly recommended that frovatriptan not be given to patients in whom unrecognized CAD is predicted by the presence of risk factors (e.g., hypertension, hypercholesterolemia, smoking, obesity, diabetes, strong family history of CAD, female with surgical or physiological menopause, or male over 40 years of age) unless a cardiovascular evaluation provides satisfactory clinical evidence that the patient is reasonably free of coronary artery and ischemic myocardial disease or other significant underlying cardiovascular disease. It should not be used within 24 hours of treatment with another 5- HT1 agonist, an ergotamine-containing or ergot-type medication, or methysergide. Ergot-containing drugs have been reported to cause prolonged vasospastic reactions. The most common adverse events were dizziness, paresthesia, headache, dry mouth, fatigue, flushing, hot or cold sensation, and chest pain. Serious cardiac events, including some that have been fatal, have occurred following the use of a 5-HT1 agonist. These events are extremely rare, and most have been reported in patients with risk factors predictive of CAD. There are no adequate and well-controlled studies in pregnant women. Pregnancy Category C. Use only if potential benefit to mother outweighs potential risk to fetus. Excretion in breast milk is unknown; use caution. Safety and effectiveness in pediatrics have not been established.

Administration: Oral.

Patient Care Implications: Take with fluids. Take at first sign of migraine attack. It does not prevent migraine. For patients with risk factors predictive of CAD who have been determined to have a satisfactory cardiovascular evaluation, it is strongly recommended that administration of the first dose be given in a physician's office.

Preparations: Tablets, 2.5 mg.

FRUCTOSE—Levulose

Description/Actions: Carbohydrate administered parenterally as a source of calories.

Preparations: Solution, 10%.

FUDR®, see Floxuridine

FULVESTRANT—Faslodex®

Description/Actions: Fulvestrant is an estrogen receptor antagonist. Fulvestrant is indicated for the treatment of hormone receptor–positive metastatic breast cancer in postmenopausal women with disease progression following antiestrogen therapy. It is approved for use only in postmenopausal women.

Precautions/Adverse Reactions: Fulvestrant is contraindicated in individuals hypersensitive to fulvestrant or any component of the formulation and in pregnant women. It should not be used in patients with bleeding diathesis or thrombocytopenia or in patients on anticoagulants. Metabolism is primarily in the liver; use with caution in patients with liver disease, and monitor closely. Pregnancy Category D. Most common adverse reactions were nausea, vomiting, constipation, diarrhea, abdominal pain, headache, back pain, vasodilation (hot flushes), and pharyngitis. Three of the most serious common effects were anemia, leukopenia, and thrombocytopenia.

Administration: Intramuscular injection.

Preparations: Injection, solution (prefilled syringe): 50 mg/ml (2.5 ml, 5 ml).

FULVICIN®, see Griseofulvin

FUNGIZONE®, see Amphotericin B

FURACIN®, see Nitrofurazone

FURADANTIN®, see Nitrofurantoin

FURAZOLIDONE—Furoxone®

Description/Actions: Anti-infective agent indicated in the treatment of bacterial or protozoal diarrhea and enteritis caused by susceptible organisms.

Preparations: Tablets, 100 mg. Liquid, 50 mg/15 ml.

FUROSEMIDE—Lasix®

Description/Actions: Is a loop diuretic indicated (a) for the treatment of edema associated with congestive heart failure, cirrhosis of the liver, and renal diseases and (b) hypertension. Is also indicated via intravenous use as adjunctive therapy in acute pulmonary edema.

Precautions/Adverse Reactions: Is contraindicated in anuria. May cause volume and electrolyte depletion. Potential for hypokalemia warrants periodic measurement of serum potassium levels. Reduction in potassium levels may increase the action and toxicity of digoxin and related glycosides. Parenteral therapy is best avoided in patients receiving aminoglycoside antibiotics because of an increased risk of ototoxicity.

Administration: Oral, intravenous, and intramuscular.

Preparations: Tablets, 20, 40, and 80 mg. Oral solution, 10 mg/ml. Ampules, vials, and syringes, 10 mg/ml.

FUROXONE®, see Furazolidone

G

GABAPENTIN—Neurontin®

Description/Actions: Antiepileptic agent indicated as adjunctive therapy in the treatment of partial seizures with and without secondary generalizations in patients over 12 years of age with epilepsy. Gabapentin is also indicated as adjunctive therapy in the treatment of partial seizures in pediatric patients age 3–12 years and for the management of postherpetic neuralgia in adults.

Precautions/Adverse Reactions: Adverse reactions include somnolence, dizziness, ataxia, nystagmus, and tremor. Patients should be cautioned not to drive or operate machinery until they have gained sufficient experience with the use of the drug to determine whether it affects their mental and/or motor performance adversely. Bioavailability is reduced by the administration of aluminum/magnesium-containing antacids, and it should be administered at least 2 hours following the antacid.

Administration: Oral.

Preparations: Capsules, 100, 300, and 400 mg. Tablets, 600 and 800 mg. Oral solution, 250 mg/5 mL.

GABITRIL®, see Tiagabine Hydrochloride

GALANTAMINE—Reminyl®, Razadyne®

Description/Actions: Galantamine is a reversible, competitive acetylcholinesterase inhibitor. It is indicated for the treatment of mild to moderate dementia of the Alzheimer's type.

Precautions/Adverse Reactions: Galantamine is contraindicated in patients with a known hypersensitivity to it or to any component of the formulation. Galantamine may cause bladder outflow obstruction and seizures. Use with caution in patients with a history of severe asthma or obstructive pulmonary disease. Use of galantamine in patients with severe hepatic and/or severe renal impairment is not recommended. Galantamine is metabolized by the cytochrome P450 enzyme system 2D6 and 3A4. Pregnancy Category B. Major adverse reactions reported during therapy with galantamine include nausea, vomiting, diarrhea, dizziness, headache, weight loss, anorexia, fatigue, abdominal pain, dyspepsia, depression, insomnia, somnolence, anemia, rhinitis, urinary tract infections, hematuria, tremor, syncope, and bradycardia. Other reported adverse reactions include chest pain, postural hypotension, hypotension, edema, cardiac failure, vertigo, convulsions, paresthesia, ataxia, flatulence, gastritis, melena, dysphagia, rectal hemorrhage, dry mouth, increased saliva, hiccup, AV block, palpitation, atrial fibrillation,

QT prolonged, bundle branch block, supraventricular tachycardia, ventricular tachycardia, hyperglycemia, increased alkaline phosphatase, epistaxis, thrombocytopenia, apathy, paranoid reaction, delirium, increased libido, incontinence, hematuria, micturition frequency, cystitis, urinary retention, nocturia, renal calculi, dehydration, aggression, upper and lower GI bleeding, and hypokalemia.

Administration: Oral, with food.

Preparations: Tablets, 4, 8, and 12 mg. Oral solution, 4 mg/mL 100 mL bottle.

GALLAMINE TRIETHIODIDE—Flaxedil®

Description/Actions: Neuromuscular blocking agent indicated as an adjunct to anesthesia to induce skeletal muscle relaxation. Also used to manage patients undergoing mechanical ventilation.

Preparations: Vials, 20 mg/ml.

GALLIUM NITRATE—Ganite®

Description/Actions: Exerts a hypocalcemic effect by inhibiting calcium resorption from bone. Indicated for the treatment of symptomatic cancer-related hypercalcemia that has not responded to adequate hydration.

Precautions/Adverse Reactions: Contraindicated in patients with severe renal impairment. May cause renal effects, and serum creatinine levels should be monitored. Concurrent use with other potentially nephrotoxic drugs (e.g., aminoglycosides, amphotericin B) may increase the risk of developing severe renal insufficiency. Other adverse reactions include hypocalcemia, transient hypophosphatemia, decreased sodium bicarbonate, anemia, decreased blood pressure, and nausea and/or vomiting.

Administration: Intravenous. The daily dose must be administered as an IV infusion over 24 hours. Adequate hydration must be maintained throughout the treatment period.

Preparations: Vials, 500 mg.

GAMMA BENZENE HEXACHLORIDE, see Lindane

GANCICLOVIR SODIUM—Cytovene®

Description/Actions: Antiviral agent that inhibits replication of herpes viruses including cytomegalovirus (CMV). Indicated for the treatment of cytomegalovirus retinitis in immunocompromised individuals, including patients with AIDS. Also indicated in transplant patients at risk for CMV disease.

Precautions/Adverse Reactions: May cause granulocytopenia and thrombocytopenia, and it is recommended that neutrophil counts and platelet counts be performed every 2 days during the period in which ganciclovir is dosed twice daily and at least weekly thereafter. Other adverse reactions include anemia, fever, rash, and abnormal liver function values. Has been reported to be teratogenic in animals and should be used during pregnancy only if the benefits outweigh the risks. Because of the mutagenic potential of ganciclovir, women of childbearing potential should be advised to use effective contraception during treatment, and male patients should be advised to practice barrier contraception during and for at least 90 days following treatment with the drug. The concurrent use of ganciclovir and zidovudine is associated with an increased risk of granulocytopenia. Seizures have been reported in some patients receiving ganciclovir and imipenem-cilastatin concurrently, so the use of these agents in combination should be avoided if possible. Probenecid may reduce the renal clearance and increase the action of ganciclovir.

Administration: Intravenous infusion (at a constant rate over a period of 1 hour) and oral, which should be taken with food.

Preparations: Vials, containing ganciclovir sodium equivalent to 500 mg ganciclovir. Capsules, 250 mg.

GANIRELIX—Antagon®

Description/Actions: Ganirelix is a gonadotropin-releasing hormone antagonist (GnRH) that is used in women receiving assisted insemination or reproductive technology (ART) procedures.

Precautions/Adverse Reactions: Ganirelix should not be given to patients who have a hypersensitivity to mannitol or ganirelix, have primary ovarian failure, or have an ovarian cyst. The drug should be given carefully to patients with either kidney or hepatic impairment. Also, ganirelix should be avoided in pregnant women, breast-feeding women, and children. Ganirelix is usually well tolerated, but some common adverse reactions are abdominal pain, headache, ovarian hyperstimulation syndrome, vaginal bleeding, menstrual irregularity, nausea, vomiting, and hot flashes.

Administration: SQ injection.

Patient Care Implications: Patients should avoid excessive alcohol or tobacco consumption during therapy. Patients with renal or hepatic impairment should be monitored carefully. A pregnancy test should be done before therapy is started. Monitor the patient by getting serum estradiol and gonadotropin levels and also conducting pelvic exams and pelvic ultrasounds.

Preparations: Syringe, 250 mcg.

GANITE®, see Gallium Nitrate

GANTANOL®, see Sulfamethoxazole

GANTRISIN®, see Sulfisoxazole

GANTRISIN ACETYL®, see Sulfisoxazole Acetyl

GARAMYCIN®, see Gentamicin

GASTROCROM®, see Cromolyn

GATIFLOXACIN—Tequin®

Description/Actions: Indicated for the treatment of infections in the following conditions: acute bacterial exacerbation of chronic bronchitis, acute sinusitis, community acquired pneumonia, uncomplicated urinary tract infections, pyelonephritis, uncomplicated urethral and cervical gonorrhea, and acute, uncomplicated rectal infections in women. Uncomplicated skin and skin-structure infections.

Precautions/Adverse Reactions: Tequin is contraindicated in persons with a history of hypersensitivity to gatifloxacin or any member of the quinolone class of antimicrobial agents. The safety and effectiveness of gatifloxacin in pediatric patients, adolescents, and pregnant or lactating women have not been established. Gatifloxacin may have the potential to prolong the QTc interval of the electrocardiogram of some patients. Due to the lack of clinical experience, gatifloxacin should be avoided in patients with known prolongation of the QTc interval, patients with uncorrected hypokalemia, and patients receiving class IA or class III antiarrhythmic agents. Quinolones may cause CNS events, including nervousness, agitation, insomnia, anxiety, nightmares, or paranoia. Caution should be used in patients with renal insufficiency. Rupture of the shoulder, hand, and Achille's tendon, or other tendons that require surgical repair or resulted in prolonged disability have been reported in patients receiving gatifloxacin. Rare cases of sensory or sensorimotor axonal polyneuropathy affecting small and/or large axons resulting in paresthesias, hypoesthesias, dysesthesias, and weakness have been reported in patients treated with quinolones.

Administration: Oral, intravenous.

Preparations: Tablets, 200 and 400 mg. IV solution, 20- and 40-ml vials, 10 mg/ml; 100- and 200-ml flexible containers, 2 mg/ml.

G-CSF, see Filgrastim

GEFITINIB—Iressa™

Description/Actions: Gefitinib is an antineoplastic agent, indicated as monotherapy for the treatment of patients with locally advanced or metastatic nonsmall-cell lung cancer after failure of both platinum-based and docetaxel chemotherapies. Its mechanism of antitumor action is not fully understood. Gefitinib inhibits intracellular phosphorylation of numerous tyrosine kinases associated with transmembrane cell surface receptors, including the tyrosine kinases associated with the epidermal growth factor receptor (EGFR). EGFR is expressed on the cell surface of many normal and cancer cells.

Precautions/Adverse Reactions: Gefitinib is contraindicated in pregnancy and in individuals hypersensitive to gefitinib or any component of the formulation. Pregnancy Category D; animal studies have demonstrated fetal harm. Excretion in breast milk unknown; breast-feeding not recommended. Rare, sometimes fatal, pulmonary toxicity has occurred. Patients present with the acute onset of dyspnea, sometimes associated with cough or low-grade fever, often becoming severe within a short time. Gefitinib is cleared primarily by the liver; therefore, gefitinib exposure may be increased in patients with hepatic dysfunction. Use caution in patients with hepatic impairment; periodic liver function testing should be considered. Most common adverse reactions were diarrhea, rash, acne, dry skin, nausea, and vomiting. Inducers of CYP3A4 activity increase metabolism of gefitinib and decrease its plasma concentrations (e.g., phenytoin, nafcillin, and phenobarbital). CYP3A4 inhibitors (e.g., cipro, clarithromycin, isoniazid, and nicardipine) inhibit metabolism of gefitinib and increase its levels. Drugs that cause significant sustained elevation in gastric pH (ranitidine or cimetidine) may reduce plasma concentrations and therefore may reduce efficacy of gefitinib. Elevation in international normalized ratio (INR) and/or bleeding events have been reported in some patients taking warfarin while on gefitinib therapy. Monitor for changes in prothrombin time or INR.

Administration: Oral.

Patient Care Implications: Take with or without food. Do not take with grapefruit juice and/or antacids 2 hours before or 2 hours after taking this medication. Advise patients to seek medical advice promptly if they develop (a) severe or persistent diarrhea, nausea, anorexia, or vomiting, as these have sometimes been associated with dehydration; (b) an onset or worsening of pulmonary symptoms; (c) an eye irritation; or (d) any persistent adverse reaction. Patients may experience loss of appetite, nausea, and vomiting (small, frequent meals, and frequent mouth care may help). Use appropriate contraceptive measures while on this medication.

Preparations: Tablet: 250 mg.

GEMCITABINE HYDROCHLORIDE—Gemzar®

Description/Actions: Antineoplastic agent. Gemcitabine in combination with paclitaxel is indicated for the first-line treatment of patients with metastatic breast cancer after failure of prior anthracycline-containing adjuvant chemotherapy, unless anthracycline is clinically contraindicated. Gemzar® is indicated in combination with cisplatin for the first-line treatment of patients with inoperable, locally advanced (stage IIIA or IIIB), or metastatic (stage IV) nonsmall-cell lung cancer. Gemzar® is indicated as first-line treatment for patients with locally advanced (nonresectable stage II or stage III) or metastatic (stage IV) adenocarcinoma of the pancreas. Gemzar® is indicated for patients previously treated with 5–FU.

Precautions/Adverse Reactions: Prolongation of infusion time beyond 30 minutes and more frequent administration than weekly dosing have been shown to increase toxicity. Side effects include myelosuppression, fever, rash, pruritis, transient elevations in serum transaminases, mild hematuria, and proteinuria. Monitor patients prior to each dose with a CBC including differential and platelet count.

Administration: Intravenous.

Preparations: Powder for injection 20 mg/ml (10 ml/50 ml).

GEMFIBROZIL—Lopid®

Description/Actions: Antihyperlipidemic agent indicated as adjunctive therapy to diet for (a) the treatment of patients with very high serum triglyceride levels (type IV or V hyperlipoproteinemia) who present a risk of abdominal pain and pancreatitis and who do not respond adequately to dietary measures and (b) reducing the risk of coronary heart disease.

Precautions/Adverse Reactions: Concomitant therapy with gemfibrozil and an HMG-CoA reductase inhibitor (simvastatin, fluvastatin, lovastatin, atorvastatin, pravastatin) is associated with an increased risk of skeletal muscle toxicity manifested as rhabdomyolysis, markedly elevated creatine kinase (CPK) levels, and myoglobinuria, leading to acute renal failure and death.

Preparations: Capsules, 300 mg. Tablets 600 mg.

GEMIFLOXACIN—Factive®

Description/Actions: Gemifloxacin is a synthetic broad spectrum antibacterial agent related to the fluoroquinolone class of antibiotics.

Gemifloxacin acts by inhibiting DNA synthesis through the inhibition of both DNA gyrase and topoisomerase IV. Gemifloxacin is indicated for the treatment of acute exacerbation of chronic bronchitis caused by *Streptococcus pneumoniae, Haemophilus influenzae, Haemophilus parainfluenzae* or *Moraxella catarrhalis* and for the treatment of community acquired pneumonia caused by *Streptococcus pneumoniae* (including multi-drug resistant strains), *Haemophilus influenzae, Moraxella catarrhalis, Mycoplasma pneumoniae, Chlamydia pneumoniae* or *Klebsiella pneumoniae.*

Precautions/Adverse Reactions: Gemifloxacin is contraindicated in patients with a known hypersensitivity to it, fluoroquinolone antibiotic agents, or to any component of the formulation. Gemifloxacin may prolong the QT interval in some patients. Gemifloxacin should be avoided in patients with a history of prolongation of the QTc interval, patients with uncorrected electrolyte disorders (hypokalemia or hypomagnesemia), and patients receiving class IA (e.g., quinidine, procainamide), or class III (e.g., amiodarone, sotalol) antiarrhythmic agents. Use with caution when giving concurrently with drugs known to prolong the QTc interval such as erythromycin, antipsychotics, and tricyclic antidepressants. Use caution when administering to patients with proarrhythmic conditions such as clinically significant bradycardia or acute myocardial ischemia. The likelihood of QTc prolongation may increase with increasing dose of the drug; therefore, the recommended dose should not be exceeded, especially in patients with renal and or hepatic impairment. QTc interval prolongation may lead to torsades de pointes. Serious and occasionally fatal hypersensitivity and or anaphylactic reactions have been reported in patients receiving gemifloxacin. Gemifloxacin should be discontinued immediately at the appearance of any sign of an immediate type 1 hypersensitivity skin rash or any other manifestation of a hypersensitivity reaction. Tendonitis and rupture of the shoulder, hand, and Achilles tendons that require surgical repair or resulted in prolonged disability have been reported in patients receiving fluoroquinolones. Gemifloxacin should be discontinued if patient experiences pain, inflammation, or rupture of a tendon. Use with caution in patients with CNS diseases such as epilepsy or patients predisposed to convulsions. Pseudomembranous colitis has been reported with the use of gemifloxacin. Coadministration of gemifloxacin and aluminum- and magnesium-containing antacids, or ferrous sulfate, multivitamin preparations containing zinc or other metal cations, or didanosine chewable/buffered tablets, or the pediatric powder for oral solution should not be taken within 3 hours before or 2 hours after taking gemifloxacin. When gemifloxacin is coadministered with sucralfate, sucralfate should be administered 2 hours after the gemifloxacin. Coadministration of gemifloxacin and theophylline, digoxin, oral contraceptives, cimetidine, omeprazole, and warfarin did not lead to clinically significant changes in the pharmacokinetics of gemifloxacin. Pregnancy Category C. No adequate and well-controlled studies in pregnant women. The safety and effectiveness of gemifloxacin in children, adolescents (less than 18 years of age), pregnant women, and lactating women have not been established. Gemifloxacin should not be used in pregnant women unless the potential benefit to the mother outweighs the risk to the fetus. Excretion in human breast milk is unknown. Most common adverse effects observed in gemifloxacin treated patients include diarrhea, rash, nausea, headache, abdominal pain, vomiting, dizziness, taste perversion, anorexia, arthralgia, constipation, dermatitis, dry mouth, dyspepsia, fatigue, flatulence, fungal infection, gastritis, genital moniliasis, hyperglycemia, insomnia, leucopenia, pruritis, somnolence, urticaria, thrombocythemia, vaginitis, anemia, asthenia, back pain, bilirubinemia, dyspnea, eczema, photosensitivity, granulocytopenia, increased GGT, leg cramps, myalgia, pharyngitis, tremor, and vertigo. Increases in AST, ALT, CPK, potassium, alkaline phosphatase, serum creatinine, and calcium have also been reported during treatment with gemifloxacin.

Administration: Oral.

Patient Care Implications: Patients should discontinue gemifloxacin and call their health care provider if they develop a rash or other sign of an allergic reaction. Gemifloxacin may cause dizziness. If this occurs, patients should be instructed not to operate an automobile or engage in activities requiring mental alertness.

Preparations: Tablets, 320 mg.

GEMTUZUMAB OZOGAMICIN—Mylotarg®

Description/Actions: Gemtuzumab is a chemotherapeutic agent that is indicated for the treatment of patients with CD33 positive acute myeloid leukemia in first relapse who are 60 years of age or older and who are not considered candidates for other cytotoxic chemotherapy.

Precautions/Adverse Reactions: Gemtuzumab is contraindicated in patients with a known hypersensitivity to gemtuzumab ozogamicin or any of its components, anti-CD33 antibody, calicheamicin derivatives, or inactive ingredients. Gemtuzumab should be administered under the supervision of physicians experienced in the treatment of acute leukemia. As there are no data to support using gemtuzumab in combination with other chemotherapeutic agents, it should only be used as single-agent therapy. Severe myelosuppression will occur in all patients. Severe hypersensitivity reactions, including anaphylaxis, infusion reactions, and pulmonary events, can occur during the infusion or within 24 hours of the start of the infusion. Postinfusion reactions characterized by fever, chills, hypotension, or dyspnea may occur during the first 24 hours after administration. Vital signs should be monitored during the infusion and for 4 hours following the infusion.

Hepatotoxicity has been reported with gemtuzumab therapy. Caution should be exercised when administering to patients with hepatic impairment. Tumor lysis syndrome may occur as a consequence of leukemic treatment. Prophylactic hydration and allopurinol should be started to prevent hyperuricemia. Leukoreduction with hydroxyurea and leukapheresis to decrease the peripheral white blood cell count to <30,000 cells/ml prior to the administration of gemtuzumab. Do not administer as an intravenous push or bolus. No formal drug interaction studies have been performed. Pregnancy Category D. There are no adequate and well-controlled studies in pregnant women. May cause fetal harm if administered to pregnant women. Excretion in human breast milk is unknown. The most common side effects observed in patients on gemtuzumab were infusion-related effects such as chills, fever, nausea, vomiting, headache, hypotension, hypertension, hypoxia, dyspnea, and hyperglycemia. Severe myelosuppression is the major toxicity associated with gemtuzumab. In clinical trials, neutropenia was observed in 98% of patients, thrombocytopenia (99%), anemia (47%), infection (28%), herpes simplex infections (22%), and 15% of patients experienced bleeding. Mucositis was observed in 35% of patients. Increased bilirubin, AST, and ALT were also observed during gemtuzumab therapy.

Administration: For intravenous infusion only.

Patient Care Implications: Vital signs should be monitored during the infusion and for 4 hours after the infusion. The solution must not be given as an intravenous push or bolus. Administer diphenhydramine and acetaminophen 1 hour prior to the start of the infusion. Gemtuzumab is light sensitive; use a UV protective bag over the IV bag during infusion. A separate IV line equipped with a low protein-binding 1.2–micron filter must be used for administration of the drug. Chemotherapeutic agent should be handled and disposed of properly.

Preparations: Powder for injection, 5 mg of lyophilized powder in 20 ml amber glass vial.

GEMZAR®—see Gemcitabine

GENOTROPIN®—see Somatropin

GENTAMICIN SULFATE—Garamycin®

Description/Actions: Aminoglycoside antibiotic indicated for the parenteral treatment of serious infections caused by gram-negative bacteria including *Pseudomonas aeruginosa.* Is also effective in the treatment of staphylococcal infections. Has also been used topically in the treatment of dermatologic and ocular infections.

Precautions/Adverse Reactions: May cause nephrotoxicity, ototoxicity, and neurotoxicity, so the concurrent or serial use of other nephrotoxic or ototoxic agents should be avoided.

Administration: Intravenous, intramuscular, intrathecal, topical, and ophthalmic.

Preparations: Vials, 40 mg/ml. Vials, syringes, and piggyback units, 60, 70, 80, 90, 100, 120, 160, and 180 mg. Vials (for intrathecal use), 2 mg/ml. Cream and ointment, 0.1%. Ophthalmic solution and ointment, 0.3%.

GENTIAN VIOLET—Methylrosaniline Chloride

Description/Actions: Anti-infective agent used topically in the treatment of dermatologic and vaginal infections.

Preparations: Solutions, 1% and 2%.

GENTRAN®, see Dextran

GEOCILLIN®, see Carbenicillin Indanyl Sodium

GEODON™, see Ziprasidone

GLEEVEC™, see Imatinib Mesylate

GLIMEPIRIDE—Amaryl®

Description/Actions: Sulfonylurea antidiabetic agent used as an adjunct to diet and exercise in noninsulin-dependent diabetes mellitus (NIDDM) in individuals who are unable to maintain glycemic control by diet and exercise alone. Also indicated for secondary failure in combination with insulin.

Precautions/Adverse Reactions: Contraindicated in ketoacidosis as this condition should be treated with insulin. Administration of oral hypoglycemic drugs has been reported to be associated with increased cardiovascular mortality as compared to treatment with diet alone or diet plus insulin. May cause hypoglycemia, dizziness, asthenia, headache, nausea, allergic skin reactions, and blood dyscrasias.

Administration: Oral once daily with breakfast or first main meal.

Preparations: Scored tablets, 1, 2, and 4 mg.

GLIPIZIDE—Glucotrol®, Glucotrol XL

Description/Actions: Sulfonylurea hypoglycemic agent indicated as an adjunct to diet for the control of hyperglycemia and its associated symptomatology in patients with non-insulin dependent diabetes mellitus, after an adequate trial of dietary therapy has proved unsatisfactory.

Precautions/Adverse Reactions: May cause hypoglycemia, so patients should be advised to contact their physician if symptoms of hypoglycemia develop. Adverse reactions include nausea, diarrhea, pruritus, and erythema. Oral hypoglycemic agents have been suggested to be associated with increased cardiovascular mortality as compared to treatment with diet alone or diet plus insulin. Corticosteroids and thiazide and other diuretics may increase blood glucose levels and necessitate an increase in dosage of glipizide. Therapy in patients also receiving a beta-adrenergic blocking agent should be monitored closely.

Administration: Oral.

Preparations: Tablets, 5 and 10 mg. Controlled-release tablets (Glucotrol XL), 5 and 10 mg.

GLIPIZIDE AND METFORMIN—Metaglip™

Description/Actions: Metaglip™ is indicated as second-line therapy for the management of type 2 diabetes when hyperglycemia cannot be managed with a sulfonylurea or metformin along with diet and exercise.

Precautions/Adverse Reactions: Metaglip™ is contraindicated in individuals with a known hypersensitivity to glipizide, other sulfonamides, metformin, or any component of the formulation. Not to be used in patients with renal disease or renal dysfunction (serum creatinine $\geq$1.5 mg/dL in males or $\geq$1.4 mg/dL in females, or creatinine clearance <60 ml/minute). Metaglip™ is contraindicated in patients with congestive heart failure requiring pharmacologic treatment and in acute or chronic metabolic acidosis, including diabetic ketoacidosis, with or without coma. Temporarily discontinue in patients undergoing radiologic studies involving intravascular administration of iodinated contrast materials, because use of such products may result in acute alteration of renal function. Discontinue Metaglip™ prior to the procedure, and hold for 48 hours subsequent to the procedure. Reinstitute only after renal function has been reevaluated and found to be normal. Use should also be suspended temporarily for any surgical procedure (except minor procedures not associated with restricted intake of food and fluids). Restart when the patient's oral intake has resumed and renal function has been evaluated as normal. Lactic acidosis is a rare but serious metabolic complication that can occur due to metformin accumulation. When it occurs, it is fatal in approximately 50% of cases. Pregnancy Category C. Most common adverse reactions were upper respiratory tract infection, headache, hypoglycemia, musculoskeletal pain, nausea, vomiting, and diarrhea.

Administration: Oral.

Preparations: Tablet (film coated), 2.5 mg/250 mg (glipizide 2.5 mg and metformin 250 mg), 2.5/500 mg (glipizide 2.5 mg and metformin 500 mg), and 5/500 mg (glipizide 5 mg and metformin 500 mg).

GLUCAGON

Description/Actions: Agent to increase blood glucose levels. Indicated for parenteral use in counteracting severe hypoglycemic reactions in diabetic patients or during insulin shock therapy in psychiatric patients. Used to facilitate radiographic examination of the GI tract.

Precautions/Adverse Reactions: Contraindicated in pheochromocytoma. Adverse reactions include GI upset and hypersensitivity reaction (urticaria, respiratory distress, hypotension).

Preparations: Vials, 1 and 10 mg.

GLUCOPHAGE® see Metformin Hydrochloride

GLUCOPHAGE® XR, see Metformin Hydrochloride

GLUCOSE, see Dextrose

GLUCOTROL®, see Glipizide

GLUCOTROL XL®, see Glipizide

GLUCOVANCE™, Combination of Glyburide and Metformin Hydrochloride. See individual discussion on Glyburide and Metformin.

GLUTAMIC ACID HYDROCHLORIDE

Description/Actions: Gastric acidifier used in the treatment of conditions associated with a deficiency of hydrochloric acid in the gastric juice.

Preparations: Capsules, 340 mg.

GLUTETHIMIDE—Doriglute®

Description/Actions: Hypnotic indicated for the short-term treatment of insomnia, sedative effect preoperatively, and during the first stage of labor.

Preparations: Tablets, 250 mg.

GLYBURIDE—DiaBeta®, Micronase®, Glynase®

Description/Actions: Sulfonylurea hypoglycemic agent indicated as an adjunct to diet to lower the blood glucose in patients with non–insulin-dependent diabetes mellitus whose hyperglycemia cannot be controlled by diet alone.

Precautions/Adverse Reactions: May cause hypoglycemia, so patients should be advised to contact their physician if symptoms of hypoglycemia develop. Adverse reactions include nausea, heartburn, epigastric fullness, pruritus, erythema, urticaria, and rash. Oral hypoglycemic agents have been suggested to be associated with increased cardiovascular mortality as compared to treatment with diet alone or diet plus insulin. Corticosteroids and thiazide and other diuretics may increase blood glucose levels and necessitate an increase in dosage of glyburide. Therapy in patients also receiving a beta-adrenergic blocking agent should be monitored closely.

Administration: Oral.

Preparations: Tablets, 1.25, 2.5, and 5 mg. Tablets, micronized, 1.5, 3, and 6 mg (Glynase PresTab).

GLYCERYL TRIACETATE, see Triacetin

GLYCERYL TRINITRATE—Former name for Nitroglycerin

GLYCINE, see Aminoacetic Acid

GLYCOPYRROLATE—Robinul®

Description/Actions: Anticholinergic agent used as adjunctive therapy in the treatment of peptic ulcer. Is also used parenterally as a preoperative antimuscarinic, intraoperatively to counteract drug induced or vagal traction reflexes with the associated arrhythmias, or to protect against the peripheral muscarinic effects of cholinergic agents given to reverse the neuromuscular blockade due to nondepolarizing muscle relaxants.

Preparations: Tablets, 1 and 2 mg. Vials, 0.2 mg/ml.

GLYNASE®, see Glyburide

GLY-OXIDE®, see Carbamide Peroxide

GM-CSF, see Sargramostim

GOLD SODIUM THIOMALATE—Myochrysine®

Description/Actions: Gold formulation indicated for the intramuscular treatment of rheumatoid arthritis.

Preparations: Ampules, 10, 25, and 50 mg.

GoLYTELY®, see Polyethylene Glycol 3350

GONADORELIN HYDROCHLORIDE—Factrel®

Description/Actions: Synthetic luteinizing hormone-releasing hormone indicated for diagnostic use in evaluating the functional capacity and response of the gonadotropes of the anterior pituitary.

Preparations: Vials, 100 mg.

GONADOTROPIN, CHORIONIC see Chorionic Gonadotropin

GOSERELIN ACETATE—Zoladex®

Description/Actions: Is a synthetic analog of gonadotropin-releasing hormone. Chronic administration leads to a sustained suppression of pituitary gonadotropins, resulting in a fall in serum testosterone levels. Indicated in the palliative treatment of advanced carcinoma of the prostate, treatment of endometriosis, and palliative treatment of advanced breast cancer in peri- and postmenopausal women. May be used in combination with Flutamide and radiation therapy for locally confined stage T2B–T4 (stage B2-C) prostatic carcinoma.

Precautions/Adverse Reactions: Is contraindicated during pregnancy. Adverse reactions include hot flashes, sexual dysfunction, decreased erections, lower urinary tract symptoms, pain, lethargy, dizziness, insomnia, anorexia, nausea, upper respiratory infection, chronic obstructive pulmonary disease, edema, congestive heart failure, rash, and sweating. When treatment is initiated, there is a transient increase in serum testosterone levels, which may cause a temporary worsening of signs and symptoms during the first few weeks of therapy.

Administration: Subcutaneous. The formulation is implanted into the upper abdominal wall and provides a continuous release of the drug over a 28-day period.

Preparations: Implant, 3.6 mg.

GRANISETRON HYDROCHLORIDE—Kytril®

Description/Actions: Is a selective blocking agent of the serotonin 5-HT$_3$ receptor type. Antiemetic indicated for the prevention of nausea and vomiting associated with initial and repeat courses of emetogenic cancer therapy, including high-dose cisplatin, radiation therapy–induced nausea and vomiting, and for the prophylaxis and treatment of postoperative nausea and vomiting.

Precautions/Adverse Reactions: Adverse reactions include headache, asthenia, somnolence, diarrhea, and constipation.

Administration: Oral and intravenous.

Preparations: Tablets, 1 mg. Vials, 1 mg.

GRANULOCYTE COLONY STIMULATING FACTOR,
see Filgrastim

GRANULOCYTE-MACROPHAGE COLONY STIMULATING FACTOR, see Sargramostim

GRIFULVIN®, see Griseofulvin Ultramicrosize

GRISACTIN®, see Griseofulvin Ultramicrosize

GRISEOFULVIN MICROSIZE—Fulvicin-U/F®, Grifulvin V®, Grisactin®. See Griseofulvin Ultramicrosize

GRISEOFULVIN ULTRAMICROSIZE—Fulvicin P/G®, Grisactin Ultra®, Gris- PEG®

Description/Actions: Antifungal agent administered orally for tinea (ringworm) infections of the skin, hair, and nails. Should not be used for superficial infection that may respond to topical antifungals.

Preparations: Microsize—Capsules and tablets, 125, 250, and 500 mg. Suspension, 125 mg/5 ml. Ultramicrosize tablets, 125, 165, 250, and 330 mg.

GRIS-PEG®, see Griseofulvin Ultramicrosize

GUAIFENESIN—Humabid LA®, Humabid Sprinkle®, Robitussin®, Sinumist SR Caplets®

Description/Actions: Expectorant indicated for the symptomatic relief of respiratory conditions characterized by dry, nonproductive cough and in the presence of mucus in the respiratory tract.

Preparations: Capsules and tablets, 100 and 200 mg. Syrup, 67 mg/5 ml, 100 mg/5 ml, and 200 mg/5 ml. Extended-release capsules/tablets, 300 and 600 mg.

GUANABENZ ACETATE—Wytensin®

Description/Actions: Antihypertensive agent that exhibits a central alpha-2 adrenergic agonist action.

Preparations: Tablets, 4 and 8 mg.

GUANADREL SULFATE—Hylorel®

Description/Actions: Antihypertensive agent indicated in the treatment of hypertension in patients who have not responded adequately to a thiazide-type diuretic.

Preparations: Tablets, 10 and 25 mg.

GUANETHIDINE MONOSULFATE—Ismelin®

Description/Actions: Antihypertensive agent indicated for the treatment of moderate and severe hypertension, and for the management of renal hypertension.

Preparations: Tablets, 10 and 25 mg.

GUANFACINE HYDROCHLORIDE—Tenex®

Description/Actions: Is a centrally acting Alpha$_2$ adrenergic receptor agonist. Indicated in the management of hypertension.

Precautions/Adverse Reactions: Adverse reactions include sedation, weakness, dizziness, dry mouth, constipation, and impotence. Patients should be advised to exercise caution when operating machinery or driving motor vehicles until it is determined that they do not become drowsy or dizzy from the medication. The potential exists for interactions with other drugs that have a central nervous system depressant action, so patients should be warned that their tolerance for alcohol and other CNS depressants may be decreased. The abrupt discontinuation of therapy may be associated with symptoms of nervousness and anxiety as well as increases in blood pressure (rebound hypertension).

Administration: Oral.

Preparations: Tablets, 1 mg.

GYNE-LOTRIMIN®, see Clotrimazole

H

HABITROL®, see Nicotine

HALAZEPAM—Paxipam®

Description/Actions: Benzodiazepine anti-anxiety agent indicated for the management of anxiety disorders or the short-term relief of the symptoms of anxiety.

Preparations: Tablets, 20 and 40 mg.

HALCINONIDE—Halog®

Description/Actions: Corticosteroid applied topically for the relief of the inflammatory and pruritic manifestations of corticosteroid-responsive dermatoses.

Preparations: Cream, 0.025% and 0.1%. Ointment and solution, 0.1%.

HALCION®, see Triazolam

HALDOL®, see Haloperidol

HALOBETASOL PROPIONATE—Ultravate®

Description/Actions: A high- to super-high-potency topical corticosteroid indicated for the relief of the inflammatory and pruritic manifestations of corticosteroid-responsive dermatoses.

Precautions/Adverse Reactions: Adverse reactions include stinging, burning, itching, dry skin, erythema, and skin atrophy. May cause suppression of the hypothalamic-pituitary- adrenal (HPA) axis and appropriate precautions should be taken (e.g., regarding the extent and duration of treatment).

Administration: Topical.

Preparations: Cream and ointment, 0.05%.

HALOG®, see Halcinonide

HALOPERIDOL—Haldol®

Description/Actions: A butyrophenone derivative indicated for (a) the management of manifestations of psychotic disorders, (b) the control of tics and vocal utterances of Tourette's disorder, and, in children who have not responded to psychotherapy or medications other than neuroleptics, (c) the treatment of severe behavior problems in children of combative, explosive hyperexcitability, and (d) the short-term treatment of hyperactive children who show excessive motor activity with accompanying conduct disorders.

Precautions/Adverse Reactions: Contraindicated in patients with parkinsonism or severe CNS depression. Adverse reactions include drowsiness and other CNS effects. Patients should be cautioned regarding activities such as driving and operating machinery, as well as interactions with other CNS-acting drugs including alcohol. Other adverse reactions include extrapyramidal reactions, tardive dyskinesia, neuroleptic malignant syndrome, and hypotension. Concomitant therapy with lithium must be closely monitored because there have been reports of an encephalopathic syndrome in some patients receiving both medications.

Administration: Oral and intramuscular.

Preparations: Tablets, 0.5, 1, 2, 5, 10, and 20 mg. Solution concentrate (as the lactate), 2 mg/ml. Ampules and vials (as the lactate), 5 mg/ml.

HALOPERIDOL DECANOATE—Haldol Decanoate®

Description/Actions: Is a long-acting parenterally administered form of haloperidol indicated in the management of patients requiring prolonged parenteral neuroleptic therapy.

Precautions/Adverse Reactions: See discussion on haloperidol.

Administration: Intramuscular. The recommended interval between doses is 4 weeks.

Preparations: Ampules, 50 and 100 mg per ml.

HALOPROGIN—Halotex®

Description/Actions: Antifungal agent indicated for the topical treatment of superficial tinea (ringworm) infections and tinea versicolor.

Preparations: Cream and solution, 1%.

HALOTESTIN®, see Fluoxymesterone

HALOTEX®, see Haloprogin

HALOTHANE—Fluothane®

Description/Actions: Inhalation general anesthetic indicated for the induction and maintenance of general anesthesia.

Preparations: Liquid, 125 and 250 ml.

HECTOROL®, see Doxercalciferol

HELIDAC®

Description/Actions: Combination agent used in treatment of active duodenal ulcer associated with *H. pylori*. Bismuth subsalicylate, metronidazole, and tetracyline.

HEMABATE®, see Carboprost Tromethamine

HEPARIN SODIUM—Liquaemin Sodium®

Description/Actions: Exhibits an anticoagulant action, in part, by inhibiting the conversion of fibrinogen to fibrin. Indicated in the prophylaxis and treatment of venous thrombosis and its extension, pulmonary embolism, peripheral arterial embolism, and atrial fibrillation with embolization. Also used in the diagnosis and treatment of acute and chronic consumptive coagulopathies, in a low-dose regimen for prevention of postoperative deep vein thrombosis and pulmonary embolism in patients undergoing major surgery, as an adjunct in the treatment of coronary occlusion with acute myocardial infarction, in the prevention of clotting in arterial and heart surgery, and in blood transfusions, extracorporeal circulation, and dialysis procedures. Used in very low doses to maintain patency of IV catheters (heparin flush).

Precautions/Adverse Reactions: May cause hemorrhage, so therapy must be closely monitored. Action may be increased by agents such as aspirin and nonsteroidal anti-inflammatory drugs.

Administration: Intravenous or deep subcutaneous. Intramuscular use should be avoided because of the danger of hematoma formation.

Preparations: Ampules and vials, 10, 100, 1000, 5000, 10,000, 20,000, and 40,000 units/ml.

HEROIN—Diacetylmorphine

Description/Actions: Narcotic analgesic not legally available in the United States.

HERPLEX®, see Idoxuridine

HESPAN®, see Hetastarch

HETASTARCH—Hespan®

Description/Actions: Plasma expander with colloidal properties approximating those of human albumin. Indicated for intravenous infusion when plasma volume expansion is desired as an adjunct in the treatment of shock due to hemorrhage, burns, surgery, sepsis, or other trauma.

Preparations: Solution, 6% in 250 and 500 cc bottles.

HEXACHLOROPHENE—pHisoHex®

Description/Actions: Anti-infective agent indicated for topical use as a surgical scrub and a bacteriostatic skin cleanser.

Preparations: Emulsion, 3%.

HEXADROL®, see Dexamethasone

HEXALEN®, see Altretamine

HEXAVITAMIN

Description/Actions: Vitamin mixture that includes Vitamins A, D, B_1, B_2, and C, and nicotinic acid. Used in the prevention and treatment of deficiencies of these vitamins.

Preparations: Capsules and Tablets.

HIBICLENS®, see Chlorhexidine Gluconate

HIBISTAT®, see Chlorhexidine Gluconate

HIPREX®, see Methenamine Hippurate

HISTAMINE PHOSPHATE

Description/Actions: Diagnostic agent used to test the ability of the gastric mucosa to produce hydrochloric acid, and in the diagnosis of pheochromocytoma.

Preparations: Ampules containing the equivalent of 0.1 and 0.2 mg histamine base/ml.

HISTRELIN ACETATE—Supprelin®

Description/Actions: Is an analog of naturally occurring gonadotropin-releasing hormone (GnRH), and is a potent inhibitor of gonadotropin secretion when administered daily in therapeutic doses. Chronic daily administration inhibits the secretion of pituitary gonadotropin, which, in turn, causes a reduction in ovarian and testicular steroid production. Indicated for the control of the manifestations of centrally mediated precocious puberty occurring before the age of 8 years in girls or 9.5 years in boys.

Precautions/Adverse Reactions: Also contraindicated in women who are or may become pregnant while receiving the drug and in nursing mothers. Adverse reactions include skin reactions at the injection site (e.g., redness, swelling, itching), vaginal bleeding, and hypersensitivity reactions.

Administration: Subcutaneous. Daily injection should be rotated through different body sites (upper arms, thighs, abdomen). Patients and their families should be informed of the need to give injections at approximately the same time each day; otherwise, the pubertal process may be reactivated. Treatment should be discontinued when the onset of puberty is desired.

Preparations: Vials (and syringes with needles) that deliver 0.6 ml of a solution containing 200 mcg/ml (120 mcg/vial), 500 mcg/ml (300 mcg/vial), or 1000 mcg/ml (600 mcg/vial).

HIVID®, see Zalcitabine

HOMATROPINE HYDROBROMIDE

Description/Actions: Anticholinergic agent for ophthalmic use. Indicated for use as a mydriatic and cycloplegic for refraction, and in the management of certain ocular inflammatory conditions. Also used orally for anticholinergic action in combination with other agents.

Preparations: Ophthalmic solutions, 2% and 5%.

HUMABID LA®, see Guaifenesin

HUMABID SPRINKLE®, see Guaifenesin

HUMALOG®, see Insulin

HUMATIN®, see Paromomycin

HUMATROPE®, see Somatropin

HUMIRA™, see Adalimunab

HUMORSOL®, see Demecarium

HUMULIN®, see Insulin

HYALURONIDASE—Wydase®

Description/Actions: Enzyme indicated as an adjuvant to increase the absorption and dispersion of other injected drugs, for hypodermoclysis, and as an adjunct in subcutaneous urography for improving resorption of radiopaque agents.

Preparations: Vials, 150 and 1500 units.

HYCAMTIN®, see Topotecan Hydrochloride

HYCODAN®, Combination of Hydrocodone and Homatropine. See individual discussion on Hydrocodone and Homatropine.

HYDELTRA®, see Prednisolone Tebutate

HYDELTRASOL®, see Prednisolone Sodium Phosphate

HYDERGINE®, see Ergoloid Mesylates

HYDRALAZINE HYDROCHLORIDE—Apresoline®

Preparations: Tablets, 10, 25, 50, and 100 mg. Injection, 20 mg/ml.

HYDREA®, see Hydroxyurea

HYDROCHLOROTHIAZIDE—Esidrix®, HydroDIURIL®, Microzide®, Oretic®

Description/Actions: Indicated in the management of hypertension, and as adjunctive therapy in edema associated with congestive heart failure, hepatic cirrhosis, and corticosteroid and estrogen therapy. Is also useful in edema due to various forms of renal dysfunction such as nephrotic syndrome.

Precautions/Adverse Reactions: May cause hypokalemia, and serum potassium levels should be determined periodically. Reduction in potassium levels may increase the action and toxicity of digoxin and related glycosides. Concurrent use with lithium is best avoided because of an increased risk of lithium toxicity. May cause hyperglycemia and hyperuricemia, and therapy in patients having diabetes or gout should be closely monitored. Excreted in breast milk. If drug therapy with hydrochlorothiazide is essential, patient should be instructed to stop nursing.

Administration: Oral.

Preparations: Tablets, 25, 50, and 100 mg. Capsules, 12.5 mg. Oral solution, 50 mg/5 ml. Concentrated oral solution, 100 mg/ml.

HYDROCODONE BITARTRATE—Hycodan®

Description/Actions: Opioid analgesic and antitussive indicated for the relief of moderate to moderately severe pain and for the relief of cough. Used in combination with other agents.

HYDROCODONE BITARTRATE WITH ACETAMINOPHEN—

Norco®, Vicodin®. See individual discussion on Hydrocodone Bitartrate and Acetaminophen.

HYDROCORTISONE—Cortisol, Cortef®, Hydrocortone®, Pandel®

Description/Actions: Corticosteroid indicated in a wide range of endocrine, rheumatic, allergic, dermatologic, respiratory, hematologic, neoplastic, and other disorders.

Preparations: Tablets, 5, 10, and 20 mg. Oral suspension (as the cypionate), 10 mg/5 ml. Vials, (as the sodium phosphate), 50 mg/ml. Vials (as the sodium succinate), 100, 250, 500, and 1000 mg. Vials (as the acetate for intralesional, intra-articular, or soft tissue injection), 25 mg/ml and 50 mg/ml. Retention enema, 100 mg. Cream, ointment, lotion, gel, aerosol for topical use (some formulations contain the acetate salt), 0.25%, 0.5%, 1%, and 2.5%. Cream and ointment (as the butyrate), 0.1%. Cream (as buteprate) and ointment (as the valerate), 0.2%.

HYDROCORTONE®, see Hydrocortisone

HYDRODIURIL®, see Hydrochlorothiazide

HYDROFLUMETHIAZIDE—Diucardin®, Saluron®

Description/Actions: Thiazide diuretic indicated as adjunctive therapy in the treatment of edema. Is also indicated in the management of hypertension.

Preparations: Tablets, 50 mg.

HYDROGEN PEROXIDE

Description/Actions: Antiseptic/cleansing agent applied to the skin and certain mucous membranes.

Preparations: Solution, 3%.

HYDROMORPHONE HYDROCHLORIDE—Dilaudid®

Description/Actions: Opioid analgesic indicated for the relief of moderate to severe pain. Has also been used to suppress cough.

Preparations: Tablets, 1, 2, 4, and 8 mg. Suppositories, 3 mg. Ampules, vials, and syringes, 1 mg/ml, 2 mg/ml, 3 mg/ml, 4 mg/ml, and 10 mg/ml.

HYDROMOX®, see Quinethazone

HYDROPHILIC OINTMENT

Description/Actions: Ointment base that is "water removable" and into which medications are often incorporated and applied.

HYDROPHILIC PETROLATUM

Description/Actions: Ointment base capable of absorbing quantities of water or aqucous solutions containing medications.

HYDROQUINONE—Eldoquin®, Lustra®

Description/Actions: A depigmenting agent indicated in ultraviolet-induced dyschromia and discoloration of the skin due to pregnancy, oral contraceptives, hormone replacement therapy, or skin trauma.

Precautions/Adverse Reactions: Do skin sensitivity test before use. If itching, vesicle formation, or excessive inflammation occurs, avoid further treatment. Avoid sun and UV light. Avoid contact with eyes. Pregnancy Category C. Adverse reactions include localized contact dermatitis (discontinue if occurs).

Administration: Topical. Discontinue if lightening effect does not occur after 2 months.

Preparations: 4% cream in 2 oz jar.

HYDROXOCOBALAMIN

Description/Actions: Vitamin B_{12} analog indicated in the parenteral treatment of pernicious anemia, dietary deficiency of vitamin B_{12}, malabsorption of vitamin B_{12}, and other situations in which there is inadequate utilization of vitamin B_{12}. Also used for the Schilling test.

Preparations: Vials, 1000 g/ml.

HYDROXYAMPHETAMINE HYDROBROMIDE

Description/Actions: Sympathomimetic amine indicated for ophthalmic use to dilate the pupil.

Preparations: Ophthalmic solution, in combination with other agents.

HYDROXYCHLOROQUINE SULFATE—Plaquenil®

Description/Actions: Antimalarial agent indicated for the treatment of acute attacks and suppression of malaria. Also used in the management of rheumatoid arthritis and lupus erythematosus in patients who have not responded satisfactorily to drugs having a lesser potential to cause serious adverse effects.

Preparations: Tablets, 200 mg.

HYDROXYPROGESTERONE CAPROATE—Duralutin®

Description/Actions: Progestin administered intramuscularly in the management of amenorrhea, abnormal uterine bleeding due to hormonal imbalance, production of secretory endometrium and desquamation, and adenocarcinoma of uterine corpus in advanced stage.

Preparations: Vials, 125 mg/ml and 250 mg/ml.

HYDROXYUREA—Hydrea®

Description/Actions: Antineoplastic agent indicated in the treatment of melanoma, chronic myelocytic leukemia, and carcinoma of the ovary. Has also been of benefit in reducing the frequency and severity of painful sickle cell crises.

Preparations: Capsules, 500 mg.

HYDROXYZINE—Atarax®, Vistaril®

Description/Actions: Exhibits sedative and antihistaminic actions. Indicated (a) for symptomatic relief of anxiety and tension associated with psychoneurosis and as an adjunct in organic disease states in which anxiety is manifested; (b) in the management of pruritus due to allergic conditions such as chronic urticaria and atopic and contact dermatoses, and in histamine-mediated pruritus; and (c) as a sedative when used as premedication and following general anesthesia.

Precautions/Adverse Reactions: Contraindicated in early pregnancy. Adverse reactions include drowsiness and other CNS effects; patients should be cautioned regarding activities such as driving and operating machinery, as well as interactions with other CNS-acting drugs including alcohol. When other CNS-depressant drugs are administered concurrently, their dosage should be appropriately reduced.

Administration: Oral and intramuscular.

Preparations: Tablets and capsules, 10, 25, 50, and 100 mg. Syrup, 10 mg/5 ml, oral suspension, 25 mg/5 ml. Vials, 25 and 50 mg/ml.

HYGROTON®, see Chlorthalidone

HYLOREL®, see Guanadrel

HYOSCINE, see Scopolamine

HYOSCYAMINE SULFATE—Anaspaz, Cystospaz®, Levbid®, Levsin®, Levsinex®

Description/Actions: Anticholinergic agent used as adjunctive therapy in the treatment of peptic ulcer. Also used in other gastrointestinal disorders, biliary and renal conditions, as a drying agent in acute rhinitis, and in the management of parkinsonism.

Preparations: Tablets, 0.125 and 0.15 mg. Controlled-release capsules, 0.375 mg. Elixir, 0.125 mg/5 ml. Drops, 0.125 mg/ml. Vials, 0.5 mg/ml.

HYPERSTAT®, see Diazoxide

HYTAKEROL®, see Dihydrotachysterol

HYTRIN®, see Terazosin

HYZAAR®, Combination drug containing Lorsartan Potassium and Hydrochlorothiazide. See individual discussion on Losartan and Hydrochlorothiazide.

I

IBRITUMOMAB TIUXETAN—Zevalin™

Description/Actions: Zevalin™ is indicated for the treatment of patients with relapsed or refractory low-grade, follicular, or transformed B-cell non-Hodgkin's lymphoma, including patients with rituximab refractory follicular non-Hodgkin's lymphoma.

Precautions/Adverse Reactions: Zevalin™ is contraindicated in patients with known type I hypersensitivity or anaphylactic reactions to murine proteins or to any component of this product, including rituximab, yttrium chloride, and indium chloride. Because rituximab is part of the regimen, consult warnings for rituximab. Fatal infusion reactions have occurred; deaths have occurred within 24 hours of rituximab infusion. Fatalities associated with an infusion reaction symptom complex that included hypoxia, pulmonary infiltrates, acute respiratory distress, myocardial infarction, ventricular fibrillation, or cardiogenic shock. These severe reactions typically occur during the first rituximab infusion, with time to onset of 30–120 minutes. These signs and symptoms may require interruption of rituximab, In 111 Zevalin™, or y 90 Zevalin administration. Y 90 Zevalin™ administration results in severe and prolonged cytopenias in most patients. It should not be given to patients with ≥25% lymphoma marrow involvement and/or impaired bone marrow reserve. Y 90 Zevalin™ should not be administered to patients with altered biodistribution of In 111 Zevalin™. The therapeutic regimen is intended as a single-course treatment and is to be used in combination with rituximab. The contents of the kit are not radioactive. Pregnancy Category D. There is a potential risk that the Zevalin™ regimen could cause toxic effects on the male and female gonads. Effective contraceptive methods should be used during treatment and for up to 12 months following the regimen. The most serious adverse reactions include infections, allergic reactions (bronchospasm and angioedema), and hemorrhage while thrombocytopenic (resulting in death). Patients who have received Zevalin™ regimen have developed myeloid malignancies and dysplasias. Most common toxicities were neutropenia, thrombocytopenia, anemia, nausea, vomiting, abdominal pain, increased cough, dyspnea, dizziness, asthenia, chills, fever, and headache. No formal drug interaction studies have been performed. Because of the frequent occurrence of severe thrombocytopenia, agents that interfere with platelet function and/or anticoagulation should be weighed against the potential increased risks of bleeding and hemorrhage. Safety and effectiveness in children have not been established.

Administration: Intravenous.

Patient Care Implications: Do not give y 90 Zevalin to patients with a platelet count <100,000/mm³. Y 90 dose should not exceed the absolute maximum allowable dose of 32.0 mCi (1184 MEq), regardless of the patient's weight. Patient should be measured by a suitable radioactivity calibration system immediately prior to administration. Proper aseptic technique and precautions for handling radioactive materials should be employed. Radiolabeling of ibritumomab with y 90 and In 111 (not included in kit) must be performed by appropriate personnel in a specialized facility. Human antimurine antibody should be done prior to treatment. If positive, the patient may have an allergic or hypersensitivity reaction when treated. Monitor for infusion-related allergic reactions. Obtain complete blood counts and platelet counts at least weekly. Platelet count must be done prior to step 2. Biodistribution of In 111 Zevalin should be assessed by imaging at 2–24 hours and at 48–72 hours postinjection, and a third image may be necessary at 90–120 hours. If biodistribution is not acceptable, the patient should not proceed to step 2. Kit is not radioactive. Do not freeze. To prepare radiolabeled injection, follow manufacturer's guidelines. Should be prepared only by individuals trained in the preparation of radiopharmaceuticals in a facility that is designated for this purpose.

Preparations: Each kit contains 4 vials for preparation of either In 111 or y 90. In 111 Zevalin kit provides for the radiolabeling of ibritumomab tiuxetan with In 111. Has 4 vials: 1 Zevalin vial containing 3.2 mg of ibritumomab tiuxetan in 2 ml of 0.9% sodium chloride solution, 1 vial containing 50 mM of sodium acetate, 1 formulation buffer vial, 1 empty reaction vial, and 4 identification labels. Y 90 Zevalin kit provides for radiolabeling of ibritumomab tiuxetan with y 90. Kit has 4 vials: 1 Zevalin vial containing 3.2 mg of ibritumomab tiuxetan in 2 ml 0.9% sodium chloride, 1 vial containing 50 mM of sodium acetate, 1 formulation buffer vial, 1 empty reaction vial, and 4 identification labels.

IBUPROFEN—Advil®, Children's Advil®, Motrin®, Children's Motrin®, Nuprin®, Pediacare Fever Liquid®, Rufen®

Description/Actions: Nonsteroidal anti-inflammatory agent that inhibits prostaglandin synthesis and is indicated for the relief of mild to moderate pain, primary dysmenorrhea, rheumatoid arthritis, osteoarthritis, and reduction of fever.

Precautions/Adverse Reactions: Should not be given to patients in whom aspirin or another NSAID causes asthma, rhinitis, urticaria, or other allergic-type reactions. May cause GI effects, so use should be avoided in patients with active GI tract disease and closely monitored in patients with a previous history of such disorders. Other adverse reactions include dizziness and rash.

Administration: Oral.

Preparations: Caplets and tablets, 100, 200, 300, 400, 600, and 800 mg. Gelcaps, 200 mg. Chewable tablets, 50 and 100 mg. Suspension, 100 mg/5 ml, oral drops 40 mg/ml and 50 mg/1.25 ml (dropperful).

IBUTILIDE FUMARATE—Corvert®

Description/Actions: Predominantly a class III antiarrhythmic agent used in the rapid conversion of atrial fibrillation or atrial flutter of recent onset to sinus rhythm. Patients with atrial arrhythmias of longer duration are less likely to respond to ibutilide. The effectiveness of ibutilide has not been determined in patients with arrhythmias of >90 days duration.

Precautions/Adverse Reactions: Administer in appropriate treatment environment as this drug may cause life-threatening arrhythmias such as sustained polymorphic ventricular tachycardia, usually in association with QT prolongation (torsades de pointes) but sometimes without QT prolongation. These arrhythmias can be reversed if treated promptly with cardioversion. An appropriate environment should include continuous ECG monitoring, personnel skilled in arrhythmia recognition, and life-support equipment. Reports of reversible heart block have been associated with ibutilide administration.

Administration: Intravenous.

Preparations: Solution, 0.1mg/ml in 10 ml vials.

ICHTHAMMOL

Description/Actions: Antibacterial agent and astringent applied topically in certain dermatologic disorders.

Preparations: Ointment, 10% and 20%.

IDAMYCIN®, see Idarubicin Hydrochloride

IDARUBICIN HYDROCHLORIDE—Idamycin®

Description/Actions: Is an anthracycline derivative that is indicated for use in combination with other antileukemic drugs (usually cytarabine) for the treatment of acute myeloid leukemia in adults.

Precautions/Adverse Reactions: May cause severe myelosuppression and should not be given to patients with preexisting bone marrow suppression induced by previous drug therapy or radiotherapy unless the benefit warrants the risk. Other adverse reactions include myocardial toxicity (e.g., congestive heart failure, arrhythmias), GI effects (e.g., nausea, vomiting, mucositis, abdominal pain, diarrhea), alopecia, dermatologic effects (e.g., rash, urticaria), pulmonary effects, mental status effects, fever, headache, neurologic effects, hyperuricemia secondary to rapid lysis of leukemic cells, and extravasation. Should not be used in pregnant women unless the benefit outweighs the risk. In patients with hepatic or renal impairment, a reduction in dosage should be considered and treatment should be closely monitored.

Administration: Intravenous. Follow vesicant procedures.

Preparations: Vials, 5 and 10 mg.

IDOXURIDINE—IDU, Herplex®, Stoxil®

Description/Actions: Antiviral agent indicated for ophthalmic use in the treatment of herpes simplex keratitis.

Preparations: Ophthalmic solution, 0.1%. Ophthalmic ointment, 0.5%.

IDU, see Idoxuridine

IFEX® see Ifosfamide

IFOSFAMIDE—Ifex®

Description/Actions: Antineoplastic agent that is an analog of cyclo-phosphamide and requires metabolic activation by liver microsomal enzymes to produce biologically active metabolites. Indicated for use in combination with other antineoplastic agents, for third line chemotherapy of germ cell testicular cancer. Should be used in combination with mesna to reduce the risk of hemorrhagic cystitis.

Precautions/Adverse Reactions: May cause leukopenia, thrombocytopenia, and urotoxic effects, especially hemorrhagic cystitis. Other adverse reactions include sedation confusion, hallucinations, alopecia, nausea, and vomiting.

Administration: Intravenous infusion (lasting a minimum of 30 minutes). Should be given with extensive hydration consisting of at least 2 liters of oral or intravenous fluid per day, and with the uroprotective agent, mesna.

Preparations: Vials, 1 and 3 g.

ILETIN®, see Insulin

ILOPAN®, see Dexpanthenol

ILOSONE®, see Erythromycin Estolate

ILOTYCIN®, see Erythromycin Base and Gluceptate

IMATINIB MESYLATE—Gleevec™

Description/Actions: Imatinib is indicated as first-line treatment of patients with chronic myeloid leukemia; for the treatment of patients with Philadelphia chromosome-positive chronic myeloid leukemia in blast crisis, accelerated phase; or for chronic phase after failure of interferon–alpha therapy. Imatinib is also indicated for the treatment of patients with kit-positive unresectable and or metastatic gastrointestinal stromal tumors.

Precautions/Adverse Reactions: Imatinib is contraindicated in patients with a known hypersensitivity to it or to any component of the formulation. Women of childbearing age should be advised not to become pregnant while on imatinib therapy. Therapy with imatinib is often associated with edema and occasionally serious fluid retention. Probability of edema was increased with higher imatinib doses and age >65 years. Severe fluid retention (pleural effusion, pericardial effusion, pulmonary edema, and ascites) has been reported. Severe superficial edema has also been reported. Imatinib may cause gastrointestinal irritation.

To minimize this effect, Gleevec should be taken with food and with a large glass of water. Hemorrhage is possible with imatinib therapy. Treatment with imatinib is associated with hematologic toxicity, namely, neutropenia or thrombocytopenia. Complete blood counts should be performed weekly for the first month, biweekly for the second month, and periodically thereafter as clinically indicated. Hepatotoxicity may occur with imatinib therapy. It may be severe. Liver function tests (transaminases, bilirubin, and alkaline phosphatase) should be monitored before initiation of therapy and monthly or as clinically indicated. Long-term safety data on treatment with imatinib are unknown; however, potential long-term toxicities include liver toxicity, renal toxicity, and immunosuppression. Imatinib is metabolized primarily by the cytochrome P450 enzyme system 3A4. Coadministration of imatinib and CYP3A4 inhibitors such as ketoconazole, itraconazole, erythromycin, and clarithromycin resulted in decreased metabolism and increased plasma levels of imatinib. Coadministration of imatinib and CYP3A4 inducers such as dexamethasone, phenytoin, carbamazepine, rifampin, phenobarbital, and St. John's Wort may reduce plasma levels of imatinib. Coadministration of imatinib and simvastatin resulted in increased plasma concentrations of simvastatin. Use caution when coadministering imatinib and drugs with a narrow therapeutic index such as cyclosporine and pimozide. Imatinib will increase serum concentrations of other drugs metabolized by CYP3A4 such as triazolebenzodiazepines, dihydropyridine calcium channel blockers, and certain HMG-CoA reductase inhibitors. Coadministration of imatinib and warfarin has resulted in decreased metabolism of warfarin. It is recommended that patients requiring anticoagulation should receive low molecular weight or standard heparin. In vitro imatinib inhibits cytochrome P450 2D6 activity at similar concentrations that affect CYP3A4 activity. Plasma concentrations of substrates of CYP2D6 are expected to increase when coadministered with imatinib. Pregnancy Category D. Women of childbearing potential are advised to avoid becoming pregnant while receiving imatinib therapy. Excretion in human breast milk is unknown. Women should be advised against breast-feeding while taking imatinib. Gleevec™ safety and efficacy have been demonstrated only in children with Philadelphia chromosome-positive (Ph+) chronic phase CML with recurrence after stem cell transplantation or resistance to interferon alpha therapy. There are no data in children under 3 years of age. The most frequently reported drug-related adverse events were nausea, vomiting, diarrhea, edema, and muscle cramps. Edema was mostly periorbital or in the lower limbs and was managed with diuretics or by reducing the dose of imatinib. Peripheral effusions, ascites, pulmonary edema, and rapid weight gain with or without superficial edema have been reported. These events appear to be dose related and were more common in the blast crisis and accelerated phase studies, and are more common in the elderly.

Neutropenia and thrombocytopenia have been associated with imatinib therapy, occurring with a higher frequency at doses ≥750 mg.

Administration: Oral.

Patient Care Implications: Imatinib should be taken with a meal and a large glass of water. Patients should be weighed and monitored regularly for signs and symptoms of fluid retention. Complete blood counts should be performed weekly for the first month, biweekly for the second month, and periodically thereafter as clinically indicated. Liver function tests should be monitored before initiation of treatment and monthly or as clinically indicated. Patients should be monitored for potential renal toxicity and immunosuppression. Female patients should be advised to avoid becoming pregnant.

Preparations: Tablets, 100 and 400 mg.

IMDUR®, see Isosorbide Mononitrate

IMIGLUCERASE—Cerezyme®

Description/Actions: Agent for Gaucher's disease. It is an analog of the human enzyme beta-glucocerebrosidase produced by recombinant technology. Indicated for long-term enzyme replacement therapy for patients with a confirmed diagnoses of type I Gaucher's disease that results in one or more of the following conditions: anemia, thrombocytopenia, bone disease, hepatomegaly, or splenomegaly.

Precautions/Adverse Reactions: Adverse reactions include headache, nausea, abdominal discomfort, dizziness, pruritus, and rash. Caution should be exercised in patients previously treated with alglucerase and who have developed antibody to alglucerase or who have exhibited symptoms of hypersensitivity to alglucerase. Anaphylactoid reactions have been reported during treatment with imiglucerase. Use caution with further treatments. Most patients have successfully completed therapy after a reduction in the rate of infusion and pretreatment with antihistamines and/or corticosteroids. Pulmonary hypertension has also been reported with the use of imiglucerase.

Administration: Intravenous. Is administered by IV infusion over 1–2 hours.

Preparations: Vials, 200 units.

IMIPENEM-CILASTATIN SODIUM—Primaxin IV®, Primaxin IM®

Description/Actions: Carbapenem antibiotic. Imipenem has a very broad spectrum of action that includes almost all gram-positive and gram-negative bacteria. Cilastatin is an enzyme inhibitor that significantly reduces the renal metabolism of imipenem, resulting in a much greater urinary recovery of the antibiotic. Indicated for intravenous use for the treatment of lower respiratory tract infections, urinary tract infections, intra-abdominal infections, gynecologic infections, bacterial septicemia, bone and joint infections, skin and skin-structure infections, endocarditis, and polymicrobic infections caused by susceptible organisms. Indicated for intramuscular use in the treatment of serious infections of mild to moderate severity for which IM therapy is appropriate.

Precautions/Adverse Reactions: Must be used cautiously, if at all, in patients who have experienced hypersensitivity reactions to a penicillin or cephalosporin. Seizures have been reported, although infrequently, and therapy must be closely supervised in patients with predisposing factors such as a history of seizures.

Administration: Intravenous and intramuscular.

Preparations: Vials and infusion bottles for intravenous use, 250 mg imipenem equivalent to 250 mg cilastatin equivalent, and 500 mg of each agent. Vials for intramuscular use, 500 mg imipenem equivalent to 500 mg cilastatin equivalent, and 750 mg of each agent.

IMIPRAMINE HYDROCHLORIDE—Tofranil®. See discussion on Imipramine Pamoate.

IMIPRAMINE PAMOATE—Tofranil-PM®

Description/Actions: Tricyclic antidepressant indicated for the relief of symptoms of depression. Oral formulation of imipramine hydrochloride is also used in the management of childhood enuresis.

Preparations: Tablets, 10, 25, and 50 mg. Capsules (pamoate), 75, 100, 125, and 150 mg. Ampules, 25 mg.

IMIQUIMOD—Aldara®

Description/Actions: Immune response modifier indicated for the treatment of external genital and perianal warts (condyloma acuminata) in individuals 12 years of age and older. Imiquimod is also indicated for the topical treatment of clinically typical, nonhyperkeratotic, nonhypertrophic actinic keratoses on the face or scalp in immunocompetent adults and for the topical treatment of biopsy confirmed, primary superficial basal cell carcinoma in immunocompetent adults with a maximum tumor diameter of 2 centimeters located on the trunk (excluding anogenital skin), neck, or extremities (excluding hands and feet) only when surgical methods are medically less appropriate and patient follow-up can be reasonably assured. Imiquimod induces mRNA encoding cytokines including interferon-alpha at the treatment site. In addition, $HPLV_1$ mRNA and HPV DNA are significantly decreased following treatment. Other therapies used to treat genital warts can cause damage to tissue and surrounding areas and imiquimod should not be applied until these areas have healed.

Precautions/Adverse Reactions: Not for use in treating urethral, intravaginal, cervical, rectal, or intra-anal human papilloma viral disease. Not for use on lesions that have not healed from other therapies (drug or surgical). Avoid sexual contact while cream is applied to skin. Avoid eyes. Do not occlude. May exacerbate inflammatory skin conditions. Concomitant use of diaphragms or condoms not recommended. Adverse reactions include local and remote reactions (e.g., erythema, erosion, itching, burning, soreness), headache, flu-like symptoms, and myalgia. Safety and efficacy in patients below the age of 12 have not been established.

Administration: Apply a thin layer to warts and rub in 3 times per week at bedtime (e.g., Mon-Wed-Fri or Tues-Thurs-Sat). Maximum usage not to exceed 16 weeks. Remove with soap and water after 6–10 hours. If local reactions occur, suspend therapy until reactions subside. When treating warts under foreskin of uncircumcised males, the foreskin should be retracted and cleansed daily. New warts may develop during therapy. Wash hands before and after application. Notify prescriber of severe skin reactions. Instruct female patients to avoid using the product in the vagina.

Preparations: Single-use packets of 5% cream (250 mg each).

IMITREX®, see Sumatriptan Succinate

IMODIUM®, see Loperamide

IMODIUM ADVANCED®—Combination Agent Loperamide and Simethicone (Opioid and Antiflatulent). See individual discussion on Loperamide and Simethicone.

IMODIUM A-D®, see Loperamide

IMURAN®, see Azathioprine

INAMRINONE—Inocor®

Description/Actions: Increases myocardial contractility and decreases preload and afterload by a direct dilating effect on vascular smooth muscle. Indicated for short-term treatment of congestive heart failure unresponsive to glycosides, diuretics, and vasodilators.

Precautions/Adverse Reactions: Contraindicated in idiopathic hypertrophic subaortic stenosis (IHSS). Correct fluid and electrolytes associated with previous aggressive diuretic therapy prior to initiating amrinone.

Adverse reactions include arrhythmias, hypotension, thrombocytopenia, and tachyphylaxis. Initiate in monitored environment.

Administration: Intravenous.

Preparations: Injection, 5 mg/ml.

INAPSINE®, see Droperidol

INDAPAMIDE—Lozol®

Description/Actions: Diuretic indicated for the treatment of hypertension and for the treatment of salt and fluid retention associated with congestive heart failure.

Preparations: Tablets, 1.25 and 2.5 mg.

INDERAL®, see Propranolol

INDINAVIR—Crixivan®

Description/Actions: Antiviral, protease inhibitor used in the treatment of HIV infection.

Precautions/Adverse Reactions: Contraindicated with concurrent use of terfenadine, astemizole, cisapride, triazolam, and midazolam. Coadministration of indinavir with sildenafil, vardenafil, or tadalafil results in increased plasma concentrations of these agents and may lead to hypotension, visual changes, and priapism. Adverse reactions include nephrolithiasis, aymptomatic hyperbilirubinemia, GI upset, abdominal pain, kidney stones, headache, fatigue, insomnia, flank pain, and dysguesia. Maintain adequate hydration (1.5 L/day). Discontinue or suspend therapy (e.g., 1–3 days) during acute nephrolithiasis or impaired hepatic function.

Administration: Oral with water on an empty stomach or with a light meal.

Preparations: Capsules, 200, 333, and 400 mg.

INDOCIN®, see Indomethacin

INDOMETHACIN—Indocin®, Indocin SR®

Description/Actions: Nonsteroidal anti-inflammatory agent that inhibits prostaglandin synthesis and is indicated in the treatment of rheumatoid arthritis, osteoarthritis, ankylosing spondylitis, acute painful shoulder, and acute gouty arthritis. Used as an alternative to surgery in the management of patent ductus arteriosus in premature neonates.

Precautions/Adverse Reactions: Should not be given to patients in whom aspirin or another NSAID causes asthma, rhinitis, urticaria, or other allergic-type reactions. Suppositories are contraindicated in patients with a history of proctitis or recent rectal bleeding. May cause GI effects and use should be avoided in patients with active GI tract disease and closely monitored in patients with a previous history of such disorders. Other reactions include headache and dizziness.

Administration: Oral, rectal, and intravenous. Should be administered with food or antacids, or immediately after meals, to reduce GI effects.

Preparations: Capsules, 25 and 50 mg. Sustained-release capsules, 75 mg. Oral suspension, 25 mg/5 ml. Suppositories, 50 mg. Injection, 1 mg vials.

InFeD®, see Iron Dextran

INFLIXIMAB—Remicade®

Description/Actions: Remicade® is indicated in combination with methotrexate for reducing signs and symptoms, inhibiting the progression of structural damage, and improving physical function in patients with moderately to severely active rheumatoid arthritis. Remicade® is also indicated for reducing the number of draining enterococcus and retrovaginal fistulas and maintaining fistula closure in patients with fistulating Crohn's disease. It is also indicated for reducing signs and symptoms in patients with active ankylosing spondylitis and for reducing signs and symptoms of active arthritis in patients with psoriatic arthritis.

Precautions/Adverse Reactions: Contraindicated in patients with allergy to murine protein. Discontinue if lupus-like syndrome with antibody formation occurs. Use cautiously in elderly. Pregnancy Category C. Use in children and nursing mothers not recommended. Tuberculosis (frequently disseminated or extrapulmonary at clinical presentation), invasive fungal infections, and other opportunistic infections have been observed in patients receiving infliximab. Some have been fatal. Patients should be evaluated for latent tuberculosis infection. Cases of histoplasmosis, listeriosis, pneumocystosis, and worsening heart failure have been reported in patients treated with infliximab. Do not initiate therapy in patients with congestive heart failure. Severe hepatic reactions, including acute liver failure, jaundice, hepatitis, and cholestasis have been reported. Some of these cases were fatal or necessitated liver transplantation. Patients with symptoms or signs of liver dysfunction should be evaluated for evidence of liver injury. If jaundice and or a marked liver enzyme elevation (e.g., ≥5 times the upper limit of normal) develops, infliximab should be discontinued.

Remicade® has been associated with reactivation of hepatitis B in patients who are chronic carriers of this virus. Serious infections including sepsis and pneumonia have been reported in patients receiving tumor necrosis blocking agents. Some of these infections have been fatal. Cases of leukopenia, neutropenia, thrombocytopenia, and pancytopenia, some with a fatal outcome, have been reported in patients receiving infliximab. Infliximab has been associated with hypersensitivity reactions that include: urticaria, dyspnea, and/or hypotension requiring hospitalization in some cases. Other adverse reactions include infusion-related reactions including cases of anaphylactic-like reactions including laryngeal/pharyngeal edema and severe bronchospasm and seizure, nausea, vomiting, fatigue, fever, pain, dizziness, bronchitis, sinusitis, rhinitis and rash. Malignancies including non-Hodgkin's lymphoma and Hodgkin's disease as well as breast, colorectal, and melanoma have been reported with infliximab therapy.

Administration: Intravenous. Reconstitute vial with 10 ml of sterile water for injection. The total dose of reconstituted product should be further diluted in 250 ml of normal saline.

Patient Care Implications: Administration of infliximab has been associated with hypersensitivity reactions. Discontinue the medication for severe reactions. Instruct patients in the signs and symptoms of infection and to promptly report onset to the prescriber.

Preparations: Powder for injection, 100 mg.

INH, see Isoniazid

INNOHEP®, see Tinzaparin

INOCOR®, see Inamrinone

INOMAX®, see Nitric Oxide

INSPRA™, see Eplerenone

INSULATARD®, see Insulin

INSULIN ASPART—Novolog®

Description/Actions: Indicated in the treatment of hyperglycemia in adult patients with diabetes mellitus. It should be used together with intermediate-acting or long-acting insulin. Insulin aspart may also be infused subcutaneously by external insulin pump.

Precautions/Adverse Reactions: Insulin aspart is contraindicated in patients with a known hypersensitivity to insulin aspart or to any component of the product. It is also contraindicated during episodes of hypoglycemia. Injection of insulin aspart should be immediately followed by a meal. It should be used in conjunction with a longer-acting insulin in type I diabetics. Hypoglycemia and hypokalemia are common adverse effects during insulin therapy. Changes in insulin therapy should be made cautiously and under medical supervision. Monitoring of blood glucose levels is recommended for all diabetics. Lipodystrophy and hypersensitivity reactions may occur at the injection site. Decreased doses of insulin aspart may be required in patients with renal or hepatic impairment. Oral antidiabetic agents, ACE inhibitors, disopyramide, fibrates, fluoxetine, monoamine oxidase inhibitors, propoxyphene, salicylates, octreotide, and sulfonamide antibiotics may increase the blood glucose-lowering effects of insulin aspart. Corticosteroids, niacin, danazol, diuretics, sympathomimetic agents, isoniazid, phenothiazine derivatives, somatropin, thyroid hormones, estrogens, and progestins may decrease the blood glucose-lowering effects of insulin aspart. Beta-blockers, clonidine, lithium salts, and alcohol may either increase or decrease the blood glucose-lowering effects of insulin aspart. Pentamidine has the potential for causing both hyperglycemia and hypoglycemia. Beta-blockers, clonidine, guanethidine, and reserpine may mask the signs of hypoglycemia. Pregnancy Category C. There are no well-controlled clinical studies on the use of insulin aspart during pregnancy. Excretion in human breast milk is unknown. Safety and efficacy in children have not been studied. The most common adverse effect observed in patients on insulin therapy is hypoglycemia. Other side effects include lipodystrophy, injection site pain, pruritis, rash, and allergic reactions.

Administration: SQ injection.

Patient Care Implications: For subcutaneous administration. Injection should immediately be followed by a meal. Insulin aspart may be mixed with NPH human insulin. When insulin aspart is mixed with NPH human insulin, the insulin aspart should be drawn up first, and the mixture should be used immediately. Insulin aspart should not be mixed with crystalline zinc insulins. Monitor patient for signs and symptoms of hypoglycemia. Rotate injection sites. Instruct patient on the proper injection technique. Insulin aspart should be stored in the refrigerator—do not freeze. Do not use insulin aspart if it has been frozen. Cartridges or vials may be kept at ambient temperature away from excessive heat or sunlight for up to 28 days. Patients should be educated on the importance of self-monitoring of blood glucose levels.

Preparations: Injection, 100 units/ml, 10 ml vials. Cartridges, 3 ml PenFill® cartridges for use with NovoPen® 3 Insulin delivery devices and Norofine® disposable needles.

INSULIN GLARGINE—Lantus®

Description/Actions: Indicated in the treatment of adult and pediatric patients with type I diabetes mellitus or adults with type II diabetes mellitus who require basal (long-acting) insulin therapy.

Precautions/Adverse Reactions: Insulin glargine is contraindicated in patients with a known hypersensitivity to insulin glargine or to any component of the product. Prolonged hypoglycemia and recovery from hypoglycemia may occur with insulin glargine. Glucose monitoring is recommended for all patients. Any changes in insulin dosage should be made cautiously and under medical supervision. Insulin glargine is not intended for intravenous administration. Lantus® must not be diluted or mixed with any other insulin or solution, as this may alter the pH and therefore the onset or duration of the insulin glargine. Lantus® requirements may be decreased in patients with renal or hepatic impairment. Lipodystrophy may occur at the injection site. Injection sites should be rotated. Insulin requirements may be altered during periods of illness, stress, or emotional disturbances. Do not use in the treatment of diabetic ketoacidosis. Oral antidiabetic agents, ACE inhibitors, disopyramide, fibrates, fluoxetine, monoamine oxidase inhibitors, propoxyphene, salicylates, octreotide, and sulfonamide antibiotics may increase the blood glucose-lowering effects of insulin glargine. Corticosteroids, niacin, danazol, diuretics, sympathomimetic agents, isoniazid, phenothiazine derivatives, somatropin, thyroid hormones, estrogens, and progestins may decrease the blood glucose-lowering effects of insulin glargine. Beta-blockers, clonidine, lithium salts, and alcohol may either increase or decrease the blood glucose-lowering effects of insulin glargine. Pentamidine has the potential for causing both hyperglycemia and hypoglycemia. Beta-blockers, clonidine, guanethidine, and reserpine may mask the signs of hypoglycemia. Pregnancy Category C. There are no well-controlled clinical studies in pregnant women. Excretion in human breast milk is unknown. Studies have shown Lantus® to be safe and effective in children 6–15 years of age with type I diabetes mellitus. The most common adverse effect observed in patients on insulin therapy is hypoglycemia. Other adverse effects include injection site pain, lipodystrophy, pruritis and rash.

Administration: SQ injection.

Patient Care Implications: Do not mix or dilute with any other insulin or solution. Monitor patients for signs and symptoms of hypoglycemia. Store unopened vials in the refrigerator. Opened 10 ml vials may be kept at room temperature for up to 28 days away from excessive heat and direct sunlight. Opened 5 ml vials may be kept at room temperature for up to 14 days away from excessive heat and direct sunlight. Use only if the solution is clear and colorless with no particles visible.

Rotate injection sites. Instruct patients on the proper injection technique. Educate patients on the importance of self-monitoring blood glucose levels.

Preparations: Injection, 100 units/ml, 10 ml vials.

INSULIN INJECTION—Regular Iletin I and II®, Humalog®, Humulin R®, Novolin R®, Velosulin®

ISOPHANE INSULIN SUSPENSION (NPH)—NPH Iletin I and II®, Insulatard NPH®, Humulin N®, Novolin N®

INSULIN ZINC SUSPENSION (LENTE)—Lente Iletin I and II®, Humulin L®, Novolin L®

INSULIN ZINC SUSPENSION, EXTENDED (Ultralente)PROTAMINE ZINC INSULIN SUSPENSION (PZI)

Description/Actions: Is the principal hormone required for proper glucose use in normal metabolic processes. Hypoglycemic agent indicated in the treatment of diabetes mellitus that cannot be properly controlled by diet alone. Also used in severe ketoacidosis or diabetic coma.

Precautions/Adverse Reactions: Hypoglycemia may result from excessive dosage. Adverse reactions include allergic responses and lipodystrophy. Corticosteroids and thiazide and other diuretics may increase blood glucose levels and necessitate an increase in insulin dosage.

Administration: Subcutaneous.

Preparations: Preparations are classified as rapid-acting (Regular, Semilente), intermediate-acting (NPH, Lente), and long-acting (PZI, Ultralente), based on the promptness, duration, and intensity of action following subcutaneous administration. Some preparations contain human insulin prepared using recombinant DNA technology (Humulin) or semisynthetically (Novolin, Insulatard, Velosulin); other preparations are derived from beef and pork sources. Vials, 100 units/ml. A concentrated solution of regular insulin containing 500 units per ml is available for the treatment of patients with insulin resistance.

INSULIN ZINC SUSPENSION, PROMPT (Semilente)

INTAL®, see Cromolyn

INTEGRILIN®, see Eptifibatide

INTERFERON ALFACON-1—Intergen®

Description/Actions: Indicated in treatment of chronic hepatitis C virus (HCV) infection in patients with compensated liver disease who have anti-HCV serum antibodies and/or presence of HCV-RNA.

Precautions/Adverse Reactions: Contraindicated in hypersensitivity to *E. coli*-derived products. Use only under the supervision of qualified MDs. Do not interchange brands. Exclude other causes of hepatitis (e.g., hepatitis B, autoimmune hepatitis). Use cautiously in cardiac disease, endocrine disorders, autoimmune disorders, leukopenia (esp. granulocytopenia), thrombocytopenia, and other myelosuppressive conditions. Withhold treatment if absolute neutrophil count <500 × 106/L or if platelet count is <50 × 109/L. Not recommended for use in severe psychiatric disorders or decompensated liver disease. Discontinue if either occurs. Not for use in pregnancy (Category C) or nursing mothers. Do pretreatment eye exams in diabetics and hypertensives. Refer to ophthalmologist if visual disturbances occur. Monitor lab values (blood counts, TSH, and T4 creatinine, albumin, triglycerides, bilirubin) before, 2 weeks after starting, and periodically thereafter. Adverse reactions include flu-like symptoms, pain, edema, psychiatric/CNS effects (e.g., depression, insomnia, dizziness), local reactions, GI upset, cardiac or upper respiratory effects, rash, alopecia, pruritis, and visual or lab abnormalities. Instruct patients in effective contraception (both males and females).

Administration: SQ injection.

Preparations: 9 and 15 mcg vials for SC injection, preservative free.

INTERFERON ALFA-2a RECOMBINANT—Roferon-A®

INTERFERON ALFA-2b RECOMBINANT—Intron A®

Description/Actions: Prepared using recombinant DNA technology. Indicated for the treatment of hairy-cell leukemia in patients 18 years of age or older and in the treatment of AIDS-related Kaposi's sarcoma in patients 18 years of age or older. Interferon alfa-2b is also indicated for the treatment of chronic hepatitis non-A, non-B/C, chronic hepatitis B, and for the intralesional treatment of condylomata acuminata (venereal or genital warts). Interferon alfa-2a is indicated in the treatment of chronic hepatitis C in patients with compensated liver disease.

Precautions/Adverse Reactions: Most patients experience flu-like symptoms (e.g., fever, headache, myalgia, chills) at the beginning of therapy; these effects can often be effectively managed with an analgesic-antipyretic such as acetaminophen. Fatigue, dizziness, and other CNS effects may occur, and patients should be cautioned about the risks of engaging in activities in which full mental and physical alertness and coordination are required.

Administration: Intramuscular and subcutaneous for hairy-cell leukemia, AIDS-related Kaposi's sarcoma, and chronic hepatitis non-A, non-B/C. Intralesional for condylomata acuminata.

Preparations: Interferon alfa-2a: Vials 3, 9, 18, and 36 million IU, and a powder formulation in vials containing 18 million IU. Interferon alfa-2b: Vials containing 3, 5, 10, 18, 25, and 50 million IU of lyophilized powder.

INTERFERON ALFA-N3 (HUMAN LEUKOCYTE DERIVED)— Alferon N®

Description/Actions: Is manufactured from pooled units of human leukocytes and is designated as a natural interferon. Antiviral agent indicated for the intralesional treatment of refractory or recurring external condylomata acuminata (genital warts) in patients 18 years of age or older.

Precautions/Adverse Reactions: Adverse reactions include flu-like symptoms (e.g., fever, headache, myalgia, chills, back pain, and insomnia).

Administration: Intralesional. The drug should be injected into the base of each wart.

Preparations: Vials, 5 million IU.

INTERFERON BETA-1A—Avonex®

Description/Actions: For the treatment of relapsing forms of multiple sclerosis to slow the accumulation of physical disability and decrease the frequency of clinical exacerbations. Interferon Beta-1A is also approved for the treatment of patients with a first multiple sclerosis (MS) attack if magnetic resonance imaging (MRI) of the brain shows abnormalities characteristic of MS.

Preparations: Powder for injection, 33 mg (6.6 million units).

INTERFERON BETA-1B—Betaseron®

Description/Actions: Produced by recombinant DNA technology and exhibits antiviral and immunoregulatory activities. Indicated for use in ambulatory patients with relapsing-remitting multiple sclerosis to reduce the frequency of clinical exacerbations and slow the accumulation of physical disability.

Precautions/Adverse Reactions: Adverse reactions include injection site reactions, flu-like symptoms, menstrual disorders, reduction in neutrophil and white blood cell counts, and elevation in SGPT levels. Use has been associated with depression and suicide attempts, and patients should be advised to immediately report symptoms of depression. Has been reported in animal studies to have abortifacient activity.

Administration: Subcutaneous, administered every other day. Sites for self-injection include arms, abdomen, hips, and thighs.

Preparations: Room temperature formulation—injectible. Vials, 0.3 mg Betaseron (9.6 million IU), plus a separate vial containing diluent.

INTERFERON GAMMA-1B—Actimmune®

Description/Actions: Prepared by recombinant DNA technology. Exhibits immunomodulatory properties and a phagocyte-activating effect, which mediates the killing of microorganisms. Indicated for reducing the frequency and severity of serious infections associated with chronic granulomatous disease.

Precautions/Adverse Reactions: Adverse reactions include flu-like symptoms (e.g., fever, headache, chills, myalgia, fatigue), which may decrease in severity as treatment continues. Some symptoms may be minimized by bedtime administration. Acetaminophen may be useful in alleviating fever and headache. May cause CNS effects (e.g., dizziness, decreased mental status) and caution should be exercised in patients with known seizure disorders and/or compromised CNS function. May cause hematologic effects (e.g., neutropenia) and caution should be exercised when used in patients with myelosuppression or when used in combination with other potentially myelosuppressive agents.

Administration: Subcutaneous. Optimum sites of injection are the right deltoid and anterior thigh. Vials should not be shaken.

Preparations: Vials, 100 mcg (3 million units).

INTERGEN, see Interferon Alfacon-1

INTERLEUKIN-2, see Aldesleukin

INTRON A®, see Interferon Alfa-2b Recombinant

INTROPIN®, see Dopamine

INVERSINE®, see Mecamylamine

INVERT SUGAR—Travert®

Description/Actions: Mixture of dextrose and fructose used intravenously for fluid and caloric replacement.

Preparations: Solution, 10%.

INVIRASE®, see Saquinavir

IODINATED GLYCEROL

Description/Actions: Mucolytic/expectorant indicated as adjunctive treatment in respiratory conditions such as bronchitis and asthma.

Preparations: Tablets, 30 mg. Elixir, 1.2%. Solution, 5%.

IODINE

Description/Actions: Antiseptic applied topically to prevent or treat dermatologic infections. Also used to disinfect the skin preoperatively. Has also been used (often as sodium iodide or potassium iodide) orally and parenterally in the management of certain thyroid conditions.

Preparations: Solution (with sodium or potassium iodide), 2% and 5% (Lugol's solution). Tincture (with sodium or potassium iodide), 2% and 5%.

IODOCHLORHYDROXYQUIN—former name of Clioquinol

IODOQUINOL—Diiodohydroxyquin, Yodoxin®

Description/Actions: Amebicide indicated in the treatment of intestinal amebiasis.

Preparations: Tablets, 210 and 650 mg.

IOPIDINE®, see Apraclonidine

IPECAC

Description/Actions: Emetic used in the management of drug overdose and in certain other poisonings.

Preparations: Syrup.

IPRATROPIUM BROMIDE—Atrovent®

Description/Actions: Is an anticholinergic agent administered by inhalation for the maintenance treatment of bronchospasm associated with chronic obstructive pulmonary disease, including chronic bronchitis and emphysema. Nasal spray is used for rhinorrhea associated with allergic and nonallergic perennial rhinitis and rhinorrhea associated with the common cold.

Precautions/Adverse Reactions: Adverse reactions include cough, exacerbation of symptoms, nervousness, dizziness, headache, nausea, gastrointestinal distress, and palpitations. Nasal spray may cause epistaxis, pharyngitis, nasal dryness, or irritation. Systemic anticholinergic effects are uncommon, but caution should be exercised in patients with narrow-angle glaucoma, prostatic hypertrophy, or bladder-neck obstruction. Teach patients to avoid use during acute bronchospasm. Patients should be warned against spraying the aerosol into their eyes, because temporary blurring of vision may result.

Administration: Oral inhalation, nasal spray.

Preparations: Metered-dose inhaler. Inhalation solution, 0.02%. Nasal spray, 0.03% aqueous solution.

IRBESARTAN—Avapro®

Description/Actions: Angiotensin II receptor antagonist indicated in the treatment of hypertension and for use in patients with type 2 diabetes for the treatment of nephropathy with an elevated serum creatinine and proteinuria (>300 mg/day) in patients with type 2 diabetes and hypertension.

Precautions/Adverse Reactions: Correct salt/volume depletion (e.g., patients vigorously treated with diuretics or those on dialysis) before beginning therapy, or use a low initial dose. Use cautiously in renal impairment, severe CHF, renal artery stenosis. Pregnancy Category C in first trimester. Pregnancy Category D in second and third trimesters. Adverse reactions include diarrhea, dyspepsia, and fatigue.

Administration: Oral.

Preparations: Tablets, 75, 150, and 300 mg.

IRON DEXTRAN—InFeD®

Description/Actions: Iron formulation indicated for the parenteral treatment of iron deficiency anemia.

Preparations: Ampules and vials, 50 mg iron/ml.

ISMELIN®, see Guanethidine

ISMO®, see Isosorbide Mononitrate

ISOETHARINE—Bronkometer®, Bronkosol®

Description/Actions: Bronchodilator administered by inhalation and indicated for bronchial asthma and for reversible bronchospasm that may occur in association with bronchitis and emphysema.

Preparations: Solution for nebulization (as the hydrochloride), numerous concentrations ranging from 0.062% to 1%. Metered dose inhaler (as the mesylate), 340 µg/metered dose.

ISOFLUROPHATE—Floropryl®

Description/Actions: Cholinesterase inhibitor indicated for ophthalmic use in the treatment of open-angle glaucoma, conditions obstructing aqueous outflow, following iridectomy, and accommodative esotropia.

Preparations: Ophthalmic ointment, 0.025%

ISOMETHEPTENE MUCATE

Description/Actions: Sympathomimetic agent used in combination with other agents in the treatment of tension and vascular headaches.

ISONIAZID—INH, Nydrazid®

Description/Actions: Antitubercular agent used in the treatment of tuberculosis and as preventive therapy in selected patients who are at risk of tubercular infection.

Preparations: Tablets, 50, 100, and 300 mg. Syrup, 50 mg/ml. Vials, 100 mg/ml.

ISOPROPYL ALCOHOL

Description/Actions: Antiseptic that is applied to the skin as isopropyl rubbing alcohol and in other formulations.

Preparations: Solutions, 70%, 91%, and 100%.

ISOPROTERENOL HYDROCHLORIDE—Isuprel®

Description/Actions: Bronchodilator indicated for the treatment of bronchospasm associated with bronchial asthma, pulmonary emphysema, bronchitis, and bronchiectasis. Also used as an adjunct in the management of shock and in the treatment of cardiac standstill or arrest, in the management of certain ventricular arrhythmias and other serious cardiac complications. May also be used in the management of bronchospasm during anesthesia.

Preparations: Solution for nebulization, 0.25% (1:400), 0.5% (1:200), and 1% (1:100). Aerosol solution and metered-dose inhalers. Sublingual tablets, 10 and 15 mg. Ampules, vials, and syringes, 0.2 mg/ml. (1:5000).

ISOPTIN®, see Verapamil

ISOPTIN SR®, see Verapamil

ISOPTO-CARBACHOL®, see Carbachol

ISORDIL®, see Isosorbide Dinitrate

ISOSORBIDE DINITRATE—Isordil®, Sorbitrate®

Description/Actions: An organic nitrate indicated for the treatment and prevention of angina pectoris.

Precautions/Adverse Reactions: Adverse reactions include headache, dizziness, hypotension, and cutaneous vasodilation with flushing.

Administration: Oral and sublingual.

Preparations: Sublingual tablets, 2.5, 5, and 10 mg. Tablets, 2.5, 5, 10, 20, 30, and 40 mg. Controlled-release tablets, 40 mg. Chewable tablets, 5 and 10 mg.

ISOSORBIDE MONONITRATE—Imdur®, Ismo®, Monoket®

Description/Actions: An organic nitrate that has a primary action of relaxation of vascular smooth muscle. Is the major active metabolite of isosorbide dinitrate. Indicated for the prevention of angina pectoris due to coronary artery disease.

Precautions/Adverse Reactions: Adverse reactions include headache, dizziness, and nausea/vomiting. May cause hypotension and should be used with caution in patients who are volume depleted or who are already hypotensive. Symptomatic hypotension may occur when used concurrently with a calcium channel-blocking agent and dosage adjustments may be necessary.

Administration: Oral.

Preparations: Tablets, 10 and 20 mg. Controlled-release tablets (Imdur®), 30, 60, and 120 mg.

ISOTRETINOIN—Accutane®

Description/Actions: Retinoid (vitamin A analog) indicated for the treatment of severe recalcitrant cystic acne. Isotretinoin should be reserved for patients with severe nodular acne who are unresponsive to conventional therapy, including systemic antibiotics. Only indicated for those female patients who are not pregnant because isotretinoin can cause severe birth defects. The Accutane® Pregnancy Prevention and Risk Management Programs, consisting of the System to Manage Accutane® Related Teratogenicity (S.M.A.R.T.) and the Accutane® Pregnancy Prevention Program (PPP) should be followed for prescribing Accutane® with the goal of preventing fetal exposure to isotretinoin.

Precautions/Adverse Reactions: May cause fetal abnormalities and must not be taken during pregnancy. Pregnancy Category X. Exercise caution when prescribing to patients with a genetic predisposition for age-related osteoporosis, a history of childhood osteoporosis, osteomalacia, or other disorders of bone metabolism, including patients diagnosed with anorexia nervosa and those on chronic drug therapy that causes drug-induced osteoporosis/osteomalacia and/or affects vitamin D metabolism such as systemic corticosteroids and any anticonvulsant. Accutane® may cause depression, psychosis, and rarely suicidal ideation, suicide attempts, suicide, and aggressive and or violent behaviors. Discontinuation of Accutane® may be insufficient; further evaluation may be necessary.

Preparations: Capsules, 10, 20, and 40 mg.

ISOVEX®, see Ethaverine

ISOXSUPRINE HYDROCHLORIDE—Vasodilan®

Description/Actions: Peripheral vasodilator used for relief of symptoms associated with cerebral vascular insufficiency, in peripheral vascular disease of arteriosclerosis obliterans, thromboangiitis obliterans, and Raynaud's disease. Has been utilized investigationally in threatened premature labor.

Preparations: Tablets, 10 and 20 mg.

ISRADIPINE—DynaCirc®

Description/Actions: A calcium channel-blocking agent that is indicated in the management of hypertension. May be used alone or concurrently with a thiazide-type diuretic.

Precautions/Adverse Reactions: Adverse reactions include dizziness, edema, palpitations, flushing, tachycardia, fatigue, and headache. Caution should be exercised when the drug is used in patients with congestive heart failure. Concurrent use with a beta-adrenergic blocking agent may be employed advantageously in some patients but may be associated with risks such as an excessive reduction in blood pressure.

Administration: Oral.

Preparations: Capsules, 2.5 and 5 mg. Controlled-release tablets, 5 and 10 mg.

ISUPREL®, see Isoproterenol

ITRACONAZOLE—Sporanox®

Description/Actions: Antifungal agent that inhibits the cytochrome P-450-dependent synthesis of ergosterol, which is a vital component of fungal cell membranes. Indicated for the treatment of blastomycosis (pulmonary and extrapulmonary) and histoplasmosis, including chronic cavitary pulmonary disease and disseminated, nonmeningeal histoplasmosis. Is indicated for these infections in both immunocompromised and non-immunocompromised patients. Also indicated for the treatment of pulmonary aspergillosis in patients who are intolerant of or who are refractory to amphotericin B therapy. Indicated for the onchomycosis of the toenail with or without fingernail involvement and in onchomycosis of the fingernail.

Precautions/Adverse Reactions: Caution must be exercised in patients who are hypersensitive to other azole antifungal agents. Concurrent use with terfenadine astemizole or cisapride is contraindicated. Adverse reactions include nausea, vomiting, diarrhea, edema, fatigue, fever, rash, headache, and hypertension. Abnormal hepatic function, including rare reports of reversible idiosyncratic hepatitis, has been experienced, and patients should be advised to report any signs or symptoms that may suggest liver dysfunction. Rare cases of serious hepatotoxicity, including liver failure and death, have been reported with itraconazole; some of the events developed within the first week of treatment. Treatment should be stopped immediately and liver function testing should be conducted in patients who develop signs and symptoms suggestive of liver disease, such as unusual fatigue, anorexia, nausea, vomiting, jaundice, dark urine, or palor stools.

Administration: Oral. Should be administered with food.

Preparations: Capsules, 100 mg. Oral solution, 10 mg/ml. Injection kit, 10 mg/ml–25 ml ampule with one 50 ml bag of 0.9% sodium chloride and filtered infusion set.

K

KADIAN®, see Morphine Sulfate

KALETRA™, see Lopinavir and Ritonavir

KANAMYCIN SULFATE—Kantrex®

Description/Actions: Aminoglycoside antibiotic primarily used in the parenteral treatment of infections caused by gram-negative bacteria. Has been used orally for the suppression of intestinal bacteria in the management of hepatic coma and in combination with other drugs to treat tuberculosis in patients resistant to conventional therapy.

Administration: IV, IM, intraperitoneal, inhalation, and irrigation.

Preparations: Vials and syringes, 75 and 500 mg and 1 g. Capsules, 500 mg.

KANTREX®, see Kanamycin

KAOLIN

Description/Actions: Adsorbent used in combination with other agents in the management of diarrhea.

KAON®, see Potassium Gluconate

KAY CIEL®, see Potassium Chloride

KAYEXALATE®, see Sodium Polystyrene Sulfonate

KEFLEX®, see Cephalexin

KEFLIN®, see Cephalothin

KEFTAB®, see Cephalexin Hydrochloride

KEFUROX®, see Cefuroxime Sodium

KEFZOL®, see Cefazolin

KEMADRIN®, see Procyclidine

KENACORT®, see Triamcinolone

KENALOG®, see Triamcinolone

KEPPRA®, see Levetiracetam

KERLONE®, see Betaxolol

KETALAR®, see Ketamine

KETAMINE HYDROCHLORIDE—Ketalar®

Description/Actions: General anesthetic administered parenterally as the sole anesthetic in certain procedures, for the induction of anesthesia prior to the administration of other general anesthetic agents, and to supplement low-potency agents such as nitrous oxide.

Preparations: Vials, 10 mg/ml, 50 mg/ml, and 100 mg/ml.

KETOCONAZOLE—Nizoral®

Description/Actions: Antifungal agent indicated for oral use in the treatment of systemic fungal infections and for the treatment of severe recalcitrant cutaneous dermatophytic infections that have not responded to topical therapy or oral griseofulvin, or in patients who are unable to take griseofulvin. Also used topically in the treatment of tinea corporis, tinea cruris, and tinea versicolor, cutaneous candidiasis, and seborrheic dermatitis. Used as a shampoo in the reduction of scaling due to dandruff.

Precautions/Adverse Reactions: Should not be used concurrently with terfenadine, astemizole, or cisapride.

Administration: Oral and topical.

Preparations: Tablets, 200 mg. Cream, 2%. Shampoo, 2%.

KETOPROFEN—Actron®, Orudis®, Oruvail®

Description/Actions: Nonsteroidal anti-inflammatory agent that inhibits prostaglandin synthesis and is indicated for the treatment of rheumatoid arthritis and osteoarthritis, mild to moderate pain, and dysmenorrhea.

Precautions/Adverse Reactions: Should not be given to patients in whom aspirin or another NSAID causes asthma, rhinitis, urticaria, or other allergic-type reactions. May cause GI effects, so use should be avoided in patients with active GI tract disease and closely supervised in patients with a previous history of such disorders. Other adverse reactions include headache, malaise, nervousness, and edema.

Administration: Oral.

Preparations: Tablets, 12.5 mg. Capsules, 25, 50, and 75 mg. Controlled-release capsules (Oruvail), 200 mg.

KETOROLAC TROMETHAMINE—Acular®, Acular LS®, Acular PF®, Toradol®

Description/Actions: A nonsteroidal anti-inflammatory drug (NSAID) that inhibits prostaglandin synthesis. Indicated for intramuscular or intravenous use for the short-term (up to 5 days) management of moderately severe, acute pain, usually in a postoperative setting. Therapy should be initiated by the IM or IV route and is to be used orally only as a continuation treatment. Treatment by any route (or combination of routes) of administration should not exceed 5 days. Indicated for ophthalmic use for the relief of itching due to seasonal allergic conjunctivitis and post-op inflammation after cataract extraction.

Precautions/Adverse Reactions: Should not be given to patients in whom aspirin or another NSAID causes asthma, rhinitis, urticaria, or other allergic-type reactions. Use is contraindicated in patients at risk of GI bleeding or other bleeding reactions, and in patients with advanced renal impairment. Adverse reactions include nausea, dyspepsia, gastrointestinal pain, and drowsiness.

Administration: Oral, intravenous, intramuscular, and ophthalmic.

Preparations: Tablets, 10 mg. Single-dose syringes, 15, 30, and 60 mg. Ophthalmic solution, 0.4% and 0.5% and as preservative free.

KETOTIFEN—Zaditor®

Description/Actions: Ketotifen is used to provide temporary relief of itching due to allergic conjunctivitis.

Precautions/Adverse Reactions: Ketotifen should be administered to contact lens wearers 10 minutes before they insert their lenses. The safety of the drug has not been established in pregnant women, breast-feeding women, and children under the age of 3. Ketotifen is usually well tolerated. Some side effects are conjuctival hyperemia, headache, rhinitis, conjunctivitis, eyelid swelling, flu syndrome, keratitis, lacrimation disorder, mydriasis, ocular pain, photophobia, and xerophthalmia.

Administration: Ophthalmic.

Patient Care Implications: Ketotifen should be used 10 minutes before patient inserts contact lens. Drug safety not established in pregnant women, breast-feeding women, and children under age 3. Do not share drops between patients, and wash hands before and after use.

Preparations: Eye drops, 5 ml bottle.

KINERET™, see Anakinra

KLARON®, see Sulfacetamide Sodium

KLONOPIN®, see Clonazepam

K-LOR®, see Potassium Chloride

KLORVESS®, see Potassium Chloride

KLOTRIX®, see Potassium Chloride

KONAKION®, see Phytonadione

K-TAB®, see Potassium Chloride

KWELL®, see Lindane

KYTRIL®, see Granisetron Hydrochloride

L

L-CARNITINE—Carnitor®, Vitacarn®

Description/Actions: Indicated in the treatment of primary systemic carnitine deficiency.

Precautions/Adverse Reactions: Adverse reactions include nausea, vomiting, abdominal cramps, diarrhea, and patient body odor. Reducing the dosage often decreases or eliminates the GI effects or drug-related odor.

Administration: Oral.

Preparations: Tablets, 330 mg. Enteral liquid, 100 mg/ml.

LABETALOL HYDROCHLORIDE—Normodyne®, Trandate®

Description/Actions: Exhibits nonselective beta-adrenergic and selective alpha 1-adrenergic-blocking actions. Indicated in the management of hypertension, and when administered intravenously, is also indicated for the treatment of severe hypertension.

Precautions/Adverse Reactions: Contraindicated in patients with bronchial asthma, overt cardiac failure, greater than first-degree heart block, cardiogenic shock, or severe bradycardia. Adverse reactions include fatigue, dizziness, nausea, and nasal stuffiness. Use is best avoided in patients with bronchospastic diseases, and therapy in diabetic patients must be closely monitored.

Administration: Oral and intravenous. Patients should be cautioned about the interruption or discontinuation of therapy; exacerbation of angina pectoris may occur following the abrupt cessation of therapy, and, when therapy is to be discontinued, the dosage should be gradually reduced over a period of 1–2 weeks.

Preparations: Tablets, 100, 200, and 300 mg. Ampules and vials, 5 mg/ml.

LAC-HYDRIN®, see Ammonium Lactate

LACTATED RINGER'S INJECTION

Description/Actions: Intravenous electrolyte replenishment solution containing sodium, potassium, calcium, chloride, and lactate.

Preparations: Solutions, 250, 500, and 1000 ml.

LACTULOSE—Cephulac®, Chronulac®

Description/Actions: Disaccharide used orally in the treatment of constipation, and orally or rectally in the prevention and treatment of portal-systemic encephalopathy, including the states of hepatic pre-coma and coma.

Preparations: Syrup, 10 g/15 ml.

LAMICTAL®, see Lamotrigine

LAMISIL®, see Terbinafine Hydrochloride

LAMIVUDINE—Epivir®, Epivir HBV®, 3TC

Description/Actions: Antiretroviral indicated in the management of HIV infection (AIDS) in combination with zidovudine. Epivir HBV® is indicated for the treatment of chronic hepatitis B associated with evidence of hepatitis B viral replication and active liver inflammation.

Precautions/Adverse Reactions: Use cautiously in patients with renal dysfunction and children with a history of, or other risk factors for, pancreatitis. Adverse reactions in adults include headache, malaise, fever, GI upset, neuropathy, dizziness, sleep or depressive disorders, rash, respiratory effects, and musculoskeletal pain. Adverse reactions in children include pancreatitis, paresthesias, and peripheral neuropathy.

Administration: Oral without regard to food.

Preparations: Tablets, 100 mg and 150 mg. Oral solution, 10 mg/ml.

LAMOTRIGINE—Lamictal®

Description/Actions: Antiepileptic drug indicated as an adjunctive therapy in the treatment of partial seizures in patients with epilepsy, as adjunct in Lennox-Gastaut Syndrome in adults, and for the treatment of inadequately controlled partial seizures in children 2 years of age or older. It is also indicated for conversion to monotherapy in adults with partial seizures who are receiving treatment with a single enzyme-inducing antiepileptic drug (EIAED) or valproate. Lamotrigine is also indicated for the maintenance treatment of Bipolar I Disorder to delay the time to occurrence of mood episodes (depression, mania, hypomania, mixed episodes) in patients treated for acute mood episodes with standard therapy. The effectiveness of Lamictal® in the acute treatment of mood episodes has not been established.

Precautions/Adverse Reactions: Use cautiously in patients with reduced renal function, impaired cardiac or hepatic function. Adverse reactions include ataxia, dizziness, headache, somnolence, nausea, vomiting, rash, and photosensitivity.

Administration: Oral without regard to meals. Abrupt discontinuation may result in an increase in seizure activity, so gradual withdrawal over 2 weeks is recommended unless safety concerns require more rapid withdrawal.

Preparations: Tablets, 25, 100, 150, and 200 mg. Chewable/dispersible tablets, 5 and 25 mg.

LAMPRENE®, see Clofazimine

LANOLIN—Wool Fat

Description/Actions: Ointment base used topically in the management of certain dermatological conditions associated with dry skin and as a vehicle into which other medications are incorporated.

LANOXICAPS®, see Digoxin

LANOXIN®, see Digoxin

LANSOPRAZOLE—Prevacid®, Prevacid® I.V., Prevacid® Solutab

Description/Actions: Indicated for short-term treatment (up to 4 weeks) of active duodenal ulcer, short-term treatment (up to 8 weeks) of erosive esophagitis, and long-term treatment of pathological hypersecretory states (e.g., Zollinger-Ellison syndrome). In combination with clarithromycin and/or amoxicillin for *H. pylori* eradication in duodenal ulcer disease, to reduce the risk of duodenal ulcer recurrence. Also indicated for the short-term treatment of symptomatic gastroesophageal reflux disease (GERD) and for the short-term treatment of erosive esophagitis in pediatric patients 1–17 years of age. Lansoprazole is also indicated for the maintenance of healed duodenal ulcers, short-term treatment of active benign gastric ulcer, short-term treatment of GERD, and for the treatment of NSAID-associated gastric ulcer in patients who continue to use NSAIDs. It is indicated for reducing the risk of NSAID-associated gastric ulcers in patients with a history of documented gastric ulcer who require the use of an NSAID.

Precautions/Adverse Reactions: Adverse reactions include diarrhea, abdominal pain, and nausea. Because it is a potent acid inhibitor, drugs that require an acidic environment may not be as well absorbed.

Administration: Oral and intravenous. May open capsules and mix intact granule with 40 ml of apple juice and inject via nasogastric tube.

Preparations: Delayed-release capsules, 15 and 30 mg. Delayed-release oral suspension packets, 15 and 30 mg. Delayed-release orally disintegrating tablets, 15 and 30 mg. Solution for injection, 30 mg vials.

LARGON®, see Propiomazine

LARIAM®, see Mefloquine

LARODOPA®, see Levodopa

LASIX®, see Furosemide

LATANOPROST—Xalatan®

Description/Actions: Latanoprost is indicated for the initial treatment of elevated intraocular pressure associated with open-angle glaucoma or ocular hypertension and for the reduction of elevated intraocular pressure in patients with open-angle glaucoma and ocular hypertension who are intolerant of other intraocular pressure-lowering medications or are insufficiently responsive to other intraocular pressure-lowering medications.

Precautions/Adverse Reactions: Use cautiously in renal or hepatic impairment. Adverse reactions include blurred vision, burning, stinging, increased pigmentation of the iris, punctate epithelial keratopathy, photophobia, upper respiratory tract infection, pain, angina, and rash. Latanoprost may gradually change eyelashes and vellus hair. These changes include increased length, thickness, pigmentation, and number of lashes or hairs and misdirected growth of eyelashes.

Administration: Ophthalmic. Remove contact lenses before use, and do not reinsert for 15 minutes afterwards. Allow at least 5 minutes between application of other topical ophthalmic agents.

Preparations: 0.005% ophthalmic solution containing benzalkonium chloride.

LEDERCILLIN VK®, see Penicillin V Potassium

LEFLUNOMIDE—Arava®

Description/Actions: Disease-modifying antirheumatic drug indicated to reduce the signs and symptoms of active rheumatoid arthritis (RA) and to retard structural damage as evidenced by X-ray erosions and joint space narrowing. Leflunomide has antiproliferative and anti-inflammatory activity.

Precautions/Adverse Reactions: Leflunomide is contraindicated in women of childbearing potential who are not using reliable contraception and in patients with significant hepatic impairment and hepatitis. Rare cases of severe liver injury, including cases with fatal outcome, have been reported during treatment with leflunomide. Most cases of severe liver injury occur within 6 months of therapy and in a setting of multiple risk factors for hepatotoxicity. Leflunomide is not recommended in patients with significant hepatic impairment or evidence of infection with hepatitis B or C viruses given the risk of increased hepatotoxicity. Leflunomide is not recommended in patients with severe immunodeficiency, bone marrow dysplasia, or severe uncontrolled infections. Rarely, severe infections including sepsis, which may be fatal, have been reported. Rare cases of pancytopenia, agranulocytosis, thrombocytopenia, Stevens-Johnson syndrome, and toxic epidermal necrolysis have been reported. Pregnancy Category X. Use in nursing mothers not recommended. Monitor liver function tests at the start of therapy to establish baseline values, and then monthly until stable, then do periodic testing. Obtain a negative pregnancy test before starting therapy. Use cautiously in patients with renal impairment, severe immunodeficiency, bone marrow dysplasia, and severe uncontrolled infections. Delay giving live vaccines. Adverse reactions include diarrhea, elevated liver enzymes, alopecia, rash, respiratory infections, hypertension, headaches, and GI upset. Leflunomide may cause immunosuppression.

Administration: Oral.

Patient Care Implications: Instruct patients that leflunomide can remain within the body for up to 2 years unless an elimination procedure is followed. Contraception must be practiced while on this medication. Both men and women who wish to engage in pregnancy should be warned that they should seek the advice of their prescriber and undergo an elimination procedure before attempting to become pregnant. Simply stopping the drug and then attempting to become pregnant may result in serious birth defects or fetal death. Aspirin, NSAIDs, and low-dose corticosteroids may be used concurrently.

Preparations: Tablets, 10, 20, and 100 mg.

LENTE INSULIN, see Insulin

LEPIRUDAN—Refludan®

Description/Actions: Indicated to treat heparin-induced thrombocytopenia and associated thromboembolic disease in order to prevent further thromboembolic complications.

Precautions/Adverse Reactions: Carefully assess risk in patients with increased risk of bleeding (e.g., recent puncture of large vessels or organ biopsy, anomaly of vessels or organs, recent cerebrovascular accident, stroke, intercerebral surgery or other neuraxial procedures, severe uncontrolled hypertension, bacterial endocarditis, advanced renal impairment, hemorrhagic diathesis, recent major surgery, recent major bleeding). Obtain baseline aPTT ratio and continue to monitor closely during therapy. Use cautiously in renal insufficiency, liver injury, and reexposure. Adverse reactions include hemorrhagic events, abnormal liver function, allergic skin reactions, infections, multiorgan failure, and ventricular fibrillation.

Administration: Intravenous.

Preparations: Vials, 50 mg.

LESCOL®, see Fluvastatin Sodium

LESCOL® XL, see Fluvastatin Sodium

LETROZOLE—Femara®

Description/Actions: Letrozole is a nonsteroid aromatase inhibitor indicated for first-line treatment of postmenopausal women with hormone receptor positive or hormone receptor unknown locally advanced or metastatic breast cancer and for the treatment of advanced breast cancer in postmenopausal women with disease progression following anti-estrogen therapy. It is also indicated for the extended adjuvant treatment of early breast cancer in postmenopausal women who have received five years of adjuvant tamoxifen therapy.

Administration: Oral.

Preparations: Tablets, 2.5 mg.

LEUCOVORIN CALCIUM—Citrovorum Factor,
    Folinic Acid, Wellcovorin®

Description/Actions: Folic acid analog indicated to prevent and treat the hematologic and other undesired effects of folic acid antagonists (e.g., methotrexate) and to counteract the effect of overdosage of these agents. Has also been used in the treatment of certain megaloblastic anemias. Is also indicated for parenteral use in combination with 5-fluorouracil to prolong survival in the palliative treatment of patients with advanced colorectal cancer.

Preparations: Tablets, 5, 10, 15, and 25 mg. Ampules, 3 mg/ml and 5 mg/ml. Vials, 50, 100, and 350 mg. Implant, 72 mg, 65 mg free base.

LEUKERAN®, see Chlorambucil

LEUKINE®, see Sargramostim

LEUPROLIDE ACETATE—Lupron®, Lupron Depot-3 month®,
    Lupron Depot-Ped®, Viadur™, Eligard®

Description/Actions: Gonadotropin-releasing hormone analog administered parenterally in the treatment of advanced prostatic cancer, endometriosis, and central precocious puberty. Also indicated for the treatment of uterine leimyomata in women who fail iron therapy. Leuprolide acetate solution is injected daily via the subcutaneous route. The depot formulation is injected via the intramuscular route once a month (Lupron Depot® 3.75 mg and 7.5 mg), once every 3 months (Lupon Depot®-3 month (11.25 and 22.5 mg) or once every 4 months (Lupron Depot®-4 month (30 mg). Viadur™ (implant formulation): One subcutaneous implant for 12 months. Must be removed after 12 months of hormonal therapy; another implant may be inserted to continue therapy.

Patient Care Implications: Patient should be counseled on the possibility of the development or worsening of depression and the occurrence of memory disorders during treatment.

Preparations: Powder for injection, 3.75 mg, 7.5 mg, 11.25 mg, and 15 mg., 22.5 mg and 30 mg. Solution for injection, 5 mg/ml. Implant, 72 mg, 65 mg free base. Suspension for injection, 45 mg.

LEUSTATIN®, see Cladribine

LEVALBUTEROL—Xopenex®, Xopenex HFA™

Description/Actions: Indicated in the prevention and treatment of bronchospasm in reversible obstructive airway disease.

Precautions/Adverse Reactions: Use cautiously in patients with cardiovascular disease (esp. coronary insufficiency, arrhythmias, hypertension), seizure disorders, diabetes, and hyperthyroidism. Pregnancy Category C. Use not recommended in nursing mothers. Adverse reactions include nervousness, tremor, infection, tachycardia, migraine, anxiety, dyspepsia, leg cramps, dizziness, cough, turbinate edema, hypokalemia, and paradoxical bronchospasm.

Administration: Inhaled via nebulizer.

Patient Care Implications: Instruct patients to seek medical attention if the drug becomes less effective, if they do not experience significant improvement within 60 minutes of treatment, if symptoms worsen, or if more drug is needed to control symptoms. Use appropriate nebulizer. Do not mix other drugs in the nebulizer with the levalbuterol. Teach patients not to exceed dosing limits and to contact the prescriber if they feel this is necessary.

Preparations: Preservative-free inhalation solution, 0.31 mg/3 ml, 0.63 mg/3 ml, and 1.25 mg/3 ml per vial. Metered dose inhaler, 15 g delivering 45 mcg/actuation.

LEVAMISOLE—Ergamisol®

Description/Actions: An immunomodulator that appears to restore depressed immune function. Indicated as adjunct treatment in combination with fluorouracil after surgical resection in patients with Dukes' stage C colon cancer.

Precautions/Adverse Reactions: May cause agranulocytosis. Use in combination with fluorouracil has been associated with neutropenia, anemia, and thrombocytopenia. Adverse reactions include nausea, vomiting, diarrhea, stomatitis, anorexia, rash and/or pruritus, flu-like symptoms, dizziness, ataxia, depression, and confusion. Disulfiram-like reactions may occur following the consumption of alcoholic beverages.

Administration: Oral.

Preparations: Tablets, 50 mg.

LEVAQUIN®, see Levofloxacin

LEVARTERENOL, see Norepinephrine

LEVATOL®, see Penbutolol

LEVBID®, see Hyoscyamine Sulfate

LEVETIRACETAM—Keppra®

Description/Actions: Levetiracetam is used as adjunctive therapy for the treatment of partial seizures.

Precautions/Adverse Reactions: Levetiracetam dosage should be adjusted in patients with renal impairment and the drug should not be stopped abruptly. The drug should also be given with caution to patients who are pregnant or breast-feeding and children under 16. Levetiracetam may affect patient's mental or motor performance, so caution should be used in operating machinery until patient knows how drug affects him or her. Some side effects are drowsiness, fatigue, difficulty breathing, ataxia, lack of coordination, agitation, anxiety, apathy, depression, hallucinations, and nervousness.

Administration: Oral.

Patient Care Implication: Levetiracetam dosage must be adjusted in patients with renal impairment, and creatinine and BUN must be monitored in all patients receiving the drug. Levetiracetam should be given cautiously to patients who are pregnant or breast-feeding and children under 16. Patients should avoid operating machinery after taking the medication.

Preparations: Oral solution, 100 mg/ml. Tablets, 250, 500, and 750 mg.

LEVOBETAXOLOL HCL OPHTHALMIC SUSPENSION 0.5%— Betaxon®

Description/Actions: Indicated for lowering intraocular pressure in patients with chronic open-angle glaucoma or ocular hypertension.

Precautions/Adverse Reactions: Levobetaxolol is contraindicated in patients with sinus bradycardia greater than a first-degree atrioventricular block, cardiogenic shock, patients with overt cardiac failure, or in patients with a hypersensitivity to levobetaxolol or to any component of the product. Some systemic absorption may occur with topically applied beta-adrenergic blocking agents. Severe respiratory and cardiac reactions including death due to bronchospasm can occur in patients with asthma. Use caution when using in patients with a history of cardiac failure or heart block. Discontinue therapy with levobetaxolol at the first sign of heart failure. Use cautiously in patients with diabetes mellitus, patients suspected of developing thyrotoxicosis, patients with myasthenic symptoms, and patients with restriction of pulmonary function. Gradually withdraw beta-adrenergic blocking agents prior to general anesthesia. Potential additive effect with concomitant administration of an orally active beta-adrenergic blocking agent. Additive hypotension and or bradycardia may occur in patients receiving concomitant therapy with catecholamine-depleting drugs such as reserpine. Use cautiously in patients using concomitant adrenergic psychotropic drugs. Pregnancy Category C. There are no adequate and well-controlled studies in pregnant women. Use during pregnancy only if the potential benefit justifies the potential risk to the fetus. Excretion in human breast milk is unknown. Safety and efficacy in pediatric patients have not been established. Most common adverse effects observed during therapy with levobetaxolol include transient ocular discomfort upon instillation (11%) and transient blurred vision (2%). Cataracts and vitreous disorders have been reported in less than 2% of patients.

Administration: Ophthalmic.

Patient Care Implications: Do not use with contact lenses in the eyes. Protect from light. Shake well before using.

Preparations: Ophthalmic suspension, 5 ml, 10 ml, and 15 ml Drop-Tainer® dispenser.

LEVOBUNOLOL HYDROCHLORIDE—Betagan®

Description/Actions: A noncardioselective beta-adrenergic blocking agent indicated for ophthalmic use in the treatment of chronic open-angle glaucoma and ocular hypertension.

Precautions/Adverse Reactions: Contraindicated in patients with bronchial asthma or severe chronic obstructive pulmonary disease, sinus bradycardia, second- and third-degree AV block, overt cardiac failure, or cardiogenic shock. Adverse reactions include transient ocular burning and stinging and systemic effects such as decrease in heart rate and blood pressure. Caution must be exercised in patients who are also taking another beta-blocker orally for another indication.

Administration: Ophthalmic.

Preparations: Ophthalmic solution, 0.25% and 0.5%.

LEVOCABASTINE HYDROCHLORIDE—Livostin®

Description/Actions: Antihistamine indicated for topical ophthalmic use for the temporary relief of the signs and symptoms of seasonal allergic conjunctivitis.

Precautions/Adverse Reactions: Adverse reactions include mild, transient stinging and burning, and headache. Contains benzalkonium chloride, so patients should be instructed not to wear soft contact lenses during treatment.

Administration: Ophthalmic.

Preparations: Ophthalmic suspension, 0.05%.

LEVOCARNITINE—Carnitor®

Description/Actions: Amino acid derivative used as replacement therapy in primary and secondary carnitine deficiency.

Precautions/Adverse Reactions: Adverse reactions include nausea, vomiting, abdominal cramps, diarrhea, and patient body odor. Reducing the dosage often decreases or eliminates the GI effects of drug-related odor.

Administration: Oral, intravenous.

Preparations: Tablets, 330 mg. Enteral liquid, 100 mg/ml. Injection, 200 mg/ml in 2.5 and 5 ml ampules.

LEVODOPA—Dopar®, Larodopa®

Description/Actions: Is converted to dopamine, which is the active pharmacologic agent. Indicated in the treatment of parkinsonism.

Precautions/Adverse Reactions: Should not be given concomitantly with a monoamine oxidase inhibitor or in patients with narrow-angle glaucoma. Should be administered cautiously in patients with severe cardiovascular or pulmonary disease, bronchial asthma, renal, hepatic, or endocrine disease. Adverse reactions include choreiform and/or dystonic movements, palpitations, orthostatic hypotension, mental changes, headache, dizziness, nausea, and vomiting. Effect may be reduced by pyridoxine, and preparations containing this vitamin should be avoided unless carbidopa is being given concomitantly with levodopa (i.e., in the combination product, Sinemet® and Sinemet CR®). Not useful for treatment of drug-induced extrapyramidal reactions.

Administration: Oral.

Preparations: Capsules and tablets, 100, 250, and 500 mg. Sinemet tablets, 10 mg/100 mg, 25 mg/100 mg, and 25 mg/250 mg carbidopa/levodopa. Sinemet CR (controlled-release) tablets, 50 mg/200 mg carbidopa/levodopa.

LEVO-DROMORAN®, see Levorphanol

LEVOFLOXACIN—Levaquin®, Quixin™

Description/Actions: Fluoroquinolone anti-infective agent indicated for the treatment of acute maxillary sinusitis, acute bacterial exacerbation of chronic bronchitis, nosocomial pneumonia, community acquired pneumonia (including multi-drug resistant strains [MDRSP]), complicated skin and skin structure infections, chronic bacterial prostatitis, complicated urinary tract infections, acute pyelonephritis, uncomplicated urinary tract infections, and inhalational anthrax.

Precautions/Adverse Reactions: Maintain adequate hydration. Use cautiously in patients with renal impairment, severe cerebral arteriosclerosis, epilepsy, and other seizure risks. Discontinue if rash, other signs of hypersensitivity, hypoglycemic reactions, phototoxicity, or tendon pain with inflammation or rupture occurs. Risk of tendon rupture may be increased in patients receiving concomitant corticosteroids, especially in the elderly. Has been associated with QT interval prolongation and torsades de pointes in patients with concurrent medical conditions or concomitant medications that may prolong the QT interval (e.g., class Ia or class III antiarrhythmic agents). Use of levofloxacin in the presence of risk factors for torsades de pointes, such as hypokalemia, significant bradycardia, and cardiomyopathy, should be avoided. Monitor blood, renal, hepatic, and hematopoetic function in prolonged use. Adverse reactions include nausea and diarrhea. Not recommended for children >18 years of age.

Administration: Oral, intravenous and ophthalmic.

Preparations: Tablets, 250 mg, 500 mg, and 750 mg. Solution for IV infusion, 25 mg/ml. Ophthalmic solution, 0.5%. Oral solution, 25 mg/ml.

LEVONORGESTREL

Description/Actions: Progestin component in certain oral contraceptive formulations.

LEVONORGESTREL AND ETHINYL ESTRADIOL—Preven®

Description/Actions: This product is a hormonal contraceptive kit containing 4 tablets of a combination oral contraceptive, one HCG pregnancy test, and detailed patient information and product labeling. The tablets are indicated for the prevention of pregnancy in women after known or suspected contraceptive failure or unprotected intercourse.

Precautions/Adverse Reactions: Contraindicated in known or suspected pregnancy, pulmonary embolism, ischemic heart disease, history of cerebrovascular accident, valvular heart disease with complications, severe hypertension, diabetes with vascular involvement, headaches with focal neurological symptoms, major surgery with prolonged immobilization, breast cancer, liver tumors, active liver disease, and over 35 y/o if a heavy smoker (more than 15 cigarettes/day). Use cautiously in patients during postpartum, in smokers, patients with cardiovascular disease, hypertension, diabetes, liver disease, ectopic pregnancy, unexplained vaginal bleeding, migraine, and conditions that may decrease GI transit time (may decrease ethinyl estradiol levels). Adverse reactions include nausea, vomiting, menstrual irregularities, breast tenderness, headache, abdominal pain/cramps, and dizziness. Contact the prescriber if vomiting occurs within 1 hour of taking the medication.

Administration: Oral. Rule out pregnancy first by using the enclosed pregnancy test kit. Take 2 tablets as soon as possible (but no longer than 72 hours after unprotected intercourse), then take the remaining 2 tablets 12 hours later.

Patient Care Implications: Instruct patients that this is not a substitute for regular contraception. The effect of repeated use (more than once in a menstrual cycle or in multiple cycles) of emergency contraception is not known. Emergency contraceptives are not as effective as some other methods of contraception. Warn patients if the pregnancy test is positive not to take the tablets. Inform patients that this medication does not prevent transmission of sexually transmitted diseases.

Preparations: Levonorgestrel 0.25 mg + Ethinyl Estradiol 0.05 mg—4 tablets and 1 urine hCG test.

LEVONORGESTREL IMPLANT—Norplant®

Description/Actions: Progestin implant system used as a contraceptive and is effective for up to 5 years.

Preparations: Kit containing 6 capsules (each containing 36 mg) and the equipment needed to implant all 6 capsules subdermally in the mid-portion of the upper arm.

LEVOPHED®, see Norepinephrine

LEVOPROME®, see Methotrimeprazine

LEVORPHANOL TARTRATE—Levo-Dromoran®

Description/Actions: Opioid analgesic indicated for the relief of moderate to severe pain.

Preparations: Tablets, 2 mg. Ampules and vials, 2 mg/ml.

LEVOTHYROXINE SODIUM—Eltroxin®, Levoxyl®, Synthroid®

Description/Actions: Is the principal hormone secreted by the normal thyroid gland. Indicated as replacement therapy for reduced or absent thyroid function.

Precautions/Adverse Reactions: Use is best avoided in patients with acute myocardial infarction, uncorrected adrenal insufficiency, and thyrotoxicosis. Must be used cautiously in patients with cardiovascular disorders and endocrine disorders such as diabetes. Adverse reactions include headache, nervousness, palpitations, tachycardia, and nausea. May increase the action of anticoagulants.

Administration: Oral, intravenous, and intramuscular.

Preparations: Tablets, 0.025, 0.05, 0.075, 0.088, 0.1, 0.112, 0.125, 0.137, 0.15, 0.175, 0.2, and 0.3 mg. Vials, 0.2 and 0.5 mg.

LEVOXYL®, see Levothyroxine Sodium

LEVSIN®, see Hyoscyamine Sulfate

LEVSINEX®, see Hyoscyamine Sulfate

LEVULAN KERASTICK®, see Aminolevulinic Acid Hydrochloride

LEVULOSE, see Fructose

LEXAPRO™, see Escitalopram Oxalate

LEXXEL®—Combination of Enalapril Maleate and Felodipine. See individual discussion on Enalapril and Felodipine.

LIBRAX®, Combination of Chlordiazepoxide and Clidinium. See individual discussion on Chlordiazepoxide and Clidinium.

LIBRITABS®, see Chlordiazepoxide

LIBRIUM®, see Chlordiazepoxide

LIDEX®, see Fluocinonide

LIDOCAINE AND PRILOCAINE CREAM—EMLA Cream®

Description/Actions: An emulsion of lidocaine and prilocaine indicated for use on normal intact skin for local analgesia and on genital mucous membranes as pretreatment for infiltration anesthesia.

Precautions/Adverse Reactions: EMLA is contraindicated in patients with a known history of sensitivity to local anesthetics of the amide type or to any other component of the product. EMLA should be used with caution in patients who may be more sensitive to the systemic effects of lidocaine and prilocaine, including acutely ill, debilitated, or elderly patients as well as those with severe hepatic disease. Application to larger areas or for longer times than those recommended could result in serious adverse effects. Adverse reactions most commonly involve application site reactions (e.g. erythema, edema, hyperpigmentation, itching, rash). Dose-related systemic reactions occur more rarely and include CNS excitation and/or depression as well as cardiovascular effects such as bradycardia, hypotension, and cardiovascular collapse.

Administration: Topical.

Preparations: Tubes, 5 and 30 g with or without Tegaderm™ dressing.

LIDOCAINE HYDROCHLORIDE—Xylocaine®

Description/Actions: Local anesthetic and antiarrhythmic agent. Used by the intravenous and intramuscular routes in the management of ventricular arrhythmias. Also administered parenterally as a local anesthetic for infiltration and nerve block, and by transtracheal and retrobulbar injection. Is also used topically during certain procedures (e.g., urological) and for dermatologic conditions. Several formulations are intended for application to the mucous membranes of the mouth and pharynx.

Preparations: Vials (for IV infusion), 0.2%, 0.4%, and 0.8%. Vials and syringes (for IV admixtures), 4%, 10%, and 20%. Ampules, vials, and syringes (for direct IV administration), 1% and 2%. Ampules and automatic injection device (for IM administration), 10%. Ampules, vials, and syringes (for infiltration and nerve block), 0.5%, 1%, 1.5%, 2%, 4%, and in combination with epinephrine. Premixed IV solutions for infusion, 2 mg/ml (0.2%), 4 mg/ml (0.4%), and 8 mg/ml (0.8%) in 250 and 500 ml containers. Ointment, 2.5% and 5%. Solution (for topical application to mucous membranes), 2%, 4%, and 10%. Jelly, 2% and ointment, 5%, both for topical application to mucous membranes.

LIME SULFUR SOLUTION, see Sulfurated Lime

LINCOCIN®, see Lincomycin

LINCOMYCIN HYDROCHLORIDE—Lincocin®

Description/Actions: Antibiotic indicated for the treatment of infections caused by susceptible gram-positive bacteria.

Preparations: Capsules, 250 and 500 mg. Vials and syringes, 300 mg/ml.

LINDANE—Gamma Benzene Hexachloride, Kwell®

Description/Actions: Parasiticide indicated in the treatment of patients with scabies and lice infestations. Contraindicated in neonates. Adverse reactions include seizures. Children are at increased risk of systemic absorption and CNS side effects. Instruct parents and/or patients to follow application instructions carefully to minimize systemic absorption and toxic effects.

Preparations: Cream, lotion, and shampoo, 1%.

LINEZOLID—Zyvox®

Description/Actions: Linezolid is indicated in the treatment of the following infections: Vancomycin resistant *Enterococcus faecium* infections, nosocomial pneumonia, complicated skin and skin-structure infections, including diabetic foot infections, without concomitant osteomyelitis, uncomplicated skin and skin-structure infections, and community acquired pneumonia.

Precautions/Adverse Reactions: Linezolid should not be taken with tyramine foods and should be used with caution in pregnant women, breast-feeding women, and hypertensive patients. Linezolid should not be given to children. The most common adverse events are diarrhea, headache, nausea, constipation, dizziness, insomnia, and rash. Other adverse events reported include pseudomembranous colitis, hypertension, dyspepsia, localized abdominal pain, pruritus, and tongue discoloration. Myelosupression, including anemia, leukopenia, pancytopenia, and thrombocytopenia, have been reported in patients receiving linezolid.

Administration: Oral, intravenous.

Patient Care Implications: Patients who are pregnant, breast-feeding, or hypertensive should be careful using the drug. Linezolid should not be given to children. Platelets should be monitored in patients receiving the medication. Monitor weekly complete blood counts for patients receiving linezolid, especially those patients receiving linezolid for longer than 2 weeks, patients with preexisting myelosuppression, patients receiving concomitant therapy with other myelosuppressive agents, and patients with a chronic infection who have received previous or concomitant antibiotic therapy.

Preparations: Tablets, 400 and 600 mg. Injection, 200 mg/100 ml, 400 mg/200 ml, 600 mg/300 ml. Oral suspension, 100 mg/5 ml, 150 ml bottle.

LIORESAL®, see Baclofen

LIOTHYRONINE SODIUM—Triiodothyronine, T3, Cytomel®, Triostat®

Description/Actions: A thyroid hormone indicated as replacement or supplemental therapy in patients with hypothyroidism, as a pituitary/thyroid-stimulating hormone suppressant in the treatment or prevention of various goiters, as a diagnostic agent, and, via parenteral use, for myxedema coma and precoma.

Preparations: Tablets, 5, 25, and 50 mcg. Vials, 10 mcg/ml (Triostat®).

LIPITOR®, see Atorvastatin

LIQUAEMIN®, see Heparin

LIQUEFIED PHENOL, see Phenol

LIQUID PETROLATUM, see Mineral Oil

LISINOPRIL—Prinivil®, Zestril®

Description/Actions: An angiotensin converting enzyme (ACE) inhibitor that is a derivative of enalaprilat, the active form of enalapril. Indicated for the treatment of hypertension and may be used alone or concomitantly with other antihypertensive agents. Also indicated as adjunctive therapy in the management of congestive heart failure in patients not responding adequately to diuretics and digitalis. Used as an adjunct to other therapies within 24 hours postMI in hemodynamically stable patients, to reduce mortality.

Precautions/Adverse Reactions: Lisinopril is contraindicated in patients with a known hypersensitivity to any component of the product, in patients with a history of angioedema related to previous treatment with an ACE inhibitor, and in patients with hereditary or idiopathic angioedema. Lisinopril should be given with caution to patients with obstruction in the outflow tract of the left ventricle. Adverse reactions include dizziness, headache, fatigue, diarrhea, upper respiratory symptoms, cough, and hyperkalemia. An excessive reduction in blood pressure may occur, particularly in patients with severe salt/volume depletion (e.g., those treated vigorously with diuretics). Angioedema has occurred infrequently, sometimes after the first dose. Coadministration of lisinopril and nonsteroidal anti-inflammatory drugs in patients with compromised renal function may result in a further deterioration of renal function. These effects are usually reversible.

Administration: Oral.

Preparations: Tablets, 2.5, 5, 10, 20, and 40 mg.

LITHANE®, see Lithium Carbonate

LITHIUM CARBONATE—Eskalith®, Lithane®, Lithium Citrate, Lithonate®

Description/Actions: Psychotherapeutic agent indicated in the acute treatment of manic episodes of manic-depressive illnesses, and as prophylaxis against their recurrence.

Preparations: Capsules and tablets, 150, 300, and 600 mg. Controlled-release tablets, 300 and 450 mg. Syrup, 300 mg/5ml.

LITHONATE®, see Lithium Carbonate

LITHOSTAT®, see Acetohydroxamic Acid

LIVER

Description/Actions: Antianemic agent used as a source of vitamin B_{12}.

Preparations: Tablets. Vials, 2, 10, and 20 mcg vitamin B_{12}/ml.

LOBELINE

Description/Actions: Smoking deterrent used as a temporary aid to break the habit of smoking cigarettes.

Preparations: Tablets, 2 mg.

LODINE®, see Etodolac

LODOSYN®, see Carbidopa

LODOXAMIDE TROMETHAMINE—Alomide®

Description/Actions: Indicated for the topical treatment of vernal keratoconjunctivitis, vernal conjunctivitis, and vernal keratitis.

Precautions/Adverse Reactions: Adverse reactions include transient burning, stinging, or discomfort upon instillation. Contains benzalkonium chloride, so patients should be instructed not to wear soft contact lenses during treatment.

Administration: Ophthalmic.

Preparations: Ophthalmic solution, 0.1%.

LOESTRIN®—Oral Contraceptive Combination of Ethinyl Estradiol and Norethindrone Acetate. See individual discussion on Ethinyl Estradiol and Norethindrone Acetate.

LOFENE®, see Diphenoxylate

LOMANATE®, see Diphenoxylate

LOMEFLOXACIN HYDROCHLORIDE—Maxaquin®

Description/Actions: Fluoroquinolone anti-infective agent that inhibits DNA gyrase and exhibits a bactericidal action against many gram-positive and gram-negative bacteria. Indicated for lower respiratory tract infections and urinary tract infections caused by susceptible organisms. Also indicated for prophylaxis (preoperatively) to reduce the incidence of urinary tract infections in the early postoperative period (3–5 days postsurgery) in patients undergoing transurethral surgical procedures.

Precautions/Adverse Reactions: Rare cases of sensory or sensorimotor axonal polyneuropathy affecting small and/or large axons resulting in paresthesias, hypoesthesias, dysesthesias, and weakness have been reported. Rupture of the shoulder, hand, Achille's tendon, or other tendons that require surgical repair or resulted in prolonged disability have also been reported. Contraindicated in patients with a known hypersensitivity to any of the fluoroquinolones or the related quinolone antibacterial agents (i.e., nalidixic acid, cinoxacin). Fluoroquinolones have caused erosion of cartilage in weight-bearing joints and other signs of arthropathy in juvenile animals, and use in children under 18, pregnant women, and women who are nursing is best avoided. Adverse reactions include nausea, diarrhea, headache, dizziness, and photosensitivity reactions. Patients should be advised to avoid excessive sunlight and artificial ultraviolet light during the period of treatment. May cause dizziness, lightheadedness, and other central nervous system effects, and patients should know how they tolerate the drug before they engage in activities that require mental alertness and coordination. Convulsions have been reported in patients receiving lomefloxacin.

Administration: Oral.

Preparations: Tablets, 400 mg.

LOMOTIL®, see Diphenoxylate Hydrochloride with Atropine Sulfate

LOMUSTINE—CCNU®, CeeNU®

Description/Actions: Antineoplastic agent indicated in the treatment of brain tumors and Hodgkin's disease.

Preparations: Capsules, 10, 40, and 100 mg.

LONITEN®, see Minoxidil

LONOX®, see Diphenoxylate

LO/OVRAL®, Oral Contraceptive Combination of Ethinyl Estradiol and Norgestrel. See individual discussion on Ethinyl Estradiol and Norgestrel.

LOPERAMIDE HYDROCHLORIDE—Imodium®, Imodium A-D®, Imodium Advanced®

Description/Actions: Antidiarrheal agent indicated for the control and symptomatic relief of acute nonspecific diarrhea and of chronic diarrhea associated with inflammatory bowel disease. Also indicated for reducing the volume of discharge from ileostomies.

Precautions/Adverse Reactions: Adverse reactions include abdominal pain, nausea, vomiting, constipation, and tiredness.

Administration: Oral.

Preparations: Capsules and caplets, 2 mg. Liquid, 1 mg/5 ml. Also as a combination agent containing loperamide HCl 2 mg and Simethicone 125 mg in a chewable tablet (Imodium Advanced®).

LOPID®, see Gemfibrozil

LOPINAVIR AND RITONAVIR—Kaletra™

Description/Actions: Kaletra™ is a coformulation of lopinavir and ritonavir. It is used in the treatment of HIV in combination with other antiretroviral agents.

Precautions/Adverse Reactions: Kaletra™ is contraindicated in patients with known hypersensitivity to any of its ingredients, including ritonavir. Breast-feeding is contraindicated while receiving Kaletra™. Certain drugs that are metabolized via the cytochrome P450 isoform CYP3A or CYP2D6 are associated with increased levels and possible serious and/or life-threatening events when administered with Kaletra™. The following drugs should *not* be used in combination with Kaletra™: flecainide, propafenone, astemizole, terfenadine, dihydroergotamine, ergotamine, methylergonovine, cisapride, pimozide, midazolam, and triazolam. Avoid concurrent use with St. John's Wort, lovastatin, and simvastatin. Coadministration of Kaletra™ with sildenafil, vardenafil, or tadalafil results in increased plasma concentrations of these agents and may lead to hypotension, visual changes, and priapism. Pancreatitis has been observed in patients on Kaletra™; use caution in patients with a history of pancreatitis. Patients with signs or symptoms of pancreatitis should be evaluated and therapy should be suspended as clinically appropriate. New onset diabetes mellitus and exacerbation of preexisting diabetes have been reported in patients receiving protease inhibitors. Use caution in patients with hepatic dysfunction; patients with underlying hepatic disease or marked elevations in transaminase prior to treatment may be at increased risk for further increases in transaminase levels. The potential of resistance/cross-resistance with other protease inhibitors is currently being evaluated. Increased bleeding has been reported in hemophilia types A and B patients treated with Kaletra™. Redistribution/accumulation of body fat has been observed in patients on antiretroviral therapy. Large increases in the concentration of total cholesterol and triglycerides have occurred in patients on Kaletra™; lipid testing should be performed prior to initiating therapy and periodically throughout treatment. Pregnancy Category C. Safety and efficacy in pediatric patients <6 months have not been established. Kaletra™ is an inhibitor of CYP3A and CYP2D6; coadministration of Kaletra™ and drugs primarily metabolized by these isoenzyme systems may result in increased plasma concentrations that could increase their therapeutic and/or adverse effects. Some adverse effects are nausea, abdominal pain, hypercholesterolemia, increased triglycerides, increased amylase, increased liver function tests, headache, insomnia, rash, and hyperglycemia.

Administration: Oral.

Preparations: Capsule: lopinavir 133.3 mg and ritonavir 33.3 mg. Solution, oral: Lopinavir 80 mg and ritonavir 20 mg per ml. Oral solution and gelatin capsules should be refrigerated (stored) at 2°–8°C (36°–46°F). If stored at room temperature (25°C or 77°F), use within 2 months.

LOPRESSOR®, see Metoprolol

LOPROX®, see Ciclopirox Olamine

LOPURIN®, see Allopurinol

LORABID®, see Loracarbef

LORACARBEF—Lorabid®

Description/Actions: Carbapenem antibiotic. Inhibits bacterial cell wall synthesis and exhibits a bactericidal action against many gram-positive and gram-negative bacteria. Indicated for upper respiratory tract infections, lower respiratory tract infections, acute maxillary sinusitis, uncomplicated skin and skin-structure infections, and urinary tract infections caused by susceptible organisms.

Precautions/Adverse Reactions: Contraindicated in patients with a known hypersensitivity to loracarbef or any of the cephalosporins. Must be used cautiously, if at all, in penicillin-sensitive patients, and use should be avoided in patients with a history of immediate and/or severe reactions to penicillins. Adverse reactions include diarrhea, nausea, vomiting, abdominal pain, rash, headache, and vaginitis.

Administration: Oral. Should be administered at least one hour before or 2 hours after a meal.

Preparations: Capsules, 200 mg. Powder for oral suspension, 100 mg/5 ml and 200 mg/5 ml.

LORATADINE—Claritin®

Description/Actions: Selectively antagonizes peripheral histamine H_1-receptors and is designated as a nonsedating antihistamine. Indicated for the relief of symptoms of seasonal allergic rhinitis and idiopathic chronic urticaria.

Precautions/Adverse Reactions: Adverse reactions include headache, somnolence, fatigue, and dry mouth, although the incidence of these effects was similar in patients receiving placebo.

Administration: Oral. Should be administered on an empty stomach.

Preparations: Tablets, 10 mg. Reditabs, 10 mg. Syrup, 1 mg/ml.

LORAZEPAM—Ativan®

Description/Actions: Benzodiazepine indicated for the management of anxiety disorders or for the short-term relief of the symptoms of anxiety and insomnia. Also indicated for parenteral use as a preanesthetic medication and in status epilepticus.

Precautions/Adverse Reactions: Contraindicated in patients with acute narrow-angle glaucoma. Adverse reactions include drowsiness and other CNS effects; patients should be cautioned regarding activities such as driving and operating machinery, as well as interactions with other CNS-acting drugs including alcohol. Can cause dependence and is included in Schedule IV.

Administration: Oral, intravenous, and intramuscular.

Preparations: Tablets, 0.5, 1, and 2 mg. Vials, 2 and 4 mg/ml. Concentrated solution, 2 mg/ml.

LORTAB®, Combination Opioid and Analgesic. Hydrocodone Bitartrate and Acetaminophen

LOSARTAN POTASSIUM—Cozaar®, Hyzaar®

Description/Actions: Angiotensin II receptor antagonist indicated in the treatment of hypertension and for use in patients with type 2 diabetes for the treatment of nephropathy with an elevated serum creatinine and proteinuria (>300 mg/day) in patients with type 2 diabetes and hypertension.

Precautions/Adverse Reactions: Adverse reactions include hypotension and dizziness. Contraindicated in pregnancy. May increase serum potassium levels. The antihypertensive effect of losartan may be diminished by concomitant administration of indomethacin.

Administration: Oral.

Preparations: Tablets, 25 and 50 mg. Available in combination formulation (Hyzaar) that contains 50 mg of losartan potassium and 12.5 mg of hydrochlorothiazide and 100 mg of losartan and 25 mg of hydrochlorothiazide.

LOTEMEX®, see Loteprednol Etabonate

Description/Actions: Anti-inflammatory agent indicated in the treatment of seasonal allergic conjunctivitis (Alrex®), steroid responsive ocular disease, and postop inflammation after ocular surgery (Lotemax®).

Precautions/Adverse Reactions: Contraindicated in ocular fungal, viral, or mycobacterial infections. Reevaluate if no improvement after 2 days. Prescribe initially and renew after 14 days only after appropriate exam. Use cautiously in corneal or scleral thinning, glaucoma, or a history of herpes simplex. Monitor IOP and for secondary infections in prolonged therapy (>10 days). Avoid abrupt cessation. Remove soft contact lenses for installation and wait 10 minutes before reinserting. Included local reactions (e.g., blurred vision, burning, itching eyes, dry eye), photophobia, headache, rhinitis, and pharyngitis. May mask or exacerbate ocular infections. Prolonged use may result in increased IOP, optic nerve damage, visual acuity and field defects, cataract formation, and corneal perforation.

Administrations: Ophthalmic.

Preparations: 2% ophthalmic suspension (contains benzakonium chloride).

LOTENSIN®, see Benazepril Hydrochloride

LOTEPREDNOL ETABONATE—Alrex®, Lotemax®

LOTREL®, Combination of Amlodipine and Benazepril. See individual discussion on Amlodipine and Benazepril.

LOTRIMIN®, see Clotrimazole

LOTRIMIN AF®, see Clotrimazole

LOTRISONE®, Combination of Clotrimazole and Betamethasone Dipropionate. See individual discussion on Clotrimazole and Betamethasone Dipropionate.

LO-TROL®, see Diphenoxylate

LOVASTATIN—Mevacor®, Altoprev®

Description/Actions: Results in a reduction of low-density lipoprotein (LDL) cholesterol and total plasma cholesterol, while high-density lipoprotein (HDL) concentrations increase. Indicated as an adjunct to diet for the reduction of elevated total and LDL cholesterol levels in patients with primary hypercholesterolemia (types IIa and IIb), when the response to diet and other nonpharmacologic measures alone has been inadequate. Also indicated to slow the progression of coronary atherosclerosis in patients with coronary heart disease.

Precautions/Adverse Reactions: Contraindicated during pregnancy and lactation because lovastatin has been reported to exhibit teratogenic effects in some animal studies. It is also contraindicated in patients with active liver disease or unexplained persistent elevations of serum transaminases. Marked persistent increases in serum transaminases may occur and it is recommended that liver function tests be performed every 4–6 weeks during the first 15 months of therapy and periodically thereafter. Adverse reactions include headache, rash, pruritus, nausea, diarrhea, constipation, abdominal pain, and myalgia. Some individuals experience myositis, so patients should be advised to report unexplained muscle pain or tenderness. Although it is not known whether lovastatin causes ocular problems, it is recommended that ophthalmologic exams be conducted before or shortly after starting therapy, and annually thereafter.

Administration: Oral.

Preparations: Tablets, 10, 20, and 40 mg (Mevacor). Extended-release tablets, 10 mg, 20 mg, 40 mg, and 60 mg (Altoprev).

LOVENOX®, see Enoxaparin

LOXAPINE—Loxitane®

Description/Actions: Antipsychotic agent indicated for the management of the manifestations of psychotic disorders.

Preparations: Capsules (as the succinate), 5, 10, 25, and 50 mg. Oral concentrate (as the hydrochloride), 25 mg/ml. Ampules and vials (as the hydrochloride and for IM use), 50 mg/ml.

LOW-QUEL®, see Diphenoxylate

LOXITANE®, see Loxapine

LOZOL®, see Indapamide

LUDIOMIL®, see Maprotiline

LUFYLLIN®, see Dyphylline

LUGOL'S SOLUTION, see Iodine

LUMIGAN®, see Bimatoprost

LUMINAL®, see Phenobarbital

LUNELLE™, Combination of Medroxyprogesterone Acetate and Estradiol Cypionate

LUPRON®, see Leuprolide

LUPRON DEPOT®, see Leuprolide

LUPRON DEPOT-PED®, see Leuprolide

LURIDE®, see Sodium Fluoride

LUSTRA®, see Hydroquinone

LUTREPULSE®, see Gonadorelin Acetate

LUVOX®, see Fluvoxamine Maleate

LUXIOL®, see Betamethasome Valerate

LYPHOCIN®, see Vancomycin

LYSODREN®, see Mitotane

M

MAALOX®, see Aluminum and Magnesium Hydroxide

MACROBID®, see Nitrofurantoin

MACRODANTIN®, see Nitrofurantoin Macrocrystals

MACRODEX®, see Dextran

MAFENIDE ACETATE—Sulfamylon®

Description/Actions: Sulfonamide anti-infective agent indicated for topical use as adjunctive therapy of patients with second- and third-degree burns.

Preparations: Cream, 8.5%.

MAGALDRATE—Riopan®

Description/Actions: Antacid indicated for the relief of hyperacidity and related symptoms.

Preparations: Tablets and chewable tablets, 480 mg. Suspension, 540 mg/ 5 ml.

MAGAN®, see Magnesium Salicylate

MAGNESIUM CARBONATE

Description/Actions: Antacid used in combination with other agents.

MAGNESIUM CHLORIDE—Slow-Mag®

Description/Actions: Magnesium supplement.

Preparations: Controlled-release tablets, 64 mg magnesium (as chloride).

MAGNESIUM CITRATE—Citrate of Magnesia

Description/Actions: Laxative used in the treatment of constipation and with other agents as a bowel evacuant in the preparation of the colon for radiologic examinations.

Preparations: Solution.

MAGNESIUM HYDROXIDE—Milk of Magnesia

Description/Actions: Antacid and laxative used alone or in combination with other agents.

Preparations: Tablets, 325 mg. Suspension.

MAGNESIUM OXIDE

Description/Actions: Used for the replacement of magnesium in various magnesium deficiencies.

Preparations: Capsules 140 mg. Tablets, 400 mg, 420 mg, and 500 mg.

MAGNESIUM SALICYLATE—Doan's Pills®, Magan®

Description/Actions: Salicylate analgesic/anti-inflammatory agent indicated for the relief of pain and the signs and symptoms of arthritic disorders.

Preparations: Tablets, 325, 545, and 600 mg.

MAGNESIUM SULFATE

Description/Actions: Laxative, anticonvulsant, and electrolyte. Used orally in the treatment of constipation, and parenterally to prevent or control convulsions. Also used parenterally as replacement therapy in the treatment of hypomagnesemia.

Preparations: Granules (to prepare solution for oral administration). Ampules and vials, 10%, 12.5%, 25%, and 50%.

MAGNESIUM TRISILICATE

Description/Actions: Antacid used in combination with other agents.

MALARONE™, see Atovaquone and Proguanil Hydrochloride

MANDELAMINE®, see Methenamine Mandelate

MANDOL®, see Cefamandole

MANNITOL—Osmitrol®

Description/Actions: Osmotic diuretic indicated in the prevention and treatment of the oliguric phase of acute renal failure following cardiovascular surgery, severe traumatic injury, surgery in the presence of severe jaundice, hemolytic transfusion reaction, to reduce intraocular pressure (IOP) and intracranial pressure (ICP). Most common adverse reaction is electrolyte imbalance, especially hyponatremia.

Administration: Intravenous, GU irrigant.

Preparations: IV injection, 5, 10, 15, and 20%. GU irrigant, 5%. Also in combination with sorbitol for GU irrigation.

MAOLATE®, see Chlorphenesin Carbamate

MAPROTILINE HYDROCHLORIDE—Ludiomil®

Description/Actions: Tetracyclic antidepressant indicated in the treatment of depression and for the relief of anxiety associated with depression.

Preparations: Tablets, 25, 50, and 75 mg.

MARCAINE®, see Bupivacaine

MAREZINE®, see Cyclizine

MARIJUANA, see Dronabinol

MARINOL®, see Dronabinol

MASOPROCOL—Actinex®

Description/Actions: Indicated for the topical treatment of actinic (solar) keratoses.

Precautions/Adverse Reactions: Adverse reactions include erythema, flaking, itching, dryness, edema, burning, and soreness. May induce sensitization (allergic contact dermatitis) and, if such reactions occur, the drug should be discontinued.

Administration: Topical.

Preparations: Cream, 10%.

MATULANE®, see Procarbazine

MAVIK®, see Trandolapril

MAXAIR®, see Pirbuterol

MAXAQUIN®, see Lomefloxacin

MAXIFLOR®, see Diflorasone

MAXIPIME®, see Cefepime

MAXIVATE®, see Betamethasone Dipropionate

MAXZIDE®, Combination of Triamterene and
Hydrochlorothiazide

MAZANOR®, see Mazindol

MAZINDOL—Mazanor®, Sanorex®

Description/Actions: Anorexiant indicated in the management of exogenous obesity as a short-term adjunct in a regimen of weight reduction based on caloric restriction.

Preparations: Tablets, 1 and 2 mg.

MEBARAL®, see Mephobarbital

MEBENDAZOLE—Vermox®

Description/Actions: Anthelmintic indicated for the treatment of pinworm, whipworm, roundworm, and hookworm infections.

Preparations: Chewable tablets, 100 mg.

MECAMYLAMINE HYDROCHLORIDE—Inversine®

Description/Actions: Antihypertensive agent indicated in the management of moderately severe to severe hypertension.

Preparations: Tablets, 2.5 mg.

MECHLORETHAMINE HYDROCHLORIDE—Mustargen®,
Nitrogen Mustard

Description/Actions: Antineoplastic agent indicated for the parenteral treatment of Hodgkin's disease, lymphosarcoma, chronic myelocytic or chronic lymphocytic leukemia, polycythemia vera, mycosis fungoides, and bronchogenic carcinoma. Also administered intrapleurally, intraperitoneally, or intrapericardially for the palliative treatment of metastatic carcinoma resulting in effusion.

Precautions/Adverse Reactions: This drug is highly toxic, and both powder and solution must be handled and administered with care. Inhalation of dust vapors and contact with skin or mucous membranes, especially those of the eyes, must be avoided. Avoid exposure during pregnancy. Due to the toxic properties of mechlorethamine, special handling procedures should be reviewed prior to handling and followed diligently. Extravasation of the drug into subcutaneous tissue results in painful inflammation.

Preparations: Vials, 10 mg.

MECLAN®, see Meclocycline

MECLIZINE HYDROCHLORIDE—Antivert®, Bonine®

Description/Actions: Exhibits antihistaminic and anticholinergic activity. Indicated for the management of nausea, vomiting, and dizziness associated with motion sickness, and in vertigo associated with diseases affecting the vestibular system.

Precautions/Adverse Reactions: Must be used with caution in patients with asthma, glaucoma, or enlargement of the prostate. Adverse reactions include drowsiness, and patients should be cautioned regarding activities such as driving and operating machinery, as well as interactions with other CNS-acting drugs including alcohol. Other adverse reactions include dry mouth.

Administration: Oral.

Preparations: Tablets, 12.5, 25, and 50 mg. Chewable tablets, 25 mg. Capsules, 15, 25, and 30 mg.

MECLOCYCLINE SULFOSALICYLATE—Meclan®

Description/Actions: Tetracycline antibiotic indicated for topical use in the treatment of inflammatory acne vulgaris.

Preparations: Cream, 1%.

MEDROL®, see Methylprednisolone

MEDROXYPROGESTERONE ACETATE—Cycrin®, Depo-Provera®, Provera®

Description/Actions: Is a derivative of progesterone and is indicated in the treatment of secondary amenorrhea, and abnormal uterine bleeding due to hormonal imbalance in the absence of organic pathology, such as fibroids or uterine cancer. Also indicated for intramuscular use as adjunctive therapy and palliative treatment of inoperable, recurrent, and metastatic endometrial carcinoma or renal carcinoma. Also indicated for intramuscular use as a long-term injectable contraceptive when administered at 3-month intervals.

Precautions/Adverse Reactions: Contraindicated in patients with hepatic dysfunction, undiagnosed vaginal bleeding, and known or suspected malignancy of breast or genital organs. May cause thromboembolic phenomena including thrombophlebitis and pulmonary embolism, and use is contraindicated in patients with a history of such disorders. Women who use Depo-Provera® may lose significant bone mineral density (BMD). Bone loss is greater with increasing duration of use and may not be completely reversible. May cause adverse effects in the fetus, and use during the first 4 months of pregnancy is not recommended. Other adverse reactions include rash, pruritus, edema, nausea, insomnia, depression, somnolence, and breakthrough bleeding.

Administration: Oral and intramuscular.

Preparations: Tablets, 2.5, 5, and 10 mg. Vials (Depo-Provera), 100 mg/ml, 150 mg/ml, and 400 mg/ml. Prefilled syringe, 150 mg/ml.

MEFENAMIC ACID—Ponstel®

Description/Actions: Nonsteroidal anti-inflammatory drug indicated for the relief of moderate pain and the treatment of primary dysmenorrhea.

Preparations: Capsules, 250 mg.

MEFLOQUINE HYDROCHLORIDE—Lariam®

Description/Actions: Acts as a blood schizonticide, but does not eliminate exoerythrocytic (hepatic phase) parasites. Indicated for the treatment of moderate acute malaria caused by susceptible strains of *Plasmodium falciparum* or *Plasmodium vivax*. Is also indicated for the prophylaxis of *Plasmodium falciparum* and *Plasmodium vivax* malaria infections.

Precautions/Adverse Reactions: The drug should not be used during pregnancy, and women of childbearing potential should use reliable contraceptive measures for the duration of mefloquine use and for 2 months after the last dose. Adverse reactions include CNS effects, so patients should be cautioned regarding activities such as driving and operating machinery, as well as interactions with other CNS-acting drugs including alcohol. Rare cases of suicidal ideation and suicide have been reported. Other adverse reactions include nausea, vomiting, diarrhea, abdominal pain, loss of appetite, headache, tinnitus, fever, chills, myalgia, and rash. Concomitant use with chloroquine may increase the risk of convulsions.

Administration: Oral. For malaria prophylaxis, therapy should be initiated one week prior to departure to an endemic area, and the drug should be administered on the same day of the week. Prophylaxis should be continued for 4 additional weeks following return. Doses of mefloquine should not be taken on an empty stomach and should be administered with at least 8 oz of water.

Preparations: Tablets, 250 mg.

MEFOXIN®, see Cefoxitin

MEGACE®, see Megestrol

MEGESTROL ACETATE—Megace®

Description/Actions: Antineoplastic agent indicated for the treatment of advanced carcinoma of the breast or endometrium. Also indicated for the treatment of anorexia, cachexia, or significant weight loss in patients with AIDS.

Preparations: Tablets, 20 and 40 mg. Suspension, 40 mg/ml.

MELLARIL®, see Thioridazine

MELOXICAM—Mobic®

Description/Actions: Mobic® is indicated for relief of the signs and symptoms of osteoarthritis and rheumatoid arthritis.

Precautions/Adverse Reactions: Meloxicam should not be given to patients who have experienced asthma, urticaria, or allergic-type reactions after taking aspirin or other NSAIDs. Severe, rarely fatal, anaphylactic-like reactions have been reported in such patients. Serious gastrointestinal toxicity such as bleeding, ulceration, and perforation of the stomach, and small or large intestine, can occur at any time. The most common adverse events reported are gastrointestinal, including abdominal pain, diarrhea, dyspepsia, flatulence, constipation, and nausea and vomiting. Less common GI effects reported are colitis, xerostomia, peptic ulcer disease, eructation, esophagitis, gastritis, and GERD. In general, anorexia may also occur. Other adverse events are allergic or respiratory reactions including ingioedema, asthma, bronchospasm, dyspnea, dizziness, flu-like symptoms, headache, rash, edema, and upper respiratory tract infections.

Administration: Oral.

Patient Care Implications: Monitor signs and symptoms of GI perforation, ulceration, and bleeding. Experience with chronic NSAID therapy in elderly and debilitated patients suggests greater potential for serious GI adverse events. Monitor liver function tests. Use of meloxicam is not recommended in patients with severe hepatic insufficiency. If clinical signs and symptoms consistent with liver disease develop, or if systemic manifestations occur (i.e., eosinophilia, rash, etc.), meloxicam should be discontinued.

Preparations: Tablets, 7.5 and 15 mg.

MELPHALAN—Alkeran®

Description/Actions: Antineoplastic agent indicated for the treatment of multiple myeloma and for the palliation of nonresectable carcinoma of the ovary. Administered by intravenous infusion for the palliative treatment of multiple myeloma when oral therapy is not appropriate.

Preparations: Tablets, 2 mg. Vials, 50 mg.

MEMANTINE—Nameda™

Description/Actions: Memantine is an N-Methyl-D-Aspartate (NMDA) receptor antagonist. It is indicated in the treatment of moderate to severe dementia of Alzheimer's disease (AD). The leading cause of dementia in the elderly is AD. Persistent activation of central nervous system NMDA receptors by the excitatory amino acid glutamate has been hypothesized to contribute to symptoms of AD. Memantine is thought to exert its effect by binding to NMDA receptors and blocking the actions of glutamate.

Precautions/Adverse Reactions: Memantine is contraindicated in individuals hypersensitive to memantine or any component of the formulation. A major route of elimination is renal; patients with moderate renal impairment should have dose reductions. Not recommended in patients with severe renal impairment. Clearance of memantine is reduced by alkaline urine. Use caution with dietary changes, patient condition, and medications that alter urine pH. Use caution with seizure disorders; has not been evaluated in patients with a seizure disorder. Pregnancy Category B. Excretion in breast milk unknown/use caution. Most common adverse effects were dizziness, hypertension, confusion, headache, constipation, and cough.

Administration: Oral.

Patient Care Implications: May be taken with or without food.

Preparations: Tablet: 5 mg, 10 mg.

MENEST®, see Estrogens, Esterified

MENOTROPINS—Pergonal®

Description/Actions: Gonadotropins (follicle-stimulating hormone [FSH] and luteinizing hormone [LH]) administered intramuscularly for the induction of ovulation and pregnancy in anovulatory women, and to stimulate spermatogenesis in men with infertility.

Preparations: Ampules, 75 IU each of FSH and LH and 150 IU each of FSH and LH.

MENTAX®, see Butenafine Hydrochloride

MENTHOL

Description/Actions: Analgesic/cooling agent included with other agents in formulations that are applied topically to the skin or throat (e.g., lozenges).

MEPERIDINE HYDROCHLORIDE—Demerol®

Description/Actions: Opioid analgesic indicated for the relief of moderate to severe pain, for preoperative medication, for support of anesthesia, and for obstetrical analgesia.

Precautions/Adverse Reactions: Adverse reactions include sedation and other CNS effects; patients should be cautioned regarding activities such as driving and operating machinery, as well as interactions with other CNS-acting drugs including alcohol. Other adverse reactions include flushing of the face, hypotension, and pain at the injection site. Is contraindicated in patients receiving a monoamine oxidase inhibitor. Can cause dependence, and formulations are covered under the provisions of the Controlled Substances Act.

Administration: Oral, intramuscular, intravenous, and subcutaneous.

Preparations: Tablets, 50 and 100 mg. Syrup, 50 mg/5 ml. Ampules, vials, and syringes, 10 mg/ml, 25 mg/ml, 50 mg/ml, 75 mg/ml, and 100 mg/ml.

MEPHENTERMINE SULFATE—Wyamine®

Description/Actions: Sympathomimetic agent indicated for the parenteral treatment of hypotension secondary to ganglionic blockade and that occurring with spinal anesthesia.

Preparations: Ampules and vials, 15 mg/ml and 30 mg/ml.

MEPHENYTOIN—Mesantoin®

Description/Actions: Anticonvulsant indicated for the control of grand mal, focal, Jacksonian, and psychomotor seizures in those patients who are refractory to less toxic anticonvulsants.

Preparations: Tablets, 100 mg.

MEPHOBARBITAL—Mebaral®

Description/Actions: Barbiturate indicated as a sedative for the relief of anxiety and tension, and as an anticonvulsant for the treatment of grand mal and petit mal epilepsy.

Preparations: Tablets 32, 50, and 100 mg.

MEPHYTON®, see Phytonadione

MEPIVACAINE HYDROCHLORIDE—Carbocaine®

Description/Actions: Local anesthetic used to produce local anesthesia by infiltration injection, peripheral nerve block, and central neural blocks by the lumbar or caudal epidural route. Also indicated for use in dental procedures.

Preparations: Vials, 1%, 1.5%, and 2%. Dental cartridges, 3%.

MEPROBAMATE—Equanil®, Meprospan®, Miltown®

Description/Actions: Antianxiety agent indicated for the management of anxiety disorders or for the short-term relief of the symptoms of anxiety.

Preparations: Tablets, 200, 400, and 600 mg. Controlled-release capsules, 200 and 400 mg.

MEPRON®, see Atovaquone

MEPROSPAN®, see Meprobamate

MEQUINOL/TRETINOIN TOPICAL SOLUTION—Solag®

Description/Actions: A solution containing 2% mequinol and 0.01% tretinoin indicated for the treatment of solar lentigines.

Precautions/Adverse Reactions: The combination of mequinol and tretinoin may cause fetal harm when administered to pregnant women. Solag Topical Solution should therefore not be used in women of childbearing potential. Solag is also contraindicated in individuals with a history of sensitivity reactions to any of its ingredients. Solag should not be administered if the patient is also taking drugs known to be photosensitizers because of the possibility of augmented phototoxicity. Caution should be used in patients with eczematous skin or a history of vitiligo. During the use of Solag, exposure of the treated area to sunlight should be avoided or minimized. Adverse reactions include erythema, burning, stinging or tingling, desquamation, pruritus, and skin irritation. Some patients experience temporary hypopigmentation of treated lesions or of the skin surrounding treated lesions.

Administration: Apply Solag to solar lentigines using the applicator top while avoiding application to the surrounding skin. Patients should not shower or bathe the treatment areas for at least 6 hours after application. When applying, avoid the eyes, mouth, paranasal sinuses, and mucous membranes.

Patient Care Implications: Solag should only be used as an adjunct to a comprehensive skin care and sun avoidance program. If a drug sensitivity, chemical irritation, or systemic adverse reaction develops, use of Solag should be discontinued. Patients require detailed instruction to obtain maximal benefits and to understand all the precautions necessary to use this drug with greatest safety.

Preparations: Topical solution, 30 ml bottle.

MERBROMIN—Mercurochrome

Description/Actions: Antiseptic that is applied topically.

Preparations: Solution, 2%.

MERCAPTOPURINE—Purinethol®

Description/Actions: Antineoplastic agent indicated in the management of leukemias.

Preparations: Tablets, 50 mg.

MERCUROCHROME®, see Merbromin

MERCURY, AMMONIATED, see Ammoniated Mercury

MEROPENEM—Merrem®

Description/Actions: Synthetic, broad spectrum carbapenem antibiotic. Bactericidal activity results from the inhibition of cell wall synthesis.

Precautions/Adverse Reactions: Contraindicated in patients who have experienced anaphylactic reactions to other carbopenems (imipenem) or to beta-lactam antibiotics. Use cautiously in patients with CNS disorders, history of seizures, or renal impairment. Monitor renal, hepatic, and hematopoietic function in long-term use. Adverse reactions include local reactions, GI upset, headache, rash, pruritus, apnea, seizures, constipation, superinfection, and pseudomembraneous colitis. Meropenem may decrease serum levels of valproic acid to subtherapeutic.

Administration: IV infusion or bolus.

Preparations: Powder for reconstitution, 500 mg and 1 g.

MERREM®, see Meropenem

MERTHIOLATE®, see Thimerosal

MESALAMINE—Asacol®, Pentasa®, Rowasa®, Canasa®

Description/Actions: Also known as 5-aminosalicylic acid (5-ASA) and is a metabolite of sulfasalazine. Indicated in the treatment of active mild to moderate distal ulcerative colitis.

Precautions/Adverse Reactions: Contraindicated in patients who are hypersensitive to the drug or to any component (e.g., sulfite) of the formulation. Adverse reactions include an acute intolerance syndrome characterized by cramping, acute abdominal pain, bloody diarrhea, and sometimes fever, headache, and a rash. Some patients experience mild hair loss.

Administration: Oral and rectal.

Preparations: Tablets, delayed release, 400 mg (Asacol®). Capsules, controlled release, 250 mg (Pentasa®). Suspension enema, 4 g/60 ml (Rowasa). Suppositories, 500 mg (Rowasa). Suppository, 1g (Canasa).

MESANTOIN®, see Mephenytoin

MESNA—Mesnex®

Description/Actions: Reacts with the urotoxic metabolites (e.g., acrolein) of ifosfamide. Uroprotective agent indicated as a prophylactic agent in reducing the incidence of hemorrhagic cystitis caused by ifosfamide.

Precautions/Adverse Reactions: Adverse reactions include nausea, vomiting, and diarrhea.

Administration: Oral and intraveneous.

Preparations: Ampules, 200 and 400 mg; 1 g. Tablets, 400 mg.

MESNEX®, see Mesna

MESORIDAZINE BESYLATE—Serentil®

Description/Actions: Phenothiazine antipsychotic agent indicated in the treatment of schizophrenia, behavioral problems in mental deficiency and chronic brain syndrome, alcoholism, and psychoneurotic manifestations.

Preparations: Tablets, 10, 25, 50, and 100 mg. Oral concentrate, 25 mg/ml. Ampules, 25 mg.

MESTINON®, see Pyridostigmine

MESTRANOL

Description/Actions: Estrogen included in combination with a progestin in various oral contraceptive formulations.

METAGLIP™, see Glipizide and Metformin

METAHYDRIN®, see Trichlormethiazide

METAMUCIL®, see Psyllium

METAPROTERENOL SULFATE—Alupent®, Metaprel®

Description/Actions: Stimulates beta-adrenergic receptors. Indicated for bronchial asthma and for reversible bronchospasm that may occur in association with bronchitis and emphysema.

Precautions/Adverse Reactions: Contraindicated in patients with cardiac arrhythmias associated with tachycardia, and should be used with caution in patients with other cardiovascular disorders. Adverse reactions include nervousness, tremor, tachycardia, palpitations, hypertension, nausea, and vomiting. Other sympathomimetic agents should not be used concurrently. Beta-adrenergic blocking agents and metaproterenol may inhibit the effect of each other.

Administration: Oral and oral inhalation.

Preparations: Tablets, 10 and 20 mg. Syrup, 10 mg/5 ml. Metered dose inhaler. Inhalant solution, 0.4%, 0.6%, and 5%.

METARAMINOL BITARTRATE—Aramine®

Description/Actions: Sympathomimetic agent indicated for parenteral administration in the prevention and treatment of the acute hypotensive state occurring with spinal anesthesia. Also used for the adjunctive treatment of hypotension due to other causes.

Preparations: Vials, 1%.

METASTRON®, see Strontium-89 Chloride

METAXALONE—Skelaxin®

Description/Actions: Skeletal muscle relaxant indicated as an adjunct to rest, physical therapy, and other measures for the relief of discomfort associated with acute, painful musculoskeletal conditions.

Preparations: Tablets, 400 mg and 800 mg.

METFORMIN HYDROCHLORIDE—Glucophage®, Glucophage® XR, Riomet™

Description/Actions: Antihyperglycemic agent indicated as monotherapy or as an adjunct to sulfonylureas or insulin in combination with diet to lower blood glucose in patients with noninsulin-dependent diabetes mellitus (NIDDM) whose diet or sulfonylurea does not result in adequate glycemic control.

Precautions/Adverse Reactions: Contraindicated in patients with renal disease and acute or chronic metabolic acidosis, CHF requiring drug treatment, and concomitant intravascular iodinated radiocontrast agent. Withhold the drug in patients undergoing radiologic studies involving iodinated contrast materials as such products may result in an acute alteration of renal function. Adverse reactions include lactic acidosis, diarrhea, nausea, vomiting, abdominal bloating, flatulence, anorexia, metallic taste, and asymptotic subnormal serum vitamin B_{12} concentrations.

Administration: Oral with meals to reduce the incidence of GI effects.

Preparations: Tablets, 500 and 850 mg, 1000 mg. Extended-release tablets, 500 mg. Oral solution, 100 mg/mL.

METHADONE HYDROCHLORIDE—Dolophine®

Description/Actions: Opioid analgesic indicated for relief of severe pain, for detoxification treatment of narcotic addiction, and for temporary maintenance treatment of narcotic addiction.

Preparations: Tablets, 5, 10, and 40 mg. Oral solution, 5 mg/5 ml and 10 mg/5 ml. Ampules and vials, 10 mg/ml.

METHAMPHETAMINE HYDROCHLORIDE—Desoxyn®

Description/Actions: Anorexiant indicated as a short-term adjunct in a regimen of weight reduction based on caloric restriction. Also used in attention deficit disorder with hyperactivity, narcolepsy, epilepsy, postencephalitic parkinsonism, and in treatment of certain depressive reactions.

Preparations: Tablets, 5 mg. Long-acting tablets, 5, 10, and 15 mg.

METHAZOLAMIDE—Neptazane®

Description/Actions: Carbonic anhydrase inhibitor indicated for adjunctive treatment of open-angle glaucoma, secondary glaucoma, and preoperatively in acute angle-closure glaucoma where delay of surgery is desired in order to lower intraocular pressure.

Preparations: Tablets, 25 and 50 mg.

METHENAMINE HIPPURATE—Hiprex®

METHENAMINE MANDELATE—Mandelamine®

Description/Actions: Urinary tract antibacterial indicated for prophylactic or suppressive treatment of frequently recurring urinary tract infections.

Preparations: Tablets, 500 mg and 1 g.

METHERGINE®, see Methylergonovine

METHICILLIN SODIUM—Staphcillin®

Description/Actions: Penicillin antibiotic indicated for the parenteral treatment of staphylococcal infections.

Preparations: Vials, 1, 4, 6, and 10 g.

METHIMAZOLE—Tapazole®

Description/Actions: Antithyroid agent indicated for the treatment of hyperthyroidism.

Preparations: Tablets, 5 and 10 mg.

METHIONINE—Pedameth®

Description/Actions: Indicated for the treatment of diaper rash in infants, and for control of odor, dermatitis, and ulceration caused by ammoniacal urine in incontinent adults.

Preparations: Capsules, 200 mg. Liquid, 75 mg/5 ml.

METHOCARBAMOL—Robaxin®

Description/Actions: Skeletal muscle relaxant indicated as an adjunct to rest, physical therapy, and other measures for the relief of discomfort associated with acute, painful musculoskeletal conditions.

Preparations: Tablets, 500 and 750 mg. Vials, 100 mg/ml.

METHOHEXITAL SODIUM—Brevital Sodium®

Description/Actions: Barbiturate general anesthetic indicated for intravenous use for induction of anesthesia, for supplementing other anesthetic agents, as anesthesia for short surgical procedures with minimum painful stimuli, or as an agent for inducing a hypnotic state.

Preparations: Vials, 500 mg, 2.5 and 5 g.

METHOTREXATE—Rheumatrex®

Description/Actions: Antineoplastic agent indicated for the treatment of gestational choriocarcinoma, in patients with chorioadenoma destruens and hydatiform mole, acute lymphocytic leukemia, meningeal leukemia, breast cancer, epidermoid cancers of the head and neck, lung cancer, lymphosarcoma, and mycosis fungoides. Also used in the symptomatic control of severe, recalcitrant, disabling psoriasis, and in the treatment of severe, active, classical, or definite rheumatoid arthritis in selected adults who have had an insufficient therapeutic response to, or are intolerant of, an adequate trial of first-line therapy, including full dose NSAIDs.

Precautions/Adverse Reactions: Methotrexate should be used only in life-threatening neoplastic diseases, or in patients with psoriasis or rheumatoid arthritis with severe, recalcitrant, disabling disease that is not adequately responsive to other forms of therapy. Patients should be closely monitored for bone marrow, liver, lung, and kidney toxicities. Methotrexate has been reported to cause fetal death and or congenital abnormalities. Not recommended for use by women of childbearing potential. Pregnant women with psoriasis or rheumatoid arthritis should not receive methotrexate. Unexpectedly severe (sometimes fatal) bone marrow suppression, aplastic anemia, and gastrointestinal toxicity have been reported with concomitant administration of methotrexate and NSAIDs. Methotrexate-induced lung disease, including acute or chronic interstitial pneumonitis, is a potentially dangerous lesion, which may occur acutely at any time during therapy. It is not always fully reversible and fatalities have been reported. Hemorrhagic enteritis and deaths from intestinal perforation may occur. Diarrhea and ulcerative stomatitis require interruption of therapy. Methotrexate may induce tumor lysis syndrome in patients with rapidly growing tumors. Severe, occasionally fatal skin reactions have been reported. Potentially fatal opportunistic infections have been reported with the use of methotrexate.

Methotrexate given concomitantly with radiotherapy may increase the risk of soft tissue necrosis and osteonecrosis.

Preparations: Tablets, 2.5 mg. Dose pack, 2.5 mg tablets (Rheumatrex). Vials, 20, 50, 100, and 250 mg. Vials, 2.5 mg/ml and 25 mg/ml.

METHOTRIMEPRAZINE—Levoprome®

Description/Actions: Analgesic administered parenterally for the treatment of moderate to severe pain in nonambulatory patients.

Preparations: Vials, 20 mg/ml.

METHOXAMINE HYDROCHLORIDE—Vasoxyl®

Description/Actions: Sympathomimetic amine indicated for parenteral use for restoring or maintaining blood pressure during anesthesia. Also used to terminate some episodes of supraventricular tachycardia.

Preparations: Ampules, 20 mg.

METHOXSALEN—Oxsoralen®, Oxsoralen-Ultra®

Description/Actions: Photoactive agent indicated for topical use with long-wave ultraviolet radiation for the repigmentation of vitiligo, and for oral use with long-wave UVA radiation for the symptomatic control of severe, recalcitrant, disabling psoriasis.

Preparations: Capsules (Oxsoralen-Ultra), 10 mg. Lotion (to be applied by a physician and not to be dispensed to patients), 1%.

METHOXYFLURANE—Penthrane®

Description/Actions: Inhalation general anesthetic usually indicated in combination with oxygen and nitrous oxide. Also used to provide analgesia in obstetrics and in minor surgical procedures.

Preparations: Bottles, 15 and 125 ml.

METHSUXIMIDE—Celontin®

Description/Actions: Anticonvulsant indicated for the control of absence (petit mal) seizures that are refractory to other drugs.

Preparations: Capsules, 150 and 300 mg.

METHYCLOTHIAZIDE—Enduron®

Description/Actions: Thiazide diuretic indicated as adjunctive therapy in edema, and in the management of hypertension.

Preparations: Tablets, 2.5 and 5 mg.

METHYLCELLULOSE—Citrucel®

Description/Actions: Laxative used in the treatment of constipation.

Preparations: Powder and liquid.

METHYLDOPA, METHYLDOPATE HYDROCHLORIDE—Aldomet®

Description/Actions: Antihypertensive agent indicated in the treatment of hypertension.

Precautions/Adverse Reactions: Contraindicated in patients with active hepatic disease because liver disorders have been associated with therapy. Other adverse reactions include sedation, headache, orthostatic hypotension, edema, bradycardia, nausea, vomiting, positive Coombs' test, and hemolytic anemia.

Administration: Oral and intravenous.

Preparations: Tablets, 125, 250, and 500 mg. Suspension, 250 mg/5 ml. Vials, 250 mg/5 ml.

METHYLENE BLUE

Description/Actions: Antiseptic and antidote. Has been used as a genitourinary antiseptic and in the management of patients with oxalate urinary tract calculi. Has also been used in the management of methemoglobinemia and as an antidote for cyanide poisoning.

Preparations: Tablets, 65 mg. Ampules, 10 mg/ml.

METHYLERGONOVINE MALEATE—Methergine®

Description/Actions: Oxytocic indicated for routine management after delivery of the placenta, postpartum atony and hemorrhage, subinvolution. Under full obstetric supervision, may be given in the second stage of labor following delivery of the anterior shoulder.

Preparations: Tablets, 0.2 mg. Ampules, 0.2 mg/ml.

METHYLIN®, see Methylphenidate

METHYLPHENIDATE HYDROCHLORIDE—Concerta™, Ritalin®, Ritalin-SR®, Methylin®

Description/Actions: Central nervous system stimulant indicated in the management of attention deficit disorder and narcolepsy.

Preparations: Tablets, 5, 10, and 20 mg. Controlled-release tablets, 20 mg. Osmotic controlled-release tablets, 18, 36, and 54 mg. Extended-release tablets, 18 mg, 36 mg, and 54 mg. Chewable tablets, 2.5 mg, 5 mg, and 10 mg. Oral solution, 5 mg/5 mL and 10 mg/5 mL.

METHYLPREDNISOLONE—Medrol®

Description/Actions: Corticosteroid indicated in a wide range of endocrine, rheumatic, allergic, dermatologic, respiratory, hematologic, neoplastic, and other disorders. Use has been reported to improve neurologic recovery in patients with acute spinal cord injury when the medication (as methylprednisolone sodium succinate) is given in the first 8 hours.

Precautions/Adverse Reactions: Contraindicated in patients with systemic fungal infections. Adverse reactions include sodium and fluid retention, potassium depletion, muscle weakness, osteoporosis, peptic ulcer, thin fragile skin, development of cushingoid state, glaucoma, cataracts, and negative nitrogen balance. May mask signs of infection and new infections may appear during use. May increase requirements for hypoglycemic agents in diabetic patients.

Administration: Oral.

Preparations: Tablets, 2, 4, 8, 16, 24, and 32 mg.

METHYLPREDNISOLONE ACETATE—Depo-Medrol®, Medrol Acetate Topical®. See discussion of Methylprednisolone.

Administration: Intramuscular, intra-articular, intralesional, and soft tissue administration. Topical.

Preparations: Vials, 20, 40, and 80 mg/ml. Ointment, 0.25% and 1%.

METHYLPREDNISOLONE SODIUM SUCCINATE—Solu-Medrol®. See discussion of Methylprednisolone.

Administration: Intravenous and intramuscular.

Preparations: Vials, 40, 125, and 500 mg, 1 and 2 g.

METHYLROSANILINE CHLORIDE, see Gentian Violet

METHYL SALICYLATE—Oil of Wintergreen

Description/Actions: Salicylate analgesic used in combination with other agents and applied topically in the management of certain dermatologic and muscular conditions.

Preparations: Lotion, liniment, and cream formulations.

METHYLTESTOSTERONE—Oreton Methyl®

Description/Actions: Androgen indicated for replacement therapy in conditions associated with a deficiency or absence of endogenous testosterone, including primary hypogonadism (e.g., testicular failure due to cryptorchidism) and hypogonadotropic hypogonadism. May be used to stimulate puberty in carefully selected males with clearly delayed puberty, and for the treatment of impotence and male climacteric symptoms when these are secondary to androgen deficiency. May also be used in women with advanced inoperable metastatic mammary cancer who are 1 to 5 years postmenopausal, and for the management of postpartum breast pain and engorgement.

Preparations: Tablets, 10 and 25 mg. Buccal tablets, 5 and 10 mg.

METHYSERGIDE MALEATE—Sansert®

Description/Actions: Indicated for the prevention or reduction of intensity and frequency of vascular headaches in patients who experience frequent and/or severe headaches. Observe for development of retroperitoneal fibrosis during long-term therapy.

Preparations: Tablets, 2 mg.

METICORTEN®, see Prednisone

METIPRANOLOL HYDROCHLORIDE—OptiPranolol®

Description/Actions: A nonselective beta-adrenergic blocking agent indicated for ophthalmic use in the treatment of ocular conditions like chronic open-angle glaucoma and ocular hypertension.

Precautions/Adverse Reactions: Contraindicated in patients with a history of bronchial asthma, severe chronic obstructive pulmonary disease, symptomatic sinus bradycardia, greater than a first degree atrioventricular block, cardiogenic shock, or overt cardiac failure. Adverse reactions include transient local discomfort, conjunctivitis, abnormal vision, and occasional systemic effects. Caution must be exercised in patients taking another beta-blocker orally for another indication.

Administration: Ophthalmic.

Preparations: Ophthalmic solution, 0.3%.

METOCLOPRAMIDE HYDROCHLORIDE—Reglan®

Description/Actions: Stimulates motility of the upper GI tract. Indicated (a) as short-term therapy for patients with symptomatic gastroesophageal reflux who fail to respond to conventional therapy, (b) for the relief of symptoms associated with diabetic gastric stasis, (c) for the prophylaxis of vomiting associated with cancer chemotherapy, (d) to facilitate small bowel intubation, and (e) to stimulate gastric emptying and intestinal transit of barium in radiological examinations.

Precautions/Adverse Reactions: Contraindicated in patients in whom the stimulation of GI motility may be dangerous (e.g., in the presence of GI hemorrhage), and in patients with epilepsy or pheochromocytoma. May cause extrapyramidal reactions and should not be used in patients receiving other drugs likely to cause such reactions. Metoclopramide produces a transient increase in plasma aldosterone. Certain patients (patients with cirrhosis or congestive heart failure) may be at risk for developing fluid retention and volume overload. If this occurs, the drug should be discontinued. Adverse reactions include drowsiness and other CNS effects. Patients should be cautioned regarding activities such as driving and operating machinery, as well as interactions with other CNS-acting drugs including alcohol. Other adverse reactions include nausea, diarrhea, visual disturbances, fluid retention, amenorrhea, gynecomastia, and impotence. There have been rare reports of an uncommon but potentially fatal symptom complex sometimes referred to as Neuroleptic Malignant Syndrome (NMS) associated with metoclopramide. Clinical manifestations of NMS include hyperthermia, muscle rigidity, altered consciousness, and evidence of autonomic instability (irregular pulse or blood pressure, tachycardia, diaphoresis, and cardiac arrhythmias).

Administration: Oral, intravenous, and intramuscular. Oral administration should be 30 minutes before meals and at bedtime.

Preparations: Tablets, 5 and 10 mg. Syrup, 5 mg/5 ml. Ampules and vials, 5 mg/ml.

METOCURINE IODIDE—Metubine Iodide®

Description/Actions: Muscle relaxant administered intravenously as an adjunct to anesthesia to induce skeletal muscle relaxation.

Preparations: Vials, 2 mg/ml.

METOLAZONE (rapidly available formulation)—Mykrox®

Description/Actions: Diuretic indicated in the management of hypertension and in the treatment of edema.

Preparations: Tablets, 0.5 (Mykrox®), 2.5, 5, and 10 mg.

METOLAZONE—Zaroxolyn®

METOPROLOL SUCCINATE—Toprol XL®

Description/Actions: A cardioselective beta-adrenergic blocking agent indicated in the management of hypertension, angina pectoris, and hemodynamically stable patients with definite or suspected acute myocardial infarction to reduce cardiovascular mortality. Metoprolol succinate is also indicated in the treatment of stable, symptomatic

NYHA class II or III heart failure of ischemic, hypertensive, or cardiomyopathic origin.

Precautions/Adverse Reactions: Contraindicated in patients with sinus bradycardia, heart block greater than first degree, cardiogenic shock, and overt cardiac failure. Adverse reactions include tiredness, dizziness, depression, bradycardia, shortness of breath, diarrhea, pruritus, and rash. Use is best avoided in patients with bronchospastic diseases, and therapy in diabetic patients must be closely monitored. Beta-blockers can precipitate or aggravate symptoms of arterial insufficiency in patients with peripheral vascular disease. Caution should be exercised in such individuals. Because of significant inotropic and chronotropic effects in patients treated with beta-blockers and calcium channel blockers of the verapamil and diltiazem type, caution should be exercised in patients treated with these agents concomitantly.

Administration: Oral and intravenous. Patients should be cautioned about the interruption or discontinuation of therapy; exacerbation of angina pectoris has occurred following the abrupt cessation of therapy, and when therapy is to be discontinued, the dosage should be gradually reduced over a period of 1–2 weeks.

Preparations: Tablets 25, 50, and 100 mg. Controlled-release tablets (Toprol XL), 25 mg, 50 mg, 100 mg, and 200 mg. Ampules and syringes, 5 mg/5 ml.

METOPROLOL TARTRATE—Lopressor®

METRODIN®, see Urofollitropin

METROGEL®, see Metronidazole

METROGEL-VAGINAL®, see Metronidazole

METRONIDAZOLE—Flagyl®, MetroGel®, MetroGel-Vaginal®, Noritate®

Description/Actions: Anti-infective agent indicated in the treatment of trichomoniasis, amebiasis, and anaerobic bacterial infections, and in the topical treatment of rosacea. Vaginal gel is indicated in the treatment of bacterial vaginosis.

Preparations: Tablets, 250 and 500 mg. Capsules, 375 mg. Extended-release tablets, 750 mg. Vials (for intravenous administration), 500 mg and 500 mg/100 ml. Gel, 0.75%. Vaginal gel, 0.75%. Cream, 1%.

METUBINE®, see Metocurine

METYRAPONE

Description/Actions: Diagnostic test of pituitary adrenocorticotropic function.

Preparations: Tablets, 250 mg.

METYROSINE—Demser®

Description/Actions: Agent for pheochromocytoma. Indicated in the treatment of patients with pheochromocytoma for preoperative preparation for surgery, management of patients when surgery is contraindicated, and the chronic treatment of patients with malignant pheochromocytoma.

Preparations: Tablets, 250 mg.

MEVACOR®, see Lovastatin

MEXILETINE HYDROCHLORIDE—Mexitil®

Description/Actions: A class IB antiarrhythmic agent that is similar to lidocaine in its electrophysiologic properties. Indicated for the suppression of symptomatic ventricular arrhythmias, including frequent premature ventricular contractions (unifocal or multifocal), couplets, and ventricular tachycardia.

Precautions/Adverse Reactions: Contraindicated in patients with cardiogenic shock or second- or third-degree AV block (unless a pacemaker is present). Adverse reactions include proarrhythmic events, GI distress, lightheadedness, tremor, and coordination difficulties.

Administration: Oral.

Preparations: Capsules, 150, 200, and 250 mg.

MEXITIL®, see Mexiletine

MEZLIN®, see Mezlocillin

MEZLOCILLIN SODIUM—Mezlin®

Description/Actions: Is bactericidal and is active against many gram-positive and gram-negative bacteria, including *Pseudomonas aeruginosa*. Is usually used in conjunction with an aminoglycoside antibiotic in the treatment of *Pseudomonas* infections.

Precautions/Adverse Reactions: Contraindicated in patients with a history of allergic reaction to any of the penicillins. Adverse reactions include hypersensitivity reactions, GI disturbances, and local reactions at the injection site.

Administration: Intravenous and intramuscular.

Preparations: Vials and infusion bottles, 1, 2, 3, 4, and 20 g.

MIACALCIN®, see Calcitonin salmon

MICARDIS®, see Telmisartan

MICARDIS® HCT, Combination of Telmisartan and Hydrochlorothiazide

MICATIN®, see Miconazole

MICONAZOLE—Monistat IV® See discussion on Miconazole Nitrate

MICONAZOLE NITRATE—Monistat 3®, Monistat 7®, Monistat-Derm®, Micatin®

Description/Actions: Antifungal agent indicated for (a) topical application in the treatment of tinea pedis, tinea cruris, tinea corporis, candidiasis, and tinea versicolor; (b) vaginal administration for vulvovaginal candidiasis; and (c) intravenous administration for systemic fungal infections.

Precautions/Adverse Reactions: Adverse reactions associated with topical and vaginal use include local irritation and itching. Adverse reactions associated with intravenous use include phlebitis, pruritus, rash, fever, nausea, and vomiting. Base contained in the vaginal suppository formulation may interact with certain rubber or latex products, such as those used in vaginal contraceptive diaphragms. Therefore, concurrent use is not recommended.

Administration: Topical, vaginal, intravenous, intrathecal, and bladder instillation.

Preparations: Cream, lotion, powder, and spray, 2%. Vaginal cream, 1%. Vaginal suppositories, 100 and 200 mg. Ampules, 10 mg/ml.

MICRO-K®, see Potassium Chloride

MICRONASE®, see Glyburide

MICRONOR®, see Norethindrone

MICROZIDE®, see Hydrochlorothiazide

MIDAMOR®, see Amiloride

MIDAZOLAM HYDROCHLORIDE—Versed®

Description/Actions: A short-acting benzodiazepine CNS depressant. Indicated (a) intramuscularly for preoperative sedation and to impair memory of perioperative events; (b) intravenously as an agent for conscious sedation prior to short diagnostic or endoscopic procedures, and in therapeutic procedures; and (c) intravenously for induction of general anesthesia, before administration of other anesthetic agents. Can also be used as a component of intravenous supplementation of nitrous oxide and oxygen (balanced anesthesia) for short surgical procedures.

Precautions/Adverse Reactions: Contraindicated in patients with acute narrow-angle glaucoma. Adverse reactions include apnea, decreased tidal volume and/or respiratory rate decrease, hypotension, and oversedation. Effects may be increased by the concurrent administration of other agents having CNS depressant, respiratory depressant, and/or hypotensive effects, and the dosage of one or both agents should be appropriately reduced. Lower dosages should be used in elderly, debilitated, and other high-risk patients.

Administration: Intravenous and intramuscular.

Preparations: Vials, 1 mg/ml and 5 mg/ml.

MIDODRINE HYDROCHLORIDE—ProAmatine®

Description/Actions: Alpha-adrenergic agonist, indicated in the treatment of orthostatic hypotension. Also used (investigational) in managing urinary incontinence.

Precautions/Adverse Reactions: Contraindicated in patients with severe heart disease, acute renal disease, urinary retention, thyrotoxicosis, pheochromocytoma, supine hypertension. Caution must be exercised in patients with diabetes. Adverse reactions include supine hypertension, bradycardia, paresthesia, pruritus (primarily of the scalp), piloerection (goose bumps), chills, dysuria, urinary frequency and urgency, and urinary retention. Use cautiously with other medications that may reduce the heart rate. Discontinue and reevaluate if the patient develops signs or symptoms of bradycardia (e.g., pulse slowing, increased dizziness, or syncope).

Administration: Oral.

Preparations: Tablets, 2.5 and 5 mg.

MIFEPREX®, see Mifepristone

MIFEPRISTONE—Mifeprex®

Description/Actions: Indicated for the medical termination of intrauterine pregnancy through the first 49 days of pregnancy.

Precautions/Adverse Reactions: Mifepristone is contraindicated in women with a known hypersensitivity to mifepristone, misoprostol, other prostaglandins, or any component of the product. It is also contraindicated in ectopic pregnancy, intrauterine device (IUD) in place, chronic adrenal failure, porphyrias, pregnancy greater than 49 days, hemorrhagic disorders, concurrent anticoagulant therapy, concurrent long-term corticosteroid therapy, undiagnosed adnexal mass, and inadequate or lack of access to medical facilities equipped to provide emergency medical care of incomplete abortion, blood transfusions, and emergency resuscitation from the first visit until discharged by the physician. In addition, mifepristone should not be used in patients unable to fully understand and comply with the treatment regimen. Women should be instructed to review the Medication Guide and Patient Agreement. Signed informed consent is required prior to treatment initiation, and a copy must be kept in the patient's file. There are no safety or efficacy data on the use of mifepristone in women with chronic medical conditions such as cardiovascular, hypertensive, hepatic, or renal disease; insulin-dependent diabetes mellitus; severe anemia; or history of heavy smoking. Women older than 35 years of age who also smoke more than 10 cigarettes per day were not included in clinical trials; therefore, treat with caution. Pregnancy termination must be confirmed by ultrasound or clinical exam. Treatment failures must be managed with surgical abortions. Vaginal bleeding is expected to last 9–16 days, but as long as 69 days has been reported. Vaginal bleeding may be severe and may require treatment with vasoconstrictors, curettage, saline infusions, and/or blood transfusions. Cases of serious bacterial infections, including very rare cases of fatal septic shock, have been reported following the use of mifepristone. Use with caution in patients with severe anemia. The effectiveness of mifepristone may be decreased if misoprostol is administered more than 2 days after mifepristone. May only be administered by qualified physicians able to assess the duration of pregnancy accurately, diagnose ectopic pregnancies, and provide surgical intervention in the event of an incomplete abortion or severe bleeding. The physician has agreed to provide these services or has made plans to provide these services through others and can assure patient access to emergency medical services. The physician must report to the manufacturer any hospitalization, transfusion, or other serious event encountered during treatment of a patient with mifepristone. No drug interaction studies have been done; however, mifepristone is metabolized by the cytochrome p450 system 3A4 and is expected to interact with drugs metabolized via the same enzyme system. Ketoconazole, itraconazole, erythromycin, and grapefruit juice may increase serum levels of mifepristone by inhibiting its metabolism. Rifampin, dexamethasone, phenytoin, phenobarbital, carbamazepine, and St. John's Wort may decrease mifepristone levels by inducing its metabolism. Mifepristone may inhibit the metabolism of drugs that are cytochrome p450 3A4 substrates. Exercise caution when coadministering with mifepristone. Pregnancy Category X. Mifepristone is used to terminate pregnancy. Excretion in human breast milk is unknown. Safety and efficacy in pediatric patients have not been established. Major adverse effects associated with mifepristone include bleeding more heavily than during a normal menstrual period (80–90%), abdominal pain/cramping (96%), nausea, vomiting, diarrhea, headache, back pain, dizziness, and fatigue.

Administration: Oral. Treatment with mifepristone requires three office visits. Signed informed consent is required by the patient prior to initiation of therapy.

Patient Care Implications: Serum human chorionic gonadotropin (HCG) levels will not adequately confirm termination of pregnancy until at least 10 days after the administration of mifepristone. Pregnancy termination must be confirmed by ultrasound and/or clinical exam. Vaginal bleeding may be heavy and require medical treatment with curettage, transfusions, vasoconstrictors, and saline infusions. Hemoglobin and hematocrit levels should be monitored. Patients should be advised to review the Medication Guide and Patient Agreement. Patients must understand the importance of completing the entire treatment schedule and returning for follow-up visits. Patients should be aware that bleeding and cramping will occur. Patients should be aware that bleeding is not proof of a complete abortion and that surgical intervention will be required for incomplete abortions. Fetal harm may occur if pregnancy is not terminated after a failed abortion with mifepristone. Physician must give the patient a phone number to call for questions or for emergencies. Patients may become pregnant again before their next menstrual period. Contraception may be resumed once termination of pregnancy is confirmed.

Preparations: Tablets, 200 mg supplied in single-dose blister packets containing 3 tablets.

MIGLITOL—Glyset®

Description/Actions: Miglitol is an antidiabetic drug indicated as an adjunct to diet in type II diabetes, alone or with a sulfonylurea.

Precautions/Adverse Reactions: Miglitol is contraindicated in ketoacidosis, inflammatory bowel disease, colonic ulceration, partial intestinal obstruction (or predisposition to such), chronic intestinal diseases associated with marked disorders of digestion, or absorption or conditions that may deteriorate from increased intestinal gas formation. Use not recommended in patients with significant renal dysfunction (serum cr >2 mg/dl), in pregnancy (Category B), and nursing mothers. Adverse reactions include flatulence, diarrhea, and abdominal pain.

Administration: Oral. Take with the first bite of each main meal.

Patient Care Implications: Whereas miglitol does not cause hypoglycemia when used alone, it can contribute to hypoglycemia when used in conjunction with sulfonylurea agents. If treatable hypoglycemia develops because of the mechanism of action of miglitol, treat with glucose instead of fructose.

Preparations: Tablets, 25, 50, and 100 mg.

MIGLUSTAT—Zavesca®

Description/Actions: Miglustat is an enzyme inhibitor used in the treatment of mild to moderate type 1 Gaucher disease when enzyme replacement therapy is not a therapeutic option. Type 1 Gaucher disease is caused by a functional deficiency of glucocerebrosidase, the enzyme that results in the degradation of the glycosphingolipid glucosylceramide. The failure of glucosylceramide to degrade results in an accumulation causing complications specific to this disease. Miglustat inhibits the enzyme needed to produce glycosphingolipids and decreases the rate to glycosphingolipid glucosylceramide formation.

Precautions/Adverse Reactions: Miglustat is contraindicated in patients who are hypersensitive to miglustat and to any component of the formulation. Cases of peripheral neuropathy have been reported; all patients should undergo baseline and repeat neurological evaluations at 6 month intervals. Those who develop numbness and tingling should have a careful reassessment of the risk/benefit of therapy. Tremor or exacerbations of existing tremor may occur; dose reduction may ameliorate the tremor. Pregnancy risk factor X. Women and men should use effective contraception during therapy. Men should maintain reliable contraceptive methods for 3 months after therapy. Excretion in breast milk unknown/breast-feeding not recommended. Use caution in renal impairment. Most common adverse effects were diarrhea (approximately 85% of patients), weight loss (65%), flatulence, abdominal pain, nausea, anorexia, headache, dizziness, tremor, and visual disturbances. Miglustat increases the clearance of imiglucerase; combination therapy is not indicated.

Administration: Oral.

Patient Care Implications: Capsules should be swallowed whole and taken at the same time each day, with or without food. May cause headache and dizziness (use caution when driving or engaging in hazardous tasks until response to drug is known). Patients may experience nausea and vomiting (small, frequent meals and good mouth care may help). Notify physician of any numbness, pain, or burning in the hands or feet, the development of tremor, or worsening of an existing tremor.

Preparations: Capsules: 100 mg

MILK OF MAGNESIA, see Magnesium Hydroxide

MILONTIN®, see Phensuximide

MILRINONE LACTATE—Primacor®

Description/Actions: Is a phosphodiesterase inhibitor and increases cardiac output by inhibiting the enzymatic hydrolysis of cAMP, resulting in both positive inotropic and vasodilating effects. Indicated for the short-term intravenous treatment of congestive heart failure.

Precautions/Adverse Reactions: Adverse reactions include ventricular arrhythmias, supraventricular arrhythmias, hypotension, angina or chest pain, and headache. Should not be used in patients with severe obstructive aortic or pulmonic valvular disease in lieu of surgical relief of the obstruction. It is recommended that it not be used in patients in the acute phase after myocardial infarction. May aggravate outflow tract obstruction in hypertrophic subaortic stenosis. If hypokalemia exists, it should be corrected with a potassium supplement before or during the use of milrinone.

Administration: Intravenous.

Preparations: Vials, milrinone lactate equivalent to 1 mg of milrinone per ml. Carpuject sterile cartridge-needle unit with Interlink System Cannula (1 mg/ml).

MILTOWN®, see Meprobamate

MINERAL OIL—Liquid Petrolatum

Description/Actions: Laxative used in the form of oil or in emulsion formulations.

MINIPRESS®, see Prazosin

MINITRAN®, see Nitroglycerin

MINOCIN®, see Minocycline

MINOCYCLINE HYDROCHLORIDE—Minocin®

Description/Actions: Tetracycline antibiotic active against many gram-positive and gram-negative bacteria, mycoplasmal, chlamydial, and rickettsial organisms, and certain spirochetes. Indicated in the treatment of respiratory and urinary tract infections and a number of other types of infections. Effective in the treatment of infections caused by *Chlamydia trachomatis* and *Ureaplasma urealyticum.* Is useful as adjunctive therapy in the management of severe acne. Is also indicated in the treatment of asymptomatic carriers of *Neisseria meningitidis.*

Precautions/Adverse Reactions: Use is best avoided during the last half of pregnancy and in childhood to the age of 8 years because of the risk of discoloration of the teeth. May cause lightheadedness, dizziness, and vertigo, and patients should be cautioned about activities such as driving or operating machinery. Other adverse reactions include nausea, vomiting, diarrhea, rash, photosensitivity reactions, and fungal superinfections. Must be used with caution in patients with impaired renal function. Absorption may be reduced by the simultaneous administration of antacids.

Administration: Oral and intravenous. May be administered orally without regard to meals.

Preparations: Capsules and tablets, 50 and 100 mg. Suspension, 50 mg/5 ml. Vials, 100 mg.

MINOXIDIL—Loniten®, Rogaine®

Description/Actions: Indicated for the treatment of hypertension that is symptomatic or associated with target organ damage and is not manageable with conventional antihypertensive regimens. Also indicated for the topical treatment of male pattern baldness of the vertex of the scalp, and female androgenetic alopecia (i.e., diffuse hair loss or thinning of the frontoparietal areas).

Preparations: Tablets, 2.5 and 10 mg (Loniten). Topical solution, 2% and 5% (Rogaine).

MINTEZOL®, see Thiabendazole

MIOSTAT®, see Carbachol

MIRADON®, see Anisindione

MIRTAZAPINE—Remeron®

Description/Actions: Antidepressant of tetracylic chemical structure indicated in the treatment of depression. Patients may begin to see improvements in 1–4 weeks.

Precautions/Adverse Reactions: Do not administer concurrently with or within 14 days of MAOIs. Use cautiously in patients with hepatic or renal dysfunction, conditions that may be exacerbated by hypotension, disease that affects hemodynamic response, history of mania or hypomania, seizure disorders, suicidal ideation, immunocompromised patients, and elderly. Antidepressants increased the risk of suicidal thinking and behavior (suicidality) in short-term studies in children and adolescents with Major Depressive Disorder (MDD) and other psychiatric disorders. Anyone considering the use of mirtazepine or any other antidepressant in a child or adolescent must balance this risk with the clinical need. Patients who are started on therapy should be observed closely for clinical worsening, suicidality, or unusual changes in behavior. Remeron® is not approved for use in pediatric patients. Adverse reactions include somnolence, increased appetite, weight gain, dizziness, nausea, dry mouth, constipation, asthenia, flu syndrome, edema, and CNS effects.

Administration: Oral.

Preparations: Tablets, 15 and 30 mg.

MISOPROSTOL—Cytotec®

Description/Actions: An analog of prostaglandin E1 that exhibits actions that protect the gastroduodenal mucosa. Indicated for the prevention of NSAID-induced gastric ulcers in patients at high risk of complications from a gastric ulcer (e.g., patients over age 60, individuals with a history of ulcer, patients taking corticosteroids).

Precautions/Adverse Reactions: Contraindicated during pregnancy because the drug exhibits an abortifacient action. Adverse reactions include diarrhea, abdominal pain, nausea, flatulence, dyspepsia, and headache. Should not be used in women of childbearing potential unless the patient requires NSAID therapy and is at high risk of developing gastric ulcers and/or associated complications.

Administration: Oral. Should be taken with a meal and the last dose of the day should be at bedtime.

Preparations: Tablets, 100 and 200 mcg.

MITHRACIN®, see Plicamycin

MITHRAMYCIN, see Plicamycin

MITOMYCIN—Mutamycin®

Description/Actions: Antineoplastic agent indicated for the parenteral treatment of disseminated adenocarcinoma of the stomach or pancreas, in combination with other agents.

Preparations: Vials, 5, 20, and 40 mg.

MITOTANE—Lysodren®

Description/Actions: Antineoplastic agent indicated in the treatment of inoperable adrenal cortical carcinoma.

Preparations: Tablets, 500 mg.

MITOXANTRONE HYDROCHLORIDE—Novantrone®

Description/Actions: Antineoplastic agent indicated in combination with other approved drug(s) (e.g., cytosine arabinoside) in the initial therapy of acute nonlymphocytic leukemia in adults. Mitoxanthrone is also indicated in the treatment of patients with secondary progressive multiple sclerosis, including progressive relapsing disease.

Precautions/Adverse Reactions: Myocardial toxicity, manifested in its most severe form by potentially fatal congestive heart failure (CHF), may occur either during therapy with mitoxantrone or months to years after termination of therapy. Secondary acute myelogenous leukemia (AML) has been reported in cancer patients treated with anthracyclines. Severe myelosuppression occurs and complete blood counts are necessary for appropriate dose adjustments. Other adverse reactions include bleeding, infection, nausea, vomiting, diarrhea, abdominal pain, stomatitis, fever, headache, alopecia, cough, dyspnea, conjunctivitis, tachycardia, and congestive heart failure. The drug may cause fetal harm when administered during pregnancy. The drug may impart a blue-green color to the urine for 24 hours after administration, and patients should be advised to expect this during the therapy.

Administration: Intravenous infusion.

Preparations: Vials, 2 mg mitoxantrone free base per ml (10 ml [20 mg], 12.5 ml [25 mg], 15 ml [30 mg]).

MITROLAN®, see Polycarbophil

MIVACRON®, see Mivacurium

MIVACURIUM CHLORIDE—Mivacron®

Description/Actions: Nondepolarizing neuromuscular blocking agent indicated as an adjunct to general anesthesia, to facilitate tracheal intubation, and to provide skeletal muscle relaxation during surgery or mechanical ventilation.

Precautions/Adverse Reactions: Use from multidose vials is contraindicated in patients with a known allergy to benzyl alcohol. Adverse reactions include transient cutaneous flushing of the face, neck, and/or chest. Must be used with caution in patients with neuromuscular disease (e.g., myasthenia gravis, myasthenic syndrome), and in patients receiving other medications that may increase and/or prolong neuromuscular block (e.g., inhalation anesthetics, aminoglycosides, quinidine, magnesium salts). May cause histamine release, and caution should be exercised in patients with clinically significant cardiovascular disease and patients with any history (e.g., asthma) suggesting a greater sensitivity to the release of histamine. Is metabolized by plasma cholinesterase, and duration of action may be markedly prolonged in the presence of genetic abnormalities of plasma cholinesterase.

Administration: Intravenous.

Preparations: Vials, 2 mg/ml. Premixed infusion in 5% Dextrose. Injection, 0.5 mg/ml. Solutions are acidic and may not be compatible with alkaline solutions having a pH greater than 8.5 (e.g., barbiturate solutions).

MOBAN®, see Molindone

MOBIC®, see Meloxicam

MOCTANIN®, see Monooctanoin

MODAFINIL—Provigil®

Description/Actions: Modafinil is indicated to improve wakefulness in patients with excessive sleepiness associated with narcolepsy, obstructive sleep apnea/hypopnea syndrome, and shift work sleep disorder.

Precautions/Adverse Reactions: Use is not recommended in patients with a history of LV hypertrophy, ischemic EKG changes, chest pain, arrhythmias, or other significant manifestations of mitral valve prolapse. Use cautiously in patients with a history of recent MI, unstable angina, hypertension, cardiovascular disease, psychosis, severe hepatic or renal impairment, and the elderly. Pregnancy Category C. Monitor patients periodically as abuse potential exists. May antagonize hormonal contraceptives. Reduce dose in the elderly. Adverse reactions include headache, infection, nausea, anxiety, depression, insomnia, and other CNS effects.

Administration: Oral.

Patient Care Implications: Instruct patients of childbearing potential who employ oral contraceptives for birth control to use alternate means of contraception. Instruct patients to avoid alcohol.

Preparations: Tablets, 100 mg and 200 (scored) mg.

MODANE®, see Bisacodyl

MODERIL®, see Rescinnamine

MODURETIC®, Combination of Amiloride and Hydrochlorothiazide

MOEXIPRIL HYDROCHLORIDE—Univasc®

Description/Actions: Angiotensin converting enzyme inhibitor used in the treatment of hypertension.

Preparations: Tablets, 7.5 and 15 mg.

MOLINDONE HYDROCHLORIDE—Moban®

Description/Actions: Antipsychotic agent indicated for the management of the manifestations of psychotic disorders.

Preparations: Tablets, 5, 10, 25, 50, and 100 mg. Oral concentrate, 20 mg/ml.

MOMETASONE FUROATE—Elocon®

Description/Actions: Topical corticosteroid indicated for the relief of the inflammatory and pruritic manifestations of corticosteroid-responsive dermatoses.

Precautions/Adverse Reactions: Adverse reactions include burning, tingling/stinging, pruritus, and signs of skin atrophy.

Administration: Topical.

Preparations: Cream, ointment, and lotion, 0.1%.

MOMETASONE FUROATE—Nasonex®

Description/Actions: Corticosteroid indicated in prophylaxis and treatment of seasonal allergic rhinitis symptoms and treatment of perennial allergic rhinitis symptoms.

Precautions/Adverse Reactions: Use not recommended in tuberculosis, varicella, vaccinia, unhealed nasal wounds, untreated fungal, bacterial, and viral infections, or ocular herpes simplex. Discontinue if nasopharyngeal candida infection occurs. If adrenal insufficiency exists following systemic corticosteroid therapy, replacement with topical corticosteroids may exacerbate symptoms of adrenal insufficiency (e.g., depression). Monitor for vision changes or if there is a history of glaucoma or cataracts. Pregnancy Category C. Cautious use in nursing mothers. Adverse reactions include headache, viral infection, pharyngitis, epistaxis, cough, upper respiratory tract infections, pain, sinusitis, and others. Instruct patients to adhere to dosing and interval recommendations. Advise patients to seek medical advice if exposed to chicken pox or measles.

Administration: Nasal.

Preparations: 50 mcg/spray in 17 g (120 sprays) metered dose, manual pump spray, and dosage counter spray. Nasal spray scent-free 50 mcg/actuation.

MONISTAT®, see Miconazole Nitrate

MONOBENZONE—Benoquin®

Description/Actions: Depigmenting agent indicated for final depigmentation in extensive vitiligo.

Preparations: Cream, 20%.

MONODOX®, see Doxycycline Monohydrate

MONOOCTANOIN—Moctanin®

Description/Actions: A solubilizing agent for treatment of cholesterol gallstones retained in the biliary tract after cholecystectomy, when other means of removing cholesterol stones in the common bile duct have failed or cannot be undertaken.

Precautions/Adverse Reactions: Contraindicated in patients with clinical jaundice, significant biliary tract infection, or with a history of recent duodenal ulcer or jejunitis. Adverse reactions include GI pain, nausea, vomiting, and diarrhea. Patients should have periodic liver function tests.

Administration: As a continuous perfusion through a catheter inserted directly into the common bile duct, or through a nasobiliary tube placed by endoscopy.

Preparations: Bottles containing 120 ml.

MONOPRIL®, see Fosinopril Sodium

MONTELUKAST—Singulair®

Description/Actions: A leukotriene antagonist indicated in prophylaxis and chronic treatment of asthma.

Precautions/Adverse Reactions: Not for primary treatment of acute attack. Not for monotherapy in treatment and management of exercise-induced bronchospasm. Monitor patients closely when withdrawing from oral steroids. Safety and efficacy in pediatric patients <12 months of age have not been established. Adverse reactions include headache, asthenia/fatigue, fever, GI disturbances, laryngitis, and pharyngitis. Instruct patients to report increased need for short-acting bronchodilators. Have appropriate rescue meds available. Continue usual regimen for exercise-induced bronchospasm prophylaxis. Pregnancy Category B.

Administration: Oral.

Preparations: Chewable tablets in cherry flavor, 4 and 5 mg. Tablets, 10 mg. 4 mg granule packets.

MONUROL®, see Fosfomycin

MORICIZINE HYDROCHLORIDE—Ethmozine®

Description/Actions: A class I antiarrhythmic agent. Indicated for the treatment of documented life-threatening arrhythmias.

Precautions/Adverse Reactions: Contraindicated in the presence of cardiogenic shock, and in patients with preexisting second- or third-degree atrioventricular block, and in patients with right bundle branch block when associated with left hemiblock unless a pacemaker is present. Adverse reactions include proarrhythmic effects, congestive heart failure, conduction abnormalities, chest pain, palpitations, dizziness, fatigue, sleep disorders, nervousness, headache, nausea, vomiting, dyspepsia, abdominal pain, paresthesias, musculoskeletal pain, blurred vision, and dyspnea.

Administration: Oral.

Preparations: Tablets, 200, 250, and 300 mg.

MORPHINE SULFATE—Astramorph PF®, Duramorph®, Kadian®, MS Contin®, MSIR®, Oramorph SR®, RMS®, Roxanol®, Roxanol SR®

Description/Actions: Opioid analgesic indicated for the relief of moderate to severe pain, for preoperative medication, to facilitate induction of anesthesia, and as an anesthetic or adjunct to anesthesia.

Precautions/Adverse Reactions: Adverse reactions include sedation and other CNS effects; patients should be cautioned regarding activities such as driving and operating machinery, as well as interactions with other CNS-acting drugs including alcohol. Other adverse reactions include constipation and hypotension. Cases of anaphylaxis, intestinal obstruction, and death have also been reported. Can cause dependence and formulations are covered under the provisions of the Controlled Substances Act.

Administration: Oral, rectal, intravenous, intramuscular, subcutaneous, epidural, intrathecal.

Preparations: Tablets, 10, 15, and 30 mg. Controlled-release tablets, 15, 30, 60, and 100 mg. (MS Contin, Oramorph SR, Roxanol SR). Sustained-release pellets in capsules, 20, 50, and 100 mg. Oral solution, 4 mg/ml, 20 mg/ml, 10 mg/5 ml, 20 mg/5 ml, and 100 mg/5 ml. Suppositories, 5, 10, 20, and 30 mg (RMS). Ampules, vials, and syringes, 2, 4, 5, 8, 10, 15, 25, and 50 mg/ml. Ampules and vials (preservative-free and can be used via epidural and intrathecal routes), 0.5 and 1 mg/ml. (Astramorph PF, Duramorph). Solution for IV injection (PCA device), 1 mg/ml, 2 mg/ml, 3 mg/ml, and 5 mg/ml.

MOTOFEN®, see Difenoxin Hydrochloride/Atropine Sulfate

MOTRIN®, see Ibuprofen

MOXIFLOXACIN HYDROCHLODIDE—Avelox®

Description/Actions: A synthetic broad spectrum fluoroquinolone antibiotic indicated for the treatment of adults with acute bacterial sinusitis, acute bacterial exacerbation of chronic bronchitis, and community acquired pneumonia.

Precautions/Adverse Reactions: Contraindicated in patients with a history of hypersensitivity to moxifloxacin or any member of the quinolone class of antimicrobial agents. The safety and effectiveness of moxifloxacin in patients less than 18 years of age and pregnant or lactating women have not been established. The drug should be avoided in patients with known prolongation of the QT interval, patients with uncorrected hypokalemia, and patients receiving class IA or class III antiarrhythmic agents, due to lack of clinical experience with the drug in these patient populations. Adverse reactions include nausea, diarrhea, dizziness, headache, abdominal pain, vomiting, taste perversion, abnormal liver function tests, and dyspepsia. Achilles and other tendon ruptures that required surgical repair or resulted in prolonged disability have been reported with moxifloxacin.

Administration: Intravenous and oral.

Preparations: Tablets, 400 mg. Injection, 400 mg/250 mL.

MS CONTIN®, see Morphine

MSIR®, see Morphine

MUCOMYST®, see Acetylcysteine

MUPIROCIN—Bactroban®

Description/Actions: Topical and intranasal antibiotic. Indicated for the topical treatment of impetigo due to *Staphylococcus aureus*, beta hemolytic *Streptococcus*, and *Streptococcus pyogenes*. Eradication of nasal colonization of methicillin-resistant *S. aureus* (MRSA) in adult patients and health care workers in certain institutional settings during outbreaks of MRSA.

Precautions/Adverse Reactions: Topical adverse reactions include burning, stinging, pain, and itching. Reactions to nasal applications include headache, rhinitis, respiratory disorder, pharyngitis, taste perversion, cough, and pruritus.

Administration: Topical, nasal.

Preparations: Ointment, 2% (15 g and 30 g). Cream, 2% (15 g and 30 g).

MUROMONAB-CD3—Orthoclone OKT$_3$®

Description/Actions: Immunosuppressant indicated for the treatment of acute allograft rejection in renal, heart, and liver transplant patients.

Precautions/Adverse Reactions: Contraindicated in patients who are in fluid overload. The most severe reaction is potentially fatal pulmonary edema, which has occurred in some patients with fluid overload prior to treatment. Patients should be evaluated for fluid overload by chest X-ray or according to the criterion of weight gain. Most patients experience fever and chills during the first 2 days of therapy. Other adverse reactions commonly encountered during the first 2 days of therapy include dyspnea, chest pain, nausea, vomiting, wheezing, diarrhea, and tremor. Therapy can result in increased susceptibility to infection. The dosage of other immunosuppressants (e.g., prednisone, azathioprine) used concomitantly should be reduced. The use of cyclosporine should be reduced or discontinued to reduce the risk of nephrotoxicity.

Administration: Intravenous.

Preparations: Ampules, 5 mg.

MUSTARGEN®, see Mechlorethamine

MUTAMYCIN®, see Mitomycin

MYAMBUTOL®, see Ethambutol

MYCELEX®, see Clotrimazole

MYCIFRADIN®, see Neomycin

MYCOBUTIN®, see Rifabutin

MYCOPHENOLATE MOFETIL—CellCept®, Myfortic®

Description/Actions: Immunosuppressant indicated in prophylaxis of organ rejection in patients receiving allogeneic renal transplants as an adjunct to cyclosporine and corticosteroids.

Precautions/Adverse Reactions: May cause neutropenia, so complete blood counts should be performed weekly for the first month, twice monthly for the second and third months, and then monthly for the first year. If neutropenia develops (absolute neutrophil count of less than 1300/mm2), treatment should be interrupted or dosage reduced. Adverse reactions include sepsis, diarrhea, vomiting, and GI tract hemorrhage. Caution must be exercised in patients with active digestive system disease. Counseling of appropriate, contraception to prevent pregnancy is recommended as the drug is contraindicated in pregnancy.

Administration: Oral and intravenous. Oral on an empty stomach. Initiate within 72 hours following transplantation. Administer IV if unable to take orally.

Preparations: Capsules, 250 mg. Tablets 500 mg. Powder for oral suspension 200 mg/ml. Powder for injection, lyophilized 500 mg. Delayed release tablets, 180 mg and 360 mg (Myfortic).

MYCOSTATIN®, see Nystatin

MYDRIACYL®, see Tropicamide

MYFORTIC®, see Mycophenolate

MYKROX®, see Metolazone

MYLANTA®, see Aluminum Hydroxide 200 mg, Magnesium Hydroxide 200 mg, Simethicone 20 mg/5 ml.

MYLANTA—Children's Tablets and Liquid. Tablets, Calcium Carbonate 400 mg; Liquid, Calcium Carbonate 400 mg/5 ml. See discussion on Calcium Carbonate.

MYLANTA AR®, see Famotidine

MYLANTA DS TABLETS®—Calcium Carbonate 700 mg, Magnesium 300 mg

MYLANTA GELCAPS®—Calcium Carbonate 550 mg, Magnesium 125 mg

MYLANTA SUPREME®—Combination Drug Containing Calcium Carbonate 400 mg and Magnesium Hydroxide 135 mg/5 ml

MYLANTA TABLETS®—Calcium Carbonate 350 mg, Magnesium Hydroxide 150 mg

MYLERAN®, see Busulfan

MYLICON®, see Simethicone

MYLOTARG®, see Gemtuzumab Oogamicin

MYOFLEX®, see Trolamine Salicylate

MYSOLINE®, see Primidone

MYTELASE®, see Ambenonium

N

NABUMETONE—Relafen®

Description/Actions: Nonsteroidal anti-inflammatory agent that exhibits analgesic, anti-inflammatory, and antipyretic actions indicated for the treatment of signs and symptoms of rheumatoid arthritis and osteoarthritis.

Precautions/Adverse Reactions: Contraindicated in patients in whom aspirin or another nonsteroidal anti-inflammatory drug induces asthma, urticaria, or other allergic-type reactions. May cause gastrointestinal effects including diarrhea, dyspepsia, abdominal pain, constipation, flatulence, nausea, vomiting, gastritis, dry mouth, and stomatitis. Use should be avoided in patients with active gastrointestinal tract disease and closely monitored in patients with a previous history of such disorders. Other adverse reactions include fluid retention, edema, dizziness, headache, pruritus, rash, tinnitus, fatigue, increased sweating, insomnia, nervousness, somnolence, and photosensitivity reactions. Use is not recommended during the third trimester of pregnancy or in nursing mothers.

Administration: Oral.

Preparations: Tablets, 500 and 750 mg.

NADOLOL—Corgard®

Description/Actions: A nonselective beta-adrenergic blocking agent indicated in the management of hypertension and angina pectoris.

Precautions/Adverse Reactions: Contraindicated in patients with bronchial asthma, sinus bradycardia, and greater than first-degree conduction block, cardiogenic shock, and overt cardiac failure. Adverse reactions include sedation, dizziness, fatigue, bradycardia, and symptoms of peripheral vascular insufficiency. Use is best avoided in patients with bronchospastic diseases, and therapy in diabetic patients must be closely monitored.

Administration: Oral. Patients should be cautioned about the interruption or discontinuation of therapy; exacerbation of angina pectoris has occurred following the abrupt cessation of therapy, and when therapy is to be discontinued, the dosage should be gradually reduced over a period of 1–2 weeks.

Preparations: Tablets, 20, 40, 80, 120, and 160 mg.

NAFARELIN ACETATE—Synarel®

Description/Actions: A synthetic agonistic analog of gonadotropin-releasing hormone. With repeated dosing, it causes a decrease in sex hormone levels. Indicated for the management of endometriosis in women 18 years of age and older, and for the treatment of central precocious puberty in children.

Precautions/Adverse Reactions: Contraindicated in pregnancy, in women who are breast-feeding, and in women with undiagnosed abnormal vaginal bleeding. Adverse reactions include hot flashes, decreased libido, vaginal dryness, headaches, and emotional lability. Although the drug usually inhibits ovulation and stops menstruation, contraception is not insured, particularly if patients miss successive doses and experience breakthrough bleeding or ovulation. Patients should use a nonhormonal method of contraception.

Administration: Nasal. Treatment of endometriosis should be started between days 2 and 4 of the menstrual cycle. Patients should be advised of the importance of having their prescription refilled in a timely manner so that they do not miss a dose. The duration of treatment should be limited to 6 months, primarily because of a concern about a loss in bone density. However, if symptoms of endometriosis recur following a 6-month course of therapy and further treatment is being considered, it is recommended that bone density be assessed before retreatment begins.

Preparations: Nasal solution, 2 mg/ml.

NAFCIL®, see Nafcillin Sodium

NAFCILLIN SODIUM—Nafcil®, Nallpen®, Unipen®

Description/Actions: Penicillin antibiotic indicated in the treatment of staphylococcal infections.

Preparations: Capsules, 250 mg. Tablets, 500 mg. Vials, 500 mg, 1, 2, and 10 g.

NAFTIFINE HYDROCHLORIDE—Naftin®

Description/Actions: Antifungal agent indicated for the topical treatment of tinea pedis, tinea cruris, and tinea corporis.

Precautions/Adverse Reactions: Adverse reactions include burning/stinging, dryness, erythema, itching, and local irritation.

Administration: Topical.

Preparations: Cream and gel, 1%.

NAFTIN®, see Naftifine

NALBUPHINE HYDROCHLORIDE—Nubain®

Description/Actions: Opioid agonist-antagonist analgesic indicated for parenteral use for the relief of moderate to severe pain. Also used as a supplement to balanced anesthesia, for preoperative and postoperative analgesia, and for obstetrical analgesia during labor and delivery.

Precautions/Adverse Reactions: Severe fetal bradycardia has been reported when nalbuphine is administered during labor. Use in pregnancy only if clearly needed.

Preparations: Ampules, vials, and syringes, 10 mg/ml and 20 mg/ml.

NALFON®, see Fenoprofen

NALIDIXIC ACID—NegGram®

Description/Actions: Anti-infective agent indicated for the treatment of urinary tract infections caused by susceptible gram-negative bacteria.

Preparations: Tablets, 250 and 500 mg, 1 g. Suspension, 250 mg/5 ml.

NALLPEN®, see Nafcillin Sodium

NALMEFENE HYDROCHLORIDE—Revex®

Description/Actions: Opioid antagonist indicated in the complete or partial reversal of effects induced by opioids and in the management of known or suspected opioid overdose. Is longer acting than naloxone.

Precautions/Adverse Reactions: Adverse reactions include nausea, vomiting, tachycardia, and hypertension. Can produce acute withdrawal symptoms in patients with physical dependence on opioids or following surgery involving high doses of opioids.

Administration: Intravenous bolus, but may be given intramuscularly or subcutaneously if venous access cannot be established.

Preparations: Ampules, 100 mcg/ml and 1 mg/ml.

NALOXONE HYDROCHLORIDE—Narcan®

Description/Actions: Opioid antagonist indicated for parenteral use for the reversal of narcotic depression induced by opioids. Is also used for the diagnosis of suspected acute opioid overdosage. Is also included in tablet formulations of pentazocine to prevent the effect of the analgesic if the product is misused by injection. Can produce acute withdrawal symptoms in patients with physical dependence on opioids or following surgery involving high doses of opioids.

Preparations: Ampules, vials, and syringes, 0.02 mg/ml and 0.4 mg/ml.

NALTREXONE HYDROCHLORIDE—ReVia®

Description/Actions: Opioid antagonist indicated to provide blockade of the pharmacologic effects of exogenously administered opioids as an adjunct to the maintenance of the opioid-free state in detoxified formerly opioid-dependent individuals. Also indicated for the treatment of alcohol dependence.

Precautions/Adverse Reactions: Naltrexone is contraindicated in patients currently dependent on opioids, including those currently maintained on opiate agonists (e.g., methadone or LAAM [levo-alpha-acetyl-methadol]).

Preparations: Tablets, 50 mg.

NANDROLONE DECANOATE—Deca-Durabolin®

Description/Actions: Anabolic steroid indicated for the parenteral management of the anemia of renal insufficiency. Adequate iron intake is required for optimal response. Should be administered deep into gluteal muscle.

Preparations: Ampules, vials, and syringes, 50 mg/ml, 100 mg/ml, and 200 mg/ml.

NANDROLONE PHENPROPIONATE—Durabolin®

Description/Actions: Anabolic steroid indicated for the parenteral treatment of metastatic breast cancer. Administer deep into gluteal muscle.

Preparations: Vials, 25 mg/ml and 50 mg/ml.

NAPHAZOLINE HYDROCHLORIDE—Privine®

Description/Actions: Decongestant indicated for nasal and ophthalmic use in the relief of congestion and related symptoms associated with various nasal and ocular conditions.

Preparations: Nasal drops and spray, 0.05%. Ophthalmic solution, 0.012%, 0.02%, 0.03%, 0.05%, 0.1%.

NAPRELAN, see Naproxen Sodium

NAPROSYN®, see Naproxen

NAPROXEN—Naprosyn®, EC Naprosyn®. See discussion on Naproxen Sodium.

NAPROXEN SODIUM—Aleve®, Anaprox®, Anaprox DS®, Naprelan®

Description/Actions: Nonsteroidal anti-inflammatory agent that inhibits prostaglandin synthesis and is indicated for the relief of mild to moderate pain, primary dysmenorrhea, rheumatoid arthritis, osteoarthritis, juvenile arthritis, ankylosing spondylitis, tendinitis and bursitis, and acute gout. Also used in the treatment of fever.

Precautions/Adverse Reactions: Should not be given to patients in whom aspirin or another NSAID causes asthma, rhinitis, urticaria, or other allergic-type reactions. May cause GI effects, and use should be avoided in patients with active GI tract disease and closely monitored in patients with a previous history of such disorders. Other adverse reactions include headache, dizziness, drowsiness, itching, skin eruptions, tinnitus, edema, and dyspnea.

Administration: Oral.

Preparations: Naproxen—Tablets, 250, 375, and 500 mg. Enteric-coated tablets, 375 and 500 mg. Suspension, 125 mg/5 ml. Naproxen sodium—Tablets, 220 (Aleve), 275 and 550 mg. Controlled-release tablets (Naprelan), 375 and 500 mg.

NARATRIPTAN—Amerge®

Description/Actions: Selective $5HT_{Ib/Id}$ receptor agonist indicated in acute treatment of migraine with or without aura, in adults. Effective in relieving the pain and other symptoms associated with migraine (e.g., nausea, photophobia). Due to its long half-life relative to other "triptans," it may be an appropriate choice for patients who have longer-lasting migraines.

Precautions/Adverse Reactions: Confirm diagnosis. Exclude underlying cardiovascular disease, supervise first dose, and consider ECG monitoring in patients with likelihood of unrecognized coronary disease. Monitor cardiovascular function in long-term intermittent use. Use cautiously in hepatic or renal dysfunction. Not recommended for use in the elderly. Contraindicated in ischemic cardiac disease, cerebrovascular disease, peripheral vascular disease, uncontrolled hypertension, severe renal or hepatic impairment, basilar or hemoplegic migraine, and within 24 hours of other 5-HT, agonist, or ergot-type drugs. Pregnancy Category C. Adverse reactions include paresthesia, dizziness, drowsiness, malaise/fatigue, and throat/neck symptoms.

Administration: Oral.

Preparations: Tablets, 1 and 2.5 mg.

NAQUA®, see Trichlormethiazide

NARCAN®, see Naloxone

NAROPIN®, see Ropivicaine Hydrochloride

NASACORT®, NASACORT AQ®, see Triamcinolone Acetonide

NASALCROM®, see Cromolyn

NASALIDE®, see Flunisolide

NASAREL®, see Flunisolide

NASCOBAL®, see Cyanocobalamin

NASONEX®, see Mometasone Furoate

NATACYN®, see Natamycin

NATAMYCIN—Natacyn®

Description/Actions: Antifungal agent indicated for ophthalmic use in the treatment of fungal blepharitis, conjunctivitis, and keratitis.

Preparations: Ophthalmic suspension, 5%.

NATEGLINIDE—Starlix®

Description/Actions: Nateglinide is indicated as monotherapy to lower blood glucose in patients with type 2 diabetes whose hyperglycemia cannot be adequately controlled by diet and exercise and who have not been chronically treated with other antidiabetic agents. Starlix® is also indicated for use in combination with metformin or a thiazolidinedione. In patients whose hyperglycemia is inadequately controlled with metformin or after therapeutic response to a thiazolidinedione. Starlix® may be added to, but not substituted for those drugs.

Precautions/Adverse Reactions: Nateglinide is contraindicated in patients with a known hypersensitivity to the drug, type I diabetes mellitus, and diabetic ketoacidosis. Hypoglycemia is a possibility with nateglinide therapy. Risk of hypoglycemia may be increased by strenuous exercise, alcohol, insufficient caloric intake, or combining with other antidiabetic agents. Use caution in patients with moderate to severe hepatic insufficiency. Glycemic control may be lost with infection, fever, trauma, or surgery, necessitating insulin therapy. Nateglinide is metabolized by the cytochrome P450 isoenzyme CYP2C9 and CYP3A4. It is an inhibitor of CYP2C9. No significant interactions were observed with the concomitant administration of glyburide, metformin, digoxin, warfarin, or diclofenac. Thiazide diuretics, corticosteroids, thyroid products, and sympathomimetic agents may decrease the hypoglycemic effect of nateglinide. Nonsteroidal anti-inflammatory agents, salicylates, monoamine oxidase inhibitors, and nonselective beta-adrenergic agents may increase the hypoglycemic effect of nateglinide. Pregnancy Category C. There are no adequate and well-controlled studies in pregnant women. Nateglinide should not be used during pregnancy. Excretion in human breast milk is unknown; therefore, nateglinide should not be administered to nursing women. Safety and efficacy in pediatric patients have not been studied. Adverse reactions observed in ≥2% of patients treated with nateglinide alone include upper respiratory infections, back pain, flu symptoms, dizziness, weight gain, arthropathy, diarrhea, accidental trauma, bronchitis, coughing, and hypoglycemia. Hyperuricemia was observed in patients treated with nateglinide alone and in combination with metformin. Hypersensitivity reactions such as rash, itching, and urticaria have been reported.

Administration: Oral.

Preparations: Tablets, 60 mg and 120 mg.

NATRECOR®, see Nesiritide Citrate

NATURETIN®, see Bendroflumethiazide

NAVANE®, see Thiothixene

NAVELBINE®, see Vinorelbine Tartrate

NEBCIN®, see Tobramycin

NEBUPENT®, see Pentamidine

NEDOCROMIL SODIUM—Tilade®

Description/Actions: Is an anti-inflammatory agent that appears to inhibit the activation of, and release of mediators (e.g., histamine) from, various inflammatory cell types associated with asthma. Indicated for maintenance therapy in the management of patients with mild to moderate bronchial asthma. Should not be used for the reversal of acute bronchospasm.

Precautions/Adverse Reactions: Adverse reactions include unpleasant taste, cough, pharyngitis, headache, upper respiratory tract infection, nausea, and vomiting.

Administration: Oral inhalation.

Preparations: Metered-dose inhaler, at least 112 metered inhalations with each actuation delivering 1.75 mg of the drug from the mouthpiece. Nebulizer solution, 0.5%.

NEDOCROMIL SODIUM OPHTHALMIC SODIUM—Alocril®

Description/Actions: Indicated for the treatment of itching associated with allergic conjunctivitis.

Precautions/Adverse Reactions: The most frequently reported adverse effect is headache. Ocular burning, irritation and stinging, unpleasant taste, and nasal congestion can also occur. More rarely, asthma, conjunctivitis, eye redness, photophobia, and rhinitis are seen.

Administration: Ophthalmic.

Preparations: Solution, 2% in 5 ml.

NEFAZODONE HYDROCHLORIDE

Description/Actions: Inhibits neuronal reuptake of serotonin and norepinephrine and indicated in the treatment of depression.

Precautions/Adverse Reactions: Nefazodone therapy has been associated with liver abnormalities ranging from asymptomatic reversible serum transaminase increases to cases of necrosis and liver failure resulting in transplant and/or death. Treatment should not be initiated in individuals with active liver disease or with elevated baseline serum transaminases. Patients should be alert for signs and symptoms of developing liver failure (jaundice, anorexia, gastrointestinal complaints, malaise, etc.) and should report them to their physician immediately. Nefazodone should be discontinued in patients with signs or symptoms suggestive of hepatocellular injury such as increased serum AST or serum ALT levels greater than 3 times the upper limit of normal. Nefazodone is contraindicated in patients who were withdrawn from therapy because of evidence of liver injury. Nefazodone is also contraindicated in patients with a known hypersensitivity to any component of the formulation or to other phenylpiperazine antidepressants. Concurrent administration of terfenadine or astemizole is contraindicated. Antidepressants increased the risk of suicidal thinking and behavior (suicidality) in short-term studies in children and adolescents with Major Depressive Disorder (MDD) and other psychiatric disorders. Anyone considering the use of nefazodone or any other antidepressant in a child or adolescent must balance this risk with the clinical need. Patients who are started on therapy should be observed closely for clinical worsening, suicidality, or unusual changes in behavior. Nefazodone is not approved for use in pediatric patients. Adverse reactions include somnolence, dizziness, lightheadedness, confusion, nausea, constipation, dry mouth, asthenia, blurred vision, abnormal vision, headache, sinus bradycardia, and orthostatic hypotension. Patients should be advised to avoid the consumption of alcoholic beverages, and cautioned about operating machinery until response is ascertained.

Administration: Oral.

Preparations: Tablets, 100, 150, 200, and 250 mg.

NEGGRAM®, see Nalidixic Acid

NELFINAVIR—Viracept®

Description/Actions: Protease inhibitor indicated in the treatment of HIV infection when antiretroviral therapy is warranted, preferably in combination with other antiretroviral agents.

Precautions/Adverse Reactions: Contraindicated with concurrent use of terfenadine, astemisole, cisapride, triazolam, or midazolam. Prescribers should review patient's drug profile and adjust accordingly prior to prescribing. Use cautiously in patients with hepatic impairment and hemophilia. Avoid use of powder in patients with phenylketonuria, as it contains phenylalanine. Adverse reactions include diarrhea, nausea, flatulence, abdominal pain, and rash.

Administration: Oral. Take with meals or light snack. Powder may be mixed in a small amount of nonacidic food or beverage (e.g., water, milk, formula) with meals. Once mixed with food or a beverage, must be used immediately or may be refrigerated for up to 6 hours.

Preparations: Tablets, 250 and 625 mg. Oral powder, 50 mg/g (contains 11.2 mg phenylalanine).

NELOVA®

Description/Actions: Oral contraceptive combination of mestranol and norethindrone.

NEMBUTAL®, see Pentobarbital

NEOMYCIN SULFATE—Mycifradin®

Description/Actions: Aminoglycoside antibiotic most often used topically, alone or in combination with other anti-infective agents, in the treatment of dermatologic, ocular, and otic infections. Has also been used orally for preoperative suppression of intestinal bacteria, for GI infections, in hepatic coma, and to reduce elevated blood cholesterol levels. Has been used as a bladder irrigant (usually with polymyxin B to prevent urinary tract infections).

Preparations: Cream and ointment, 0.5%. Tablets, 500 mg. Oral solution, 125 mg/5 ml.

NEORAL®, see Cyclosporine

NEOSAR®, see Cyclophosphamide

NEOSTIGMINE METHYLSULFATE—Prostigmin®

Description/Actions: Anticholinesterase indicated for the symptomatic control of myasthenia gravis. Methylsulfate derivative is administered parenterally and is also indicated for the prevention and treatment of postoperative distention and urinary retention, and to reverse the effects of nondepolarizing neuromuscular blocking agents (e.g., tubocurarine).

Preparations: Tablets, 15 mg. Ampules and vials, 1:4000, 1:2000, and 1:1000.

NEO-SYNEPHRINE®, see Phenylephrine

NEOTHYLLINE®, see Dyphylline

NEPTAZANE®, see Methazolamide

NESACAINE®, see Chloroprocaine

NESIRITIDE CITRATE—Natrecor®

Description/Actions: Natrecor® is indicated for the intravenous treatment of patients with acutely decompensated congestive heart failure, who have dyspnea at rest or with minimal activity.

Precautions/Adverse Reactions: Nesiritide should not be used as primary therapy for patients with cardiogenic shock or in patients with a systolic blood pressure <90 mmHg. Avoid using nesiritide in patients suspected of having or known to have low cardiac filling pressures. Not recommended for use in patients with significant valvular stenosis, restrictive or obstructive cardiomyopathy, constrictive pericarditis, pericardial tamponade, or other conditions in which cardiac output is dependent upon venous return, or for patients suspected to have low cardiac filling pressures. There is an increased incidence of symptomatic hypotension in patients receiving oral angiotensin converting enzyme (ACE) inhibitors and nesiritide. Pregnancy Category C. Use in pregnancy only if the potential benefit justifies the potential risk to the fetus. Excretion in human breast milk is unknown. Safety and efficacy in pediatric patients have not been established. Adverse reactions noted in at least 3% of the patients treated with nesiritide include hypotension, ventricular tachycardia, nonsustained ventricular tachycardia, ventricular extra systoles, headache, back pain, dizziness, anxiety, and nausea. The dose-limiting effect of nesiritide is hypotension. Use cautiously in patients with systolic blood pressure <100 mmHg at baseline, as the rate of symptomatic hypotension may be increased in this patient population. Hypotension may be prolonged. Administer only in settings where blood pressure can be monitored closely. Dosage reductions and/or discontinuation of the drug may be warranted in patients who develop hypotension.

Administration: Intravenous.

Patient Care Implications: Monitor blood pressure closely during nesiritide administration.

Preparations: Powder for injection, 1.5 mg, single-use vials.

NETILMICIN SULFATE—Netromycin®

Description/Actions: Aminoglycoside antibiotic indicated for parenteral use, primarily in the treatment of infections caused by gram-negative bacteria.

Preparations: Vials, 100 mg/ml.

NETROMYCIN®, see Netilmicin

NEUPOGEN®, see Filgrastim

NEURONTIN®, see Gabapentin

NEUTRA-PHOS K®, see Potassium Phosphate

NEUTREXIN®, see Trimetrexate Glucuronate

NEVIRAPINE—Viramune®

Description/Actions: Indicated in combination with nucleoside analog in the treatment of HIV-1 infected adults who have experienced clinical and/or immunologic deterioration.

Precautions/Adverse Reactions: Severe, life-threatening, and, in some cases, fatal hepatotoxicity, particularly in the first 18 weeks, has been reported. In some cases, patients presented with nonspecific prodromal signs or symptoms of hepatitis and progressed to hepatic failure. These events are often associated with rash. Female gender and higher CD4 counts at initiation of therapy place patients at increased risk; women with CD4 counts >250 cells/mm^3, including pregnant women, receiving nevirapine in combination with other antiretrovirals for the treatment of HIV infection, are at the greatest risk. Severe life-threatening skin reactions, including Stevens-Johnson syndrome, toxic epidermal necrolysis, and hypersensitivity reactions characterized by rash, constitutional findings, and organ dysfunction, including fatal cases, have occurred. It is essential to monitor patients closely during the first 18 weeks of therapy to detect potentially life-threatening hepatotoxicity or skin reactions.

Administration: Oral.

Preparations: Tablets, 200 mg (scored). Oral suspension, 50 mg/5 ml.

NEXIUM™, see Esomeprazole

NIACIN, see Nicotinic Acid

NIACIN AND LOVASTATIN—Advicor™

Description/Actions: Advicor™ is indicated for the treatment of primary hypercholesterolemia (heterozygous familial and nonfamilial) and mixed lipidemia (Frederickson types IIa and IIb).

Precautions/Adverse Reactions: Advicor™ is contraindicated in patients with active liver disease or unexplained persistent elevations of serum transaminases, active peptic ulcer disease, arterial bleeding, or pregnancy. It should not be substituted for equivalent doses of immediate-release (crystalline) niacin. Cases of severe hepatic toxicity, including fulminant hepatic necrosis, have occurred in patients who have substituted sustained-release niacin products for immediate-release niacin. It should be used with caution in patients who consume substantial quantities of alcohol and/or have a past history of liver disease. Niacin and lovastatin have been associated with abnormal liver tests. Use with caution in patients with unstable angina or in the acute phase of MI, especially when such patients also are receiving vasoactive drugs such as nitrates, calcium channel blockers, or adrenergic-blocking agents. Use with caution in patients predisposed to gout because elevated uric acid levels have occurred with niacin therapy. HMG-CoA reductase inhibitors cause myopathy, manifested as muscle pain or weakness associated with elevated creatine kinase. Rhabdomyolysis, with or without acute renal failure, has occurred with HMG-CoA reductase inhibitors. Risk of myopathy increased with concomitant therapy with drugs metabolized by the cytochrome P450 isoform 3A4, which increase levels of lovastatin. Niacin is excreted through the kidneys and should be used with caution in patients with renal dysfunction. Niacin extended-release tablets have been associated with slight reductions in platelet counts and prolongation in PT. Pregnancy Category X. Because of the HMG-CoA reductase inhibitor's ability to decrease synthesis of cholesterol and possibly other products of the cholesterol biosynthesis pathway, Advicor™ is contraindicated in women who are pregnant and in lactating mothers. Cholesterol and other products of the cholesterol biosynthesis pathway are essential components for fetal development. Most common adverse effect was flushing, which may be accompanied by symptoms of dizziness, tachycardia, palpitations, shortness of breath, sweating, and chills. Other common adverse reactions were headache, pain, pruritus, rash, nausea, diarrhea, and back pain.

Administration: Oral.

Patient Care Implications: Obtain liver function tests and total cholesterol profile prior to therapy. LFTs monitored every 6–12 weeks for the first 6 months, then at 6-month intervals. Lipid determination should be performed at intervals no less than 4 weeks and dosage adjusted according to patient's response. Monitor blood glucose.

Flushing may be reduced by pretreatment with aspirin (taken up to 30 minutes prior to dose) or other NSAIDs. Flushing, pruritus, and GI distress are reduced by slowly increasing the dose of niacin and avoiding administration on an empty stomach. Advise patient of risk of myopathy and to report unexplained muscle pain, tenderness, or weakness promptly. If taking with bile acid–binding resins, 4 to 6 hours should elapse. Avoid ingestion of alcohol or hot drinks at the time of administration to minimize flushing. Do not administer with grapefruit juice because of the increase in lovastatin concentrations. Discontinue therapy temporarily for elective major surgery, acute medical or surgical conditions, or if patient experiences an acute or serious condition predisposing to renal failure secondary to rhabdomyolysis.

Preparations: Tablets, extended-release niacin and immediate-release lovastatin: niacin, 500 mg, and lovastatin, 20 mg; niacin, 750 mg, and lovastatin, 20 mg; niacin, 1000 mg, and lovastatin, 20 mg.

NIACINAMIDE, see Nicotinamide

NIASPAN, see Nicotinic Acid

NICARDIPINE HYDROCHLORIDE—Cardene®, Cardene IV®

Description/Actions: A calcium channel-blocking agent that is indicated for the treatment of hypertension and for the management of chronic stable angina.

Precautions/Adverse Reactions: Contraindicated in patients with advanced aortic stenosis. Adverse reactions include flushing, headache, edema of the feet, asthenia, palpitations, dizziness, tachycardia, and nausea. Some angina patients experience increased anginal symptoms.

Administration: Oral and intravenous.

Preparations: Capsules, 20 and 30 mg. Sustained-release capsules, 30, 45, and 60 mg. Ampules, 2.5 mg/ml.

NICLOSAMIDE—Niclocide®

Description/Actions: Anthelmintic indicated for the treatment of tapeworm infections caused by beef, fish, and dwarf tapeworms.

Preparations: Tablets, 500 mg.

NICODERM®, see Nicotine

NICORETTE®, see Nicotine Polacrilex

NICORETTE DS®, see Nicotine Polacrilex

NICOTINAMIDE—Niacinamide

Description/Actions: Vitamin analog (of nicotinic acid) used in the prophylaxis and treatment of pellagra.

Preparations: Tablets, 50, 100, 125, 250, and 500 mg. Vials, 100 mg/ml.

NICOTINE—Habitrol®, Nicoderm®, Nicoderm CQ®, Nicotrol®, Nicotrol NS®, ProStep®

Description/Actions: Nicotine is contained in a multilayered transdermal system that provides systemic delivery of the drug following its application to intact skin. Indicated as an aid to smoking cessation as part of a comprehensive behavioral smoking cessation program.

Precautions/Adverse Reactions: Contraindicated during the immediate postmyocardial infarction period, and in patients with life-threatening arrhythmias or severe or worsening angina pectoris. Adverse reactions include headache, insomnia, tachycardia, erythema, pruritus, and burning at application sites.

Administration: Topical, nasal spray.

Preparations: Transdermal systems, 7, 14, and 21 mg absorbed in 24 hours (Habitrol®, Nicoderm®), 11 and 22 mg absorbed in 24 hours (ProStep®), and 5, 10, and 15 mg absorbed in 16 hours (Nicotrol). Nasal spray, 0.5 mg/spray (Nicotrol NS). Inhalation system, 10 mg (4 mg delivered), contains menthol.

NICOTINE POLACRILEX—Nicorette®, Nicorette DS®

Description/Actions: Nicotine is bound to an ion exchange resin in a chewing gum base and is absorbed through the buccal mucosa as the gum is chewed. Indicated as a temporary aid to the cigarette smoker seeking to give up his or her smoking habit while participating in a behavioral modification program.

Precautions/Adverse Reactions: Contraindicated in patients during the immediate postmyocardial infarction period, and in patients with life-threatening arrhythmias or severe or worsening angina pectoris. Should be used with caution in patients with dental problems, or with dentures, dental caps, or partial bridges to which the gum may stick and cause damage. Adverse reactions include jaw muscle ache, hiccups, nausea, vomiting, and pharyngitis.

Administration: Buccal.

Preparations: Chewing gum pieces, 2 and 4 mg.

NICOTINIC ACID—Niacin, Niaspan®, Nicobid®, Slo-Niacin®, Vitamin B₃

Description/Actions: Vitamin used to correct nicotinic acid deficiency, and in the prevention and treatment of pellagra. Has been used as adjunctive therapy in patients with significant hyperlipidemia.

Preparations: Tablets, 25, 50, 100, 125, 250, and 500 mg. Controlled-release capsules, 125, 250, 375, 400, 500, 750, and 1000 mg. Elixir, 50 mg/5 ml. Vials, 100 mg/ml.

NICOTROL®, Nicotrol® NS, see Nicotine

NIFEDIPINE—Adalat®, Adalat CC®, Procardia®, Procardia XL®

Description/Actions: Is a calcium channel- blocking agent that is indicated in the treatment of (a) vasospastic angina, (b) chronic stable angina in patients who remain symptomatic despite adequate doses of beta-adrenergic blocking agents and/or organic nitrates or who cannot tolerate these agents, and (c) hypertension.

Precautions/Adverse Reactions: Adverse reactions include hypotension, flushing, peripheral edema, dizziness, nervousness, and muscle cramps. Although usually well tolerated, concurrent therapy with a beta-adrenergic blocking agent should be closely monitored because of an increased possibility of hypotension, congestive heart failure, or exacerbation of angina.

Administration: Oral.

Preparations: Capsules, 10 and 20 mg. Controlled-release tablets, 30, 60, and 90 mg.

NILSTAT®, see Nystatin

NIMODIPINE—Nimotop®

Description/Actions: A calcium channel-blocking agent that prevents or relieves the spasm following subarachnoid hemorrhage, thereby reducing the risk of severe ischemic neurologic deficits. Indicated for the improvement of neurologic deficits due to spasm following subarachnoid hemorrhage from ruptured congenital intracranial aneurysms in patients who are in good neurologic condition.

Precautions/Adverse Reactions: Adverse reactions include decreased blood pressure, headache, nausea, and bradycardia.

Administration: Oral. Therapy should be initiated within 96 hours of the subarachnoid hemorrhage. If the capsules cannot be swallowed (e.g., at the time of surgery, or if the patient is unconscious), a hole should be made in both ends of the capsule with an 18 gauge needle, and the contents of the liquid-filled capsule withdrawn into a syringe. The contents should then be emptied into the patient's in situ nasogastric tube and washed down the tube with 30 ml of normal saline (0.9%).

Preparations: Capsules, 30 mg.

NIMOTOP®, see Nimodipine

NIPENT®, see Pentostatin

NIRAVAM™, see Alprazolam

NISOLDIPINE—Sular®

Description/Actions: Calcium channel blocker indicated in the treatment of hypertension as monotherapy or as an adjunct to other antihypertensives.

Precautions/Adverse Reactions: Use cautiously in patients with hypotension, heart failure, hepatic impairment, and coronary artery disease. Adverse reactions include peripheral edema, headache, dizziness, pharyngitis, vasodilation, sinusitis, palpitations, chest pain, nausea, rash, increased angina, and MI (rare).

Administration: Oral. Do not crush, chew, divide, or take with a high-fat meal or grapefruit juice.

Preparations: Extended-release tablets, 10, 20, 30, and 40 mg.

NITAZOXANIDE—Alinia™

Description/Actions: Nitazoxanide is a synthetic antiprotozoal. Nitazoxanide oral suspension is indicated in the treatment of diarrhea caused by *Giardia lamblia* and *Cryptosporidium parvum* in patients 1–11 years of age. Alinia™ tablets are indicated for the treatment of diarrhea caused by *Giardia lamblia* in patients 12 years of age and older.

Precautions/Adverse Reactions: Nitazoxanide is contraindicated in patients hypersensitive to nitazoxanide or any of the formulation's components. Most common adverse events were abdominal pain, diarrhea, vomiting, and headache.

Administration: Oral, with food.

Preparations: Powder for oral suspension, 100 mg/5 ml (60 ml). Tablets, 500 mg.

NITISINONE—Orfadin®

Description/Actions: Nitisinone inhibits 4–hydroxyphenylpyruvate di-oxygenase, used for the treatment of hereditary tyrosinemia type 1 (HT-1). HT-1 is a disease of the pediatric population. This disorder is characterized by progressive liver failure, increased risk of hepatocellular carcinoma, coagulopathy, painful neurologic crises, and renal tubular dysfunction resulting in rickets.

Precautions/Adverse Reactions: Nitisinone is contraindicated in patients with a hypersensitivity to nitisinone or any component of the formulation. Because it inhibits tyrosine catabolism, it must be used with dietary restriction of tyrosine and phenylalanine. Inadequate restriction can result in toxic effects to the eyes, skin, and nervous system. Plasma tyrosine levels should be kept below 500 μmol/L to avoid toxic effects to the eyes (corneal ulcers, corneal opacities, keratitis, conjunctivitis, eye pain, and photophobia), skin (painful hyperkeratotic plaques on the soles and palms), and nervous system (variable degrees of mental retardation and developmental delay). Slit-lamp exam of the eyes should be performed prior to initiation of treatment. Pregnancy Category C. Excretion in breast milk unknown; use caution. Most frequent adverse reactions were hepatic neoplasm, liver failure, conjunctivitis, corneal opacity, thrombocytopenia, and leucopenia. Leucopenia and thrombocytopenia are dose dependent; decreasing dose resulted in normalization of platelet and WBC counts.

Administration: Oral.

Preparations: Capsule, 2, 5, and 10 mg.

NITRIC OXIDE—INOmax®

Description/Actions: INOmax, in conjunction with ventilatory support and other appropriate agents, is indicated for the treatment of term and near-term (>34 weeks) neonates with hypoxic respiratory failure associated with clinical or echocardiographic evidence of pulmonary hypertension, where it improves oxygenation and reduces the need for extracorporeal membrane oxygenation.

Precautions/Adverse Reactions: INOmax should not be used in the treatment of neonates known to be dependent on right-to-left shunting of blood. Abrupt discontinuation of INOmax may lead to worsening oxygenation and increasing pulmonary arterial pressure. Adverse reactions include hypotension, withdrawal syndrome, atelectasis, hematuria, hyperglycemia, sepsis, infection, cellulitis, and stridor. INOmax should be administered with monitoring for PaO_2, methemoglobin, and NO_2.

Administration: 20 ppm maintained up to 14 days or until the underlying oxygen desaturation has resolved and the neonate is ready to be weaned from INOmax therapy. Additional therapies should be used to maximize oxygen delivery.

Preparations: Aluminum cylinders, 100 and 800 ppm.

NITRO-BID®, see Nitroglycerin

NITRODISC®, see Nitroglycerin

NITRO-DUR®, see Nitroglycerin

NITROFURANTOIN—Furadantin®, Macrobid®. See discussion on Nitrofurantoin Macrocrystals.

NITROFURANTOIN MACROCRYSTALS—Macrodantin®

Description/Actions: Urinary tract antibacterial agent indicated for urinary tract infections caused by susceptible strains of *E. coli, Proteus* species, *Klebsiella* species, *Enterobacter* species, *S. aureus,* and enterococci.

Precautions/Adverse Reactions: Contraindicated in patients with significantly impaired renal function, in pregnancy at term, and in infants under 1 month of age. Adverse reactions include nausea, vomiting, pulmonary reactions, dizziness, drowsiness, headache, peripheral neuropathy, anemia, pruritus, and urticaria.

Administration: Oral. Should be administered with food.

Preparations: Tablets, 50 and 100 mg. Suspension, 25 mg/5 ml. Capsules (macrocrystals), 25, 50, and 100 mg. Capsules (Macrobid), 100 mg (25 mg macrocrystals and 75 mg monohydrate).

NITROFURAZONE—Furacin®

Description/Actions: Anti-infective agent used topically for adjunctive therapy of patients with second- and third-degree burns, and in skin grafting where bacterial contamination may cause graft rejection and/or donor site infection.

Preparations: Cream and soluble dressing, 0.2%.

NITROGARD®, see Nitroglycerin

NITROGEN MUSTARD, see Mechlorethamine

NITROGLYCERIN (see list of preparations below for trade names)

Description/Actions: An organic nitrate indicated for the prophylaxis and treatment of patients with angina pectoris.

Precautions/Adverse Reactions: Adverse reactions include headache, dizziness, hypotension, palpitation, and cutaneous vasodilation with flushing.

Administration: Sublingual, translingual, transmucosal, oral, topical, and transdermal.

Preparations: Sublingual tablets (Nitrostat®), 0.15, 0.3, 0.4, and 0.6 mg. Translingual metered dose spray for oral use (Nitrolingual®), 0.4 mg/dose. Transmucosal (buccal) tablets (Nitrogard®), 1, 2, and 3 mg. Sustained-release capsules (Nitro-Bid®, Nitroglyn®), 2.5, 6.5, and 9 mg. Ointment (Nitro-Bid®, Nitrol®, Nitrostat®), 2%. Transdermal systems (Minitran®, Nitro-Dur®, Nitro-disc®), Transderm-Nitro®, Deponit®, 2.5, 5, 7.5, 10, and 15 mg/24 hours.

NITROGLYCERIN, INTRAVENOUS—Nitro-Bid IV®, Tridil®

Description/Actions: Administered intravenously for (a) control of blood pressure in perioperative hypertension, (b) congestive heart failure associated with acute myocardial infarction, (c) treatment of angina pectoris, and (d) production of controlled hypotension during surgical procedures.

Preparations: Ampules and vials, 0.5, 0.8, 5, and 10 mg/ml.

NITROGLYN®, see Nitroglycerin

NITROL®, see Nitroglycerin

NITROLINGUAL®, see Nitroglycerin

NITROPRESS®, see Sodium Nitroprusside

NITROSTAT®, see Nitroglycerin

NITROUS OXIDE—Laughing Gas

Description/Actions: Anesthetic gas usually used in conjunction with other anesthetics.

NIX®, see Permethrin

NIZATIDINE—Axid®

Description/Actions: A histamine H_2-receptor antagonist indicated for the treatment of active duodenal ulcer, for maintenance therapy for duodenal ulcer patients, for benign gastric ulcer, and for gastroesophageal reflux disease including erosive esophagitis.

Precautions/Adverse Reactions: Adverse reactions include somnolence, sweating, and urticaria. Patients receiving high doses of aspirin may experience increased salicylate levels when nizatidine is given concurrently.

Administration: Oral.

Preparations: Capsules, 150 and 300 mg. Oral solution, 15 mg/mL.

NIZORAL®, see Ketoconazole

NODOZ®, see Caffeine

NOLAHIST®, see Phenindamine

NOLVADEX®, see Tamoxifen

NONOXYNOL-9—Emko®

Description/Actions: Spermicide used in contraceptive formulations.

Preparations: Vaginal foam, jelly, gel, cream, and suppositories.

NORCO®, see Hydrocodone Bitartrate with Acetaminophen

NORCURON®, see Vecuronium

NOREPINEPHRINE BITARTRATE—Levarterenol, Levophed®

Description/Actions: Sympathomimetic agent having inotropic stimulating and peripheral vasoconstricting actions. Indicated for the restoration of blood pressure in controlling certain acute hypotensive states, and as an adjunct in the treatment of cardiac arrest and profound hypotension.

Preparations: Ampules, 1 mg/ml.

NORETHINDRONE—Micronor®, Norlutin®, Nor-QD®

NORETHINDRONE ACETATE—Norlutate®

Description/Actions: Progestin indicated in the treatment of amenorrhea, in abnormal uterine bleeding due to hormonal imbalance (e.g., uterine cancer), and in endometriosis. Used in combination with an estrogen in oral contraceptive formulations and in progestin-only oral contraceptive formulations.

Preparations: Tablets, 0.35 mg norethindrone for use as an oral contraceptive. Tablets, 5 mg.

NORETHYNODREL

Description/Actions: Progestin used in combination with an estrogen in various oral contraceptive formulations.

NORFLEX®, see Orphenadrine Citrate

NORFLOXACIN—Chibroxin®, Noroxin®

Description/Actions: Fluoroquinolone antibacterial agent indicated for the treatment of adults with complicated and uncomplicated urinary tract infections caused by susceptible strains. Also indicated for uncomplicated urethral and cervical gonorrhea, and prostatitis caused by *E. coli.* Indicated for ophthalmic use for ocular infections caused by susceptible bacteria.

Precautions/Adverse Reactions: Adverse reactions include nausea, headache, and dizziness. Because the drug may cause CNS effects, patients should be cautioned about engaging in activities that require mental alertness or coordination. The drug has caused arthropathy in immature animals, and it is recommended that norfloxacin not be used in children or pregnant women.

Administration: Oral and ophthalmic.

Preparations: Tablets, 400 mg. Ophthalmic solution, 0.3%.

NORGESTIMATE/ETHINYL ESTRADIOL—Ortho-Cyclen®, Ortho Tri-Cyclen®, Ortho Tri-Cyclen Lo®

Description/Actions: Is a progestin/estrogen combination oral contraceptive that acts primarily by the suppression of gonadotropins and inhibition of ovulation. Norgestimate exhibits a highly selective progestational action and minimal androgenicity. Indicated for the prevention of pregnancy in women who elect to use oral contraceptives as a method of contraception.

Precautions/Adverse Reactions: Contraindicated in women who have thrombophlebitis or a thromboembolic disorder, a past history of such disorders, cerebral vascular or coronary artery disease, known or suspected carcinoma of the breast, carcinoma of the endometrium or other known or suspected estrogen-dependent neoplasia, undiagnosed abnormal genital bleeding, cholestatic jaundice of pregnancy or jaundice with prior oral contraceptive use, hepatic adenomas or carcinomas, or known or suspected pregnancy. Adverse reactions include bleeding irregularities (e.g., breakthrough bleeding, spotting, changes in menstrual flow), gastrointestinal effects (e.g., nausea, vomiting, abdominal cramps), fluid retention, melasma, rash, reduced tolerance to carbohydrates, and vaginal candidiasis. Women should be strongly advised not to smoke because of the increased risk of cardiovascular effects.

Administration: Oral. Administered once a day at about the same time each day.

Preparations: Tablets (monophasic formulation), 0.25 mg of norgestimate, and 35 mcg of ethinyl estradiol in 21-day and 28-day regimens. Tablets (triphasic formulation), graduated doses of 0.18, 0.215, and 0.25 mg of norgestimate with each dosage used in 7 tablets in combination with 35 mcg of ethinyl estradiol, in 21-day and 28-day regimens. Tablets (triphasic formulation), graduated doses of 0.18, 0.215, and 0.25 mg of norgestimate with each dosage used in 7 tablets in combination with 25 mcg of ethinyl estradiol, in a 21-day regimen.

NORGESTREL—Ovrette®

Description/Actions: Progestin used alone as an oral contraceptive and also in combination with an estrogen in various oral contraceptive formulations.

Preparations: Tablets, 0.075 mg.

NORINYL®

Description/Actions: Oral contraceptive combination of ethinyl estradiol or mestranol with norethindrone.

NORITATE®, see Metronidazole

NORLESTRIN®

Description/Actions: Oral contraceptive combination of ethinyl estradiol with norethindrone acetate.

NORLUTATE®, see Norethindrone Acetate

NORLUTIN®, see Norethindrone

NORMIFLO®, see Ardeparin

NOR-MIL®, see Diphenoxylate

NORMODYNE®, see Labetalol

NOROXIN®, see Norfloxacin

NORPACE®, see Disopyramide

NORPLANT®, see Levonorgestrel Implant

NORPRAMIN®, see Desipramine

NOR-QD®, see Norethindrone

NORTRIPTYLINE HYDROCHLORIDE—Aventyl®, Pamelor®

Description/Actions: Tricyclic antidepressant indicated for the relief of symptoms of depression.

Preparations: Capsules, 10, 25, 50, and 75 mg. Oral solution, 10 mg/ 5 ml.

NORVASC®, see Amlodipine Besylate

NORVIR®, see Ritonavir

NORZINE®, see Thiethylperazine

NOSCAPINE

Description/Actions: Antitussive used in combination with other agents in the treatment of various respiratory conditions.

NOVAFED®, see Pseudoephedrine

NOVANTRONE®, see Mitoxantrone

NOVOBIOCIN SODIUM—Albamycin®

Description/Actions: Antibiotic used in selected infections when primary less toxic anti-infective agents are not effective or are contraindicated.

Preparations: Capsules, 250 mg.

NOVOCAIN®, see Procaine

NOVOLIN®, see Insulin

NOVOLOG®, see Insulin Aspart

NOVOPEN®

Description/Actions: Insulin delivery device that uses penfill insulin cartridges.

NPH INSULIN®, see Insulin

NUBAIN®, see Nalbuphine

NUMORPHAN®, see Oxymorphone

NUPERCAINAL®, see Dibucaine

NUPRIN®, see Ibuprofen

NUROMAX®, see Doxacurium Chloride

NUTROPIN DEPOT®, see Somatropin

NUTROPIN®, see Somatropin

NuvaRing®, see Ethinyl Estradiol and Etonogestrel

NYDRAZID®, see Isoniazid

NYSTATIN—Mycostatin®, Nilstat®

Description/Actions: Antifungal agent indicated in the treatment of cutaneous, mucocutaneous, vaginal, oral, and intestinal infections caused by *Candida albicans* and other *Candida* species.

Preparations: Tablets, 500,000 units. Troches, 200,000 units. Oral suspension, 100,000 units/ml. Vaginal tablets, 100,000 units. Cream, ointment, and powder, 100,000 units/g.

NYTOL®, see Diphenhydramine

O

OCTREOTIDE ACETATE—Sandostatin®

Description/Actions: Exhibits actions that are similar to those of the natural hormone somatostatin. Suppresses the secretion of growth hormone, serotonin, and the gastroenteropancreatic (GEP) peptides—gastrin, vasoactive intestinal peptide (VIP), insulin, glucagon, secretin, motilin, and pancreatic polypeptide. Indicated for the treatment of the symptoms of two types of gastroenteropancreatic carcinoma. Suppresses or inhibits the severe diarrhea and flushing episodes associated with metastatic carcinoid tumors, and is indicated for the treatment of profuse watery diarrhea associated with vasoactive intestinal peptide-secreting tumors. Also indicated in the treatment of acromegaly.

Precautions/Adverse Reactions: Adverse reactions include nausea, diarrhea, loose stools, abdominal discomfort, vomiting, cholelithiasis, and pain at the injection site. May cause hyperglycemia or hypoglycemia, and, in patients with diabetes, it may be necessary to adjust the dosage of insulin or oral hypoglycemic agent. May alter the absorption of nutrients, as well as medications that are administered orally.

Administration: Intravenous and subcutaneous.

Preparations: Ampules (1 ml), 0.05, 0.1, 0.2, and 0.5 mg.

OCUCLEAR®, see Oxymetazoline

OCUFEN®, see Flurbiprofen Sodium

OCUFLOX®, see Ofloxacin

OCUPRESS®, see Carteolol

OFLOXACIN—Floxin®, Floxin IV®, Floxin Otic®, Ocuflox®, Floxin® Otic, Floxin® Otic SINGLES®

Description/Actions: Fluoroquinolone anti-infective agent that exhibits a bactericidal action against many gram-positive and gram-negative bacteria. Indicated for the treatment of lower respiratory tract infections, acute, uncomplicated urethral and cervical gonorrhea, chlamydial urethritis and cervicitis, skin and skin-structure infections, urinary tract infections, and prostatitis. Also indicated for ophthalmic use in the treatment of bacterial conjunctivitis and corneal ulcers. Floxin® Otic is indicated for the treatment of otitis externa, chronic suppurative otitis media and acute otitis media.

Precautions/Adverse Reactions: Has caused arthropathy and damage to weight-bearing joints in immature animals, and its use in children under the age of 18, pregnant women, and women who are nursing is best avoided. Adverse reactions include nausea, headache, diarrhea, phototoxicity reactions, and hypersensitivity reactions. May cause dizziness, lightheadedness, insomnia, and other central nervous system effects, and patients should know how they tolerate the drug before they engage in activities (e.g., driving) that require mental alertness and coordination.

Administration: Oral, intravenous, and ophthalmic. The drug should not be taken with food.

Preparations: Tablets, 200, 300, and 400 mg. Vials, 200 and 400 mg. Ophthalmic solution (Ocuflox), 0.3%, bottles 5 mL and 10 ml. Otic Solution (Floxin Otic Singles), 0.3%, 0.25mL single dispensing container.

OGEN®, see Estropipate

OIL OF WINTERGREEN, see Methyl Salicylate

OLANZAPINE—Zyprexa®, Zydis®, Zyprexa® IM

Description/Actions: Oral olanzapine is indicated for the treatment of schizophrenia. It is also indicated for the treatment of acute mixed or manic episodes associated with Bipolar I Disorder, and the combination of oral olanzapine with lithium or valproate is indicated for the short-term treatment of acute manic episodes associated with Bipolar I Disorder. Olanzapine intramuscular is indicated for the treatment of agitation associated with schizophrenia and Bipolar I mania.

Precautions/Adverse Reactions: Use cautiously in cardio- or cerebrovascular disease, hypovolemia, dehydration, seizures, Alzheimer's disease, hepatic impairment, prostatic hypertrophy, narrow-angle glaucoma, history of paralytic ileus, breast cancer, patients at risk of aspiration pneumonia, and the elderly and debilitated. Elderly patients with dementia-related psychosis treated with atypical antipsychotic drugs are at an increased risk of death compared to placebo. Most deaths appeared to be either cardiovascular (e.g., heart failure, sudden death) or infectious (e.g., pneumonia) in nature. Olanzapine is not approved for the treatment of patients with dementia-related psychosis. Adverse reactions include somnolence, dizziness, constipation, weight gain, personality disorder, akathisia, rhinitis, postural hypotension, tachycardia, headache, fever, abdominal pain, cough, pharyngitis, nervousness, joint pain, and peripheral edema. May cause tardive dyskinesia or neuroleptic malignant syndrome.

Administration: Oral.

Preparations: Tablets, 2.5, 5, 7.5, 10, and 15 mg. Orally disintegrating tablets, 5, 10, 15, and 20 mg. Injection, 10 mg vials.

OLMESARTAN MEDOXOMIL—Benicar™

Description/Actions: Olmesartan is a selective AT1 subtype angiotensin II receptor antagonist. Olmesartan blocks the vasoconstrictor effects of angiotensin II by selectively blocking the binding of angiotensin II to the AT1 receptor in vascular smooth muscle. Olmesartan is used in the treatment of hypertension. It may be used alone or in combination with other antihypertensive agents.

Precautions/Adverse Reactions: Olmesartan is contraindicated in individuals with a hypersensitivity to olmesartan or any component of the formulation and in those with hypersensitivity to other angiotensin II receptor antagonists. Also contraindicated in patients with primary hyperaldosteronism or bilateral renal artery stenosis and in women who are in their second and third trimester of pregnancy. Pregnancy Category C (first trimester) and D (second and third trimesters). The drug should be discontinued as soon as possible when pregnancy is detected. Most common adverse reactions were dizziness, headache, hyperglycemia, diarrhea, and back pain.

Administration: Oral, with or without food.

Preparations: Tablet (film coated), 5, 20, and 40 mg.

OLOPATADINE HYDROCHLORIDE—Patanol®

Description/Actions: Antiallergic agent indicated in temporary prevention of itching of the eye due to allergic conjunctivitis.

Precautions/Adverse Reactions: Adverse reactions include headache, ocular effects (including burning/stinging, dry eye, foreign body sensation, hyperemia, keratitis, lid edema, pruritus), asthenia, cold syndrome, pharyngitis, rhinitis, sinusitis, and taste perversion. Use proper instillation techniques, being careful not to contaminate the dropper tip. Not for use with contact lenses.

Administration: Ophthalmic.

Preparations: 0.1% ophthalmic solution containing benzalkonium chloride.

OLSALAZINE SODIUM—Dipentum®

Description/Actions: Is converted in the colon into 2 molecules of 5-aminosalicylic acid (5-ASA, also known as mesalamine). Exhibits a topical anti-inflammatory action in the colon. Indicated for the maintenance of remission of ulcerative colitis in patients who are intolerant of sulfasalazine.

Precautions/Adverse Reactions: Contraindicated in patients who are hypersensitive to the salicylates. Adverse reactions include diarrhea, abdominal pain or cramps, nausea, dyspepsia, bloating, headache, fatigue, depression, rash, and arthralgia. Use should be monitored closely in patients with impaired renal function.

Administration: Oral. Should be administered with food to reduce the possibility of GI adverse reactions.

Preparations: Capsules, 250 mg.

OLUX, see Clobetasol Propionate

OMALIZUMAB—Xolair®

Description/Actions: Omalizumab is an anti-asthmatic monoclonal antibody, used for the treatment of adults and children 12 years of age and older with moderate to severe persistent asthma whose symptoms are inadequately controlled with inhaled corticosteroids. Omalizumab inhibits the binding of IgE to the high-affinity IgE receptor on the surface of mast cells and basophils. The decrease of surface-bound IgE limits the activation and release of mediators in the allergic response.

Precautions/Adverse Reactions: Omalizumab should not be administered to patients who have experienced a severe hypersensitivity reaction to omalizumab. It is not used to control acute asthma symptoms; it is for use in patients with a documented reactivity to a perennial aeroallergen and with symptoms uncontrolled by inhaled corticosteroids. Anaphylaxis has occurred within 2 hours of the first or subsequent administration; have appropriate medications for the treatment of hypersensitivity reactions. Malignant neoplasms have been reported with use in short-term studies. Safety and efficacy in children <12 years of age have not been established. Systemic or inhaled corticosteroids should not be abruptly discontinued upon initiation of omalizumab therapy. Dosing is based on pretreatment of IgE serum levels and body weight. IgE levels remain elevated up to 1 year following treatment; therefore, levels taken during treatment cannot be used as a dosage guide. Pregnancy Category B. No adequate and well-controlled studies in pregnant women; use only if clearly needed. Use caution in nursing women. Most common adverse effects were severe injection site reactions, arthralgia, leg pain, dizziness, upper respiratory tract infection, sinusitis, viral infection, and headache.

Administration: Subcutaneous

Patient Care Implications: Report immediately any reaction at injection site or signs of allergic response. May cause dizziness; use caution when driving or engaging in hazardous tasks until response to drug is known. Tell patient not to decrease dose or to stop taking any other asthma medications unless instructed by physician.

Preparations: Injection, preservative-free powder for reconstitution: 150 mg.

OMEPRAZOLE—Prilosec®, Zegerid™

Description/Actions: Inhibits the enzyme system known as the acid or proton pump at the secretory surface of the gastric parietal cell. Blocks the final step of acid production and is a potent inhibitor of gastric acid secretion. Indicated for the short-term treatment (4–8 weeks) of symptomatic gastroesophageal reflux disease, the maintenance treatment of healed erosive esophagitis, the long-term treatment of pathological hypersecretory conditions (e.g., Zollinger-Ellison syndrome), and the short-term treatment of active duodenal ulcer. Also used in treatment of active duodenal ulcer associated with *H. pylori* infection in combination with clarithromycin.

Precautions/Adverse Reactions: Adverse reactions include headache, diarrhea, abdominal pain, and nausea.

Administration: Oral. The drug should be taken before eating and capsules should be swallowed whole and not be opened, chewed, or crushed.

Preparations: Delayed-release capsules, 10, 20, and 40 mg. Powder for oral suspension, 20 mg and 40 mg.

OMNICEF®, see Cefdinir

OMNIPEN®, see Ampicillin

ONCASPAR®, see Pegaspargase

ONCOVIN®, see Vincristine

ONDANSETRON HYDROCHLORIDE—Zofran®, Zofran ODT

Description/Actions: Is a selective blocking agent of the serotonin 5-HT$_3$ receptor type. Indicated for the prevention of nausea and vomiting associated with initial and repeat courses of emetogenic cancer chemotherapy, including high-dose cisplatin. Also indicated for the prevention of postoperative nausea and vomiting.

Precautions/Adverse Reactions: Adverse reactions include diarrhea, headache, constipation, and elevations of hepatic enzyme levels.

Administration: Oral and intravenous.

Preparations: Tablets, 4, 8, and 24 mg. Oral disintegrating tablets 4 and 8 mg. Oral solution, 4 mg/5 ml. Vials, 2 mg/ml in 2 ml single-dose vials and 20 ml multidose vials; 32 mg/50 ml (premixed) in single-dose containers.

ONTAK®, see Denileukin Diftitox

OPHTHAINE®, see Proparacaine

OPIUM

Description/Actions: Mixture of alkaloids including morphine and codeine. Various formulations are used in the management of pain, cough, and diarrhea.

Preparations: Tincture, 10% (opium tincture, deodorized).

OPTIMINE®, see Azatadine

OPTIPRANOLOL® see Metipranolol

OPTIVAR®, see Azelastine

ORALET®, see Fentanyl Citrate

ORAMORPH SR®, see Morphine Sulfate

ORAP®, see Pimozide

ORATROL®, see Dichlorphenamide

ORETIC®, see Hydrochlorothiazide

ORETON METHYL®, see Methyltestosterone

ORFADIN®, see Nitisinone

ORGARAN®, see Danaparoid Sodium

ORINASE®, see Tolbutamide

ORLISTAT—Xenical®

Description/Actions: Orlistat works by inhibiting the absorption of dietary fat. It is indicated as an adjunct to a reduced calorie diet in obesity management, including weight loss and weight maintenance, to reduce the risk of weight regain after loss. Use in patients with an initial body mass index of ≥ 30 kg/m² or ≥ 27 kg/m² in the presence of other risk factors (e.g., hypertension, diabetes, dyslipidemia).

Precautions/Adverse Reactions: Orlistat is contraindicated in chronic malabsorption syndrome and cholestasis. Use cautiously in hypertoxaluria and calcium oxalate nephrolithiasis. Weight loss may affect doses needed for antidiabetic drugs. Pregnancy Category B. Not recommended for use in nursing mothers. Adverse reactions may include GI effects (oily spotting, flatus with discharge, fecal urgency, fatty/oily stools, oily evacuation, increased defecation, and fecal incontinence).

Administration: Oral.

Patient Care Implications: Instruct patients to eat a balanced reduced calorie diet with about 30% of calories from fat. Spread daily fat intake over

3 meals. GI side effects may decrease over time. Higher doses do not add benefit. Orlistat may reduce the absorption of fat-soluble vitamins.

Preparations: Capsules, 120 mg.

ORNADE®, Combination of Chlorpheniramine and Phenylpropanolamine

ORPHENADRINE CITRATE—Norflex®

Description/Actions: Skeletal muscle relaxant indicated as an adjunct to rest, physical therapy, and other measures for the relief of discomfort associated with acute painful musculoskeletal conditions.

Preparations: Tablets, 100 mg. Ampules, 60 mg. Extended-release tablets, 100 mg.

ORTHO-CEPT®, see Desogestrel/Ethinyl Estradiol

ORTHO-CYCLEN®, see Norgestimate/Ethinyl Estradiol

ORTHO-EVRA™, see Ethinyl Estradiol and Norelgestromin

ORTHO-NOVUM®

Description/Actions: Oral contraceptive combination of ethinyl estradiol or mestranol with norethindrone.

ORTHO TRI-CYCLEN®, see Norgestimate/Ethinyl Estradiol

ORTHO TRI-CYCLEN LO®, see Norgestimate/Ethinyl Estradiol

ORTHOCLONE OKT3®, see Muromonab-CD3

ORUDIS®, see Ketoprofen

ORUVAIL®, see Ketoprofen

OS-CAL®, see Calcium Carbonate

OSELTAMIVIR—Tamiflu®

Description/Actions: Oseltamivir acts as a neuraminidase inhibitor for the treatment of influenza A and B.

Precautions/Adverse Reactions: Oseltamivir dosage has to be adjusted in patients with renal impairment. Also, the drug should not be administered to children under 1, pregnant women, and breast-feeding women. The most common complaints are nausea and vomiting. Other common side effects are bronchitis, insomnia, vertigo, diarrhea, abdominal pain, dizziness, headache, cough, and fatigue. Arrythmias, confusion, and seizures have also been reported.

Administration: Oral.

Patient Care Implications: Oseltamivir dosage should be adjusted in patients with renal impairment. For patients with creatinine clearance of 10–30 ml/min, the dosage should be reduced to 75 mg PO once a day for 5 days. The drug should not be administered to children under 18, pregnant women, and breast-feeding women.

Preparations: Tablet, 75 mg. Oral suspension, 12 mg/ml.

OSMITROL®, see Mannitol

OTRIVIN®, see Xylometazoline

OVRAL®

Description/Actions: Oral contraceptive combination of ethinyl estradiol and norgestrel.

OVRETTE®, see Norgestrel

OVULEN®

Description/Actions: Oral contraceptive combination of mestranol and ethynodiol diacetate.

OXACILLIN SODIUM—Prostaphlin®

Description/Actions: Penicillin antibiotic indicated in the treatment of staphylococcal infections.

Preparations: Capsules, 250 and 500 mg. Powder for oral solution, 250 mg/5 ml when reconstituted. Vials, 250 and 500 mg, 2, 4, and 10 g.

OXALIPLATIN—Eloxatin™

Description/Actions: Oxaliplatin is an antineoplastic agent that undergoes nonenzymatic conversion to several active derivatives that covalently bind with macromolecules and thus inhibit DNA replication and transcription. Oxaliplatin is indicated for use in combination with 5-fluorouracil (5-FU) and leucovorin (LV) for adjuvant treatment of stage III colon cancer patients who have undergone complete resection of the primary tumor. It is also indicated for use in combination with 5-FU/LV for the treatment of advanced carcinoma of the colon or rectum.

Precautions/Adverse Reactions: Oxaliplatin should not be administered to patients with a known allergy to platinum compounds or oxaliplatin. Anaphylactic-like reactions have been reported and may occur within minutes of administration. Oxaliplatin has been associated with pulmonary fibrosis, which may be fatal. If unexplained respiratory symptoms such as nonproductive cough, dyspnea, crackles, or radiological pulmonary infiltrates occur, oxaliplatin should be discontinued until further pulmonary investigation excludes interstitial lung disease or pulmonary fibrosis. Oxaliplatin is associated with two types of neuropathy. One is an acute, reversible, primarily peripheral, sensory neuropathy that occurs within hours or 1 to 2 days. It resolves within 14 days and frequently recurs with further dosing. The second type of neuropathy is a persistent (>14 days), primarily peripheral, sensory neuropathy that is usually characterized by paresthesias, dysesthesias, or hypoesthesias but may also include deficits in proprioception that can interfere with daily activities. The most common adverse effects were peripheral sensory neuropathies, fatigue, neutropenia, nausea, emesis, and diarrhea. Pregnancy Category D.

Administration: IV infusion.

Preparations: Injection, preservative-free lyophilized powder for reconstitution: 50 and 100 mg.

OXAMNIQUINE—Vansil®

Description/Actions: Antiparasitic agent indicated in the treatment of infections caused by *Schistosoma mansoni*.

Preparations: Capsules, 250 mg.

OXANDRIN®, see Oxandrolone

OXAPROZIN—Daypro®

Description/Actions: Nonsteroidal anti-inflammatory agent that inhibits prostaglandin synthesis and exhibits analgesic, anti-inflammatory, and antipyretic actions. Indicated for acute and long-term use in the management of osteoarthritis and rheumatoid arthritis.

Precautions/Adverse Reactions: Contraindicated in patients with the syndrome of nasal polyps, angioedema, and bronchospastic reactivity to aspirin or another nonsteroidal anti-inflammatory drug. May cause gastrointestinal effects including nausea, dyspepsia, constipation, diarrhea, abdominal pain/distress, anorexia, flatulence, and vomiting. Use should be avoided in patients with active gastrointestinal tract disease and closely monitored in patients with a previous history of such disorders. Use is not recommended during the third trimester of pregnancy. May prolong bleeding time and concurrent use with warfarin should be closely monitored.

Administration: Oral.

Preparations: Caplets, 600 mg.

OXAZEPAM—Serax®

Description/Actions: Benzodiazepine indicated for the management of anxiety disorders or for the short-term relief of the symptoms of anxiety. Also useful in anxiety associated with depression and in alcoholics experiencing alcohol withdrawal.

Precautions/Adverse Reactions: Adverse reactions include drowsiness and other CNS effects; patients should be cautioned regarding activities such as driving and operating machinery, as well as interactions with other CNS-acting drugs including alcohol. Can cause dependence and is included in Schedule IV.

Administration: Oral.

Preparations: Capsules and tablets, 10, 15, and 30 mg.

OXCARBAZEPINE—Trileptal®

Description/Actions: Oxcarbazepine is an antiepileptic/anticonvulsant indicated for use as monotherapy or adjunctive therapy in the treatment of partial seizures in adults and children ages 4–16 with epilepsy.

Precautions/Adverse Reactions: Oxcarbazepine is contraindicated in patients with a hypersensitivity to oxcarbazepine or any component of the formulation. Its use has been associated with central nervous system-related adverse events, most of which were cognitive symptoms including psychomotor slowing, difficulty with concentration, speech or language problems, somnolence or fatigue, and coordination abnormalities, including ataxia and gait disturbances. Clinically significant hyponatremia can develop while on therapy; monitoring of serum sodium levels should be considered for patients during maintenance therapy. Use with caution in patients with previous hypersensitivity to carbamazepine—a cross-sensitivity occurs in 25–30%. Concurrent use with hormonal contraceptives may render this method of contraception less effective (nonhormonal contraceptive measures are recommended). Pregnancy Category C. There are no adequate well-controlled clinical studies in pregnant women; however, oxcarbazepine is closely structurally related to carbamazepine (teratogenic in humans). Should be used during pregnancy only if the potential benefit justifies the potential risk to the fetus. Oxcarbazepine and its active metabolite are excreted in human breast milk; the decision to utilize oxcarbazepine in nursing women must be based on the potential adverse effects in the nursing infant and take into account the importance of the drug to the mother. Some adverse effects are somnolence, headache, ataxia, fatigue, vertigo, vomiting, nausea, abdominal pain, tremor, dyspepsia, abnormal gait, hyponatremia, and diplopia.

Administration: Oral.

Patient Care Implications: Inform patients who have exhibited hypersensitivity reactions to carbamazepine that there is the possibility (25–30%) of cross-sensitivity reactions with oxcarbazepine. Inform patients of childbearing age that hormonal contraceptives may be less effective while on oxcarbazepine (see precaution section). Use caution if alcohol is taken with oxcarbazepine, due to the possible additive sedative effects. Early in therapy it may cause dizziness and somnolence—advise patients not to drive or operate heavy machinery until they have gained experience on oxcarbazepine to determine if it will adversely affect their ability to drive or operate heavy machinery.

Preparations: Suspension, oral: 300 mg/5 ml (250 ml). Tablet: 150 mg, 300 mg, and 600 mg.

OXICONAZOLE NITRATE—Oxistat®

Description/Actions: A topically applied antifungal agent that is indicated for the topical treatment of tinea pedis, tinea cruris, and tinea corporis.

Precautions/Adverse Reactions: Adverse reactions include itching, burning, and irritation.

Administration: Topical.

Preparations: Cream, 1%. Lotion, 1%.

OXISTAT®, see Oxiconazole

OXSORALEN®, see Methoxsalen

OXSORALEN-ULTRA®, see Methoxsalen

OXTRIPHYLLINE—Choline Theophyllinate, Choledyl®

Description/Actions: Bronchodilator indicated for relief of bronchial asthma and for reversible bronchospasm associated with chronic bronchitis and emphysema.

Preparations: Tablets, 100 and 200 mg. Syrup, 50 mg/5 ml. Elixir, 100 mg/5 ml.

OXYBENZONE

Description/Actions: Sunscreen used in combination with other agents in sunscreen formulations.

OXYBUTYNIN CHLORIDE—Ditropan®, Ditropan XL®

Description/Actions: Antispasmodic indicated for the relief of symptoms associated with voiding in patients with uninhibited neurogenic and reflex neurogenic bladder. Also indicated in the treatment of nocturia, frequent urination, urgency, and incontinence.

Precautions/Adverse Reactions: Oxybutynin is contraindicated in patients with a know hypersensitivity to it or to any component of the formulation. Oxybutynin is contraindicated in patients with urinary retention, gastric retention or uncontrolled narrow angle glaucoma and in patients who are at risk for these conditions. Use with caution in patients with hepatic or renal impairment, clinically significant bladder outflow obstruction, and gastrointestinal obstructive disorders. Use with caution in patients with ulcerative colitis, intestinal atony, and myasthenia gravis. Oxybutynin should be used with caution in patients who have gastrointestinal reflux disease and who are currently taking drugs (such as biphosphonates) that can cause or exacerbate esophagitis. Pregnancy Category B. Excretion in human breast milk is unknown. Most common side effects associated with the use of oxybutynin include: dry mouth, blurred vision, constipation, somnolence, dizziness, diarrhea, urinary tract infections and headache. Other reported side effects include: insomnia, nervousness, abdominal pain, hypertension, palpitation, vasodilation, flatulence, gastrointestinal reflux, upper respiratory infection, cough, dry skin, rash, impaired urination, tachycardia, hallucinations, cycloplegia, mydriasis, impotence and suppression of lactation. Heat prostration (fever and heat stroke) may occur because of decreased sweating.

Preparations: Tablets, 5 mg. Extended-release tablets, 5 and 10 mg. Syrup, 5 mg/5 ml. Transdermal patch, 36 mg of oxybutynin delivering 3.9 mg of oxybutynin/day (Oxytrol™).

OXYCODONE AND ACETAMINOPHEN

Description/Actions: Acetaminophen and oxycodone are used together to treat moderate to severe pain due to cancer, dental procedures, headache, back pain, arthralgias, and myalgias. The combination of these two drugs produces additive analgesia as compared to the same doses of either agent alone.

Precautions/Adverse Reactions: Acetaminophen-oxycodone should be used cautiously in patients with GI disease, including GI obstruction or ileus, ulcerative colitis, or preexisting constipation. It should not be administered to patients who are hypersensitive to oxycodone or acetaminophen. Oxycodone is contraindicated in patients who have or are suspected of having paralytic ileus. Caution should also be used in patients with asthma or severe pulmonary disease, head trauma, cardiac arrhythmias, hypotension, hypovolemia, renal impairment, hepatic disease, or anemia. Oxycodone may cause psychologic dependence, which may lead to substance abuse in a small percentage of patients. Abrupt discontinuation of prolonged acetaminophen-oxycodone therapy can result in withdrawal symptoms. Patients should be tapered off gradually to avoid a withdrawal reaction. Adverse reactions include respiratory depression, GI effects, and hepatic and renal toxicity.

Administration: Oral.

Preparations: Tablets, 2.5/325 mg, 5/325 mg, 5/500 mg, 7.5/325 mg, 7.5/500 mg, 10/325 mg, 10/650 mg. Capsules, 5/500 mg. Oral solution, 5 ml–5/325 mg.

OXYCODONE HYDROCHLORIDE—Oxycontin®, Oxyfast®, Roxicodone®

OXYCODONE TEREPHTHALATE

Description/Actions: A centrally acting opioid analgesic indicated for the relief of moderate to moderately severe pain.

Precautions/Adverse Reactions: Adverse reactions include sedation and other CNS effects; patients should be cautioned regarding activities such as driving and operating machinery, as well as interactions with other CNS-acting drugs including alcohol. Other adverse reactions include constipation, nausea, and vomiting. Can cause dependence and formulations are covered under the provisions of the Controlled Substances Act.

Administration: Oral.

Preparations: Tablets, 5 mg. Controlled-release tablets, 10, 20, 40, and 80 mg. Solution, 5 mg/5 ml. Concentrated oral solution, 20 mg/ml.

OXYFAST®, see Oxycodone

OXYGEN

Description/Actions: Gas administered by inhalation in situations in which there is insufficient oxygen available to tissues.

Preparations: Gas

OXYMETAZOLINE HYDROCHLORIDE—Afrin®, Ocuclear®

Description/Actions: Decongestant administered topically in the form of nose drops or a nasal spray, and as an ophthalmic solution for the relief of redness of the eye due to minor eye irritations.

Preparations: Drops, 0.025%. Drops and spray, 0.05%.

OXYMETHOLONE—Anadrol-50®

Description/Actions: Anabolic steroid indicated in the treatment of anemias caused by deficient red cell production.

Preparations: Tablets, 50 mg.

OXYMORPHONE HYDROCHLORIDE—Numorphan®

Description/Actions: Opioid analgesic indicated for parenteral and rectal use for the relief of moderate to severe pain.

Preparations: Ampules and vials, 1 mg/ml and 1.5 mg/ml. Suppositories, 5 mg.

OXYTETRACYCLINE HYDROCHLORIDE—Terramycin®

Description/Actions: Tetracycline antibiotic indicated for the treatment of infections caused by susceptible organisms.

Preparations: Capsules, 250 mg. Ampules and vials (for intramuscular use), 50 mg/ml and 125 mg/ml. Formulations including polymyxin B sulfate are used topically for the treatment of ocular, dermatologic, and vaginal infections.

OXYTOCIN—Pitocin®, Syntocinon®

Description/Actions: Oxytocic hormone indicated for parenteral use to initiate or improve uterine contractions (e.g., when it is desirable to induce labor), and to produce uterine contractions during the third stage of labor and to control postpartum bleeding or hemorrhage. Also used in the form of a nasal spray for initial milk letdown.

Preparations: Ampules, 5 and 10 units. Vials, 10 units/ml. Syringes, 10 units. Nasal spray, 40 units/ml.

OXYTROL™, see Oxybutynin Chloride

P

PABA, see Para-aminobenzoic Acid

PACLITAXEL—Taxol®

Description/Actions: Antineoplastic agent indicated for the treatment of metastatic carcinoma of the ovary and metastatic carcinoma of the breast, after failure of first-line or subsequent chemotherapy.

Precautions/Adverse Reactions: Contraindicated in patients who are hypersensitive to the drug or to polyoxyethylated castor oil (Cremophor EL—a solubilizing agent included in the formulation), and in patients with a history of such reactions to other drugs that are available in formulations containing polyoxyethylated castor oil. Is also contraindicated in patients with baseline neutropenia of <1500 cells/mm3. May cause myelosuppression (neutropenia, thrombocytopenia, anemia) and the resultant risks of infection and bleeding; frequent peripheral blood counts should be performed. Therapy must be closely monitored when other drugs causing myelosuppression are used concurrently or sequentially. Use has been associated with a high incidence of hypersensitivity reactions, and patients should be premedicated with a corticosteroid (e.g., dexamethasone), antihistamine (e.g., diphenhydramine), and a histamine H2-receptor antagonist (e.g., cimetidine). Other adverse reactions include peripheral neuropathy, hypotension, bradycardia, severe conduction abnormalities, arthralgia/myalgia, nausea, vomiting, diarrhea, mucositis, alopecia, and hepatic effects. Metabolism may be inhibited by the concurrent administration of ketoconazole. Women of childbearing potential should be advised to avoid becoming pregnant during treatment with the drug.

Administration: Intravenous. The concentrated solution of paclitaxel may extract the plasticizer DEHP from plasticized polyvinyl chloride (PVC) equipment or devices used to prepare solutions for infusion. Contact of the concentrate with such equipment or devices is not recommended, and diluted solutions should be stored in bottles (glass, polypropylene) or plastic bags (polypropylene, polyolefin) and administered through polyethylene-lined administration sets. The diluted solution should be administered through an inline filter with a microporous membrane not greater than 0.22 microns. Gloves should be worn when handling and preparing the solutions.

Preparations: Vials, 30 mg/5 ml (paclitaxel concentrate).

PALIVIZUMAB—Synagis®

Description/Actions: Palivizumab is an immunomodulator (antiviral monoclonal antibody) indicated in the prevention of serious lower respiratory tract infections caused by respiratory syncytial virus (RSV) in pediatric patients at high risk for RSV disease. RSV disease is the leading cause of pneumonia and bronchiolitis in infants.

Precautions/Adverse Reactions: Anaphylaxis and anaphylactoid reactions have occurred during therapy with palivizumab. Have epinephrine available for treatment of acute allergic reactions. Adverse reactions include vomiting, diarrhea, local reactions, erythma, upper respiratory infections, otitis media, rhinitis, rash, pain, hernia, SGOT increases, and pharyngitis.

Administration: Give by IM injection in the anterolateral thigh.

Patient Care Implications: Do not administer in the gluteal muscle because of the risk of sciatic nerve damage. Volumes of over 1 ml should be administered in divided doses. The first dose should be administered prior to the start of the season. Patients should continue to receive the medication throughout the season, including those who contract RSV. This product is not indicated for the treatment of established RSV. As with all IM injections, caution should be used when administering to patients with coagulation disorders.

Preparations: Vial, 50 mg for injection after reconstitution. Liquid solution, 50 mg and 100 mg vials.

PALONOSETRON—Aloxi™

Description/Actions: Palonosetron is an antiemetic and antinauseant agent used in the prevention of acute and delayed chemotherapy-induced nausea and vomiting. It is thought that chemotherapeutic agents produce nausea and vomiting by releasing serotonin from the enterochromaffin cells of the small intestine and that the released serotonin then activates $5-HT_3$ receptors located on vagal afferents to initiate the vomiting reflex. Palonosetron is a selective $5-HT_3$ receptor antagonist, blocking serotonin, both peripherally on vagal nerve terminals and centrally in the chemoreceptor trigger zone.

Precautions/Adverse Reactions: Palonosetron is contraindicated in individuals hypersensitive to palonosetron or any component of the formulation. Hypersensitivity reactions may occur in patients who have exhibited hypersensitivity to other selective $5-HT_3$ receptor antagonists. Use with caution in patients with congenital QT syndrome or other risk factors for QT prolongation (e.g., electrolyte abnormalities, diuretics, or anti-arrhythmics). Pregnancy Category B. Excretion in breast milk unknown/breast-feeding not recommended. Most common side effects were headache, constipation, diarrhea, dizziness, and fatigue.

Administration: Intravenous.

Patient Care Implications: Report immediately any chest pain, respiratory difficulty, pain or itching at infusion site. May cause dizziness or weakness; use caution when driving or engaging in hazardous tasks until response to drug is known.

Preparation: Injection, solution: 0.05 mg/ml (5 mL).

PAMELOR®, see Nortriptyline

PAMIDRONATE DISODIUM—Aredia®

Description/Actions: Inhibits bone resorption; adsorbs to calcium phosphate in bone and may directly block dissolution of this mineral component of bone. Indicated in conjunction with adequate hydration (to restore the urine output to about 2 liters per day) for the treatment of moderate or severe hypercalcemia associated with malignancy, with or without bone metastases. Also indicated for the treatment of Paget's disease and management of osteolytic bone lesions associated with multiple myeloma.

Precautions/Adverse Reactions: Contraindicated in patients who are hypersensitive to the drug or to etidronate. Adverse reactions include low-grade fever, infusion site reactions (redness, swelling, pain), fluid overload, generalized pain, hypertension, abdominal pain, anorexia, constipation, nausea, vomiting, urinary tract infection, bone pain, anemia, hypokalemia, hypomagnesemia, and hypophosphatemia. Serum calcium, electrolytes, phosphate, magnesium, and creatinine, and complete blood count, differential, and hematocrit/hemoglobin must be closely monitored.

Administration: Intravenous infusion.

Preparations: Vials, 30, 60, and 90 mg.

PAMINE®, see Methscopolamine

PANADOL®, see Acetaminophen

PANCREASE®, see Pancrelipase

PANCREATIN

Description/Actions: Digestive enzyme often used in combination with other agents as a digestive aid.

PANCRECARB MS-8®—Pancreatic Enzymes—Lipase 8000 units, Amylase 40,000 units, Protease 45,000 units

PANCRELIPASE—Pancrease®, Viokase®, Zymase®

Description/Actions: Digestive enzyme representing a standardized pancreatic enzyme concentrate that is indicated as a digestive aid in the treatment of disorders associated with pancreatic insufficiency.

Preparations: Capsules, tablets, and powder.

PANCURONIUM BROMIDE—Pavulon®

Description/Actions: Nondepolarizing neuromuscular blocking agent indicated for parenteral use as an adjunct to general anesthesia, to facilitate tracheal intubation, and to provide skeletal muscle relaxation during surgery or mechanical ventilation.

Preparations: Ampules and vials, 1 mg/ml and 2 mg/ml.

PANDEL®, see Hydrocortisone

PANIXINE DISPERDOSE™, see Cephalexin

PANMYCIN®, see Tetracycline

PANTOPRAZOLE SODIUM—Protonix®

Description/Actions: Proton pump inhibitor indicated in the short-term treatment (up to 8 weeks) of erosive esophagitis associated with gastroesophageal reflux disease (GERD). For those patients who have not healed after 8 weeks of therapy, an additional 8-week course of Protonix may be considered.

Precautions/Adverse Reactions: The safety and efficacy of Protonix for maintenance therapy (e.g., beyond 16 weeks) have not been established. Protonix is contraindicated in patients with known hypersensitivity to any component of the formulation. Adverse effects include headache, diarrhea, flatulence, abdominal pain, rash, eructation, insomnia, and hyperglycemia.

Administrations: Intravenous and oral.

Patient Care Implications: Protonix delayed-release tablets should be swallowed whole, with or without food in the stomach. Patients should be cautioned that tablets should not be split, chewed, or crushed. Use in-line filter for intravenous administration.

Preparations: Delayed-release tablets, 20 and 40 mg. Powder for injection, 40 mg.

PAPAVERINE HYDROCHLORIDE—Pavabid®

Description/Actions: Vasodilator indicated for the relief of cerebral and peripheral ischemia associated with arterial spasm and myocardial ischemia complicated by arrhythmias.

Preparations: Tablets, 30, 60, 100, 200, and 300 mg. Controlled-release capsules, 150 mg. Ampules, 30 mg/ml.

PARA-AMINOBENZOIC ACID—PABA, Potaba®

Description/Actions: Has been used orally in the treatment of conditions such as scleroderma, dermatomyositis, and Peyronie's disease, and topically as a sunscreen and protectant.

Preparations: Capsules and tablets (as the potassium salt), 500 mg. Packets (as the potassium salt), 2 g. Powder.

PARA-AMINOSALICYLIC ACID, see Aminosalicylate Sodium

PARAFLEX®, see Chlorzoxazone

PARAFON FORTE DSC®, see Chlorzoxazone

PARALDEHYDE

Description/Actions: Sedative-hypnotic and anticonvulsant used in some patients with delirium tremens and other psychiatric states characterized by excitement. Has been used in the emergency treatment of tetanus, eclampsia, and status epilepticus.

Preparations: Liquid that has been administered orally and rectally. Ampules and vials, 1 g/ml.

PARAMETHADION

Description/Actions: Anticonvulsant indicated for the control of absence (petit mal) seizures that are refractory to treatment with other drugs.

Preparations: Capsules, 150 and 300 mg. Oral solution, 300 mg/ml.

PARAPLATIN®, see Carboplatin

PARCOPA™, see Carbidopa

PAREGORIC—Camphorated Opium Tincture

Description/Actions: Analgesic and antidiarrheal. Contains opium alkaloids and is used in the treatment of diarrhea and in conditions associated with pain.

Preparations: Liquid containing the equivalent of 2 mg of morphine per 5 ml.

PARICALCITOL—Zemplar®

Description/Actions: Paricalcitol is a synthetic vitamin D analog. Vitamin D and paricalcitol have been shown to reduce parathyroid levels. Paricalcitol is indicated for the prevention and treatment of secondary hyperparathyroidism associated with chronic renal failure.

Precautions/Adverse Reactions: Paricalcitol should not be administered to patients with evidence of vitamin D toxicity, hypercalcemia, or with hypersensitivity to any of the components of this product. Adverse reactions include chills, sepsis, palpitation, nausea, edema, and pneumonia.

Administration: Intravenous.

Patient Care Implications: Instruct patients about the importance of adhering to a dietary regimen of calcium supplementation and phosphorous restriction. Teach patients about the necessity of frequent follow-up blood work to ensure proper dosing of the drug is achieved.

Preparations: Vial, 5 mcg/ml.

PARLODEL®, see Bromocriptine

PARNATE®, see Tranylcypromine

PAROMOMYCIN SULFATE—Humatin®

Description/Actions: Anti-infective agent indicated in the treatment of intestinal amebiasis. Has also been used as adjunctive therapy in the management of hepatic coma.

Preparations: Capsules, 250 mg.

PAROXETINE HYDROCHLORIDE—Paxil®, Paxil CR®

Description/Actions: Is a selective serotonin reuptake inhibitor. Indicated for the treatment of depression, panic disorders, social anxiety disorders, obsessive-compulsive disorders, and post-traumatic stress disorders. Paxil® CR is also indicated for the treatment of Premenstrual Dysphoric Disorder and for the treatment of social anxiety disorder.

Precautions/Adverse Reactions: Contraindicated in patients taking a monoamine oxidase inhibitor (MAOI) or thioridazine. Antidepressants increased the risk of suicidal thinking and behavior (suicidality) in short-term studies in children and adolescents with Major Depressive Disorder (MDD) and other psychiatric disorders. Anyone considering the use of paroxetine or any other antidepressant in a child or adolescent must balance this risk with the clinical need. Patients who are started on therapy should be observed closely for clinical worsening, suicidality, or unusual changes in behavior. Paxil® is not approved for use in pediatric patients. Adverse reactions include nausea, dry mouth, asthenia, somnolence, dizziness, insomnia, tremor, nervousness, sweating, ejaculatory disturbance, and other male genital disorders. May decrease appetite, resulting in weight loss. Should not be used concomitantly with an MAOI, or during either the 14-day period following discontinuation of treatment with an MAOI or the 14-day period preceding initiation of treatment with an MAOI. Concomitant use with tryptophan is not recommended. Dosage should be tapered prior to discontinuation of therapy.

Administration: Oral.

Preparations: Tablets, 10, 20, 30, and 40 mg. Suspension 10 mg/5 ml. Controlled-release tablets, 12.5, 25, and 37.5 mg.

PARSIDOL®, see Ethopropazine

PAS, see Aminosalicylate Sodium

PATANOL®—see Olopatadine Hydrochloride

PATHILON®, see Tridihexethyl Chloride

PATHOCIL®, see Dicloxacillin

PAVABID®, see Papaverine

PAVULON®, see Pancuronium

PAXAREL®, see Acetylcarbromal

PAXIL®, see Paroxetine Hydrochloride

PAXIL CR®, see Paroxetine Hydrochloride

PAXIPAM®, see Halazepam

PBZ®, see Tripelennamine

PCE®, see Erythromycin Base

PECTIN
Description/Actions: Adsorbent used in combination with agents such as kaolin for the treatment of diarrhea.

PEDAMETH®, see Methionine

PEDIALYTE®
Description/Actions: Fluid and electrolyte replacement. A liter contains dextrose 25 g (fructose 5 g, in fruit flavors), sodium 45 mEq, potassium 20 mEq, chloride 35 mEq, citrate 30 mEq with 100 calories.

Preparations: Liquid and freezer pops.

PEDIAZOLE®, Combination of Erythromycin Ethylsuccinate and Sulfisoxazole

PEG, see Polyethylene Glycol

PEGADEMASE BOVINE—Adagen®
Description/Actions: Also known as PEGADA, is prepared by attaching numerous strands of polyethylene glycol (PEG) to adenosine deaminase (ADA) of bovine origin. Indicated for enzyme replacement therapy for ADA deficiency in patients with severe combined immunodeficiency disease (SCID) who are not suitable candidates for—or who have failed—bone marrow transplantation.

Precautions/Adverse Reactions: Contraindicated in patients with severe thrombocytopenia. Adverse reactions include headache and pain at injection site.

Administration: Intramuscular.

Preparations: Vials, 250 units/ml.

PEGANONE®, see Ethotoin

PEGASPARGASE—Oncaspar®

Description/Actions: Is a modified form of L-asparaginase (derived from *E. coli*) that is produced by conjugating units of monomethoxypolyethylene glycol (PEG) to the enzyme. Causes a rapid depletion of asparagine resulting in the destruction of leukemic cells that are unable to synthesize asparagine. Indicated for patients with acute lymphoblastic leukemia who require L-asparaginase in their treatment regimen, but have developed hypersensitivity to the native forms of L-asparaginase. Is generally used in combination with other chemotherapeutic agents.

Precautions/Adverse Reactions: Contraindicated in patients with a history of pancreatitis or who have had significant hemorrhagic events associated with prior asparaginase therapy. Is less likely than asparaginase to cause hypersensitivity reactions but may cause immediate and life-threatening anaphylaxis. May cause pancreatitis, and frequent serum amylase determinations should be obtained to detect early evidence of pancreatitis. Thrombosis may occur, and, if possible, the concurrent use of other drugs that may increase the risk of bleeding (e.g., warfarin, aspirin, NSAIDs) should be avoided. Other adverse reactions include hyperglycemia, liver function abnormalities, nausea, vomiting, fever, and malaise.

Administration: Intravenous or intramuscular. The vials should not be shaken.

Preparations: Vials, 3,750 IU in 5 ml.

PEGASYS®, see Peginterferon Alfa-2a

PEGINTERFERON ALFA-2a—Pegasys®

Description/Actions: Peginterferon alfa-2a is indicated for the treatment of chronic hepatitis C, alone or in combination with ribavirin, in patients who have compensated liver disease and have not been previously treated with interferon alpha.

Precautions/Adverse Reactions: Peginterferon alfa-2a is contraindicated in patients with a known hypersensitivity to peginterferon alfa-2a or any of its components, interferon alfa, or polyethylene glycol (PEG). It should not be used in patients with autoimmune hepatitis, hepatic decompensation (Child-Pugh class B and C), or previous treatment with interferon, and in neonates and infants because it contains benzyl alcohol. Life-threatening or fatal neuropsychiatric reactions such as suicide, suicide ideation, depression, relapse of drug addiction, and drug overdose may manifest in patients. Avoid use in severe psychiatric disorders. Must use caution in patients with a history of depression. Serious and severe bacterial infections, some fatal, have been observed. Dyspnea, pulmonary infiltrates, pneumonia, bronchiolitis obliterans, interstitial pneumonitis, and sarcoidosis, some resulting in respiratory failure and/or patient deaths, may be induced or aggravated by peginterferon alfa-2a. Ulcerative colitis and hemorrhagic/ischemic colitis, sometimes fatal, have been observed. Discontinue immediately if abdominal pain, bloody diarrhea, and fever develop. Treatment should be suspended if signs of pancreatitis are seen. Peginterferon may induce or aggravate decrease or loss of vision, retinopathy, including macular edema, retinal artery or vein thrombosis, retinal hemorrhages and cotton wool spots, optic neuritis, and papilledema. Pregnancy Category C. There are no adequate or well-controlled studies in pregnant women. Very high doses are abortifacient in Rhesus monkeys and are assumed to have abortifacient potential in humans. Excretion into breast milk is unknown; breast-feeding not recommended during treatment. Most common adverse reactions are headache, fatigue, pyrexia, insomnia, depression, dizziness, nausea, diarrhea, abdominal pain, neutropenia, myalgia, impaired concentration, and arthralgia.

Administration: Monotherapy: Subcutaneous injection.

Preparations: Injection, solution: 180 mcg/ml (1.2 ml). Store in refrigerator (2°C to 8°C). Do not freeze or shake; protect from light. Vials are for single use only. Discard any unused portion.

PEGVISOMANT—Somavert®

Description/Actions: Pegvisomant is an analog of human growth hormone (GH) that has been structurally altered to act as a GH receptor antagonist. Pegvisomant selectively binds to GH receptors where it blocks the binding of endogenous GH and interferes with GH signal transduction. This results in decreased serum concentrations of insulin-like growth factor-I (IGF-I) and other GH-responsive proteins. Pegvisomant is indicated for the treatment of acromegaly in patients resistant to or unable to tolerate other therapies.

Precautions/Adverse Reactions: Pegvisomant is contraindicated in patients hypersensitive to pegvisomant or any of its components.

GH opposes the effects of insulin on carbohydrate metabolism by decreasing insulin sensitivity. Monitor diabetic patients carefully and reduce doses of anti-diabetic drugs as needed. In clinical studies, patients on opioids often needed higher serum pegvisomant concentrations to achieve appropriate IGF-I suppression compared with patients not receiving opioids. A state of functional GH deficiency may result; observe carefully for the clinical signs and symptoms of a GH-deficient state. Serum IGF-I concentrations should be monitored and maintained within the age-adjusted normal range. Elevation of liver tests were reported; use caution with hepatic disease and monitor LFTs. Pregnancy Category B. No adequate and well-controlled studies; use only if clearly needed during pregnancy. Excretion in breast milk unknown/use caution. Most common adverse reactions are pain, diarrhea, nausea, abnormal liver function tests, injection site reaction, infections, hypertension, chest pain, peripheral edema, and dizziness.

Administration: Subcutaneous.

Patient Care Implications: Inform patients to discontinue immediately and contact their physician if they become jaundiced. May cause dizziness. Use caution with driving or operating heavy machinery until response to drug is known.

Preparations: Injection, powder for reconstitution. Preservative free: 10 mg, 15 mg, 20 mg vial.

PEMIROLAST—Alamast®

Description/Actions: Pemirolast is used for the relief of ophthalmic pruritus due to allergic conjunctivitis.

Precautions/Adverse Reactions: The most frequent adverse effects associated with pemirolast ophthalmic solution were generally mild and included headache, rhinitis, cold/flu symptoms, burning, dry eye, foreign body sensation, and ocular discomfort. Other, nonocular adverse events included were back pain, bronchitis, cough, dysmenorrhea, fever, sneezing, nasal congestion, and sinusitis.

Administration: Ophthalmic.

Patient Care Implications: Do not touch the eyelids or surrounding areas with the dropper tip to prevent contamination of the dropper tip and solution. Keep the bottle tightly closed when not in use. Patients should not wear contact lens if their eye is red. Patients should wait at least 10 minutes after instilling Alamast before they insert their contact lenses.

Preparations: 0.1% ophthalmic solution, in 10 ml dropper bottles.

PEMOLINE—Cylert®

Description/Actions: Central nervous system stimulant indicated in the treatment of attention deficit disorder.

Preparations: Tablets, 18.75, 37.5, and 75 mg. Chewable tablets, 37.5 mg.

PENBUTOLOL SULFATE—Levatol®

Description/Actions: A nonselective beta-adrenergic blocking agent with mild intrinsic sympathomimetic activity. Indicated in the treatment of hypertension.

Precautions/Adverse Reactions: Contraindicated in patients with bronchial asthma, cardiogenic shock, severe bradycardia, and second- and third-degree atrioventricular conduction block. Adverse reactions include headache, dizziness, fatigue, and nausea. Use is best avoided in patients with bronchospastic diseases, and therapy in diabetic patients must be closely monitored.

Administration: Oral. Patients should be cautioned about the interruption or discontinuation of therapy; exacerbation of angina pectoris has occurred following the abrupt cessation of therapy, and, when therapy is to be discontinued, the dosage should be gradually reduced over a period of 1 to 2 weeks.

Preparations: Tablets, 20 mg.

PENCICLOVIR—Denavir®

Description/Actions: Antiviral agent indicated for the treatment of topical recurrent herpes simplex labialis (cold sores) on the lips and face in adults. Topical cream form of the active component of the oral antiviral prodrug famciclovir.

Precautions/Adverse Reactions: Contraindicated in patients with previous and significant adverse reactions to famciclovir. Do not use on mucous membranes or near eyes. Use cautiously in the immunocompromised patient. Adverse reactions include headache and mild skin irritation.

Administration: Topical.

Preparations: 1% cream.

PENETREX®, see Enoxacin

PENICILLAMINE—Cuprimine®, Depen®

Description/Actions: Chelating agent indicated in the treatment of Wilson's disease, cystinuria, and in patients with severe, active rheumatoid arthritis who have failed to respond to an adequate trial of conventional therapy.

Preparations: Capsules and tablets, 125 and 250 mg.

PENICILLIN G POTASSIUM

Description/Actions: Penicillin antibiotic active against gram-positive and gram-negative cocci, gram-positive and selected gram-negative bacilli, and certain spirochetes.

Precautions/Adverse Reactions: Contraindicated in patients with a history of allergic reaction to any of the penicillins. Adverse reactions include hypersensitivity reactions.

Administration: Intravenous, intramuscular, and oral.

Preparations: Tablets, 200,000, 250,000 and 400,000 units. Oral solution, 400,000 units/5 ml. Vials, 200,000, 500,000, 1, 5, 10, and 20 million units.

PENICILLIN G SODIUM

Preparations: Vials, 5 million units.

PENICILLIN V POTASSIUM—Beepen VK®, Betapen VK®, Ledercillin VK®, Pen-Vee K®, VCillin K®, Veetids®

Description/Actions: Penicillin antibiotic primarily active against gram-positive bacteria and is commonly used in conditions such as respiratory tract infections caused by susceptible organisms (e.g., streptococci).

Precautions/Adverse Reactions: Contraindicated in patients with a history of allergic reaction to any of the penicillins. Adverse reactions include hypersensitivity reactions, rash, and nausea.

Administration: Oral. May be administered without regard to meals.

Preparations: Solution, 125 mg/5 ml.

PENLAC NAIL LACQUER®, see Cicloprox

PENTAERYTHRITOL TETRANITRATE

Description/Actions: Antianginal agent used in the prophylactic treatment of angina pectoris.

Preparations: Tablets, 10, 20, and 40 mg. Controlled-release tablets, 80 mg.

PENTAGASTRIN—Peptavlon®

Description/Actions: Diagnostic agent for evaluation of gastric acid secretory function.

Preparations: Ampules, 0.25 mg/ml.

PENTAM 300®, see Pentamidine Isethionate

PENTAMIDINE ISETHIONATE—NebuPent®, Pentam 300®

Description/Actions: Antiprotozoal agent indicated for parenteral use in the treatment of *Pneumocystis carinii* pneumonia and for use via inhalation in the prevention of *Pneumocystis carinii* pneumonia in high-risk human immunodeficiency virus (HIV)–infected patients.

Preparations: Vials, 300 mg. Vials for aerosol use, 300 mg.

PENTASA®, see Mesalamine

PENTAZOCINE—Talwin®

Description/Actions: Opioid agonist-antagonist analgesic indicated for the relief of moderate to severe pain, as an analgesic during labor, as a sedative prior to surgery, and as a supplement in balanced anesthesia.

Preparations: Tablets (as the hydrochloride with naloxone hydrochloride), 50 mg (Talwin Nx®). Ampules, vials, and syringes (as the lactate), 30 mg/ml.

PENTAZOCINE HYDROCHLORIDE AND ACETAMINOPHEN— Talacen®

Description/Actions: Acetaminophen and pentazocine are used together to treat mild to moderate pain. This combination produces a greater analgesic effect than when either is used alone. Also, this combination might cause fewer adverse reactions than do equianalgesic doses of either agent alone.

Precautions/Adverse Reactions: Pentazocine is not recommended for use in the elderly due to the potential for increased CNS side effects, such as confusion and hallucinations. Adverse effects are those of the individual drug components.

Administration: Oral.

Preparations: Caplets and tablets, pentazocine 25 mg/acetaminophen 650 mg.

PENTHRANE®, see Methoxyflurane

PENTOBARBITAL SODIUM—Nembutal®

Description/Actions: Barbiturate sedative hypnotic used in the management of anxiety and insomnia. Also used parenterally as a preanesthetic medication and for the emergency control of acute convulsive episodes.

Preparations: Capsules, 50 and 100 mg. Elixir, pentobarbital acid equivalent to 20 mg of the sodium salt/5 ml. Suppositories, 30, 60, 120, and 200 mg. Vials and syringes, 50 mg/ml.

PENTOSAN POLYSULFATE SODIUM—Elmiron®

Description/Actions: Bladder protectant indicated in relief of bladder pain or discomfort associated with interstitial cystitis. A semisynthetic, low molecular weight, heparin-like compound that exerts both anticoagulant and fibrinolytic effects.

Precautions/Adverse Reactions: Use cautiously in bleeding disorders or conditions associated with an increased risk of bleeding (e.g., surgery, coagulopathy, aneurysm, hemophilia, GI ulceration, polyps, diverticulitis), in patients with a history of heparin-induced thrombocytopenia, hepatic insufficiency, and splenic disorders. Additive effects may be expected when administered with other anticoagulant drugs, such as warfarin or heparin, and possible similar effects when administered with aspirin or thrombolytics. Adverse reactions include alopecia, GI disturbances, headache, rash, abdominal pain, liver function abnormalities, dizziness, hemorrhage, or increased bleeding times.

Administration: Oral. Take with water 1 hour before or 2 hours after meals.

Preparations: Capsules, 100 mg.

PENTOSTATIN—Nipent®

Description/Actions: Antineoplastic agent indicated as single-agent treatment for adult patients with alpha-interferon-refractory hairy cell leukemia.

Precautions/Adverse Reactions: May cause myelosuppression (e.g., neutropenia), and, in patients with infections, efforts should be made to control the infection before treatment is initiated or resumed. Other adverse reactions include gastrointestinal effects (e.g., nausea, vomiting, anorexia, diarrhea), respiratory effects (e.g., increased cough, upper respiratory infection), nervous system effects (e.g., fatigue, neurologic disorders), fever, infection, pain, elevated hepatic function tests, genitourinary disorders, headache, allergic reactions, chills, myalgia, and rash. May cause fetal harm if administered during pregnancy. Concurrent use with fludarabine phosphate is not recommended because of the risk of pulmonary toxicity.

Administration: Intravenous.

Preparations: Vials, 10 mg.

PENTOTHAL®, see Thiopental

PENTOXIFYLLINE—Trental®

Description/Actions: A xanthine derivative that decreases the viscosity and improves the flow properties of blood. Indicated for the treatment of intermittent claudication on the basis of chronic occlusive arterial disease of the limbs.

Precautions/Adverse Reactions: Contraindicated in patients who have previously exhibited intolerance to a xanthine derivative (e.g., caffeine, theophylline). Adverse reactions include nausea.

Administration: Oral.

Preparations: Controlled-release tablets, 400 mg.

PEN-VEE K®, see Penicillin V Potassium

PEPCID®, see Famotidine

PEPCID AC®, see Famotidine

PEPCID RFD®, see Famotidine

PEPTAVLON®, see Pentagastrin

PEPTO-BISMOL®, see Bismuth Subsalicylate

PERCOCET®, Combination of Oxycodone and Acetaminophen

PERCODAN®, Combination of Oxycodone and Aspirin

PERGOLIDE MESYLATE—Permax®

Description/Actions: An ergot derivative that acts by stimulating dopamine receptors. Indicated as an adjunctive treatment to levodopa/carbidopa in the management of Parkinson's disease.

Precautions/Adverse Reactions: Patients treated with pergolide have reported falling asleep while engaged in activities of daily living, including the operation of motor vehicles, which sometimes resulted in accidents. Adverse reactions include somnolence, drowsiness, dyskinesia, dizziness, hallucinations, fatigue, insomnia, nausea, constipation, diarrhea, dyspepsia, rhinitis, and orthostatic hypotension. Effectiveness may be decreased by dopamine antagonists (e.g., phenothiazines, haloperidol) or metoclopramide.

Administration: Oral.

Preparations: Tablets, 0.05, 0.25, and 1 mg.

PERGONAL®, see Menotropins

PERIACTIN®, see Cyproheptadine

PERIDEX®, see Chlorhexidine Gluconate

PERMAPEN®, see Benzathine Penicillin G

PERMAX®, see Pergolide

PERMETHRIN—Elimite®, Nix®

Description/Actions: A synthetic pyrethroid that is indicated for the single-application treatment of infestation with *Pediculus humanus* var. *capitis* (the head louse) and its nits (eggs), and for the single-application treatment of scabies. Also indicated for prophylaxis during epidemic (20% of an institutional population are infected or immediate household contacts).

Precautions/Adverse Reactions: Contraindicated in patients with a known hypersensitivity to any synthetic pyrethroid or pyrethrin, or to chrysanthemums. Adverse reactions include itching, mild burning or stinging, tingling, numbness, or scalp rash.

Administration: Topical.

Preparations: Cream, 5%. Cream rinse, 1% (for head lice infestation). Lotion, 1%.

PERMITIL®, see Fluphenazine

PEROXIDE, see Hydrogen Peroxide

PERPHENAZINE—Trilafon®

Description/Actions: Phenothiazine antipsychotic agent and antiemetic.

Preparations: Tablets, 2, 4, 8, and 16 mg. Controlled-release tablets, 8 mg. Oral concentrate, 16 mg/5 ml. Ampules, 5 mg/ml.

PERSANTINE®, see Dipyridamole

PERSANTINE IV®, see Dipyridamole

PERTOFRANE®, see Desipramine

PERUVIAN BALSAM

Description/Actions: Local irritant used topically in various dermatologic disorders.

PETROLATUM

Description/Actions: Ointment base used as a vehicle for various topically applied medications. Sometimes used topically as a protective agent.

PHAZYME®, see Simethicone

PHENACEMIDE—Phenurone®

Description/Actions: Anticonvulsant indicated for the control of severe epilepsy, particularly mixed forms of complex partial (psychomotor) seizures, refractory to other drugs.

Preparations: Tablets, 500 mg.

PHENAZOPYRIDINE HYDROCHLORIDE—Azo-Standard®, Pyridium®

Description/Actions: Urinary tract analgesic indicated for the symptomatic relief of pain, burning, urgency, frequency, and other discomforts arising from irritation of the lower urinary tract mucosa. Causes a reddish orange discoloration of the urine and patients should be advised of this effect.

Preparations: Tablets, 100 and 200 mg.

PHENDIMETRAZINE TARTRATE—Bontril®

Description/Actions: Anorexiant indicated in the management of exogenous obesity as a short-term adjunct in a regimen of weight reduction based on caloric restriction.

Preparations: Capsules and tablets, 35 mg. Controlled-release capsules, 105 mg.

PHENELZINE SULFATE—Nardil®

Description/Actions: Monoamine oxidase inhibitor indicated for the treatment of depression.

Preparations: Tablets, 15 mg.

PHENERGAN®, see Promethazine

PHENINDAMINE TARTRATE—Nolahist®

Description/Actions: Antihistamine indicated in the management of allergic disorders.

Preparations: Tablets, 25 mg.

PHENIRAMINE MALEATE

Description/Actions: Antihistamine used in combination with other agents in the management of allergic and related disorders.

PHENOBARBITAL

PHENOBARBITAL SODIUM—Luminal Sodium®

Description/Actions: A CNS depressant indicated (a) for anxiety-tension states, (b) for insomnia, (c) as a long-term anticonvulsant for the treatment of tonic-clonic and cortical focal seizures, (d) in the symptomatic control of acute convulsions (e.g., tetanus, status epilepticus), (e) as a preanesthetic sedative, and (f) in other situations associated with anxiety.

Precautions/Adverse Reactions: Adverse reactions include drowsiness and other CNS effects. Patients should be cautioned regarding activities such as driving and operating machinery, as well as interactions with other CNS-acting drugs including alcohol. Can cause dependence and is included in Schedule IV.

Administration: Oral, intravenous, and intramuscular.

Preparations: Tablets, 8, 15, 30, 60, and 100 mg. Capsules, 15 mg. Elixir, 20 mg/5 ml. Injection dosage forms (phenobarbital sodium), 30, 60, 65, and 130 mg/ml.

PHENOL—Carbolic Acid

Description/Actions: Antipruritic, topical anesthetic, antiseptic, and caustic. Used topically in the management of various dermatologic conditions, and in certain other formulations (e.g., throat lozenges, mouthwashes, and gargles) that are utilized for a local effect.

Preparations: Solutions and lotions (with other agents for dermatologic use), 0.5–1%. Liquefied phenol is phenol maintained in a liquid condition by the presence of 10% water; is used as a source of phenol for preparing various formulations.

PHENOLSULFONPHTHALEIN

Description/Actions: Diagnostic agent used in evaluating renal function.

Preparations: Ampules, 6 mg/ml.

PHENOXYBENZAMINE HYDROCHLORIDE—Dibenzyline®

Description/Actions: Alpha-adrenergic receptor- blocking agent indicated in the management of pheochromocytoma to control episodes of hypertension and sweating.

Preparations: Capsules, 10 mg.

PHENSUXIMIDE—Milontin®

Description/Actions: Anticonvulsant indicated for the control of absence (petit mal) seizures in conjunction with other anticonvulsants when other forms of epilepsy coexist with petit mal.

Preparations: Capsules, 500 mg.

PHENTERMINE—Adipex®, Fastin®, Ionamin®

Description/Actions: Anorexiant indicated in the management of exogenous obesity as a short-term adjunct in a regimen of weight reduction based on caloric restriction.

Precautions/Adverse Reactions: Contraindicated in atherosclerosis, cardiovascular disease, hypertension, hyperthyroidism, glaucoma, agitation, drug or alcohol abuse, during or within 14 days of MAOIs. Discontinue if dyspnea, angina pectoris, syncope, lower extremity edema, or other symptoms of primary pulmonary hypertension occur. Discontinue after a few weeks as tolerance to anorectic effect occurs. Use cautiously in diabetes. Prescribe limited supply to prevent overdose. Pregnancy Category C. Use in nursing mothers not recommended. Can cause CNS overstimulation, dizziness, palpitation, psychosis, dry mouth, GI disturbance, urticaria, impotence, primary pulmonary hypertension, and/or regurgitant cardiac valvular disease.

Preparations: Capsules and tablets (as the hydrochloride), 8, 15, 30, and 37.5 mg. Capsules (as the resin complex), 15 and 30 mg.

PHENTOLAMINE MESYLATE—Regitine®

Description/Actions: Alpha-adrenergic-blocking agent indicated for parenteral use to prevent or control hypertensive episodes in patients with pheochromocytoma, for the prevention or treatment of dermal necrosis and sloughing following intravenous administration or extravasation of norepinephrine, and for the diagnosis of pheochromocytoma.

Preparations: Vials, 5 mg.

PHENURONE®, see Phenacemide

PHENYLEPHRINE HYDROCHLORIDE—Neo-Synephrine®

Description/Actions: Used topically in the management of nasal congestion, and in ocular conditions in which decongestant and vasoconstrictor actions are needed. Included as a decongestant in combination with other agents in orally administered formulations. Also used parenterally in the treatment of vascular failure in shock, shock-like states, drug-induced hypotension, or hypersensitivity. Is also utilized parenterally to overcome paroxysmal supraventricular tachycardia, to prolong spinal anesthesia, and as a vasoconstrictor in regional analgesia.

Preparations: Nasal drops and spray, 0.125%, 0.25%, 0.5%, and 1%. Nasal jelly, 0.5%. Ophthalmic solution, 0.12%, 2.5%, and 10%. Ampules, 1%. Injection, 10 mg/ml.

PHENYLTOLOXAMINE CITRATE

Description/Actions: Antihistamine used in combination with other agents in the management of allergic and related disorders.

PHENYTOIN—Dilantin®

Description/Actions: Anticonvulsant indicated for the control of tonic-clonic and psychomotor (grand mal and temporal lobe) seizures, and prevention and treatment of seizures occurring during or following neurosurgery. Also indicated for parenteral administration in the control of status epilepticus of the grand mal type. Has also been used intravenously in the management of certain arrhythmias (e.g., digitalis-induced arrhythmias), and orally in the treatment of trigeminal neuralgia.

Precautions/Adverse Reactions: Adverse reactions include nystagmus, ataxia, slurred speech, confusion, nausea, vomiting, rash, gingival hyperplasia, hirsutism, and hematologic effects. Effect may be reduced by chronic alcohol abuse and products containing calcium ions (e.g., antacids).

Administration: Oral, intravenous, and intramuscular. Oral formulations containing phenytoin sodium, extended, may be used for once-a-day dosing. When therapy is to be discontinued, it should be done gradually as the abrupt withdrawal of therapy in epileptic patients may precipitate status epilepticus.

Preparations: Capsules (phenytoin sodium, extended), 30 and 100 mg. Chewable infatabs, 50 mg. Oral suspension, 30 and 125 mg/5 ml.

PHISOHEX®, see Hexachlorophene

PhosLo®, see Calcium Acetate

PHOSPHALGEL®, see Aluminum Phosphate Gel

PHOSPHOLINE IODIDE®, see Echothiophate Iodide

PHOTOPLEX®, see Butyl Methoxydibenzoylmethane/Padimate 0

PHYLLOCONTIN®, see Aminophylline

PHYSOSTIGMINE—Eserine, Antilirium®

Description/Actions: Cholinesterase inhibitor indicated for ophthalmic use in the treatment of glaucoma, and for parenteral use to reverse the central nervous system effects caused by excessive dosages of anticholinergic drugs including the tricyclic antidepressants.

Preparations: Ophthalmic solution (as salicylate), 0.25% and 0.5%. Ophthalmic ointment (as sulfate), 0.25%. Ampules and syringes (as salicylate), 1 mg/ml.

PHYTONADIONE—Vitamin K$_1$, AquaMEPHYTON®, Konakion®, Mephyton®

Description/Actions: Vitamin K analog indicated for the management of anticoagulant-induced prothrombin deficiency, and for the management of hypoprothrombinemia secondary to other conditions or drug therapies (e.g., salicylates, antibiotics). Is also used parenterally in the prophylaxis and therapy of hemorrhagic disease of the newborn.

Precautions/Adverse Reactions: Severe reactions, including fatalities, have occurred during and immediately after intravenous injection of phytonadione even when precautions have been taken to dilute the phytonadione and to avoid rapid infusion. Severe reactions (hypersensitivity or anaphylaxis including shock, and cardiac and/or respiratory arrest), including fatalities, have also been reported following intramuscular administration. The intravenous and intramuscular routes of administration should be reserved for those situations where the subcutaneous route is not feasible and the potential risk is considered justified.

Administration: Whenever possible, phytonadione should be given by the subcutaneous route.

Preparations: Tablets, 5 mg. Ampules and vials, 2 mg/ml and 10 mg/ml.

PILOCARPINE HYDROCHLORIDE—Salagen®

Description/Actions: Miotic indicated for ophthalmic use in the treatment of glaucoma, and to counter the effect of cycloplegics and mydriatics. Also indicated for oral use for the treatment of symptoms of xerostomia from salivary gland hypofunction caused by radiotherapy for cancer of the head and neck.

Preparations: Ophthalmic solutions, 0.25%, 0.5%, 1%, 2%, 3%, 4%, 5%, 6%, 8%, and 10%. Ophthalmic gel, 4%. Ocular therapeutic systems, release 20 or 40 mcg pilocarpine per hour for one week. Tablets (Salagen), 5 mg.

PIMECROLIMUS—Elidel®

Description/Actions: Pimecrolimus is indicated for short-term and intermittent long-term therapy of mild to moderate eczema (atopic dermatitis) in patients not responsive to conventional therapy or when conventional therapy is deemed inadvisable.

Precautions/Adverse Reactions: Pimecrolimus is contraindicated in patients with Netherton's syndrome. It should not be applied to areas of active cutaneous viral infections. Patients with atopic dermatitis are predisposed to superficial skin infections, thereby increasing the risk of varicella zoster, herpes simplex viral infections, and eczema herpeticum. Clinical infections at the treatment sites should be cleared first before use of pimecrolimus. It is prudent to minimize or avoid natural or artificial sunlight exposure. It is not recommended for use in pediatric patients <2 years of age. There are no data to support its use in immunocompromised patients. There are no well-controlled studies in pregnant women. Pregnancy Category C. Use only if clearly needed. Excretion in breast milk is unknown; therefore, breast-feeding is not recommended. The most common side effects were a temporary, mild to moderate warm feeling or burning at the application site. Most application-site reactions did not last more than 5 days. Other common adverse effects were headache and cold-like symptoms. Cases of lymphadenopathy were reported. These cases were usually related to infections and noted to resolve upon appropriate antibiotic therapy. Consider discontinuation if lymphadenopathy occurs.

Administration: Topical.

Patient Care Implications: Patients should wash their hands after applying if hands are not an area for treatment. There is low systemic exposure via topical route; systemic drug interactions are not expected. Do not use occlusive dressings; this increases moisture, thereby increasing absorption.

Preparations: Cream, topical: 1% (15, 30, 60, and 100 g).

PIMOZIDE—Orap®

Description/Actions: Neuroleptic agent indicated for the suppression of motor and phonic tics in patients with Tourette's disorder who have failed to respond satisfactorily to standard treatment.

Preparations: Tablets, 2 mg.

PINDOLOL—Visken®

Description/Actions: A nonselective beta-adrenergic blocking agent with intrinsic sympathomimetic activity that is indicated in the management of hypertension.

Precautions/Adverse Reactions: Contraindicated in patients with bronchial asthma, overt cardiac failure, cardiogenic shock, second- and third-degree heart block, and severe bradycardia. Adverse reactions include dizziness, fatigue, insomnia, edema, nausea, and muscle and joint pain. Use is best avoided in patients with bronchospastic diseases, and therapy in diabetic patients must be closely monitored.

Administration: Oral. Patients should be cautioned about the interruption or discontinuation of therapy and, when therapy is to be discontinued, the dosage should be gradually reduced over a period of 1 to 2 weeks.

Preparations: Tablets, 5 and 10 mg.

PIOGLITAZONE—Actos®

Description/Actions: Pioglitazone is used for the treatment of NIDDM.

Precautions/Adverse Reactions: Pioglitazone should be administered with caution in patients with hepatic impairment. The drug should not be given to patients with increased baseline liver enzymes of ALT >2.5 times the upper limit of normal. Pioglitazone should be discontinued if jaundice occurs. Pioglitazone should also be used carefully in heart failure and peripheral edema patients because the drug can cause volume expansion. Drug should not be used in pregnant women, breast-feeding women, and children. Some side effects are headache, hyperglycemia, myalgia, pharyngitis, sinusitis, tooth disorder, weight gain, upper respiratory infection, and decreases in hemoglobin and hematocrit.

Administration: Oral.

Patient Care Implications: Pioglitazone should not be used in pregnant women, breast-feeding women, and children. Patients with hepatic disease should have liver enzymes monitored before initiation of drug and every 2 months after initiation. Pioglitazone should be discontinued if jaundice occurs. Pioglitazone should also be used carefully in heart failure and peripheral edema patients.

Preparations: Tablet, 15 mg, 30 mg, 45 mg.

PIPECURONIUM BROMIDE—Arduan®

Description/Actions: Nondepolarizing neuromuscular blocking agent. Acts by competing for cholinergic receptors at the motor end plate, resulting in a block of neuromuscular transmission. Indicated as an adjunct to general anesthesia to provide skeletal muscle relaxation during surgery. Can also be used to provide skeletal muscle relaxation for endotracheal intubation. Has a long duration of action and is only recommended for procedures anticipated to last 90 minutes or longer.

Precautions/Adverse Reactions: May cause excessive skeletal muscle weakness resulting in respiratory insufficiency and apnea. Action may be antagonized by neostigmine. Must be used with caution in patients with myasthenia gravis or myasthenic syndrome, and in patients receiving other medications that may intensify or produce neuromuscular block on their own (e.g., inhalation anesthetics, aminoglycosides, quinidine, magnesium salts). Other adverse reactions include bradycardia, hypotension, and hypertension.

Administration: Intravenous.

Preparations: Vials, 10 mg.

PIPERACILLIN SODIUM—Pipracil®

Description/Actions: Bactericidal penicillin antibiotic active against many gram-positive and gram-negative bacteria, including *Pseudomonas aeruginosa.* Is often used in conjunction with an aminoglycoside antibiotic in the treatment of *Pseudomonas* infections. Is also used for surgical prophylaxis.

Precautions/Adverse Reactions: Contraindicated in patients with a history of allergic reactions to any of the penicillins. Adverse reactions include hypersensitivity reactions, GI disturbances, and local reactions at the injection site.

Administration: Intravenous and intramuscular.

Preparations: Vials and infusion bottles, 2, 3, 4, and 40 g.

PIPERACILLIN SODIUM/TAZOBACTAM SODIUM—Zosyn®

Description/Actions: Is a combination of the penicillin antibiotic piperacillin with a beta-lactamase inhibitor tazobactam. By inhibiting beta-lactamase enzymes, tazobactam extends the spectrum of action of piperacillin to include certain bacteria that are not susceptible to piperacillin alone. Indicated for the treatment of the following infections caused by piperacillin-resistant, beta-lactamase-producing strains of the bacteria designated: community acquired pneumonia caused by *Haemophilus influenzae*; appendicitis (complicated by rupture or abscess), and peritonitis caused by *E. coli, Bacteroides fragilis, B. ovatus, B. thetaiotamicron,* or *B. vulgatus*; postpartum endometritis or pelvic inflammatory disease caused by *E. coli*; and uncomplicated and complicated skin and skin-structure infections, including cellulitis, cutaneous abscesses, and ischemic/diabetic foot infections caused by *Staphylococcus aureus.*

Precautions/Adverse Reactions: Contraindicated in patients with a history of allergic reaction to any of the penicillins, cephalosporins, or beta-lactamase inhibitors. Adverse reactions include diarrhea, constipation, nausea, dyspepsia, headache, insomnia, rash, pruritus, and hemolytic anemia. Should not be administered in the same solution with an aminoglycoside antibiotic.

Administration: Intravenous.

Preparations: Vials, 2.25, 3.375, and 4.5 grams, which provide 2, 3, and 4 g of piperacillin and 0.25, 0.375, and 0.5 g of tazobactam, respectively.

PIPERAZINE CITRATE—Antepar®

Description/Actions: Anthelmintic indicated in the treatment of pinworm and roundworm infections.

Preparations: Tablets, equivalent to 250 mg of piperazine hexahydrate. Syrup, equivalent to 500 mg piperazine hexahydrate/5 ml.

PIPERAZINE ESTRONE SULFATE, see Estropipate

PIPOBROMAN—Vercyte®

Description/Actions: Antineoplastic agent indicated in the treatment of polycythemia vera and the treatment of chronic granulocytic leukemia in patients refractory to busulfan.

Preparations: Tablets, 25 mg.

PIPRACIL®, see Piperacillin

PIRBUTEROL ACETATE—Maxair®

Description/Actions: Stimulates beta₂ adrenergic receptors and is indicated for the prevention and reversal of bronchospasm in patients with reversible bronchospasm including asthma.

Precautions/Adverse Reactions: Adverse reactions include nervousness, tremor, headache, dizziness, palpitations, tachycardia, cough, and nausea. Should be used with caution in patients with cardiovascular disorders, hyperthyroidism, diabetes mellitus, or convulsive disorders. Other beta-adrenergic aerosol bronchodilators should not be used concomitantly. It should be administered with caution to patients being treated with a tricyclic antidepressant or monoamine oxidase inhibitor.

Administration: Oral inhalation.

Preparations: Metered-dose inhaler. Each actuation delivers the equivalent of 0.2 mg pirbuterol.

PIROXICAM—Feldene®

Description/Actions: Nonsteroidal anti-inflammatory agent that inhibits prostaglandin synthesis and is indicated in the treatment of rheumatoid arthritis and osteoarthritis.

Precautions/Adverse Reactions: Should not be given to patients in whom aspirin or another NSAID causes asthma, rhinitis, urticaria, or other allergic-type reactions. May cause GI effects and use should be avoided in patients with active GI tract disease, and closely monitored in patients with a previous history of such disorders. Other adverse reactions include rash, edema, and decreases in hemoglobin and hematocrit. Has a long duration of action and may accumulate with continued use. Particular caution should be exercised in elderly patients.

Administration: Oral.

Preparations: Capsules, 10 and 20 mg.

PITOCIN®, see Oxytocin

PITRESSIN®, see Vasopressin

PITUITARY, POSTERIOR

Description/Actions: Hormones of the posterior pituitary administered parenterally to control postoperative ileus, to stimulate expulsion of gas prior to pyelography, as an aid to achieve hemostasis in surgery, and for treating enuresis of diabetes insipidus. Has also been used by nasal inhalation for the control of diabetes insipidus.

Preparations: Ampules, 20 units/ml. Capsules to be used for intranasal inhalation, 40 mg.

PLACIDYL®, see Ethchlorvynol

PLAQUENIL®, see Hydroxychloroquine

PLASBUMIN®, see Albumin

PLATINOL®, see Cisplatin

PLAVIX®, see Clopidogrel

PLENDIL®, see Felodipine

PLICAMYCIN—Mithramycin, Mithracin®

Description/Actions: Antineoplastic agent indicated for intravenous use in the treatment of testicular carcinoma. Also used in the treatment of symptomatic patients with hypercalcemia and hypercalciuria associated with a variety of advanced neoplasms.

Preparations: Vials, 2500 μg.

PODOFILOX—Condylox®

Description/Actions: Antimitotic indicated in the treatment of external genital warts. Not for use on mucous membrane or perianal warts. Local reactions (e.g., burning, inflammation, erosion, pain, itching, bleeding) and headache may occur.

Administration: Topical.

Preparations: 0.5% topical solution and gel.

PODOPHYLLIN, see Podophyllum Resin

PODOPHYLLUM RESIN—Podophyllin

Description/Actions: Resin applied topically for the removal of benign epithelial growths such as common warts, and also in certain other dermatologic disorders.

Preparations: Liquid, 25%, often in tincture of benzoin.

POLARAMINE®, see Dexchlorpheniramine

POLYCARBOPHIL—Equalactin®, FiberCon®, Mitrolan®

Description/Actions: Hydrophilic agent used in the treatment of constipation or diarrhea by regulating intestinal water and promoting well-formed stools.

Preparations: Chewable tablets, 500 mg.

POLYCILLIN®, see Ampicillin

POLYCITRA®, see Potassium Citrate

POLYETHYLENE GLYCOL—Miralax

Description/Actions: Miralax is an osmotic laxative indicated in the treatment of occasional constipation. It works by causing water to be retained in the stool. Unlike stimulant laxatives, it works on the stool rather than the colon.

Precautions/Adverse Reactions: Miralax is contraindicated in a bowel obstruction. It may increase the incidence of diarrhea in the elderly. Avoid prolonged, frequent, or excessive use. Adverse reactions include nausea, abdominal bloating, cramping, flatulence, and diarrhea.

Administration: Oral. Dissolve 17 g in 8 oz of water and drink promptly.

Patient Care Implications: Inform patients the first bowel movement should occur in 2–4 days after taking. Report unusual cramps, bloating, or diarrhea to the prescriber. Instruct patients in lifestyle changes that promote regular bowel movements such as regular exercise, high-fiber diet, and adequate hydration. Do not exceed the recommended dose, as this may result in severe diarrhea and dehydration. Discontinue if a rash, hives, or other symptoms of allergy occur.

Preparations: Powder for reconstitution.

POLYETHYLENE GLYCOLS—PEG, Carbowax®

Description/Actions: Ointment and suppository bases used as vehicles for active medications.

POLYETHYLENE GLYCOL 3350—Colyte®, GoLYTELY®

Description/Actions: Osmotic agent used with electrolytes for bowel cleansing prior to colonoscopy and barium enema X-ray examination.

Preparations: Powder for oral solution.

POLYMYXIN B SULFATE—Aerosporin®

Description/Actions: Antibiotic used in the treatment of infections caused by gram-negative bacteria. Administered parenterally in the treatment of infections caused by bacteria such as *Pseudomonas aeruginosa* when less toxic drugs are ineffective or contraindicated. Also indicated for ophthalmic use. Is most frequently employed in combination with other antibiotics (e.g., neomycin) in the topical management of dermatologic, otic, and ophthalmic infections, and also as a genitourinary irrigant.

Preparations: Vials, 500,000 units. Powder for ophthalmic solution, 500,000 units.

POLYMYXIN E®, see Colistin Sulfate

POLYTHIAZIDE—Renese®

Description/Actions: Thiazide diuretic indicated as adjunctive therapy in edema and in the management of hypertension.

Preparations: Tablets, 1, 2, and 4 mg.

PONSTEL®, see Mefenamic Acid

PONTOCAINE®, see Tetracaine

PORACTANT ALFA—Curosurf®

Description/Actions: Poractant alfa is used in the treatment of neonatal respiratory distress syndrome.

Precautions/Adverse Reactions: Poractant alfa should not be administered to patients with porcine hypersensitivity or to pregnant women. Also, patients should be monitored carefully for oxygenation because the drug can cause respiratory changes, and ventilatory support should be modified accordingly. Some side effects are transient episodes of hypotension, sinus bradycardia, oxygen desaturation, and endotracheal tube blockage. If these problems occur then the drug should be discontinued, the problems should be alleviated, and then the drug should be initiated again.

Administration: Intrathecal injection.

Patient Care Implications: Poractant alfa should not be used in patients with porcine hypersensitivity or in pregnant women. The drug should only be given under strict supervision of clinicians experienced in intubation, ventilators, and care of premature babies. Also, before initiation of poractant alfa, a patient should be checked for metabolic acidosis, anemia, hypoglycemia, hypotension, and hypothermia. If these problems exist, they should be corrected before the drug is started. Patient should have ABGs and chest X-rays checked while taking poractant alfa.

Preparations: Solution, 80 mg/ml, 1.5 and 3.0 ml.

POSTERIOR PITUITARY, see Pituitary, Posterior

POSTURE®, see Calcium Phosphate, Tribasic

POTABA®, see Para-aminobenzoic Acid

POTASSIUM ACETATE

Description/Actions: For intravenous potassium replacement.

Preparations: Vials, 40 mEq, 120 mEq.

POTASSIUM CHLORIDE, INTRAVENOUS

Preparations: Ampules and vials, 10, 20, 30, 40, 60, and 90 mEq.

POTASSIUM CHLORIDE, ORAL (see list of preparations below for trade names)

Description/Actions: Potassium supplement indicated for patients with hypokalemia, in digitalis intoxication, in patients with hypokalemic familial periodic paralysis, and for the prevention of potassium depletion when the dietary intake of potassium is inadequate.

Precautions/Adverse Reactions: Is contraindicated in patients with hyperkalemia; should not be used concomitantly with a potassium-sparing diuretic because of the increased risk of hyperkalemia. Solid dosage forms (e.g., tablets) have caused lesions of the small intestine and serious GI complications; these formulations should be reserved for those patients who cannot tolerate or refuse to take liquid or effervescent potassium preparations, or for patients in whom there is a problem of compliance with these preparations. Other adverse reactions include nausea and vomiting.

Administration: Oral.

Preparations: Liquid (e.g., Kay Ciel®, Klorvess®, 20 and 40 mEq/ml). Powder (e.g., Kay Ciel®, K-Lor®), 15, 20, and 25 mEq/packet. Controlled-release tablets and capsules (e.g., Slow-K®, Klotrix ®, K-Tab®, Micro-K®), 8 and 10 mEq.

POTASSIUM CITRATE—Polycitra®, Urocit-K®

Description/Actions: Alkalinizing agent and potassium replacement agent. Has been used to alkalinize the urine to reduce the risk of calculi in the urinary tract, as an adjunct to uricosuric agents in gout therapy, and to correct the acidosis of certain renal tubular disorders.

Preparations: Tablets, 540 mg. Syrup, 550 mg/5 ml with sodium citrate and citric acid.

POTASSIUM GLUCONATE—Kaon®

Description/Actions: Potassium replacement agent.

Preparations: Tablets, 5 mEq. Liquid, 20 mEq/15 ml.

POTASSIUM IODIDE

Description/Actions: Expectorant and is also used as adjunctive therapy in other respiratory conditions. Has also been used for thyroid blocking in radiation emergencies, in the treatment of thyrotoxic crisis, and as an adjunct with other antithyroid drugs in preparation for thyroidectomy.

Preparations: Enteric-coated tablets, 300 mg. Solution, 500 mg/15 ml. Saturated solution of potassium iodide (SSKI), 1 g/ml.

POTASSIUM PHOSPHATE—Neutra-Phos-K®

Description/Actions: Phosphorus-replacement products.

Preparations: Capsules and powder concentrate are both utilized to prepare liquid for oral administration. Vials, 3 mM phosphate/ml for intravenous administration.

POVIDONE-IODINE—Betadine®

Description/Actions: Anti-infective agent utilized for topical, vaginal, and perineal application.

Preparations: Numerous formulations including topical solution and ointment.

PRALIDOXIME CHLORIDE—Protopam®

Description/Actions: Cholinesterase reactivator indicated as an antidote in the treatment of poisoning due to pesticides and chemicals of the organophosphate class that have anticholinesterase activity, and in the control of overdosage by anticholinesterase drugs used in the treatment of myasthenia gravis. Atropine should be administered after ventilation is established.

Preparations: Vials, 1 g.

PRAMOXINE HYDROCHLORIDE—Tronolane®, Tronothane®

Description/Actions: Local anesthetic indicated for topical use for the temporary relief of pain and itching associated with dermatologic conditions, as well as hemorrhoids and other anorectal disorders.

Preparations: Cream, 1%. Suppositories, 1%.

PRANDIN®, see Repaglinide

PRAVACHOL®, see Pravastatin

PRAVASTATIN SODIUM—Pravachol®

Description/Actions: Reduces cholesterol biosynthesis in the liver by acting as a competitive inhibitor of 3-hydroxy-3-methylglutaryl-coenzyme A (HMGCoA) reductase. Produces a significant reduction in total and low-density lipoprotein (LDL) cholesterol concentrations, a modest reduction in triglyceride concentrations, and an increase in high-density lipoprotein (HDL) cholesterol concentrations. Indicated as an adjunct to diet for the reduction of elevated total and LDL cholesterol concentrations in patients with primary hypercholesterolemia (Type IIa and IIb) when the response to a diet restricted in saturated fat and cholesterol has not been adequate. Also indicated to reduce the risk of MI, reduce the risk of undergoing myocardial revascularization procedures, and reduce the risk of cardiavascular mortality with no increase in death from noncardiovascular causes in hypercholesterolemia without clinically evident coronary heart disease. Also indicated for the treatment of heterozygous familial hypercholesterolemia in children ages 8 and older.

Precautions/Adverse Reactions: Contraindicated in patients with active liver disease or unexplained persistent elevations in liver function tests. Is also contraindicated in pregnant women and nursing mothers. Adverse reactions include headache, rash, influenza, myalgia, myopathy, and, rarely, rhabdomyolysis. Patients should be advised to promptly report unexplained muscle pain, tenderness, or weakness. Because of the possibility of an increased risk of skeletal muscle reactions, the concurrent use of clofibrate, cyclosporine, erythromycin, gemfibrozil, or niacin (in lipid-lowering doses) is best avoided. When either cholestyramine or colestipol is used concomitantly, pravastatin should be administered at least 1 hour before or at least 4 hours after the administration of the other agent. Increases in serum transaminases may occur, and it is recommended that liver function tests be performed prior to the initiation of therapy, prior to the elevation of the dose, and when otherwise clinically indicated. Should any increase in AST or ALT of 3 times the upper limit of normal or greater persist, withdrawal of pravastatin therapy is recommended.

Administration: Oral. Should be administered at bedtime.

Preparations: Tablets, 10, 20, 40, and 80 mg.

PRAZEPAM—Centrax®

Description/Actions: Benzodiazepine indicated for the management of anxiety disorders or for the short-term relief of the symptoms of anxiety.

Precautions/Adverse Reactions: Contraindicated in patients with acute narrow-angle glaucoma. Adverse reactions include drowsiness and other CNS effects; patients should be cautioned regarding activities such as driving or operating machinery, as well as interactions with other CNS-acting drugs including alcohol. Can cause dependence, and is included in Schedule IV.

Administration: Oral.

Preparations: Capsules, 5, 10, and 20 mg. Tablets, 10 mg.

PRAZIQUANTEL—Biltricide®

Description/Actions: Antiparasitic agent indicated for the treatment of schisto-somiasis and other trematode infections by Chinese liver fluke.

Preparations: Tablets, 600 mg.

PRAZOSIN HYDROCHLORIDE—Minipress®

Description/Actions: Indicated in the treatment of hypertension. Investigational studies have suggested it to be useful in refractory congestive heart failure and in the management of Raynaud's vasospasm.

Precautions/Adverse Reactions: Prazosin is contraindicated in patients with a known hypersensitivity to quinazolines, prazosin, or any component of the formulation. May cause syncope with sudden loss of consciousness, usually attributable to an excessive postural hypotensive effect. Risk may be reduced by limiting the initial dose of the drug to 1 mg, and by subsequently increasing the dosage slowly. Adverse reactions include dizziness, drowsiness, and other CNS effects. Patients should be cautioned regarding activities such as driving and operating machinery, as well as interactions with other CNS-acting drugs including alcohol. Other adverse reactions include palpitations and nausea. The concurrent use of a beta-adrenergic blocking agent may increase the risk of hypotension.

Administration: Oral.

Preparations: Capsules and tablets, 1, 2, and 5 mg.

PRECEDEX®, see Dexmedetomidine Hydrochloride Injection

PRECOSE®, see Acarbose

PREDNICARBATE—Dermatop®

Description/Actions: Corticosteroid applied topically for the relief of the manifestations of corticosteroid-responsive dermatoses.

Preparations: Cream, 0.1%.

PREDNISOLONE ACETATE

Preparations: Vials (for IM, intralesional, intra-articular, or soft tissue injection), 25 mg/ml, 50 mg/ml, and 100 mg/ml. Ophthalmic suspension, 0.12%, 0.125%, 1%.

PREDNISOLONE—Delta-Cortef®

Description/Actions: Corticosteroid indicated in a wide range of endocrine, rheumatic, allergic, dermatologic, respiratory, hematologic, neoplastic, and other disorders.

Preparations: Tablets, 5 mg. Syrup, 15 mg/5 ml. Oral solution, 5 mg/ml.

PREDNISOLONE SODIUM PHOSPHATE—Hydeltrasol®

Preparations: Oral liquid, 5 mg/5 ml. Vials (for IV, IM, intralesional, intra-articular, or soft tissue injection), 20 mg/ml. Ophthalmic solution, 0.125%, 0.5%, and 1%.

PREDNISOLONE TEBUTATE—Hydeltra-TBA®

Preparations: Vials (for intralesional, intra-articular, or soft tissue injection) 20 mg/ml.

PREDNISONE—Deltasone®, Meticorten®

Description/Actions: Corticosteroid indicated in a wide range of endocrine, rheumatic, allergic, dermatologic, respiratory, hematologic, neoplastic, and other disorders.

Precautions/Adverse Reactions: Contraindicated in patients with systemic fungal infections. Adverse reactions include sodium and fluid retention, potassium depletion, muscle weakness, osteoporosis, peptic ulcer, thin fragile skin, development of cushingoid state, glaucoma, cataracts, and negative nitrogen balance. May mask signs of infection, and new infections may appear during use. May increase requirements for hypoglycemic agents in diabetic patients.

Administration: Oral.

Preparations: Tablets, 1, 2.5, 5, 10, 20, and 50 mg. Oral solution, 5 mg/5 ml. Oral solution (concentrate), 5 mg/ml. Syrup, 5 mg/5 ml.

PREMARIN®, see Estrogens, Conjugated

PREMPHASE®, Combination of Conjugated Estrogens and Medroxyprogesterone Acetate

PREMPRO®, Combination of Conjugated Estrogens and Medroxyprogesterone Acetate

PREPIDIL®, see Dinoprostone

PREVACID®, see Lansoprazole

PREVACID® I.V., see Lansoprazole

PREVACID® SOLUTAB, see Lansoprazole

PREVPAC®—Combination Agent Lansoprazole, Amoxicillin, and Clarithromycin (pump inhibitor and antibiotics)

PRILOCAINE HYDROCHLORIDE—Citanest®

Description/Actions: Local anesthetic administered by injection for infiltration, peripheral nerve block, central neural block, and in dental procedures.

Preparations: Ampules and vials, 1%, 2%, and 3%. Dental cartridges, 4%.

PRILOSEC®, see Omeprazole

PRIMACOR®, see Milrinone Lactate

PRIMAQUINE PHOSPHATE

Description/Actions: Antimalarial agent used to prevent relapses of infections caused by *Plasmodium vivax* and *P. ovale* and to prevent attack after departure from areas where *P. vivax* and *P. ovale* are endemic (often administered during the last 2 weeks of chloroquine prophylaxis).

Preparations: Tablets, 26.3 mg.

PRIMATENE MIST®, see Epinephrine

PRIMAXIN IV®, see Imipenem-Cilastatin Sodium

PRIMAXIN IM®, see Imipenem-Cilastatin Sodium

PRIMIDONE—Mysoline®

Description/Actions: Anticonvulsant indicated in the control of grand mal, psychomotor, and focal epileptic seizures.

Preparations: Tablets, 50, 125, and 250 mg. Suspension, 250 mg/5 ml.

PRINCIPEN®, see Ampicillin

PRINIVIL®, see Lisinopril

PRINZIDE®, Combination of Lisinopril and Hydrochlorothiazide

PRISCOLINE®, see Tolazoline

PRIVINE®, see Naphazoline

PROAMATINE®, see Midodrine Hydrochloride

PRO-BANTHINE®, see Propantheline

PROBENECID—Benemid®

Description/Actions: Uricosuric agent indicated for the treatment of hyperuricemia associated with gout and gouty arthritis and to treat the hyperuricemia secondary to thiazide therapy. Has also been used to increase the plasma levels and activity of the penicillin derivatives.

Preparations: Tablets, 500 mg.

PROCAINAMIDE HYDROCHLORIDE—Procanbid®, Pronestyl®, Pronestyl-SR®, Procan SR®

Description/Actions: Indicated in the treatment of premature ventricular contractions and ventricular tachycardia, atrial fibrillation, and paroxysmal atrial tachycardia; also useful in preventing recurrence of certain arrhythmias after conversion to sinus rhythm by other drugs or procedures.

Precautions/Adverse Reactions: Contraindicated in patients with complete heart block or lupus erythematosus, and in patients sensitive to procaine or other ester-type local anesthetics. May cause worsening of symptoms in patients with myasthenia gravis. Adverse reactions include proarrhythmic effects, hypotension (particularly after parenteral administration), nausea, vomiting, diarrhea, dizziness, weakness, pruritus, flushing, lupus erythematosus-like syndrome, and positive antinuclear antibody (ANA) test.

Administration: Oral, intravenous, and intramuscular.

Preparations: Capsules and tablets, 250, 375, and 500 mg. Sustained-release tablets, 250, 500, 750, and 1000 mg. Vials, 100 and 500 mg/ml.

PROCAINE HYDROCHLORIDE—Novocain®

Description/Actions: Local anesthetic administered by injection for infiltration anesthesia, peripheral nerve block, spinal anesthesia, and for rectal anesthesia in proctology.

Preparations: Ampules and vials, 1% and 2%. Ampules (for spinal anesthesia), 10%.

PROCAINE PENICILLIN G—Crysticillin®, Wycillin®

Description/Actions: Penicillin antibiotic administered intramuscularly and having an extended duration of action. Used in the treatment of streptococcal, gonococcal, and selected other infections.

Preparations: Vials and syringes, 300,000, 500,000, 600,000, 1,200,000, and 2,400,000 units.

PROCANBID®, see Procainamide HCl

PROCAN SR®, see Procainamide

PROCARBAZINE HYDROCHLORIDE—Matulane®

Description/Actions: Antineoplastic agent having monoamine oxidase inhibitory activity. Indicated for use in combination with other antineoplastic drugs for the treatment of Stage III and IV Hodgkin's disease.

Preparations: Capsules, 50 mg.

PROCARDIA®, see Nifedipine

PROCARDIA XL®, see Nifedipine

PROCHLORPERAZINE—Compazine®

Description/Actions: Indicated for the control of severe nausea and vomiting, and for the management of manifestations of psychotic disorders.

Precautions/Adverse Reactions: Adverse reactions include drowsiness and other CNS effects. Patients should be cautioned regarding activities such as driving and operating machinery, as well as interactions with other CNS-acting drugs including alcohol. Other adverse reactions include extrapyramidal reactions, tardive dyskinesia, blurred vision, skin reactions, and hypotension. May lower the convulsive threshold necessitating dosage adjustments of anticonvulsants. May interfere with thermoregulatory mechanisms, and must be used cautiously in persons who will be exposed to extreme heat; the risk of complications is increased in patients who are also taking other medications having anticholinergic activity.

Administration: Oral, rectal, intravenous, and intramuscular.

Preparations: Tablets (as the maleate), 5, 10, and 25 mg. Sustained-release capsules (as the maleate), 10, 15, and 30 mg. Syrup (as the edisylate), 5 mg/5 ml. Suppositories, 2.5, 5, and 25 mg. Ampules, vials, and syringes (as the edisylate), 5 mg/ml.

PROCRIT®, see Epoetin Alfa

PROCYCLIDINE HYDROCHLORIDE—Kemadrin®

Description/Actions: Antiparkinson agent indicated in the treatment of parkinsonism and drug-induced extrapyramidal effects.

Preparations: Tablets, 5 mg.

PROFENAL®, see Suprofen

PROGESTASERT®, see Progesterone

PROGESTERONE—Progestasert®

Description/Actions: Progestin used intramuscularly in the management of conditions such as amenorrhea and functional uterine bleeding. Intrauterine system has been used for contraception.

Preparations: Vials (aqueous solution and in oil), 25 mg/ml, 50 mg/ml, and 100 mg/ml. Intrauterine system, 38 mg, provides contraceptive effectiveness for a period of 1 year.

PROGLYCEM®, see Diazoxide

PROGRAF®, see Tacrolimus

PROKINE®, see Sargramostim

PROLASTIN®, see Alpha₁-Proteinase Inhibitor (human)

PROLEUKIN®, see Aldesleukin

PROLIXIN®, see Fluphenazine

PROLOPRIM®, see Trimethoprim

PROMAZINE HYDROCHLORIDE—Sparine®

Description/Actions: Phenothiazine antipsychotic agent indicated in the management of the manifestations of psychotic disorders.

Preparations: Tablets, 25, 50, and 100 mg. Vials and syringes, 25 mg/ml and 50 mg/ml.

PROMETHAZINE HYDROCHLORIDE—Phenergan®

Description/Actions: Phenothiazine antihistamine indicated for allergic disorders, motion sickness, preoperative, postoperative, or obstetric sedation, postoperative pain as an adjunct to analgesics, and the prevention and control of nausea and vomiting associated with certain types of surgery.

Precautions/Adverse Reactions: Promethazine is contraindicated for use in pediatric patients less than 2 years of age because of the potential for fatal respiratory depression. Post marketing cases of respiratory depression including fatalities have been reported with the use of promethazine in pediatric patients less than 2 years of age. Caution should be exercised when administering to pediatric patients 2 years of age and older. It is recommended that the lowest effective dose of promethazine be used in pediatric patients 2 years of age and older and that concomitant administration of other drugs with respiratory depressant effects be avoided.

Preparations: Tablets and suppositories, 10, 12.5, 25, and 50 mg. Syrup, 6.25 and 25 mg/5 ml. Ampules and vials, 25 and 50 mg/ml.

PRONESTYL®, see Procainamide

PROPAFENONE HYDROCHLORIDE—Rythmol®

Description/Actions: A class IC antiarrhythmic agent that also has local anesthetic activity, beta-adrenergic blocking activity, and a weak calcium channel-blocking effect. Indicated for the treatment of documented life-threatening arrhythmias, prolonged recurrence of paroxysmal atrial fibrillation/flutex, or paroxysmal supraventricular tachycardia (PSVT) associated with disabling symptoms in patients without structural heart disease.

Precautions/Adverse Reactions: Contraindicated in the presence of uncontrolled congestive heart failure, cardiogenic shock, sinoatrial, atrioventricular, and intraventricular disorders of impulse generation and/or conduction in the absence of an artificial pacemaker, bradycardia, marked hypotension, bronchospastic disorders, and electrolyte imbalance. Adverse reactions include proarrhythmic effects, congestive heart failure, conduction abnormalities, nausea and/or vomiting, unusual (e.g., metallic) taste, constipation, dizziness, fatigue, and dyspnea.

Administration: Oral.

Preparations: Tablets, 150, 225, and 300 mg.

PROPANTHELINE BROMIDE—Pro-Banthine®

Description/Actions: Anticholinergic agent indicated as adjunctive therapy in the treatment of peptic ulcer.

Preparations: Tablets, 7.5 and 15 mg.

PROPARACAINE HYDROCHLORIDE—Ophthaine®

Description/Actions: Local anesthetic indicated for ophthalmic use.

Preparations: Ophthalmic solution, 0.5%.

PROPECIA®, see Finasteride

PROPINE®, see Dipivefrin

PROPIOMAZINE HYDROCHLORIDE—Largon®

Description/Actions: Phenothiazine indicated for parenteral use for relief of restlessness and apprehension, preoperatively, during surgery, or during labor.

Preparations: Ampules and syringes, 20 mg/ml.

PROPOFOL—Diprivan®

Description/Actions: Has a rapid onset of action, and the recovery from anesthesia is usually prompt. Indicated as an intravenous anesthetic agent that can be used for both induction and/or maintenance of anesthesia as part of a balanced anesthetic technique for inpatient and outpatient surgery. Also indicated for continuous sedation and control of stress responses in intubated or respiratory-controlled adult patients in intensive care units.

Precautions/Adverse Reactions: Adverse reactions include excitatory reactions (e.g., spontaneous movement, twitching, tremor, myoclonus), hypotension, bradycardia, apnea, nausea, vomiting, and reactions at the injection site. Other CNS depressants can increase the depression induced by propofol and may also result in more pronounced decreases in blood pressure.

Administration: Intravenous

Preparations: Vials, 10 mg/ml. Is a white, oil-in-water emulsion that is isotonic.

PROPOXYPHENE HYDROCHLORIDE—Darvon®

PROPOXYPHENE NAPSYLATE—Darvon-N®

Description/Actions: Indicated for the relief of mild to moderate pain.

Precautions/Adverse Reactions: Adverse reactions include sedation and other CNS effects. Patients should be cautioned regarding activities such as driving and operating machinery, as well as interactions with other CNS-acting drugs including alcohol. Can cause dependence and is included in Schedule IV.

Administration: Oral.

Preparations: Capsules, 65 mg. Tablets (Darvon-N), 50 and 100 mg.

PROPRANOLOL HYDROCHLORIDE—Inderal®, Inderal LA®

Description/Actions: A nonselective beta-adrenergic blocking agent indicated in the treatment of hypertension, angina pectoris, and cardiac arrhythmias (i.e., supraventricular arrhythmias, ventricular tachycardias, tachyarrhythmias of digitalis intoxication, and resistant tachyarrhythmias due to excessive catecholamine action during anesthesia). Also indicated to reduce cardiovascular mortality in patients who have survived the acute phase of myocardial infarction, in the management of hypertrophic subaortic stenosis, in pheochromocytoma, and for the prophylaxis of common migraine headache.

Precautions/Adverse Reactions: Contraindicated in patients with cardiogenic shock, sinus bradycardia and greater than first-degree block, bronchial asthma, and congestive heart failure. Acute increases in blood pressure have occurred after insulin-induced hypoglycemia in patients on propranolol. Cutaneous reactions, including

Stevens-Johnson syndrome, toxic epidermal necrolysis, exfoliative dermatitis, erythema multiforme, and urticaria, have been reported with the use of propranolol. Hypersensitivity reactions including anaphylactic/anaphylactoid reactions have been reported in patients receiving propranolol. Adverse reactions include weakness, light-headedness, depression, bradycardia, paresthesia of hands, arterial insufficiency (e.g., Raynaud type), nausea, and diarrhea. Use is best avoided in patients with bronchospastic diseases, and therapy in diabetic patients must be closely monitored.

Administration: Oral and intravenous. Patients should be cautioned about the interruption or discontinuation of therapy; exacerbation of angina pectoris has occurred following the abrupt cessation of therapy, and, when therapy is to be discontinued, the dosage should be gradually reduced over a period of several weeks.

Preparations: Tablets, 10, 20, 40, 60, and 90 mg. Long-acting capsules (Inderal LA), 60, 80, 120, and 160 mg. Oral solution, 4, 8, and 80 mg/ml. Ampules, 1 mg/ml.

PROPYLENE GLYCOL

Description/Actions: Solvent used as part of the vehicle in certain pharmaceutical formulations.

PROPYLHEXEDRINE—Benzedrex®

Description/Actions: Nasal decongestant administered by inhalation.

Preparations: Inhaler, 250 mg.

PROPYLTHIOURACIL

Description/Actions: Antithyroid agent used in the treatment of hyperthyroidism.

Preparations: Tablets, 50 mg.

PROSCAR®, see Finasteride

ProSom®, see Estazolam

PROSTACYCLIN®, see Epoprostenol

PROSTAGLANDIN E$_2$, see Dinoprostone

PROSTAGLANDIN F$_2$ ALPHA, see Dinoprost Tromethamine

PROSTAGLANDIN 12® (PG 12), see Epoprostenol

PROSTAGLANDIN X® (PGX), see Epoprostenol

PROSTAPHLIN®, see Oxacillin Sodium

ProStep®, see Nicotine

PROSTIGMIN®, see Neostigmine

PROSTIN E$_2$, see Dinoprostone

PROSTIN F$_2$ ALPHA, see Dinoprost Tromethamine

PROSTIN 15M®, former name for Carboprost Tromethamine

PROSTIN VR PEDIATRIC®, see Alprostadil

PROTAMINE SULFATE

Description/Actions: Heparin antagonist indicated for intravenous use in the treatment of heparin overdosage and to neutralize heparin received during dialysis, cardiopulmonary bypass, and other procedures.

Preparations: Ampules, 10 mg/ml.

PROTAMINE ZINC INSULIN, see Insulin

PROTIRELIN—Relefact TRH®, Thypinone®

Description/Actions: Thyrotropin-releasing hormone used intravenously as an adjunctive agent in the diagnostic assessment of thyroid function.

Preparations: Ampules, 0.5 mg.

PROTONIX®, see Pantoprazole Sodium

PROTOPAM®, see Pralidoxime

PROTOPIC®, see Tacrolimus

PROTRIPTYLINE HYDROCHLORIDE—Vivactil®

Description/Actions: Tricyclic antidepressant indicated in the treatment of symptoms of depression.

Preparations: Tablets, 5 and 10 mg.

PROTROPIN®, see Somatrem

PROVENTIL®—Proventil HFA®, see Albuterol

PROVERA®, see Medroxyprogesterone

PROZAC®, see Fluoxetine

PROZAC®, WEEKLY™, see Fluoxetine

PSEUDOEPHEDRINE HYDROCHLORIDE—Efidac/24®, Novafed®, Sudafed®

PSEUDOEPHEDRINE SULFATE—Afrinol®

Description/Actions: A sympathomimetic agent indicated for the temporary relief of nasal congestion due to the common cold and allergic disorders.

Precautions/Adverse Reactions: Should not be used concurrently with a monoamine oxidase inhibitor. Use is best avoided in patients with advanced arteriosclerosis, symptomatic cardiovascular disease, moderate to severe hypertension, hyperthyroidism, or diabetes. Adverse reactions include restlessness, dizziness, insomnia, palpitations, tachycardia, and blood pressure elevation.

Administration: Oral.

Preparations: Tablets, 30 and 60 mg. Controlled-release capsules and tablets, 120 and 240 mg. Liquid, 15 and 30 mg/5 ml. Drops, 7.5 mg/0.8 ml.

PSYLLIUM—Metamucil®

Description/Actions: Bulk laxative used in the treatment and prevention of constipation. Used in the management of chronic watery diarrhea. Contraindicated with abdominal pain, nausea, or vomiting (especially when associated with fever), serious adhesions, and dysphagia. Diabetics and cardiacs should read product labels to see which manufacturers include sugar, aspartame, and sodium in their formulations.

Preparations: Powder, effervescent powder, granules, chewable dosage form.

PULMOZYME®, see Dornase alfa

PULMICORT RESPULES™, see Budesonide

PULMICORT TURBUHALER®, see Budesonide

PURINETHOL®, see Mercaptopurine

PYRANTEL PAMOATE—Antiminth®

Description/Actions: Anthelmintic indicated for the treatment of pinworm and roundworm infections.

Preparations: Oral suspension, 50 mg/ml.

PYRAZINAMIDE

Description/Actions: Antitubercular agent used in combination with other antitubercular agents in patients in whom therapy with the primary agents has not been satisfactory.

Preparations: Tablets, 500 mg.

PYRETHRINS—A-200 Pyrinate®, RID®, Rid Mousse®

Description/Actions: Pediculicide indicated for topical use in the treatment of head lice, body lice, and pubic (crab) lice infestations.

Preparations: Liquid, gel, and shampoo, 0.17%, 0.3%, 0.33%. Topical scalp foam.

PYRIDIUM®, see Phenazopyridine

PYRIDOSTIGMINE BROMIDE—Mestinon®

Description/Actions: Cholinesterase inhibitor used in the treatment of myasthenia gravis. Also used parenterally as a reversal agent or antagonist to nondepolarizing muscle relaxants such as the curariform drugs.

Preparations: Tablets, 60 mg. Controlled-release tablets, 180 mg. Syrup, 60 mg/5 ml. Ampules, 5 mg/ml.

PYRIDOXINE—Vitamin B_6

Description/Actions: Vitamin indicated for the treatment and prevention of pyridoxine deficiency resulting from inadequate diet or use of drugs (e.g., isoniazid) that deplete pyridoxine. May also be useful in certain seizure disorders and anemias that are related to pyridoxine deficiency.

Preparations: Tablets, 10, 25, 50, 100, 200, 250, and 500 mg. Extended-release tablets, 100, 200, and 500 mg. Vials, 100 mg/ml.

PYRILAMINE MALEATE

Description/Actions: Antihistamine used in the management of allergic and related disorders, and as an aid in the relief of insomnia.

Preparations: Tablets and capsules, 25 mg.

PYRIMETHAMINE—Daraprim®

Description/Actions: Antimalarial agent indicated for the prophylaxis of malaria and in treating infections caused by chloroquine-resistant plasmodia. Also used as an adjunct to sulfonamide in the treatment of toxoplasmosis.

Preparations: Tablets, 25 mg.

Q

QUAZEPAM—Doral®

Description/Actions: Benzodiazepine indicated for the treatment of insomnia characterized by difficulty in falling asleep, frequent nocturnal awakenings, and/or early morning awakenings. Due to accumulation, may give larger doses for 1–2 nights, then decrease.

Precautions/Adverse Reactions: Contraindicated in pregnancy. Adverse reactions include daytime sedation, headache, fatigue, dizziness, dry mouth, and dyspepsia. Patients should be cautioned regarding activities such as driving and operating machinery, as well as interactions with other CNS-acting drugs including alcohol. Can cause dependence, and is included in Schedule IV.

Administration: Oral.

Preparations: Tablets, 7.5 and 15 mg.

QUELICIN®, see Succinylcholine

QUESTRAN®, see Cholestyramine

QUESTRAN LIGHT®, see Cholestyramine

QUETIAPINE—Seroquel®

Description/Actions: Quetiapine is indicated for the treatment of schizophrenia and for the treatment of acute manic episodes associated with Bipolar I Disorder, as either monotherapy or adjunct therapy to lithium or divalproex.

Precautions/Adverse Reactions: Contraindicated in hypersensitivity or lactation. Use cautiously in cardiovascular disease, cerebrovascular disease, dehydration or hypovolemia (increased risk of hypotension), history of seizures, Alzheimer's dementia, ≥65 y/o, hepatic impairment, hypothyroidism, history of suicide attempt. Pregnancy Category C. Safety not established for children. Hepatic enzyme elevations usually occurred within the first 3 weeks of treatment and promptly returned to prestudy levels with ongoing treatment. In hepatic impairment, adjust dosing downwards. Adverse reactions include dizziness, weight gain, leukopenia, flu-like syndrome, anorexia, constipation, dry mouth, dyspepsia, palpitations, peripheral edema, postural hypotension, cough, dypsnea, pharyngitis, ear pain, rhinitis, cognitive impairment, extrapyramidal symptoms, sedation, and tardive dyskinesia.

Administration: Oral.

Preparations: Tablets, 25, 100, and 200 mg.

QUINACRINE HYDROCHLORIDE

Description/Actions: Antimalarial agent that has been used in the prevention and treatment of malaria. Acts as suppressive agent and controls clinical attacks of malaria, but is not a true prophylactic agent and does not produce a radical cure. Use as an antimalarial has been largely superseded by more effective and less toxic drugs. Also used in the treatment of giardiasis and tapeworm infections. Has been utilized via intrapleural administration in patients who experience recurrent pneumothorax.

Preparations: Tablets, 100 mg.

QUINAGLUTE®, see Quinidine Gluconate

QUINAMM®, see Quinine Sulfate

QUINAPRIL HYDROCHLORIDE—Accupril®

Description/Actions: An angiotensin converting enzyme (ACE) inhibitor that is a prodrug. Following oral administration, is converted to its active metabolite, quinaprilat. Indicated for the treatment of hypertension and may be used alone or in combination with a thiazide diuretic. Also indicated as adjunctive therapy in the management of congestive heart failure when added to conventional therapy, including a diuretic or digitalis.

Precautions/Adverse Reactions: Contraindicated in patients who are hypersensitive to the drug and in patients with a history of angioedema related to previous treatment with an ACE inhibitor. Adverse reactions include headache, dizziness, fatigue, cough, nausea, and abdominal pain. May cause an elevation in serum potassium levels; the risk of hyperkalemia is increased in patients also taking a potassium-sparing diuretic, a potassium supplement, and/or a potassium-containing salt substitute. May cause symptomatic postural hypotension. There have been infrequent reports of angioedema of the face, extremities, lips, tongue, glottis, and larynx, especially following the first dose. Patients should be told to report immediately any symptoms suggesting angio-edema and to stop taking the drug. When used during the second and third trimesters of pregnancy, ACE inhibitors have been reported to be associated with the development of neonatal hypertension, renal failure, and skull hypoplasia. Therefore, use during pregnancy should be avoided. May increase serum lithium levels, so concurrent therapy should be closely monitored. Absorption is reduced when administered with a high-fat meal, and the drug is best administered apart from meals.

Administration: Oral.

Preparations: Tablets, 5, 10, 20, and 40 mg.

QUINAPRIL/HYDROCHLOROTHIAZIDE—Accuretic®

Description/Actions: Quinapril/hydrochlorothiazide are used together orally to treat hypertension.

Precautions/Adverse Reactions: Quinapril/hydrochlorothiazide is contra-indicated in patients with a history of ACE inhibitor-induced angioede-ma, hereditary angioedema, or idiopathic angioedema because of the drug's tendency to cause angioedema. Quinapril/hydrochlorothiazide should be used with caution in patients with hepatic disease, renal disease, renal failure, or renal impairment because thiazides may cause hepatic coma or azotemia in these patients. Quinapril/hydrochloro-thiazide should also not be given to pregnant women, breast-feeding women, or children. Patients should have magnesium, calcium, potas-sium, and glucose levels in normal ranges before initiating drug. Some side affects of the drug are cough, headache, somnolence, orthostatic hypotension, electrolyte disturbances, and angioedema.

Administration: Oral.

Patient Care Implications: Quinapril/hydrochlorothiazide should not be administered to pregnant women, breast-feeding women, or children. Also, the drug should be given with caution to patients with hepatic and renal impairment. Blood glucose, creatinine/BUN, electrolytes, and uric acid should be monitored in patients receiving the drug.

Preparations: Tablets, 10/12.5 quinapril/hydrochlorothiazide, 20/12.5, 20/25.

QUINESTROL—Estrovis®

Description/Actions: Estrogen indicated in the treatment of moderate to severe vasomotor symptoms associated with menopause, atrophic vaginitis, kraurosis vulvae, female hypogonadism, female castration, and primary ovarian failure.

Preparations: Tablets, 100 mcg.

QUINETHAZONE—Hydromox®

Description/Actions: Diuretic indicated as adjunctive therapy in edema and in the management of hypertension.

Preparations: Tablets, 50 mg.

QUINIDINE GLUCONATE—Quinaglute®

Description/Actions: Antiarrhythmic agent indicated in the prevention and treatment of a number of ventricular, atrial, and junctional (nodal) arrhythmias, and in the parenteral treatment of life-threatening *Plasmodium falciparum* malaria.

Preparations: Controlled-release tablets, 324 and 330 mg. Vials, 80 mg/ml.

QUINIDINE POLYGALACTURONATE—Cardioquin®

Description/Actions: Antiarrhythmic agent indicated in the prevention and treatment of a number of ventricular, atrial, and junctional (nodal) arrhythmias.

Preparations: Tablets, 275 mg.

QUINIDINE SULFATE

Description/Actions: Antiarrhythmic agent indicated in the prevention and treatment of a number of ventricular, atrial, and junctional (nodal) arrhythmias.

Preparations: Capsules and tablets, 100, 200, and 300 mg. Controlled-release tablets, 300 mg. Ampules, 200 mg/ml.

QUININE SULFATE—Quinamm®

Description/Actions: Antimalarial agent used in the treatment of chloroquine-resistant infections. Also used in the prevention and treatment of nocturnal leg cramps.

Preparations: Capsules and tablets, 130, 200, 260, 300, and 325 mg.

QUIXIN™®, see Levofloxacin

QVAR™®, see Beclomethasone

R

RABEPRAZOLE—Aciphex®

Description/Actions: Rabeprazole is a gastric proton pump inhibitor indicated for the treatment of gastroesophageal reflux disease (GERD), peptic ulcer disease, Zollinger-Ellison syndrome for the treatment of daytime and nighttime heartburn, and other symptoms associated with GERD and for the eradication of *helicobacter pylori*. It has also been effective in the management of gastric ulcer.

Precautions/Adverse Reactions: Rabeprazole should be administered with caution in patients who are pregnant or breast-feeding. The safety of the drug has not been established in children. Rabeprazole could require dosage adjustments in patients with severe hepatic disease. Rabeprazole has few side effects, but some are headache, malaise, nausea/vomiting, diarrhea, dizziness, rashes, elevation of serum gastrin (which can lead to carcinoid tumors), and elevated hepatic enzymes.

Administration: Oral.

Patient Care Implications: Rabeprazole should be administered with caution in patients who are pregnant or breast-feeding. The drug may require dosage adjustments in patients with severe hepatic disease. Liver enzymes should be checked while patient is on the medication.

Preparations: Tablets, 20 mg.

RALOXIFENE HCL—Evista®

Description/Actions: Raloxifene is a selective estrogen receptor modulator (SERM) indicated in the prevention of osteoporosis in postmenopausal women. Clinical data indicate that raloxifene has estrogen-like effects on bone (increase in BMD) and on lipid (decrease in total and LDL cholesterol levels) metabolism.

Precautions/Adverse Reactions: Contraindicated in pregnancy (Category X) or in women who may become pregnant and in women with active, or a history of, venous thrombophlebitis. Not for use in premenopausal women. Not recommended with concomitant systemic estrogen therapy. Use cautiously in hepatic dysfunction. Discontinue 72 hours before and during prolonged immobilization and resume when fully ambulatory. Adverse reactions include hot flashes, leg cramps, and venous thromboembolic events (rare). Instruct patients in calcium and Vitamin D rich diet and supplement if inadequate. Add weight-bearing exercise and modify other risk factors as appropriate. Inform patients to avoid prolonged restrictions of movement during travel.

Administration: Oral.

Preparations: Tablets, 60 mg.

RAMIPRIL—Altace®

Description/Actions: An angiotensin-converting enzyme (ACE) inhibitor that is a prodrug. Following oral administration, is converted to its active metabolite, ramiprilat. Indicated for the treatment of hypertension and may be used alone or in combination with a thiazide diuretic. Treatment for CHF in stabilized patients post-MI has been found to reduce mortality.

Precautions/Adverse Reactions: Adverse reactions include headache, dizziness, fatigue, and cough. May cause an elevation in serum potassium levels; the risk of hyperkalemia is increased in patients also taking a potassium-sparing diuretic, a potassium supplement, and/or a potassium-containing salt substitute. May cause symptomatic postural hypotension. There have been infrequent reports of angioedema of the face, extremities, lips, tongue, glottis, and larynx, especially following the first dose. Patients should be told to report immediately any symptoms suggesting angioedema and to stop taking the drug. When used during the second and third trimesters of pregnancy, ACE inhibitors have been reported to be associated with the development of neonatal hypertension, renal failure, and skull hypoplasia. Use during pregnancy should be avoided. May increase serum lithium levels and concurrent therapy should be closely monitored.

Administration: Oral. If necessary, the capsules may be opened and the contents sprinkled on a small amount of applesauce or mixed in apple juice or water.

Preparations: Capsules, 1.25, 2.5, 5, and 10 mg.

RANICLOR™, see Cefaclor

RANITIDINE HYDROCHLORIDE—Zantac®, Zantac® 150 EFFERdose®

Description/Actions: A histamine H_2 receptor antagonist that inhibits gastric acid secretion. Indicated (a) in the short-term treatment of active duodenal ulcer; (b) for maintenance therapy for duodenal ulcer patients at reduced dosage after healing of acute ulcers; (c) for the treatment of pathological hypersecretory conditions (e.g., Zollinger-Ellison syndrome); (d) in the short-term treatment of active, benign gastric ulcer; (e) in the treatment of gastroesophageal reflux disease; and (f) in the treatment of erosive esophagitis, and in the maintenance treatment of healed erosive esophagitis.

Precautions/Adverse Reactions: Adverse reactions include headache and GI effects.

Administration: Oral, intravenous, and intramuscular.

Preparations: Tablets, 75, 150, and 300 mg. Geldose capsules, 150 and 300 mg. Efferdose tablets and granules, 150 mg. Syrup, 15 mg/ml. Vials, 25 mg/ml and 50 mg/100 ml containers. Tablets, 150 mg.

RAPACURONIUM—Raplon®

Description/Actions: Rapacuronium is used as an adjunct to general anesthesia for endotracheal intubation and surgical procedures.

Precautions/Adverse Reactions: Rapacuronium should be administered with caution in patients who have renal impairment, hepatic impairment, obesity, pulmonary disease, underlying neuromuscular disease, dehydration, electrolyte imbalance, acid/base imbalance, burns, cerebral palsy, muscle trauma, and malignant hyperthermia. The drug should be avoided in patients who are pregnant, breast-feeding, or under 1 month of age. Also any patients with a condition that would be exacerbated by histamine release should be monitored. Some adverse effects are erythema, bronchospasm, flushing, sinus tachycardia, sinus bradycardia, muscle paralysis, apnea, dyspnea, and respiratory depression. Hypotension is the most common adverse side effect.

Administration: Intravenous.

Patient Care Implications: The drug should be avoided in patients who are pregnant, breast-feeding, or under 1 month of age. Also any patients with a condition that would be exacerbated by histamine release should be monitored. The patient should have ABGs, peripheral nerve stimulation, serum electrolytes, and serum magnesium checked while on the medication. Rapacuronium should be given only after the patient is unconscious.

Preparations: Vials, 100 mg/5 ml, 200 mg/10 ml.

RAPAMUNE®, see Sirolimus

RAPLON®, see Rapacuronium

RASBURICASE—Elitek™

Description/Actions: Rasburicase is a recombinant urate-oxidase enzyme. It is indicated for the initial management of plasma uric acid levels in pediatric patients with leukemia, lymphoma, and solid tumor malignancies who are receiving anticancer therapy expected to result in tumor lysis and subsequent elevation of plasma uric acid.

Precautions/Adverse Reactions: Rasburicase is contraindicated in patients with a known hypersensitivity to it or to any component of the formulation. It is contraindicated in individuals with glucose-6–phosphate dehydrogenase (G6PD) deficiency and in patients with a known history of anaphylaxis or hypersensitivity reactions, hemolytic reactions, or methemoglobinemia. Patients at high risk for G6PD deficiency should be screened prior to initiation of therapy with rasburicase. Rasburicase should be immediately and permanently discontinued in any patient developing a serious hypersensitivity reaction, hemolysis, or methemoglobinemia. Rasburicase is immunogenic and can elicit antibodies that inhibit its activity. Time to detection of antibodies ranged from 1–6 weeks after rasburicase exposure and lasted up to 494 days. Pregnancy Category C. Most serious adverse reactions caused by rasburicase were allergic reactions including anaphylaxis (<1%), rash (1%), hemolysis (<1%), and methemoglobinemia (<1%). Most commonly observed serious adverse reactions include fever (5%), neutropenia (2%), neutropenia with fever (4%), respiratory distress (3%), sepsis (3%), and mucositis (2%). Other serious adverse reactions observed in <1% of patients include acute renal failure, arrhythmias, cardiac arrest, cardiac failure, cellulitis, cerebrovascular disorder, chest pain, convulsions, cyanosis, dehydration, diarrhea, hemorrhage, hot flashes, ileus, infection, intestinal obstruction, myocardial infarction, pancytopenia, paresthesia, pneumonia, pulmonary edema, pulmonary hypertension, retinal hemorrhage, rigors, thrombophlebitis, and thrombosis. Less serious adverse reactions include vomiting (50%), fever (46%), nausea (27%), headache (26%), abdominal pain (20%), constipation (20%), diarrhea (20%), mucositis (15%), and rash (13%).

Administration: IV infusion.

Preparations: Powder for injection, 3 × 1.5 mg rasburicase vials with 3 × 1.0 mL ampules of diluent.

RAUDIXIN®, see Rauwolfia Serpentine

RAZADYNE®, see Galantamine

REBETOL®, see Ribavirin

REFLUDAN®, see Lepirudan

REGITINE®, see Phentolamine

REGLAN®, see Metoclopramide

REGRANEX®, see Becaplermin

RELA®, see Carisoprodol

RELAFEN®, see Nabumetone

RELENZA®, see Zanamivir

RELPAX®, see Eletriptan Hydrobromide

REMERON®, see Mirtazapine

REMINYL®, see Galantamine

REMODULIN™, see Treprostinil

RENESE®, see Polythiazide

RENOVA®, see Tretinoin

REOPRO®, see Abciximab

REPAGLINIDE—Prandin®

Description/Actions: Antidiabetic agent chemically unrelated to the sulfonylureas. Its action is dependent upon functioning beta cells in the pancreatic islets. Compared to other oral antidiabetic agents, repaglinide has a quick onset of action and a short duration of action. Following oral administration, peak plasma levels occur within 1 hour, and it is rapidly eliminated from the blood with a half-life of about 1 hour. It is indicated as an adjunct to diet and exercise for patients with type 2 diabetes and as monotherapy or in combination with metformin, rosiglitazone, or pioglitazone for the treatment of type 2 diabetes.

Precautions/Adverse Reactions: Contraindicated in type I diabetes and diabetic ketoacidosis. Titrate carefully in renal or hepatic dysfunction. Use cautiously in the elderly, debilitated, malnourished, stressed, and in patients with adrenal or pituitary insufficiency. Increases the risk of hypoglycemia. Monitor for initial effect and for secondary failure. Pregnancy Category C. Not recommended for use in nursing mothers. Patients taking repaglinide should not start taking gemfibrozil; patients taking gemfibrozil should not start taking repaglinide. Concomitant use may result in enhanced and prolonged blood glucose lowering effects of repaglinide. Patients taking repaglinide and gemfibrozil should not take itraconazole. Adverse reactions include hypoglycemia, upper respiratory infection, headache, diarrhea, constipation, arthralgia, back or chest pain. Oral antidiabetics may increase the risk of cardiovascular mortality. Instruct patients to adhere to diet and exercise programs. Test blood glucose and HbA1C regularly. Inform patients about management of hypoglycemia and explain primary vs. secondary failure.

Administration: Oral.

Preparations: Tablets, 0.5, 1, and 2 mg.

RESCRIPTOR®, see Delavirdine Mesylate

RESCULA®, see Unoprostone

RESERPINE—Serpasil®

Description/Actions: Rauwolfia alkaloid indicated in the treatment of hypertension and for the relief of symptoms in agitated psychotic states. Has been used parenterally in acute hypertensive and psychiatric conditions.

Preparations: Tablets, 0.1, 0.25, and 1 mg. Ampules, 2.5 mg/ml.

RESORCINOL

Description/Actions: Antipruritic, anti-infective, and keratolytic agent used topically with other agents in the treatment of seborrheic dermatitis, acne, and other dermatologic conditions.

RESTORIL®, see Temazepam

RETAVASE®, see Reteplase

RETEPLASE—Retavase®

Description/Actions: Thrombolytic indicated to improve ventricular function post acute myocardial infarction (MI), to reduce the incidence of congestive heart failure.

Precautions/Adverse Reactions: Contraindicated in patients with a history of cerebral vascular accident, active internal bleeding, intracranial or intraspinal surgery or trauma within the past 2 months, intracranial neoplasm, arteriovenous malformation or aneurysm, bleeding diathesis, severe uncontrolled hypertension, and history of severe allergic reactions to altaplase, anistreplase, or streptokinase. Use cautiously in patients with hypertension, recent major surgery, obstetrical delivery, organ biopsy, previous puncture of noncompressible vessel, GU or GI bleeding or trauma, high risk of left-heart thrombus, subacute bacterial endocarditis, acute pericarditis, hemostatic defects, severe renal or hepatic dysfunction, cerebrovascular disease, hemorrhagic ophthalmic conditions, septic thrombophlebitis or occluded AV cannula at seriously infected sites, and patients over 75 years of age. Cholesterol embolization and/or reperfusion arrhythmias may occur. Avoid IM injections, noncompressible punctures, and unnecessary handling of patients. Minimize venipuncture. Check puncture sites. Adverse reactions include bleeding (including intracranial hemorrhage) and reperfusion arrhythmias.

Administration: Intravenous.

Preparations: Powder for IV injection supplied with 2 ml diluent (preservative-free). 10.8 units/vial.

RETIN-A®, see Tretinoin

RETINOIC ACID, see Tretinoin

RETROVIR®, see Zidovudine

REVERSOL®, see Edrophonium

REVEX®, see Nalmefene Hydrochloride

RÉV-EYES®, see Dapiprazole Hydrochloride

R-GENE®, see Arginine

ReVia®, see Naltrexone Hydrochloride

RHEOMACRODEX®, see Dextran

RHEUMATREX®, see Methotrexate

RHINOCORT®, see Budesonide

RHO(D) IMMUNE GLOBULIN—RhoGAM®

Description/Actions: Immune globulin administered intramuscularly to prevent Rh immunization in Rh negative individuals exposed to Rh positive red blood cells. Indicated in pregnancy and other obstetric conditions when it is known or suspected that fetal red cells have entered the circulation of an Rh negative mother unless the fetus or the father can be shown conclusively to be Rh negative. Also indicated for any Rh negative female of childbearing age who receives a transfusion of Rh positive red blood cells or whole blood, or components prepared from Rh positive blood.

Preparations: Vials and syringes.

RHOGAM®, see Rho(D) immune Globulin

RIBAVIRIN—Virazole®, Rebetol®

Description/Actions: Antiviral agent indicated for the aerosol treatment of carefully selected hospitalized infants and young children with severe lower respiratory tract infections due to respiratory syncytial virus (RSV).

Precautions/Adverse Reactions: Should not be used in infants requiring assisted ventilation because the drug may precipitate on the valves and tubing of the respirator and interfere with safe and effective ventilation. Is teratogenic in animals and, although presently indicated only in infants and young children, its potential value for viral infections in adults warrants recognition of the contraindication to its use during pregnancy.

Administration: Aerosol, delivered to an infant oxygen hood (or administered by face mask or oxygen tent if necessary). Is administered using a small-particle aerosol generator (model SPAG-2), and other aerosol-generating devices should not be used.

Preparations: Vials, 6 g. Oral solution, 40 mg/mL.

RIBOFLAVIN—Vitamin B₂

Description/Actions: Vitamin indicated in the prevention and treatment of riboflavin deficiency.

Preparations: Tablets, 10, 25, 50, and 100 mg.

RID®, see Pyrethrins

RIDAURA®, see Auranofin

RID MOUSSE®, see Pyrethrins

RIFABUTIN—Mycobutin®

Description/Actions: Is active against *Mycobacterium avium* and *Mycobacterium intracellulare*, which comprise *Mycobacterium avium* complex

(MAC). Indicated for the prevention of disseminated *Mycobacterium avium* complex (MAC) disease in patients with advanced human immunodeficiency virus (HIV) infection.

Precautions/Adverse Reactions: Contraindicated in patients who are hypersensitive to rifampin. Adverse reactions include rash, gastrointestinal intolerance, neutropenia, flu-like syndrome, arthralgia, hepatitis, and a brown-orange discoloration of urine, feces, saliva, sputum, perspiration, tears, and skin, as well as permanent staining of soft contact lenses. May increase the activity of hepatic enzymes and reduce the effect of other therapeutic agents that are metabolized by these enzyme systems. Patients using oral contraceptives should be advised to use nonhormonal or additional methods of birth control while taking rifabutin. Should not be administered to patients with active tuberculosis because of the possibility of the development of tuberculosis that is resistant both to rifabutin and rifampin.

Administration: Oral.

Preparations: Capsules, 150 mg.

RIFADIN®, see Rifampin

RIFADIN IV®, see Rifampin

RIFAMPIN—Rifadin®, Rifadin IV®, Rimactane®

Description/Actions: Antitubercular agent indicated in the treatment of tuberculosis. Also indicated for the treatment of asymptomatic carriers of *Neisseria meningitidis*. Has a broad spectrum of action and is useful in the treatment of staphylococcal infections, Legionnaires' disease, leprosy, and other infections.

Preparations: Capsules, 150 and 300 mg. Vials, 600 mg.

RIFAPENTINE—Priftin®

Description/Actions: Rifapentine is a drug structurally related to rifampin indicated in the treatment of susceptible pulmonary tuberculosis.

Precautions/Adverse Reactions: Perform baseline liver enzymes including bilirubin, CBC, and platelet count. Use cautiously in patients with hepatic impairment. Monitor liver functions before and every 2–4 weeks during therapy. Discontinue if signs of liver disease occur or worsen. Do periodic susceptibility tests for persistently positive cultures. Consider pyridoxine supplements in adolescents, malnourished, or those at risk for neuropathy (e.g., alcoholics, diabetics). If used in the last few weeks of pregnancy, monitor clotting parameters in the mother and infant (may need vitamin K). Adverse reactions include hyperuricemia, proteinuria, increased serum transaminases, lymphopenia, pyuria, urinary casts, hematuria, rash, arthralgia, pruritus, neutropenia, pain, GI upset, anemia, hepatitis, hyperbilirubinemia, and pseudomembranous colitis.

Administration: Oral.

Patient Care Implications: Rifapentine must always be administered with at least one other antituberculosis drug to which the isolate is susceptible. Inform the patient that the dosing schedule must be strictly followed and that doses are not to be skipped. Explain the concepts of resistance and the role the patient plays in prevention. Caution the patient to finish out the course of therapy and not to stop treatment when symptoms subside. Instruct patient to avoid alcohol during therapy. Advise the patient that the drug may produce a reddish coloration of the urine, sweat, sputum, and tears. Contact lenses may become permanently stained. Oral contraceptives may be affected by use of this medication, and other means of pregnancy prevention should be employed.

Preparations: Tablets, 150 mg.

RILUZOLE—Rilutek®

Description/Actions: Used in the treatment of amyotrophic lateral sclerosis (ALS) to extend survival or time to tracheostomy. The etiology and pathogenesis are not known, but it has been hypothesized that motor neurons, made vulnerable through either genetic predisposition or environmental factors, are injured by glutamate. Riluzole's pharmacologic properties include an inhibitory effect on glutamate release, among others, which may account for its effect on ALS.

Precautions/Adverse Reactions: Neutropenia may develop, usually within the first 2 months of treatment. Warn patients to report febrile illnesses as a trigger for prompt checking of white blood cell counts. Use cautiously in patients with a history of abnormal liver function tests. Elevation of serial LFTs (especially bilirubin) should preclude use of riluzole. Use cautiously in patients with impaired renal function. Adverse reactions include asthenia, nausea, dizziness, diarrhea, anorexia, vertigo, somnolence, circumoral paresthesia (dose-related), decreased lung function, abdominal pain, pneumonia, and vomiting.

Administration: Oral.

Preparations: Tablets, 50 mg.

RIMACTANE®, see Rifampin

RIMANTADINE HYDROCHLORIDE—Flumadine®

Description/Actions: Antiviral agent indicated for the prophylaxis and treatment of illness caused by various strains of influenza A virus in adults and for prophylaxis in children age 1 year and over.

Precautions/Adverse Reactions: Contraindicated in patients who are hypersensitive to the drug or to amantadine. Adverse reactions include insomnia, dizziness, nervousness, fatigue, headache, nausea, vomiting, anorexia, dry mouth, and abdominal pain.

Administration: Oral.

Preparations: Tablets, 100 mg. Syrup, 50 mg/5 ml.

RIMEXOLONE—Vexol®

Description/Actions: Ophthalmic preparation containing benzalkonium chloride used in the treatment of postoperative inflammation and anterior uveitis.

Precautions/Adverse Reactions: Contraindicated in epithelial herpes simplex keratitis and other viral or fungal infections, including vaccinia and varicella. Do not use in the presence of ocular mycobacterial, fungal, or untreated purident infections. Use cautiously with ocular hypertension/glaucoma, optic nerve damage, and defects in visual acuity and visual fields. Posterior subcapsular cataract formation or fungal invasion may occur with prolonged use. May mask secondary ocular infections. Corneal or scleral thinning may occur. Monitor intraocular pressures. Adverse reactions include blurred vision, discharge, discomfort, ocular pain, increased intraocular pressure, foreign body sensation, hyperemia, and pruritus.

Administration: Ophthalmic.

Preparations: Ophthalmic suspension, 5 and 10 ml.

RIMSO 50®, see Dimethyl Sulfoxide

RINGER'S INJECTION

Description/Actions: Intravenous electrolyte replacement solution containing sodium, potassium, calcium, and chloride.

Preparations: Solution, 500 and 1000 ml.

RIOMET™, see Metformin

RIOPAN®, see Magaldrate

RISENDRONATE—Actonel®

Description/Actions: Risendronate is used for the treatment of Paget's disease in certain patients and for the prevention and treatment of postmenopausal osteoporosis.

Precautions/Adverse Reactions: Risendronate should not be administered to patients with renal failure (creatinine clearance <30 ml/min). Hypocalcemia or other bone abnormalities should be corrected before initiating drug therapy. Risendronate should not be given or used with caution in pregnant women, breast-feeding women, children <18 years old, or patients with GI disease. Some adverse effects are iritis, hypocalcemia, hypophosphatemia, diarrhea, abdominal pain, bone pain, and headache.

Administration: Oral. Take ≤30 minutes before first food or drink (except water). Avoid lying down for 30 minutes after taking to reduce possibility of GI side effects.

Preparations: Tablets, 5 mg, 30 mg, and 35 mg.

RISPERDAL®, see Risperidone

RISPERDAL® CONSTA™, see Risperidone

RISPERDAL® M-TAB™, see Risperidone

RISPERIDONE—Risperdal®, Risperdal® Consta™, Risperdal® M-Tab™

Description/Actions: Risperidone is indicated for the treatment of schizophrenia. It is also indicated as monotherapy or in combination with lithium or valproate for the short-term treatment of acute manic or mixed episodes associated with Bipolar I Disorder.

Precautions/Adverse Reactions: Adverse reactions include extrapyramidal symptoms, insomnia, agitation, anxiety, headache, constipation, abdominal pain, tachycardia, and rhinitis. Patients should be cautioned about driving or operating hazardous machinery until they are reasonably certain that the drug does not affect them adversely. Caution should also be exercised in patients taking other centrally acting drugs, and patients should be advised to avoid the consumption of alcoholic beverages. May cause orthostatic hypotension, especially during the initial dose-titration period, and the initial dose should not exceed 1 mg twice daily to reduce the risk. May lengthen the QT interval, so caution should be exercised in patients with risk factors for this complication (e.g., bradycardia, use of other drugs that prolong the QT interval). May antagonize the effects of levodopa.

Cerebrovascular adverse events (e.g., stroke, transient ischemic attack), including fatalities, were reported in elderly patients with dementia-related psychosis. Risperidone has not been shown to be safe or effective in the treatment of patients with dementia-related psychosis.

Administration: Oral.

Preparations: Tablets, 0.25, 0.5, 1, 2, 3, and 4 mg. Long-acting injection, 25, 37.5, and 50 mg. Orally disintegrating tablets, 0.5, 1, and 2 mg. Oral solution, 1 mg/mL.

RITALIN®, see Methylphenidate

RITALIN SR®, see Methylphenidate

RITODRINE HYDROCHLORIDE—Yutopar®

Description/Actions: Uterine relaxant indicated in the management of preterm labor in suitable patients for the purpose of prolonging gestation. Continue IV for 12–24 hours after contractions cease, and begin PO 30 minutes before IV is stopped.

Preparations: Tablets, 10 mg. Ampules, vials, and syringes, 10 mg/ml and 15 mg/ml.

RITONOVIR—Norvir®

Description/Actions: Antiviral/protease inhibitor used in treatment of HIV infection, either as monotherapy or in combination with other nucleoside analogs or protease inhibitors.

Precautions/Adverse Reactions: Use cautiously in patients with impaired hepatic function. Adverse reactions include GI upset, asthenia, abdominal pain, headache, anorexia, paresthesias, taste perversion, fever, hyperlipidemia, dizziness, rash, throat irritation, malaise, somnolence, insomnia, and sweating. Due to increased plasma concentrations of various agents, and large increases in concentrations of highly metabolized sedatives and hypnotics, the coadministration of ritonovir with such agents is contraindicated, and prescribers should verify a patient's full drug profile prior to prescribing this agent.

Administration: Oral with meals.

Preparations: Capsules, 100 mg. Oral solution, 80 mg/ml.

RIVASTIGMINE TARTRATE—Exelon®

Description/Actions: Indicated in the treatment of mild to moderate dementia of the Alzheimer's type.

Precautions/Adverse Reactions: Rivastigmine is contraindicated in patients with a known hypersensitivity to rivastigmine, or other carbamate derivatives, or to any other component of the product. Significant gastrointestinal adverse reactions, including nausea, vomiting, anorexia, and weight loss (females > males), have been observed during therapy with rivastigmine. Cholinesterase inhibitors have been shown to increase gastric acid secretion; therefore, patients should be monitored for the development of peptic ulcers or gastrointestinal bleeding. Rivastigmine is likely to potentiate the effects of succinylcholine-type muscle relaxation during anesthesia. Use cautiously in patients with sick sinus syndrome or other supraventricular cardiac conduction conditions. Use cautiously in patients with a history of asthma or obstructive pulmonary disease. Monitor patients for urinary obstruction and/or seizures due to increased cholinergic activity. Rivastigmine is metabolized through hydrolysis by esterases with minimal metabolism via the cytochrome P450 system; therefore, no significant drug interactions are expected with drugs metabolized via this system. Anticholinergics: rivastigmine has the potential to interfere with the activity of anticholinergic agents. Other cholinesterase inhibitors: rivastigmine, may potentiate the effects of these agents. Pregnancy Category B. There are no adequate or well-controlled studies in pregnant women. Rivastigmine should be used during pregnancy only if the potential benefit justifies the potential risk to the fetus. Excretion in human breast milk is unknown. Rivastigmine has no indication for use in nursing mothers. There are no adequate or well-controlled studies documenting safety or efficacy of rivastigmine in children. Most common adverse reactions occurring in at least 5% of patients treated with rivastigmine include nausea, vomiting, anorexia, dyspepsia, weight loss, and asthenia. Other adverse effects observed include increased sweating, syncope, accidental trauma, fatigue, malaise, influenza-like symptoms, hypertension, headache, somnolence, tremor, abdominal pain, constipation, flatulence, insomnia, confusion, depression, hallucinations, urinary tract infections, and rhinitis. Monitor for GI effects.

Administration: Oral with food.

Preparations: Capsules, 1.5, 3, 4.5, and 6 mg. Oral solution, 2 mg/ml.

RIZATRIPTAN BENZOATE—Maxalt®, Maxalt MLT®

Description/Actions: A selective 5-HT$_{1B/1D}$ antimigraine medication indicated for an acute migraine attack with or without an aura.

Precautions/Adverse Reactions: Rizatriptan is contraindicated in ischemic heart disease, coronary artery vasospasm, uncontrolled hypertension, other significant cardiovascular disease, basilar or hemiplegic migraine, within 24 hours of other 5-HT1 agonists or ergo-type drugs, and during or within 2 weeks after discontinuing MAOIs. Confirm diagnosis prior to prescribing rizatriptan. Reevaluate if angina or ischemic symptoms occur or if no response after the first dose. Exclude underlying cardiovascular disease, supervise first dose, and consider ECG monitoring in patients with a likelihood of undiagnosed coronary disease. Monitor cardiovascular function in long-term intermittent use. Use cautiously in patients with hepatic dysfunctions and on dialysis. Pregnancy Category C. Adverse reactions include asthenia, somnolence, dizziness, paresthesis, chest/throat pressure or other pain, dry mouth, nausea, and headache.

Administration: Oral. Concomitant propanalol use: 5 mg; max 3 doses in a day.

Patient Care Implications: Instruct patients that this medication is for use during acute attack and does not reduce the frequency or severity of attacks. Advise patients to take the medication during the aura or immediately when the attack starts. Inform patients to notify the prescriber immediately if chest pain/tightness occurs during use and to withhold any further doses until evaluated by the prescriber. Tell patients that lying down in a quiet, darkened room may help to further relieve the headache.

Preparations: Maxalt—tablets, 5 and 10 mg. Maxalt MLT—orally disintegrating peppermint flavored tablets, 5 and 10 mg.

RMS®, see Morphine

ROBAXIN®, see Methocarbamol

ROBIMYCIN®, see Erythromycin Base

ROBINUL®, see Glycopyrrolate

ROBITUSSIN®, see Guaifenesin

ROCALTROL®, see Calcitriol

ROCEPHIN®, see Ceftriaxone

ROCURONIUM BROMIDE—Zemuron®

Description/Actions: Nondepolarizing neuromuscular blocking agent indicated for inpatients and outpatients as an adjunct to general anesthesia to facilitate both rapid sequence and routine tracheal intubation and to provide skeletal muscle relaxation during surgery or mechanical ventilation.

Precautions/Adverse Reactions: Severe anaphylactic reactions to neuromuscular blocking agents including Zemuron® have been reported. These reactions have, in some cases, been life threatening. Special precautions should be taken in patients who have had previous anaphylactic reactions to other neuromuscular blocking agents, as cross-reactivity has been reported in this class of drugs. Must be used with caution in patients with neuromuscular disease (e.g., myasthenia gravis) and in patients receiving other medications that may increase or prolong neuromuscular block. Action may be enhanced by the prior administration of succinylcholine, and rocuronium should not be administered until recovery from succinylcholine has been observed.

Administration: Intravenous.

Preparations: Vials, 10 mg/ml.

ROFERON-A®, see Interferon alfa-2a Recombinant

ROGAINE®, see Minoxidil

ROMAZICON®, see Flumazenil

ROPIVACAINE HYDROCHLORIDE—Naropin®

Description/Actions: Long-acting local anesthetic indicated in local or regional anesthesia or surgery and management of acute pain, including the pain of obstetrical procedures.

Precautions/Adverse Reactions: Contraindicated in patients with known hypersensitivity to any local anesthetic of this type (i.e., bupivacaine, lidocaine, mepivacaine). Adverse reactions include hypotension, fetal bradycardia, nausea, bradycardia, vomiting, parasthesia, and back pain. Carefully monitor vital signs including cardiovascular and respiratory status and level of consciousness after each injection. Oxygen and resuscitative equipment should be available. Use cautiously in patients with severe hepatic or renal impairment and impaired cardiovascular function.

Administration: Administer as infiltrate, block or epidural or intermittent bolus.

Preparations: Injection, 2, 5, 7.5, and 10 mg/ml.

ROSIGLITAZONE—Avandia®

Description/Actions: Antidiabetic agent indicated as an adjunct to diet and exercise in type II diabetes, for monotherapy, or added to metformin.

Precautions/Adverse Reactions: Do not use for treatment of type I diabetes or diabetic ketoacidosis. Do not start therapy in active liver disease or if ALT is >2.5 × ULN. Monitor transaminases at baseline and every 2 months for the first 12 months, then periodically. Discontinue if ALT is >3 × ULN or if jaundice occurs. Not for use in patients with a history of troglitazone-associated juandice. Use cautiously in patients with a history of liver disease. Rosiglitazone can cause fluid retention, which may exacerbate or lead to heart failure. Not recommended for use in patients with New York Heart Association (NYHA) class 3 and 4. Patients should be monitored for signs and symptoms of heart failure. Rosiglitazone may cause resumption of premenopausal ovulation in anovulatory patients with a risk of an unintended pregnancy. Pregnancy Category C. Adverse reactions include upper respiratory tract infection, edema, weight gain, anemia, and changes in serum lipid levels.

Administration: Oral.

Patient Care Implications: Instruct patients to continue following their diet and exercise to control diabetes. This drug does not eliminate the need for these other measures. Tell the patient to call the physician immediately if (s)he notes darkening of the urine or yellow color to skin or the whites of the eyes.

Preparations: Tablets, 2, 4, and 8 mg.

ROSIGLITAZONE AND METFORMIN—Avandamet™

Description/Actions: Avandamet™ is indicated as an adjunct to diet and exercise to improve glycemic control in patients with type 2 diabetes who are already treated with combination rosiglitazone and metformin or who are not adequately controlled on metformin alone. Avandamet™ is not appropriate for initial therapy of type 2 diabetes.

Precautions/Adverse Reactions: Avandamet™ is contraindicated in patients with a known hypersensitivity to rosiglitazone or metformin; patients with congestive heart failure (CHF) requiring pharmacologic treatment; patients with renal disease or renal dysfunction (serum creatinine levels = 1.5 mg/dL [males], = 1.4 mg/dL [females], or abnormal creatinine clearance); and in patients with acute or chronic metabolic acidosis, including diabetic ketoacidosis, with or without coma. Lactic acidosis is a rare but serious metabolic complication that can occur due to metformin accumulation. When it occurs, it is fatal in approximately 50% of cases. Lactic acidosis may also occur in association with a number of pathophysiological conditions, including diabetes mellitus and whenever there is significant tissue hypoperfusion and hypoxemia. Stop treatment in the presence of any condition associated with hypoxemia, dehydration, or sepsis. Intravascular contrast studies with iodinated materials can lead to acute alteration of renal function and have been associated with lactic acidosis in patients receiving metformin. Temporarily discontinue Avandamet™ prior to any intravascular radiocontrast study and for any surgical procedure (except minor procedures not associated with restricted intake of food and fluids) and hold for 48 hours subsequent to the procedure. Reinstate drug after renal function has been reevaluated and found to be normal. Impaired hepatic function has been associated with some cases of lactic acidosis. Avandamet™ should not be initiated if the patient exhibits clinical evidence of active liver disease or increased serum transaminase levels (ALT >2.5 times upper limit of normal) at baseline. Therapy with rosiglitazone may result in ovulation in some premenopausal anovulatory women. These patients may be at an increased risk for pregnancy. Adequate contraception in premenopausal women is recommended. Most common adverse reactions were diarrhea, upper respiratory tract infection, headache, anemia, and sinusitis. Pregnancy Category C.

Administration: Oral.

Preparations: Tablets, 1 mg/500 mg (rosiglitazone 1 mg and metformin 500 mg), 2 mg/500 mg (rosiglitazone 2 mg and metformin 500 mg), 2 mg/1000 mg (rosiglitazone 2 mg and metformin 1000 mg), 4 mg/500 mg (rosiglitazone 4 mg and metformin 500 mg), 4 mg/1000 mg (rosiglitazone 4 mg and metformin 1000 mg). Store at 25°C (77°F); excursions permitted to 15–30°C (59–86°F). Dispense in a tight, light-resistant container.

ROSUVASTATIN CRESTOR®

Description/Actions: Rosuvastatin is a synthetic lipid-lowering agent. Rosuvastatin is a selective and competitive inhibitor of HMG-CoA reductase, the rate-limiting enzyme that converts 3–hydroxy-3–methylglutaryl coenzyme A to mevalonate, a precursor of cholesterol. Rosuvastatin produces its lipid modifying effects in two ways. First, it increases the number of hepatic LDL receptors on the cell surface to enhance uptake and catabolism of LDL. Second, it inhibits hepatic synthesis of VLDL, which reduces the total number of VLDL and LDL particles. Rosuvastatin is indicated as adjunct to diet to reduce elevated total cholesterol, LDL-C, Apo B, non-HDL-C, and triglyceride levels, and to increase HDL-C in patients with primary hypercholesterolemia (heterozygous familial and nonfamilial) and mixed dyslipidemia (Fredrickson type IIa and IIb); as adjunct to diet for the treatment of patients with elevated serum triglyceride levels (Fredrickson type IV), to reduce LDL-C, total cholesterol, and Apo B in patients with homozygous familial hypercholesterolemia as an adjunct to other lipid lowering treatments (e.g., LDL apheresis) or if such treatments are unavailable.

Precautions/Adverse Reactions: Rosuvastatin is contraindicated in patients with a known hypersensitivity to it or to any component of the formulation. Rosuvastatin is contraindicated in patients with active liver disease or with unexplained persistent elevations of serum transaminases, pregnancy, and breast-feeding. Liver function tests should be performed before and at 12 weeks following both the initiation of therapy and any elevation of dose and semiannually thereafter. Liver enzyme changes generally occur in the first 3 months of treatment with rosuvastatin. Patients who develop increased transaminase levels should be monitored until the abnormalities have resolved. Should an increase in ALT or AST of >3 times the upper limit of normal persist, reduction of dose or withdrawal of rosuvastatin is recommended. Rare cases of rhabdomyolysis with acute renal failure secondary to myoglobinuria have been reported with rosuvastatin. Treatment-related myopathy defined as muscle aches or muscle weakness in conjunction with increases in CK values greater than 10x the upper limit of normal was reported in up to 0.1% of patients taking rosuvastatin. Rosuvastatin should be used with caution in patients with predisposing factors for myopathy such as renal impairment, advanced age, and hypothyroidism. Risk of myopathy may be increased with concurrent administration of other lipid-lowering therapies or cyclosporine. Rosuvastatin therapy should temporarily be withheld in any patient with an acute, serious condition suggestive of myopathy or predisposing to the development of renal failure secondary to rhabdomyolysis (e.g., sepsis, hypotension, major surgery, trauma, severe metabolic, endocrine, and electrolyte disorders, or uncontrolled seizures). Before instituting therapy with rosuvastatin, an attempt should be made to control hypercholesterolemia with appropriate diet and exercise, weight reduction in obese patients, and treatment of underlying medical problems. Coadministration of rosuvastatin and ketoconazole, erythromycin, itraconazole, and fluconazole did not lead to any significant changes in rosuvastatin plasma concentrations. Coadministration of rosuvastatin and cyclosporine resulted in increased serum rosuvastatin concentrations. Coadministration of rosuvastatin and warfarin resulted in increases in the International Normalized Ratio (INR). INR levels should be monitored. Coadministration of rosuvastatin and digoxin resulted in no changes to digoxin plasma concentrations. Coadministration of fenofibrate and/or niacin with rosuvastatin may increase risk of myopathy. Coadministration of rosuvastatin and gemfibrozil may lead to increased serum levels of rosuvastatin. Coadministration of oral contraceptives and rosuvastatin resulted in an increase in plasma concentrations of ethinyl estradiol and norgestrel. Pregnancy Category X. Rosuvastatin may cause fetal harm when administered to a pregnant woman. Rosuvastatin is contraindicated in women who are or may become pregnant. There are no adequate and well-controlled studies in pregnant women. Excretion in human breast milk is unknown. Safety and efficacy in pediatric patients have not been established. Most common adverse effects observed in patients treated with rosuvastatin include: myalgia, constipation, asthenia, abdominal pain, and nausea. Other reported adverse effects include: pharyngitis, angina, headache, diarrhea, dyspepsia, back pain, flu syndrome, urinary tract infections, rhinitis, sinusitis, chest pain, infection, pelvic pain, hypertension, vasodilatation, palpitation, gastroenteritis, flatulence, periodontal abscess, gastritis, diabetes mellitus, anemia, ecchymosis, peripheral edema, arthritis, arthralgia, dizziness, insomnia, paresthesia, depression, anxiety, vertigo, neuralgia, bronchitis, increased cough, dyspnea, pneumonia, asthma, rash, pruritus, elevated CPK, transaminases, alkaline phosphatase, bilirubin, and thyroid function abnormalities. Urticaria, angioedema, kidney failure, myositis, pancreatitis, photosensitivity, myopathy, and rhabdomyolysis have also been reported.

Administration: Oral.

Patient Care Implications: Patients should be advised to promptly report unexplained muscle pain, tenderness, or weakness, particularly if accompanied by malaise or fever. Rosuvastatin therapy should be discontinued if markedly elevated CK levels occur or myopathy is diagnosed or suspected. When taking with an aluminum and magnesium hydroxide combination antacid, the antacid should be taken at least 2 hours after rosuvastatin administration.

Preparations: Tablets, 5 mg, 10 mg, 20 mg, and 40 mg.

ROWASA®, see Mesalamine

ROXANOL®, see Morphine

ROXANOL SR®, see Morphine

ROXICODONE®, see Oxycodone

RUBEX®, see Doxorubicin

RUFEN®, see Ibuprofen

RYTHMOL®, see Propafenone

S

SAFFLOWER OIL

Description/Actions: Nutritional supplement used in the management of patients requiring caloric supplementation.

Preparations: Emulsion.

SALAGEN®, see Pilocarpine Hydrochloride

SALFLEX®, see Salsalate

SALICYLAMIDE

Description/Actions: Analgesic used in the management of mild to moderate pain.

Preparations: Tablets, 325 and 667 mg.

SALICYLIC ACID

Description/Actions: Keratolytic agent used topically as an aid in the removal of excessive keratin in hyperkeratotic skin disorders, including warts. Also used in combination with other agents in a number of dermatologic conditions, including acne.

Preparations: Cream, ointment, liquid, gel, and plaster in concentrations ranging from 1% to 60%.

SALMETEROL XINAFOATE—Serevent®, Serevent® Discus

Description/Actions: Is a selective beta-2-adrenergic receptor agonist that is administered by oral inhalation. Has a long duration of action that permits twice-daily administration. Indicated for long-term, twice-daily (morning and evening) administration in the maintenance treatment of asthma and in the prevention of bronchospasm in patients 12 years of age and older with reversible obstructive airway disease, including patients with symptoms of nocturnal asthma, who require regular treament with inhaled, short-acting beta-2-adrenergic agonists. Is also indicated for the prevention of exercise-induced bronchospasm and maintenance treatment of COPD-associated bronchospasm (including emphysema and chronic bronchitis). Patients must also be provided with a short-acting inhaled beta-2-adrenergic agonist (e.g., albuterol) for the treatment of symptoms that occur despite twice-daily use of salmeterol. Should not be used to treat acute symptoms.

Precautions/Adverse Reactions: Adverse reactions include headache, tremor, cough, and dizziness. Should be used with caution in patients with coronary insufficiency, cardiac arrhythmias, and hypertension, and in patients being treated with a tricyclic antidepressant or a monoamine oxidase inhibitor. Should not be used to treat acute symptoms. Data from a large placebo controlled safety study that was stopped early suggest that salmeterol may be associated with rare serious asthma episodes or asthma-related deaths. Salmeterol should not be initiated in patients with significantly worsening or acutely deteriorating asthma, which may be life threatening. Patients on salmeterol must also have a short-acting bronchodilator (e.g., albuterol) for use as needed for acute symptoms.

Administration: Oral inhalation.

Preparations: Powder for inhalation, 50 mg/blister. Serevent® Discus 50 mcg/actuation.

SALSALATE—Disalcid®, Salflex®

Description/Actions: Salicylate analgesic/anti-inflammatory agent indicated for the relief of the signs and symptoms of rheumatoid arthritis, osteoarthritis, and related disorders.

Preparations: Capsules and tablets, 500 and 750 mg.

SALT, see Sodium Chloride

SALURON®, see Hydroflumethiazide

SANDIMMUNE®, see Cyclosporine

SANDOSTATIN®, see Octreotide

SANOREX®, see Mazindol

SANSERT®, see Methysergide

SANTYL®, see Collagenase

SAQUINAVIR—Fortovase®, Invirase®

Description/Actions: Antiviral (HIV protease inhibitor) indicated in the management of advanced HIV infection in combination with zidovudine, and/or other nucleoside analogs.

Precautions/Adverse Reactions: Use cautiously in patients with hepatic impairment. Adverse reactions include diarrhea, abdominal discomfort, nausea, asthenia, and rash.

Administration: Oral with food.

Preparations: Capsules, 200 mg. Tablet, 500 mg.

SARAFEM™, see Fluoxetine Hydrochloride

SARGRAMOSTIM—Leukine®, Prokine®

Description/Actions: A human granulocyte-macrophage colony–stimulating factor (GM-CSF) produced by recombinant DNA technology. Accelerates bone marrow recovery after autologous bone marrow transplantation. Indicated for acceleration of myeloid recovery in patients with non-Hodgkin's lymphoma, acute lymphoblastic leukemia, and Hodgkin's disease undergoing autologous bone marrow transplantation. Also indicated for patients who have undergone allogeneic or autologous bone marrow transplantation in whom engraftment is delayed or has failed.

Precautions/Adverse Reactions: Contraindicated in patients with excessive leukemic myeloid blasts in the bone marrow or peripheral blood (greater than 10%). Adverse reactions include diarrhea, asthenia, rash, malaise, transient supraventricular arrhythmias, peripheral edema, and pleural and/or pericardial effusion. May cause dyspnea and special attention should be given to respiratory symptoms during or immediately following infusion, especially in patients with preexisting lung disease. Caution must be exercised in patients with any malignancy with myeloid characteristics because of the possibility that the drug may act as a growth factor for the tumor.

Administration: Intravenous. Should be administered not less than 24 hours after the last dose of chemotherapy and 12 hours after the last dose of radiotherapy.

Preparations: Vials, 250 and 500 mcg.

SCOPOLAMINE HYDROBROMIDE—Hyoscine, Transderm-Scop®

Description/Actions: Anticholinergic agent indicated for parenteral use for preanesthetic medication, for obstetric amnesia in conjunction with analgesics, and for calming delirium. Also used orally and transdermally for the prevention of nausea and vomiting associated with motion sickness. Also indicated for ophthalmic use to produce cycloplegia and mydriasis.

Preparations: Capsules, 0.25 mg. Transdermal therapeutic system, 1.5 mg (used over a period of 3 days). Ampules and vials, 0.3 mg/ml, 0.4 mg/ml, 1 mg/ml. Ophthalmic solution, 0.25%.

SECOBARBITAL SODIUM—Seconal®

Description/Actions: Barbiturate used parenterally as a preanesthetic and for the emergency control of certain acute convulsive episodes.

Preparations: Vials and syringes, 50 mg/ml.

SECONAL®, see Secobarbital

SECTRAL®, see Acebutolol

SELEGILINE HYDROCHLORIDE—Eldepryl®

Description/Actions: Also known as deprenyl, it acts as a selective inhibitor of monoamine oxidase type B. Indicated as an adjunct to levodopa/carbidopa in the management of Parkinson's disease.

Precautions/Adverse Reactions: Adverse reactions include nausea, abdominal pain, dry mouth, dizziness, fainting, confusion, hallucinations, and vivid dreams. Does not inhibit monoamine oxidase type A at the recommended dosage level, and is not likely to interact with the sympathomimetic amines and tyramine-containing foods that can cause hypertensive reactions when used concurrently with a nonselective monoamine oxidase inhibitor. However, the recommended dosage level should not be exceeded, as the selectivity of selegiline is reduced with increasing daily doses. Concomitant use of selegiline with meperidine should be avoided.

Administration: Oral.

Preparations: Capsules, 5 mg.

SELENIUM SULFIDE—Selsun®

Description/Actions: Antiseborrheic agent indicated for topical use in the treatment of dandruff and seborrheic dermatitis of the scalp and in the management of tinea versicolor.

Preparations: Lotion shampoo, 1% and 2.5%.

SELSUN®, see Selenium Sulfide

SEMI-LENTE INSULIN, see Insulin

SEMPREX-D®, see Acrivastine/Pseudoephedrine Hydrochloride

SENNA CONCENTRATE—Senokot®

Description/Actions: Laxative used in the prevention and treatment of constipation.

Preparations: Tablets, granules, syrup, liquid, and suppositories.

SENOKOT®, see Senna Concentrate

SEPTOCAINE™, see Articaine Hydrochloride and Epinephrine

SEPTRA®, see Trimethoprim-sulfamethoxazole

SERAX®, see Oxazepam

SERENTIL®, see Mesoridazine

SEREVENT®, see Salmeterol Xinafoate

SEREVENT® DISCUS, see Salmeterol Xinafoate

SEROMYCIN®, see Cycloserine

SEROPHENE®, see Clomiphene

SEROQUEL®, see Quetiapine

SEROSTIM®, see Somatropin

SERPASIL®, see Reserpine

SERTACONAZOLE—Ertaczo™

Description/Actions: Sertaconazole is a topical imidazole antifungal agent. Sertaconazole alters fungal cell wall membrane permeability and inhibits the CYP450–dependent synthesis of ergosterol. Ergosterol is a key component of the cell membrane of fungi and lack of this component leads to fungal cell injury, primarily by leakage of key constituents in the cytoplasm from the cell. Sertaconazole is indicated for the topical treatment of interdigital tinea pedis in immunocompetent patients 12 years of age and older, caused by *Trichophyton rubrum, Trichophyton mentagrophytes* and *Epidermophyton floccosum.*

Precautions/Adverse Reactions: Sertaconazole is contraindicated in patients hypersensitive to sertaconazole, other imidazoles, or any component of the formulation. Sertaconazole is for external use only, not for ophthalmic or intravaginal use. Discontinue if sensitivity or chemical irritation occurs. Diagnosis of the disease should be confirmed either by direct microscopic examination of infected superficial epidermal tissue or by culture. Pregnancy risk factor C; use only if clearly needed during pregnancy. Most common adverse effects were burning, contact dermatitis, dry skin, and skin tenderness.

Administration: Topical.

Patient Care Implications: Make sure skin is dry before applying. Do not use occlusive dressings. Wash hands after applying. Avoid contact with eyes, nose, mouth, and other mucous membranes.

Preparations: Cream, 2%.

SERTRALINE HYDROCHLORIDE—Zoloft®

Description/Actions: Is a serotonin reuptake inhibitor. Indicated for the treatment of depression, panic disorder, obsessive-compulsive disorder (OCD), post-traumatic stress disorder (PTSD), premenstrual dysphoric disorder (PMDD), and for the acute and long-term treatment of social anxiety disorder.

Precautions/Adverse Reactions: In short-term studies in children and adolescents with Major Depressive Disorder (MDD) and other psychiatric disorders, antidepressants increased the risk of suicidal thinking and behavior (suicidality). Anyone considering the use of sertraline or any other antidepressant in a child or adolescent must balance this risk with the clinical need. Patients who are started on therapy should be observed closely for clinical worsening, suicidality, or unusual changes in behavior. Zoloft® is not approved for use in pediatric patients except for patients with obsessive-compulsive disorder (OCD). Adverse reactions include nausea, diarrhea, dyspepsia, dizziness, tremor, insomnia, somnolence, dry mouth, increased sweating, and sexual dysfunction in male patients (primarily ejaculatory delay). May decrease appetite, resulting in significant weight loss. Concomitant use with a monoamine oxidase inhibitor (MAOI) or use within 14 days of treatment with an MAOI may result in serious, potentially fatal reactions (hyperthermia, rigidity, myoclonus, autonomic instability, with fluctuating vital signs and extreme agitation, which may proceed to delirium and coma). Sertraline should be stopped at least 14 days prior to MAOI therapy. Concomitant administration of sertraline and pimozide is contraindicated.

Administration: Oral.

Preparations: Tablets, 25, 50, and 100 mg. Oral concentrate, 20 mg/ml.

SEVELAMER HCL—Renagel®

Description/Actions: Sevelamer is a phosphate-binding agent indicated for the reduction of serum phosphates in end-stage renal disease (ESRD).

Precautions/Adverse Reactions: This agent is contraindicated in hypophosphotemia and bowel obstruction. Use cautiously in patients with dysphagia, swallowing disorders, severe GI motility disorders, and major GI tract surgery. Monitor serum calcium, bicarbonate, and chloride. Sevelamer may cause reductions in vitamins E, K, and folic acid, and levels should be monitored. It may bind with other agents, so, when administering with drugs that have a narrow therapeutic index, separate dosing by at least 1 hour before or 3 hours after sevelamer. Adverse reactions include nausea, constipation, diarrhea, flatulence, and dyspepsia.

Administration: Oral. Swallow whole with meals; do not crush, chew, or open.

Patient Care Implications: Instruct patients that this medication is an adjunct to diet and does not eliminate the need for dietary restrictions. Sevelamer has also been associated with decreases in total serum cholesterol and low-density lipoprotein cholesterol. It is not absorbed systemically.

Preparations: Capsules, 403 mg. Tablets, 400 and 800 mg.

SEVOFLURANE®—Ultane®

Description/Actions: Halogenated volatile anesthetic that provides rapid induction and emergence from anesthesia in inpatient and outpatient surgery.

Precautions/Adverse Reactions: May cause malignant hyperthermia and is contraindicated in patients who are hypersensitive to the drug or other halogenated agents. Adverse reactions include agitation, somnolence, cough, breath holding, laryngospasm, airway obstruction, tachycardia, bradycardia, hypotension, nausea, and vomiting.

Administration: Inhalation.

Preparations: Liquid, 250 ml.

SHOHL'S SOLUTION MODIFIED®, see Sodium Citrate

SILDENAFIL CITRATE—Viagra®

Description/Actions: An oral tablet indicated for the treatment of erectile dysfunction (ED).

Precautions/Adverse Reactions: Contraindicated with concomitant organic nitrates or nitric oxide donors. Use cautiously in anatomical penile deformation, predisposition to priapism, or patients for whom sexual activity is inadvisable or contraindicated. Avoid use in bleeding disorders, active peptic ulceration, concomitant erectile dysfunction treatment, or retinosis pigmentosa. Not indicated for use in women, children, or newborns. Adverse reactions include headache, flushing, dyspepsia, nasal congestion, UTI, abnormal vision (color tinge to vision, increased light sensitivity, blurred vision), diarrhea, dizziness, and rash. Concomitant administration of sildenafil with alpha blockers may lead to symptomatic hypotension. Sildenafil doses above 25 mg should not be taken within 4 hours of taking an alpha blocker.

Administration: Take 1 dose as needed about 1 hour before sexual activity at a frequency of up to once daily.

Preparations: Tablets, 25, 50, and 100 mg.

SILVADENE®, see Silver Sulfadiazine

SILVER NITRATE

Description/Actions: Anti-infective agent and cauterizing and caustic agent. Indicated for ophthalmic use in the prevention of gonococcal ophthalmia neonatorum. Has been used topically in the treatment of burns. Also has been used topically for its caustic and cauterizing actions in the treatment of certain dermatologic problems (e.g., warts).

Preparations: Ophthalmic solution, 1%. Ointment and solutions for topical use.

SILVER SULFADIAZINE—Silvadene®

Description/Actions: Anti-infective agent used topically as an adjunct for the prevention and treatment of wound sepsis in patients with second- and third-degree burns.

Preparations: Cream, 1%.

SIMETHICONE—Mylicon®, Phazyme®

Description/Actions: Antiflatulent indicated for relief of the painful symptoms of excess gas in the digestive tract.

Preparations: Tablets, 40, 50, 60, 80, and 95 mg. Chewable tablets, 125 mg. Capsules, 125 mg. Drops, 40 mg/0.6 ml.

SIMVASTATIN—Zocor®

Description/Actions: Is a prodrug that is converted to its active form following administration. Produces a significant reduction in total and low-density lipoprotein (LDL) cholesterol concentrations, a modest reduction in triglyceride concentrations, and an increase in high-density lipoprotein (HDL) cholesterol concentrations. Indicated as an adjunct to diet for the reduction of elevated total and LDL cholesterol concentrations in patients with primary hypercholesterolemia (type IIa and IIb) when the response to a diet restricted in saturated fat and cholesterol and other nonpharmacological measures has not been adequate. Simvastatin is indicated, along with diet, to reduce the risk of total mortality (by reducing CHD death), nonfatal MI, and stroke, and to reduce the need for coronary and noncoronary revascularization procedures in patients at high risk of coronary events because of existing CHD, diabetes, peripheral vascular disease, or history of stroke or other cerebrovascular disease.

Precautions/Adverse Reactions: Contraindicated in patients with active liver disease or unexplained persistent elevations of serum transaminases.

Is also contraindicated in pregnant women and nursing mothers. Increases in serum transaminases may occur, and it is recommended that liver function tests be monitored before treatment begins, every 6 weeks for the first 3 months, every 8 weeks during the remainder of the first year, and periodically thereafter (at about 6-month intervals). Adverse reactions include constipation, flatulence, dyspepsia, myalgia, myopathy, and, rarely, rhabdomyolysis. Patients should be advised to promptly report unexplained muscle pain, tenderness, or weakness. The risk of myopathy/rhabdomyolysis is dose related. The risk of myopathy/rhabdomyolysis is increased by concomitant administration of amiodarone or verapamil. In patients taking amiodarone or verapamil with simvastatin, the dose should not exceed 20 mg/day. The risk of myopathy/rhabdomyolysis is increased when simvastatin is given with itraconazole, ketoconazole, erythromycin, clarithromycin, HIV protease inhibitors, nefazodone or large quantities of grapefruit juice (>1 quart/day). If treatment with these drugs is unavoidable, simvastatin should be stopped during the course of treatment. The dose of simvastatin should not exceed 10 mg/day when given with cyclosporine, gemfibrozil, other fibrates, or niacin (>1 g/day).

Administration: Oral. Should be administered at bedtime.

Preparations: Tablets, 5, 10, 20, and 40 mg.

SINEMET—Combination of Levodopa and Carbidopa

SINEMET CR—Combination of Levodopa and Carbidopa (controlled-release)

SINEQUAN, see Doxepin

SINGULAIR, see Montelukast

SINUMIST SR CAPLETS, see Guaifenesin

SIROLIMUS—Rapamune®

Description/Actions: Sirolimus is used as an immunosuppressant in combination with cyclosporine and prednisone as prophylaxis for kidney transplant rejection.

Precautions/Adverse Reactions: The safety and efficacy of sirolimus as immunosuppressive therapy have not been established in liver or lung transplant patients; therefore, such use is not recommended. The use of sirolimus in combination with cyclosporine or tacrolimus in de novo liver transplant recipients was associated with an increase in hepatic artery thrombosis leading to graft loss or death. Sirolimus should be administered with caution in patients with high cholesterol or triglycerides, an active infection, pregnancy, breast-feeding, or liver disease. Increased susceptibility to infection and the possible development of lymphoma and malignancy, especially of the skin, may result from immunosuppression. Mild to moderate hepatic impairment requires dosage adjustments. Some side effects are lymphocele, hyperlipidemia, azotemia, hypertension, rash, and epistaxis.

Administrations: Oral.

Patient Care Implications: The drug should be avoided in patients who are pregnant or breast-feeding. Sirolimus should also be given cautiously in patients with high cholesterol or triglycerides, an active infection, or liver disease. Drug should be given in a facility equipped with supportive medical services. CBC, serum cholesterol, serum creatinine/BUN, serum lipid, and serum potassium must be monitored while patient is on medication.

Preparations: Oral solution, 1 mg/ml. Tablet, 1 mg.

SKELAXIN, see Metaxalone

SKELID®, see Tiludronate

SLO-BID, see Theophylline

SLO-NIACIN, see Nicotinic Acid

SLO-PHYLLIN, see Theophylline

SLOW-FE®, see Ferrous Sulfate, Exsiccated

SLOW-K®, see Potassium Chloride

SLOW-MAG®, see Magnesium Chloride

SODIUM ASCORBATE, see Vitamin C

SODIUM BENZOATE AND SODIUM PHENYLACETATE—
Ucephan®

Description/Actions: Are metabolically active compounds that decrease elevated blood ammonia concentrations in patients with inborn errors of ureagenesis. Indicated as adjunctive therapy (with dietary management [low protein diet] and amino acid supplementation) for the prevention and treatment of hyperammonemia in the chronic management of patients with urea cycle enzymopathies.

Precautions/Adverse Reactions: Adverse reactions include nausea and vomiting. Because of the sodium content of the product, the possibility of hypernatremia exists, and caution should be exercised in patients with congestive heart failure, severe renal insufficiency, and in clinical states in which there is sodium retention with edema.

Administration: Oral. Ucephan is a concentrated solution and must be diluted before use. Because sodium phenylacetate has a lingering odor, care should be taken in mixing and administering the drug to minimize contact with skin and clothing.

Preparations: Oral solution, 10% sodium benzoate and 10% sodium phenylacetate.

SODIUM BICARBONATE—Baking Soda

Description/Actions: Antacid and alkalinizer. Used orally as a gastric antacid and urinary alkalinizer. Administered intravenously in the management of metabolic acidosis and to alkalinize the urine in the treatment of certain drug intoxications.

Preparations: Tablets, 325 and 650 mg. Vials and syringes, 4%, 4.2%, 5%, 7.5%, and 8.4%.

SODIUM BIPHOSPHATE

Description/Actions: Laxative often used in combination with sodium phosphate. Has also been used as a urinary acidifier.

SODIUM BORATE—Collyrium

Description/Actions: Antiseptic and buffer indicated for ophthalmic use for flushing or irrigating the eye to remove loose foreign material.

Preparations: Ophthalmic solution.

SODIUM CELLULOSE PHOSPHATE—Calcibind®

Description/Actions: Indicated for absorptive hypercalciuria type I with recurrent calcium oxalate or calcium phosphate nephrolithiasis.

Preparations: Powder, 2.5 g packets.

SODIUM CHLORIDE—Salt

Description/Actions: Used intravenously to replace fluid and electrolytes, as a genitourinary irrigant, as an abortifacient, for ophthalmic use in the treatment and diagnosis of ocular conditions, and for intranasal use to restore moisture and alleviate discomfort in certain nasal conditions.

Preparations: Solutions for intravenous infusion, 0.45%, 0.9% (normal saline), 3%, 5%. Vials for intravenous admixtures, 50 mEq, 100 mEq, and 625 mEq. Solutions for genitourinary irrigation, 0.45% and 0.9%. Solutions for inducing abortion, 20%. Ophthalmic solution or ointment, 2% and 5%. Nose drops and spray, 0.4% and 0.65%.

SODIUM CITRATE—Bicitra®, Shohl's Solution Modified®

Description/Actions: Alkalinizing agent useful in conditions in which the maintenance of an alkaline urine is desirable, and in the alleviation of chronic metabolic acidosis such as results from chronic renal insufficiency.

Preparations: Solution, 500 mg/5 ml with citric acid. Also available in formulations with potassium citrate and citric acid.

SODIUM FLUORIDE—Luride®

Description/Actions: Indicated for prevention of dental caries and certain dental procedures. Has been investigated for possible value in the treatment of osteoporosis.

Preparations: Tablets, 0.25, 0.5, and 1 mg fluoride. Drops, rinse, and gel.

SODIUM HYPOCHLORITE

Description/Actions: Anti-infective agent and bleaching agent.

Preparations: Solution.

SODIUM IODIDE

Description/Actions: Used in thyroid disorders. May be used adjunctively with an antithyroid drug in certain hyperthyroid patients. Radioactive form (sodium iodide I 131) has been used in the management of hyperthyroidism and selected cases of thyroid carcinoma.

Preparations: Solution.

SODIUM LACTATE

Description/Actions: Administered intravenously in the treatment of metabolic acidosis.

Preparations: Vials, 50 mEq. Solution (for IV use), 167 mEq/l (⅙ molar).

SODIUM LAURYL SULFATE

Description/Actions: Surfactant used in the preparation of certain pharmaceutical formulations and to enhance the distribution/penetration of some topically applied drugs.

SODIUM MORRHUATE

Description/Actions: Sclerosing agent used in the intravenous treatment of small uncomplicated varicose veins of the lower extremities. May be useful as a supplement to venous ligation to obliterate residual varicose veins.

Preparations: Ampules and vials, 50 mg/ml.

SODIUM NITROPRUSSIDE—Nitropress®

Description/Actions: Antihypertensive agent indicated for intravenous use for the immediate reduction of blood pressure of patients in hypertensive crisis and in the treatment of cardiac pump failure or cardiogenic shock. Also used to produce controlled hypotension during anesthesia in order to reduce bleeding in surgical procedures.

Preparations: Vials, 50 mg.

SODIUM OXYBATE—Xyrem®

Description/Actions: Sodium oxybate is gamma hydroxybutyric acid (GHB), a known drug of abuse. Sodium oxybate is indicated for the treatment of cataplexy in patients with narcolepsy. Sodium oxybate oral solution is available only to prescribers and patients enrolled in the Xyrem® Patient Success Program.

Precautions/Adverse Reactions: Sodium oxybate is contraindicated in individuals with a hypersensitivity to sodium oxybate or any component of the formulation. It should not be used with ethanol and other CNS depressants, or in patients with succinic semialdehyde dehydrogenase deficiency. Sodium oxybate may impair respiratory drive; use caution with compromised respiratory function. Sodium oxybate may cause confusion, psychosis, paranoia, hallucinations, agitation, and depression; use caution in patients with a history of depression or suicide attempt. Pregnancy Category B. Most common adverse reactions were headache, nausea, dizziness, pain, somnolence, pharyngitis, infection, viral infection, accidental injury, diarrhea, urinary incontinence, vomiting, confusion, sleepwalking, depression, abnormal dreams, and abdominal pain.

Administration: Oral, on empty stomach.

Preparations: Solution, oral: 500 mg/ml (180 ml). Kit contains 2 dosing cups and a measuring device.

SODIUM PERBORATE

Description/Actions: Antiseptic and cleansing agent included in some dentifrices.

SODIUM PHOSPHATE—Visicol™

Description/Actions: Laxative often used in combination with sodium biphosphate. Also administered intravenously as a source of phosphate.

Preparations: Vials, 3 mM phosphate. Tablet, 1.5 g (total sodium phosphate)

SODIUM POLYSTYRENE SULFONATE—Kayexalate®

Description/Actions: Cation-exchange resin indicated for the treatment of hyperkalemia.

Preparations: Powder and suspension.

SODIUM SALICYLATE

Description/Actions: Salicylate analgesic indicated for the relief of mild to moderate pain and inflammation.

Preparations: Enteric-coated tablets, 325 and 650 mg. Ampules, 1 g/10 ml.

SODIUM SULFATE

Description/Actions: Laxative sometimes used in combination with other agents.

SODIUM TETRADECYL SULFATE—Sotradecol®

Description/Actions: Sclerosing agent administered intravenously in the treatment of small uncomplicated varicose veins of the lower extremities.

Preparations: Ampules, 1% and 3%.

SODIUM THIOSALICYLATE

Description/Actions: Salicylate analgesic/anti-inflammatory agent used parenterally in the management of acute gout, musculoskeletal disorders, and rheumatic fever.

Preparations: Ampules and vials, 50 mg/ml.

SODIUM THIOSULFATE—Tinver®

Description/Actions: Used in the topical treatment of tinea versicolor and other dermatologic conditions including acne. Has also been used parenterally as adjunctive therapy in the management of cyanide toxicity and in the treatment of arsenic poisoning.

Preparations: Lotion, 25%. Ampules, 1 g/10 ml.

SOLAG®, Mequinol/Tretinoin Topical Solution

SOLGANAL®, see Aurothioglucose

SOLU-CORTEF®, see Hydrocortisone (as Sodium Succinate)

SOLU-MEDROL®, see Methylprednisolone Sodium Succinate

SOMA®, see Carisoprodol

SOMATREM—Protropin®

Description/Actions: Indicated for the long-term treatment of children who have growth failure due to a lack of adequate endogenous growth hormone secretion.

Precautions/Adverse Reactions: Contraindicated in patients with closed epiphyses or when there is evidence of any progression of underlying intracranial lesion. Patients may experience glucose intolerance. Concurrent use of a glucocorticoid may inhibit the effect of somatrem. Some patients develop persistent antibodies to growth hormone.

Administration: Intramuscular.

Preparations: Vials, 5 and 10 mg.

SOMATROPIN—Humatrope®, Genotropin®, Nutropin®, Serostim®

Description/Actions: Somatropin is indicated for the long-term treatment of children who have growth failure due to Turner's Syndrome or an inadequate secretion of normal endogenous growth hormone or chronic renal insufficiency up to the time of renal transplantation, and in adults who have a deficiency in growth hormone. Indicated in AIDS wasting or cachexia (Serostim®), as somatropin has been shown to increase lean body mass and significantly increase body weight. Also indicated in growth failure associated with chronic renal insufficiency in children up to the time of renal transplant.

Precautions/Adverse Reactions: Growth hormone is contraindicated in patients with Prader-Willi syndrome who are severely obese or have severe respiratory impairment or sleep apnea or unidentified respiratory infection. Contraindicated in patients with closed epiphyses or when there is evidence of growth of intracranial lesions. Patients may experience glucose intolerance. Concurrent use of a glucocorticoid may inhibit the effect of somatropin. Some patients develop antibodies to growth hormone. Reevaluate AIDS patient if weight loss persists after 2 weeks of therapy. Give concomitant antiviral therapy. Discontinue if carpal tunnel syndrome persists after dosage reduction. Perform periodic fundoscopic exams.

Administration: Intramuscular.

Preparations: Vials, 5 and 10 mg.

SOMINEX®, see Diphenhydramine

SONATA®, see Zaleplon

SORBITOL

Description/Actions: Urologic irrigant indicated for use in transurethral prostatic resection or other transurethral surgical procedures.

Preparations: Solutions, 3% and 3.3%.

SORBITRATE®, see Isosorbide Dinitrate

SORIATANE®, see Acitretin

SOTALOL HYDROCHLORIDE—Betapace®, Betapace AF™

Description/Actions: Exhibits noncardioselective beta-adrenergic blocking activity and prolongs cardiac repolarization. Indicated for the treatment of documented life-threatening ventricular arrhythmias such as sustained ventricular tachycardia.

Precautions/Adverse Reactions: Contraindicated in patients with bronchial asthma, sinus bradycardia, second- and third-degree AV block, unless a functioning pacemaker is present, congenital or acquired long QT syndromes, cardiogenic shock, and uncontrolled congestive heart failure. May cause proarrhythmic events (e.g., torsades de pointes), the risk of which may be increased by excessive prolongation of the QT interval, history of cardiomegaly or congestive heart failure, reduction in heart rate, and reduction in serum potassium and/or magnesium. Should not be used in patients with hypokalemia or hypomagnesemia prior to the correction of the imbalance. Concurrent use with other agents known to prolong the QT interval is best avoided. Because of its beta-blocking activity, should be used with caution in patients with diabetes, bronchospastic diseases, sick sinus syndrome associated with symptomatic arrhythmias, a history of anaphylactic reactions to a variety of allergens, and patients suspected of developing thyrotoxicosis.

When sotalol is administered concurrently with a beta-2-receptor agonist (e.g., terbutaline), the dosage of the latter agent may have to be increased.

Administration: Oral.

Preparations: Tablets, 80, 120, 160, and 240 mg.

SOTRADECOL®, see Sodium Tetradecyl Sulfate

SPARFLOXACIN—Zagam®

Description/Actions: Quinolone antibiotic indicated in the treatment of susceptible infections including community acquired pneumonia and acute bacterial exacerbation of chronic bronchitis. Although cross-resistance with other fluoroquinolones may be observed, certain bacterial isolates resistant to fluoroquinolones may be susceptible to sparfloxacin.

Precautions/Adverse Reactions: Contraindicated in patients with a history of hypersensitivity to quinolones (i.e., levofloxacin, loxacin, ciprofloxacin, norfloxacin) or photosensitivity. Instruct patients to refrain from exposure to sun or UV light (direct or indirect) during or 5 days after treatment. Concomitant use of several agents may contraindicate use of sparfloxacin, so prescribers should review the patient's full profile and adjust the medication regimen accordingly. Not recommended for use in patients with hypokalemia, significant bradycardia, CHF, myocardial ischemia, atrial fibrillation, or other pro-arrhythmic conditions. Use cautiously in patients with renal insufficiency. Maintain adequate hydration. Cautious use is recommended in patients with severe cerebral arteriosclerosis, epilepsy, and other conditions that predispose to seizures or that lower seizure threshold. Not recommended in children <18 years of age due to arthropathy. Discontinue if phototoxicity, rash or tendon pain, inflammation, or rupture occurs. Adverse reactions include photosensitivity, GI upset, headache, dizziness, insomnia, pruritus, taste perversion, QTc interval prolongation, flatulence, vasodilation, and convulsions.

Administration: Oral.

Preparations: Tablets, 200 mg.

SPARINE®, see Promazine

SPASMOJECT®, see Dicyclomine Hydrochloride

SPECTAZOLE®, see Econazole

SPECTINOMYCIN HYDROCHLORIDE—Trobicin®

Description/Actions: Antibiotic indicated for intramuscular use in the treatment of acute gonorrheal urethritis and proctitis in the male and acute gonorrheal cervicitis and proctitis in the female.

Preparations: Vials, 2 and 4 g.

SPECTRACEF™, see Cefditoren Pivoxil

SPECTROBID®, see Bacampicillin

SPIRONOLACTONE—Aldactone®

Description/Actions: Potassium-sparing diuretic that is an aldosterone antagonist. Indicated in the management of edematous conditions, hypertension, primary hyperaldosteronism, and hypokalemia.

Preparations: Tablets, 25, 50, and 100 mg.

SPORANOX®, see Itraconazole

SSKI®, see Potassium Iodide

STADOL®, see Butorphanol

STADOL NS®, see Butorphanol

STANOZOLOL—Winstrol®

Description/Actions: Anabolic steroid indicated prophylactically to decrease the frequency and severity of attacks of angioedema in patients with hereditary angioedema and in selected cases of aplastic anemia to increase hemoglobin.

Preparations: Tablets, 2 mg.

STAPHCILLIN®, see Methicillin

STARLIX®, see Nateglinide

STATICIN®, see Erythromycin Base

STAVUDINE—Zerit®, Zerit® XR

Description/Actions: Antiviral agent indicated in advanced HIV infection in patients who have had prolonged prior zidovudine therapy.

Precautions/Adverse Reactions: Lactic acidosis and severe hepatomegaly with steatosis, including fatal cases, have been reported with the use of nucleoside analogs alone or in combination, including stavudine and other antiretrovirals. Fatal and nonfatal pancreatitis has occurred during therapy when stavudine was part of a combination regimen that included didanosine, with or without hydroxyurea in both treatment-naïve and treatment-experienced patients, regardless of the degree of immunosuppression. Fatal lactic acidosis has been reported in pregnant women who receive the combination stavudine and didanosine with other antiretroviral agents. The combination of stavudine and didanosine should be used with caution during pregnancy and is recommended only if the potential benefit clearly outweighs the potential risk. May cause peripheral neuropathy, so patients should be advised to report symptoms such as tingling, burning, pain, or numbness in the hands or feet. Other adverse reactions include diarrhea, nausea, vomiting, abdominal pain, headache, chills/fever, asthenia, myalgia, and rash.

Administration: Oral.

Preparations: Capsules, 15, 20, 30, and 40 mg. Oral solution, 1 mg/ml after reconstitution. Extended-release tablets, 37.5, 50, 75, and 100 mg.

STELAZINE®, see Trifluoperazine

STILPHOSTROL®, see Diethylstilbestrol Diphosphate

STIMATE®, see Desmopressin Acetate

STOXIL®, see Idoxuridine

STRATTERA®, see Atomoxetine Hydrochloride

STREPTASE®, see Streptokinase

STREPTOKINASE—Streptase®

Description/Actions: Thrombolytic enzyme indicated for parenteral use for the lysis of thrombi in the management of pulmonary embolism, deep vein thrombosis, arterial thrombosis and embolism, arteriovenous cannulae occlusion, and coronary artery thrombosis. Also indicated for intravenous use for acute myocardial infarction.

Preparations: Vials, 250,000, 750,000, and 1,500,000 IU.

STREPTOMYCIN SULFATE

Description/Actions: Aminoglycoside antibiotic indicated in the parenteral treatment of tuberculosis and selected other infections caused by susceptible organisms.

Preparations: Vials, 1 and 5 g.

STREPTOZOCIN—Zanosar®

Description/Actions: Antineoplastic agent indicated in the management of metastatic islet cell carcinoma of the pancreas.

Precautions/Adverse Reactions: Use cautiously in renal or hepatic disease, patients with active infections or bone marrow suppression. Adverse reactions include nausea, vomiting, nephrotoxicity, and phlebitis at the IV site.

Administration: Intravenous.

Preparations: Vials, 1 g.

STRONTIUM-89 CHLORIDE—Metastron®

Description/Actions: Is a radiopharmaceutical that decays by beta emission. Selectively concentrates in bone mineral, and greater concentrations accumulate in primary bone tumors and in areas of metastatic involvement than can accumulate in normal bone. Has a slow onset of action (7–20 days) and a long duration of action (6 months). Indicated for the relief of bone pain in patients with painful skeletal metastases.

Precautions/Adverse Reactions: May suppress the bone marrow, so peripheral blood cell counts should be monitored at least every two weeks. Patients should discontinue calcium medications for about 2 weeks prior to receiving the drug. May cause fetal harm, and women of childbearing potential should be advised to avoid becoming pregnant. Because the drug is radioactive, caution must be observed in handling and administering the drug, and patients should be instructed to observe appropriate cautions during the first week after the treatment.

Administration: Intravenous. Is administered by slow intravenous injection over 1–2 minutes.

Preparations: Vials, 4 millicuries (mCi).

SUBLIMAZE®, see Fentanyl Citrate

SUBOXONE®, see Buprenorphine and Naloxone

SUBUTEX®, see Buprenorphine

SUCCIMER—Chemet®

Description/Actions: Is a chelating agent that binds with lead and increases the urinary excretion of lead. Indicated for the treatment of lead poisoning in children with blood lead levels above 45 mg/dl. Use should always be accompanied by identification and removal of the source of the lead exposure.

Precautions/Adverse Reactions: Adverse reactions include gastrointestinal effects (e.g., nausea, vomiting, diarrhea), increases in serum transaminases, and rash. Should be used with caution in patients with compromised renal function. Patients should be adequately hydrated. Elevated blood lead levels and associated symptoms may return rapidly after discontinuation of the drug.

Administration: Oral. In young children who cannot swallow capsules, the drug can be administered by separating the capsule and sprinkling the medicated beads on a small amount of soft food or putting them in a spoon and following with fruit drink.

Preparations: Capsules, 100 mg.

SUCCINYLCHOLINE CHLORIDE—Anectine®, Quelicin®, Sucostrin®

Description/Actions: Depolarizing skeletal muscle relaxant for intravenous use as an adjunct to general anesthesia, to facilitate endotracheal intubation, and to provide skeletal muscle relaxation during surgery or mechanical ventilation.

Preparations: Ampules and vials, 20 mg/ml, 50 mg/ml, and 100 mg/ml. Vials, 500 mg and 1 g.

SUCOSTRIN®, see Succinylcholine Chloride

SUCRALFATE—Carafate®

Description/Actions: Is an aluminum complex of sucrose sulfate indicated in the short-term treatment of duodenal ulcer and for maintenance therapy for duodenal ulcer.

Precautions/Adverse Reactions: Adverse reactions include constipation. Simultaneous administration with other agents should be separated by an interval of at least 2 hours.

Administration: Oral. Should be administered on an empty stomach.

Preparations: Tablets, 1 g. Suspension, 1 g/10 ml.

SUDAFED®, see Pseudoephedrine

SUFENTA®, see Sufentanil

SUFENTANIL CITRATE—Sufenta®

Description/Actions: Opioid analgesic/anesthetic indicated as an analgesic adjunct in the maintenance of balanced general anesthesia, and as a primary anesthetic agent for the induction and maintenance of anesthesia with 100% oxygen in patients undergoing major surgical procedures.

Preparations: Ampules, 50 µg/ml.

SULAMYD®, see Sulfacetamide

SULAR®, see Nisoldipine

SULCONAZOLE NITRATE—Exelderm®

Description/Actions: An imidazole antifungal agent indicated for the topical treatment of tinea pedis, tinea cruris, tinea corporis, and tinea versicolor.

Precautions/Adverse Reactions: Adverse reactions include itching, burning, stinging, and redness.

Administration: Topical.

Preparations: Cream, 1%. Solution, 1%.

SULFABENZAMIDE

Description/Actions: Sulfonamide anti-infective agent used in combination with other agents in the topical management of vaginal infections.

SULFACETAMIDE SODIUM—Sulamyd sodium®, Klaron®

Description/Actions: Sulfonamide anti-infective agent indicated for ophthalmic use in the treatment of conjunctivitis, corneal ulcers, and other superficial ocular infections, and as adjunctive treatment in the management of trachoma. Also used topically in certain bacterial infections of the skin and seborrheic dermatitis, and in combination with other agents in the topical management of vaginal infections.

Preparations: Ophthalmic solution, 10%, 15%, and 30%. Ophthalmic ointment, 10%. Lotion, 10%.

SULFADIAZINE

Description/Actions: Sulfonamide anti-infective agent indicated in the treatment of infections caused by susceptible organisms.

Preparations: Tablets, 500 mg.

SULFADOXINE AND PYRIMETHAMINE

Description/Actions: Sulfonamide anti-infective agent used in combination (Fansidar®) with pyrimethamine to achieve a synergistic effect in the prevention and treatment of malaria caused by chloroquine-resistant plasmodia.

Precautions/Adverse Reactions: Fatalities associated with the administration of Fansidar® have occurred due to severe reactions, including Stevens-Johnson syndrome and toxic epidermal necrolysis. Fansidar® prophylaxis must be discontinued at the first appearance of skin rash, if a significant reduction in the count of any formed blood elements is noted, or upon the occurrence of active bacterial or fungal infections. Repeated prophylactic use of Fansidar® is contraindicated in patients with renal or hepatic failure or with blood dyscrasias. Hypersensitivity to pyrimethamine, sulfonamides, or any other ingredient in the formulation. Fansidar® is also contraindicated in pediatric patients less than 2 months of age, in patients with documented megaloblastic anemia due to folate deficiency, and for the prophylactic use of malaria during pregnancy, at term and during the nursing period.

Preparations: Tablets, 500 mg with 25 mg of pyrimethamine.

SULFAMERAZINE

Description/Actions: Sulfonamide anti-infective agent used in combination with other sulfonamides.

SULFAMETHAZINE

Description/Actions: Sulfonamide anti-infective agent used in combination with other sulfonamides.

SULFAMETHIZOLE—Thiosulfil Forte®

Description/Actions: Sulfonamide anti-infective agent indicated for the treatment of urinary tract infections.

Preparations: Tablets, 500 mg.

SULFAMETHOXAZOLE—Gantanol®

Description/Actions: Sulfonamide anti-infective agent indicated for the treatment of infections caused by susceptible organisms.

Preparations: Tablets, 500 mg and 1 g. Suspension, 500 mg/5 ml.

SULFAMYLON®, see Mafenide

SULFANILAMIDE—AVC®

Description/Actions: Sulfonamide anti-infective agent used in the topical management of vaginal infections.

Preparations: Vaginal cream, 15%. Vaginal suppositories, 1.05 g.

SULFAPYRIDINE

Description/Actions: Used in the treatment of dermatitis herpetiformis.

Preparations: Tablets, 500 mg.

SULFASALAZINE—Azulfidine®

Description/Actions: Agent for ulcerative colitis indicated in the treatment of mild to moderate ulcerative colitis and as adjunctive therapy in severe ulcerative colitis, and for the prolongation of the remission period between acute attacks of ulcerative colitis. Also indicated in rheumatoid arthritis that has not responded adequately to salicylates or other NSAIDs.

Preparations: Tablets and enteric-coated tablets, 500 mg. Oral suspension, 250 mg/5 ml.

SULFATHIAZOLE

Description/Actions: Sulfonamide anti-infective agent used in combination with other agents in the topical management of vaginal infections.

SULFINPYRAZONE—Anturane®

Description/Actions: Uricosuric agent indicated in the treatment of chronic gouty arthritis and intermittent gouty arthritis.

Preparations: Tablets, 100 mg. Capsules, 200 mg.

SULFISOXAZOLE—Gantrisin®

SULFISOXAZOLE ACETYL

Description/Actions: Sulfonamide anti-infective agent. Primarily used in the treatment of urinary tract infections and is useful in certain other infections.

Preparations: Tablets, 500 mg. Suspension (acetyl), 500 mg/5 ml.

SULFISOXAZOLE DIOLAMINE—Gantrisin®

Description/Actions: Sulfonamide anti-infective agent used in the treatment of ocular infections.

Preparations: Ophthalmic solution and ointment, 4%.

SULFUR

Description/Actions: Used topically, usually in combination with other agents, in the treatment of acne, seborrheic dermatitis, and other dermatologic conditions.

SULFURATED LIME—Lime Sulfur Solution, Vlemasque®

Description/Actions: Used topically in the treatment of acne and other dermatologic conditions.

Preparations: Cream, 6%. Topical solution.

SULINDAC—Clinoril®

Description/Actions: Nonsteroidal anti-inflammatory agent that inhibits prostaglandin synthesis and is indicated in the treatment of rheumatoid arthritis, osteoarthritis, ankylosing spondylitis, acute painful shoulder, and acute gouty arthritis.

Precautions/Adverse Reactions: Should not be given to patients in whom aspirin or another NSAID causes asthma, rhinitis, urticaria, or other allergic-type reactions. May cause GI effects, so use should be avoided in patients with active GI tract disease and closely monitored in patients with a previous history of such disorders. Other adverse reactions include dizziness, headache, edema, and rash. Should not be used concomitantly with dimethyl sulfoxide (DMSO).

Administration: Oral.

Preparations: Tablets, 150 and 200 mg.

SUMATRIPTAN SUCCINATE—Imitrex®

Description/Actions: Is a selective 5-hydroxytryptamine1 (5-HT$_1$) receptor agonist that causes vasoconstriction of intracranial blood vessels. Indicated for the acute treatment of migraine attacks with or without aura and cluster headaches.

Precautions/Adverse Reactions: Contraindicated in patients with ischemic heart disease (angina pectoris, history of myocardial infarction, or documented silent ischemia), Prinzmetal's angina, signs or symptoms consistent with ischemic heart disease, or uncontrolled hypertension. Should not be used concomitantly with ergotamine-containing preparations. Adverse reactions include pain or redness at the injection site, atypical sensations (e.g., sensations of warmth, tingling or paresthesia, pressure, burning, numbness, tightness), dizziness, weakness, neck pain/stiffness, jaw discomfort, flushing, chest discomfort, and transient increases in blood pressure. May cause vasospasm that may be additive to that caused by ergot-containing drugs, and it is recommended that the two agents not be administered within 24 hours of each other.

Administration: Subcutaneous, oral and nasal spray.

Preparations: Tablets, 25 and 50 mg. Vials, 6 mg. Unit-of-use syringes, 6 mg. Imitrex SELFdose system kit that contains two unit-of-use syringes with 6 mg each and a SELFdose unit (a push-button autoinjector). Nasal spray, 5 and 20 mg/spray.

SUMYCIN®, see Tetracycline

SUPPRELIN®, see Histrelin Acetate

SUPRANE®, see Desflurane

SUPRAX®, see Cefixime

SUPROFEN—Profenal®

Description/Actions: Nonsteroidal anti-inflammatory drug indicated for the inhibition of intraoperative miosis.

Precautions/Adverse Reactions: Caution should be exercised in the treatment of patients having a history of sensitivity to aspirin or another nonsteroidal anti-inflammatory drug.

Administration: Ophthalmic.

Preparations: Ophthalmic solution, 1%.

SURMONTIL®, see Trimipramine

SURVANTA®, see Beractant

SUTILAINS—Travase®

Description/Actions: Proteolytic enzymes applied topically as an adjunct for wound debridement of second- and third-degree burns, pressure ulcers, incisional, traumatic, and pyogenic wounds, and ulcers secondary to peripheral vascular disease.

Preparations: Ointment, 82,000 casein units/g.

SYMMETREL®, see Amantadine

SYNALAR®, see Fluocinolone

SYNALGOS-DC®, Combination of Dihydrocodeine, Aspirin, and Caffeine

SYNERCID®, see Dalfopristin/Quinupristin

SYNAREL®, see Nafarelin Acetate

SYNTHROID®, see Levothyroxine

SYNTOCINON®, see Oxytocin

SYPRINE®, see Trientine

T

TACARYL®, see Methdilazine

TACE®, see Chlorotrianisene

TACRINE HYDROCHLORIDE—Cognex®

Description/Actions: Also known as tetrahydroaminoacridine (THA). Is a reversible cholinesterase inhibitor that elevates acetylcholine concentrations in the cerebral cortex. Indicated for the treatment of mild to moderate dementia of the Alzheimer's type.

Precautions/Adverse Reactions: Contraindicated in patients previously treated with tacrine who developed treatment-associated jaundice confirmed by elevated total bilirubin greater than 3 mg/dl. May increase serum transaminase levels (e.g., alanine aminotransferase [ALT]) and cause liver toxicity. Serum transaminase levels should be monitored every 2 weeks for the first 16 weeks, then monthly for 2 months, then every 3 months thereafter. Other adverse reactions include nausea, vomiting, diarrhea, dyspepsia, anorexia, myalgia, and ataxia. Cognex® may have vagotonic effects on the sinoatrial and atrioventricular nodes possibly leading to bradycardia and or heart block. These effects may be particularly harmful to patients with conduction abnormalities, bradyarrhythmias, or a sick sinus syndrome, but may also occur in patients without known preexisting cardiac disease.

Administration: Oral. Administer at least 1 hour before meals.

Preparations: Capsules, 10, 20, 30, and 40 mg.

TACROLIMUS—Prograf®, Protopic®

Description/Actions: Immunosuppressant indicated for the prophylaxis of organ rejection in patients receiving allogeneic liver transplants. It is recommended that it be used concomitantly with adrenal corticosteroids.

Precautions/Adverse Reactions: Contraindicated in patients who are hypersensitive to the drug, or to polyoxyl 60 hydrogenated castor oil (HCO-60) that is included in the parenteral formulation as a solubilizing agent. May cause nephrotoxicity; patients with impaired renal function should receive lower doses, and caution should be exercised when it is used in patients who are also receiving other drugs that may cause nephrotoxicity (e.g., aminoglycosides). Should not be used concurrently with cyclosporine, and it is recommended that tacrolimus or cyclosporine should be discontinued at least 24 hours prior to initiating the other. May cause hyperkalemia; serum potassium concentrations should be monitored, and the concurrent use of potassium-sparing diuretics should be avoided. Other adverse reactions include tremor, headache, hypertension, hyperglycemia, diarrhea, nausea, vomiting, abdominal pain, hypomagnesemia, anemia, pain, fever, and asthenia. Anaphylactic reactions have been experienced by some patients receiving the parenteral formulation, which may be due to the castor oil derivative used as the solubilizing agent. The parenteral formulation should be used only in patients who are unable to take the capsule formulation. Patients receiving the drug intravenously should be under continuous observation for at least the first 30 minutes following the start of the intravenous infusion and at frequent intervals thereafter.

Administration: Oral and intravenous infusion. Should be administered no sooner than 6 hours after transplantation. Patients should be converted from the intravenous to the oral formulation as soon as oral therapy can be tolerated. The parenteral formulation must be diluted and the diluted infusion solution should be stored in glass or polyethylene containers and should be discarded after 24 hours.

Preparations: Capsules, 1 and 5 mg. Ampules, 5 mg/ml. Topical ointment, 0.03% and 0.1%.

TADALAFIL—Cialis®

Description/Actions: Tadalafil is an oral treatment for erectile dysfunction. It is a selective inhibitor of cyclic guanosine monophosphate (cGMP)-specific phosphodiesterase type 5 (PDE5). Tadalafil does not directly cause penile erections, but affects the response to sexual stimulation. The physiologic mechanism of erection of the penis involves release of nitric oxide (NO) in the corpus cavernosum during sexual stimulation. NO then activates the enzyme guanylate cyclase, which results in increased levels of cGMP, producing smooth muscle relaxation and inflow of blood to the corpus cavernosum. Tadalafil enhances the effect of NO by inhibiting PDE5, which is responsible for degradation of cGMP in the corpus cavernosum. When sexual stimulation causes local release of NO, inhibition of PDE5 by tadalafil causes increased levels of cGMP.

Precautions/Adverse Reactions: Tadalafil is contraindicated in patients with a hypersensitivity to tadalafil or any component of the formulation, concurrent use of organic nitrates, and concurrent use of alpha-adrenergic antagonists (except tamsulosin 0.4 mg/day). When used in conjunction with nitrates, it may be associated with severe hypotension, myocardial infarction, and possibly death. Tadalafil may increase hypotensive effect of antihypertensive agents; use caution when administered with antihypertensives. There is a degree of cardiac risk associated with sexual activity; it should not be used in men for whom sexual activity is inadvisable as a result of their underlying cardiovascular status. Before prescribing tadalafil it is important to note renal and hepatic function and if patients are on potent inhibitors of cytochrome P450 3A4 (CYP3A4). Also, tadalafil has mild systemic vasodilatory properties that may result in transient decreases in blood pressure. Patients with significant left ventricular outflow obstruction or severely impaired autonomic control of blood pressure may be particularly sensitive to the actions of vasodilators. Tadalafil should be used with caution in patients who have conditions that might predispose them to priapism (such as sickle cell anemia, multiple myeloma, or leukemia) or in patients with anatomical deformation of the penis (such as angulation, cavernosal fibrosis, or Peyronie's disease). Safety and efficacy have not been studied in patients with the following conditions; therefore, use in these patients is not recommended: arrhythmias, hypotension, uncontrolled hypertension, unstable angina or angina during intercourse, cardiac failure (NYHA Class II or greater), recent myocardial infarction, stroke within the last 6 months, and in patients with bleeding disorders or significant active peptic ulceration. Most common adverse reactions were headache, dizziness, dyspepsia, flushing, back pain, myalgia, and nasal congestion.

Administration: Oral.

Patient Care Implications: Patients who experience cardiac symptoms upon initiation of sexual activity should be advised to refrain from further activity and seek attention. Patients must be made aware of the contraindication of tadalafil with regular or intermittent use of organic nitrates and advised blood pressure could suddenly drop to an unsafe level, resulting in dizziness, syncope, or even a heart attack or stroke. If priapism is not treated promptly, irreversible damage to the erectile tissue can occur. Patients with priapism lasting > than 4 hours, whether painful or not, should seek emergency medical attention.

Advise that the use of alcohol may increase the risk of hypotension and orthostasis. May be taken with or without food.

Preparations: Tablets: 5 mg, 10 mg, 20 mg.

TAGAMET®, see Cimetidine

TAGAMET HB®, see Cimetidine

TALACEN®, see Pentazocine Hydrochloride and Acetaminophen

TALWIN®, see Pentazocine

TAMBOCOR®, see Flecainide

TAMIFLU®, see Oseltamivir

TAMOXIFEN CITRATE—Nolvadex®

Description/Actions: Antineoplastic agent indicated in the treatment of metastatic breast cancer in postmenopausal women, and in premenopausal women as an alternative to oophorectomy or ovarian radiation. Is also used in combination with cytotoxic agents following radical or modified radical mastectomy to delay recurrence of surgically curable breast cancer in postmenopausal women. Is also indicated for adjuvant treatment for axillary node-negative breast cancer, advanced breast cancer in men, and for reduction of incidence of breast cancer in high risk women. Approved for use in girls 2–10 years of age with McCune-Albright Syndrome.

Precautions/Adverse Reactions: For women with ductal carcinoma in situ and women at high risk for breast cancer, serious and life-threatening events associated with tamoxifen in the risk reduction setting, including uterine malignancies, stroke, and pulmonary embolism. Some of these were fatal.

Preparations: Tablets, 10 and 20 mg.

TAMSULOSIN HYDROCHLORIDE—Flomax®

Description/Actions: An alpha-adrenergic antagonist indicated in benign prostatic hyperplasia, resulting in an improvement in urine flow and a reduction in the symptoms of BPH.

Precautions/Adverse Reactions: Rule out prostate cancer. Use cautiously in patients with syncope. Adverse reactions include abnormal ejaculation, postural hypotension, dizziness, rhinitis, cough, somnolence, sinusitis, amblyopia, decreased libido, insomnia, and syncope. Tamsulosin has also been associated with priapism.

Administration: Oral. Do not crush, chew, or open caps. Take ½ hour after the same meal each day.

Preparations: Capsules, 0.4 mg.

TAO®, see Troleandomycin

TAPAZOLE®, see Methimazole

TARGRETIN®, see Bexarotene

TARKA®—Combination ACE Inhibitor (Trandolapril) and Calcium Channel Blocker (Verapamil)

TASMAR®, see Tolcapone

TAVIST®, see Clemastine

TAVIST-D®, Combination of Clemastine and Phenylpropanolamine

TAXOL®, see Paclitaxel

TAXOTERE®, see Docetaxel

TAZAROTENE—Tazorac®

Description/Actions: Tazarotene is indicated for the treatment of mild to moderate facial acne vulgaris or atable plaque psoriasis affecting up to 20% of the body surface area and as an adjunctive agent for use in the mitigation (palliation) of facial fine wrinkling, facial mottled hyperpigmentation and hypopigmentation, and benign facial lentigines in patients who use comprehensive skin care and sunlight avoidance programs.

Precautions/Adverse Reactions: Contraindicated in pregnancy (Category X). Obtain a reliable negative pregnancy test within 2 weeks before starting therapy. Do not use on broken, eczematous, or sunburned skin. Warn patients about sun sensitivity. Avoid sun and UV light; use adequate sun protection. Increased irritation may occur in extreme weather (e.g., wind, cold). Discontinue if excessive irritation occurs. Adverse reactions include pruritus, burning, stinging, erythema, worsening of psoriasis, irritation, skin pain, desquamation, and other local reactions.

Administration: Topical.

Preparations: 0.05 and 0.1% aqueous gel. 0.1% cream.

TAZICEF®, see Ceftazidime

TAZIDIME®, see Ceftazidime

TAZORAC®, see Tazarotene

TECZEM®, Combination Agent Enalapril Maleate and Diltiazem Maleate (ACE Inhibitor and Calcium Channel Blocker)

TEGASEROD MALEATE—Zelnorm™

Description/Actions: Tegaserod is a 5-HT$_4$ receptor partial agonist that binds with high affinity to human 5-HT$_4$ receptors. Tegaserod is indicated for the short-term treatment of women with irritable bowel syndrome (IBS) whose primary bowel symptom is constipation. Women with this medical condition suffer from abdominal pain or discomfort, bloating, and constipation. Zelnorm® is also indicated for the treatment of chronic idiopathic constipation in patients less than 65 years of age.

Precautions/Adverse Reactions: Contraindicated in individuals who are hypersensitive to tegaserod or any component of its formulation or who have severe renal impairment, moderate or severe hepatic impairment, a history of bowel obstruction, symptomatic gall bladder disease, suspected sphincter of Oddi dysfunction, or abdominal adhesions. Pregnancy Category B. Most common adverse reactions were headache, abdominal pain, dizziness, and diarrhea. A majority of patients reported diarrhea as a single episode. Diarrhea occurred during the first week of therapy and resolved with continued therapy. Serious consequences of diarrhea, including hypovolemia, hypotension, and syncope, have been reported. In some cases, these complications have required hospitalization. Tegaserod should be discontinued immediately in patients who develop severe diarrhea, hypotension, or syncope, and therapy should not be initiated in patients who are currently experiencing or frequently experience diarrhea.

Administration: Oral, on empty stomach.

Preparations: Tablets, 2 and 6 mg. Protect from moisture. Store at 25°C (77°F); excursions permitted to 15–30°C (59–86°F).

TEGOPEN®, see Cloxacillin

TEGRETOL®, see Carbamazepine

TELDRIN®, see Chlorpheniramine

TELMISARTAN—Micardis®

Description/Actions: Telmisartan is an angiotensin II receptor antagonist indicated as monotherapy or as an adjunct to other antihypertensives.

Precautions/Adverse Reactions: Contraindicated in pregnancy (Category C in first trimester; Category D in the second and third trimesters) and in nursing mothers. Correct hypovolemia before beginning therapy or monitor closely. Use cautiously in hepatic insufficiency, biliary obstruction, severe renal impairment, CHF, renal artery stenosis, and dialysis (monitor for orthostasis). Adverse reactions include back pain, upper respiratory infection, sinusitis, diarrhea, and pharyngitis.

Administration: Oral.

Patient Care Implications: Instruct patients that medication controls but does not cure hypertension. Tell patients to take the medication at the same time daily even if feeling well, as hypertension frequently occurs without any perceived symptomatology. Caution patients to avoid sudden changes in position to decrease the incidence of orthostatic hypotension.

Preparations: Tablets, 40 and 80 mg.

TEMARIL®, see Trimeprazine

TEMAZEPAM—Restoril®

Description/Actions: Benzodiazepine indicated for the management of insomnia.

Precautions/Adverse Reactions: Contraindicated during pregnancy. Adverse reactions include residual sedation and other CNS effects upon awakening. Patients should be cautioned regarding activities such as driving and operating machinery, as well as interactions with other CNS acting drugs including alcohol. Can cause dependence, and is included in Schedule IV.

Administration: Oral.

Preparations: Capsules and tablets, 7.5, 15, and 30 mg. Capsule 22.5 mg.

TEMODAR®, see Temozolomide

TEMOVATE®, see Clobetasol Propionate

TEMOZOLOMIDE—Temodar®

Description/Actions: Temozolomide is used to treat recurrent anaplastic astrocytomas.

Precautions/Adverse Reactions: Temozolomide should not be administered to patients with severe bone marrow suppression, dacarbazine hypersensitivity, pregnant women, breast-feeding women, or children under 3 years of age. The drug should be given with caution to patients with hepatic or renal impairment. Also, if the patient has a platelet count <50,000/mm3, then IM injection should not be administered. Some side effects are nausea, vomiting, headache, fatigue, myelosuppression, constipation, diarrhea, abdominal pain, anorexia, infections, fever, seizures, dizziness, insomnia, paresthesias, somnolence, confusion, Cushing's syndrome, anxiety, back pain, depression, myalgia, pruritus, incontinence, and weight gain.

Administration: Oral.

Patient Care Implications: The drug should not be administered to patients with severe bone marrow suppression, dacarbazine hypersensitivity, pregnant women, breast-feeding women, or children under 3 years of age. The drug should be given with caution to patients with hepatic or renal impairment. Also, if the patient has a platelet count <50,000/mm3, then IM injection should not be administered. A CBC with a differential should be checked during treatment. Contact or inhalation of temozolomide powder should be avoided. Temozolomide capsules should not be opened.

Preparations: Capsules, 5, 20, 100, and 250 mg.

TEMPRA®, see Acetaminophen

TENECTEPLASE—TNKase™

Description/Actions: Tenecteplase is a thrombolytic agent used in the management of acute myocardial infarction for the lysis of thrombi in the coronary vasculature to restore perfusion and reduce mortality.

Precautions/Adverse Reactions: Tenecteplase is contraindicated in patients with a hypersensitivity to tenecteplase or any component of its formulation. It is also contraindicated in the following situations because of an increased risk of bleeding: active internal bleeding, history of cerebrovascular accident, intracranial or intraspinal surgery or trauma within 2 months, intracranial neoplasm, arteriovenous malformation, aneurysm, bleeding diathesis, and severe uncontrolled hypertension. Bleeding is the potential complication during therapy—if serious bleeding occurs (not controlled by local pressure), concomitant heparin or antiplatelet agents should be discontinued. For the following conditions, the risk of bleeding is higher with the use of tenecteplase and should be weighed against the benefits: recent major surgery, cerebrovascular disease, recent gastrointestinal or genitourinary bleeding, recent trauma, hypertension (systolic BP ≥180 mm Hg and/or diastolic BP ≥110 mm Hg), suspected left heart thrombus, acute pericarditis, subacute bacterial endocarditis, hemostatic defects, severe hepatic dysfunction, pregnancy, diabetic hemorrhagic retinopathy, hemorrhagic ophthalmic conditions, septic thrombophlebitis, patients receiving anticoagulation therapy (i.e., warfarin sodium), recent administration of GP IIb/IIIa inhibitors, and advanced age. Coronary thrombolysis may result in reperfusion arrhythmias. Venipunctures should be performed carefully and only when necessary. Use caution with readministration of tenecteplase (possible antibody formation). Rare reports of cholesterol embolism have been reported. Pregnancy Category C. Administer to pregnant women only if the potential benefits justify the potential risk to the fetus. Excretion into the breast milk is unknown. Exercise caution when administering to a nursing woman. Safety and efficacy have not been established in pediatric patients. Some adverse effects are bleeding (minor), hematoma, stroke, gastrointestinal hemorrhage, epistaxis, genitourinary bleeding, and pharyngeal bleeding.

Administration: Intravenous.

Patient Care Implications: Tenecteplase should be reconstituted using the supplied 10 ml syringe with TwinPak™ dual cannula device and the 10 ml sterile water for injection (follow directions supplied within the kit). The reconstituted solution is incompatible with dextrose solutions. Dextrose-containing lines must be flushed with a saline solution before and after administration. Monitor for bleeding and avoid IM injections.

Preparations: Powder for injection, 50 mg.

TENEX®, see Guanfacine

TENIPOSIDE—Vumon®

Description/Actions: Antineoplastic agent that is a derivative of podophyllotoxin, also known as VM-26. Indicated for use in combination with other anticancer agents for induction therapy in patients with refractory childhood acute lymphoblastic leukemia.

Precautions/Adverse Reactions: Contraindicated in patients who are hypersensitive to etoposide or polyoxyethylated castor oil (Cremophor EL), a solubilizing agent included in the formulation. Adverse reactions include myelosuppression (leukopenia, neutropenia, thrombocytopenia, anemia), mucositis, diarrhea, nausea, vomiting, infection, alopecia, and bleeding. Hypersensitivity reactions to the drug or to polyoxyethylated castor oil may occur, so patients should be under continuous observation for at least 60 minutes following the start of the intravenous infusion and at frequent intervals thereafter. Transient hypotension has occurred following rapid intravenous administration, so the drug should be administered only by slow intravenous infusion, lasting at least 30–60 minutes. Patients of childbearing potential should be advised to avoid becoming pregnant during treatment. Should not be used in nursing mothers.

Administration: Intravenous. Administered as an IV infusion over at least a 30- to 60-minute period; should not be given by rapid IV injection.

Preparations: Ampules, 50 mg/ml (teniposide for injection concentrate).

TENOFOVIR DISOPROXIL FUMARATE—Viread™

Description/Actions: Tenofovir disoproxil fumarate is indicated in combination with other antiretroviral agents for the treatment of HIV-1 infection.

Precautions/Adverse Reactions: Lactic acidosis and severe hepatomegaly with steatosis, including fatal cases, have been reported with the use of nucleoside analogs alone or in combination with other antiretrovirals. The majority of cases have been in women. Exercise caution when administering nucleoside analogs to any patient with known risk factors for liver disease. Cases have also occurred in patients with no known risk factors. Tenofovir should not be administered to patients with renal insufficiency (creatinine clearance <60 ml/minute). Coadministration of tenofovir with drugs that reduce renal function or compete for active tubular secretion such as cidofovir, acyclovir, valacyclovir, ganciclovir, and valganciclovir may increase serum concentrations of tenofovir and/or increase the concentration of other renally eliminated drugs. When administered with didanosine, tenofovir should be administered 2 hours before or 1 hour after administration of didanosine. Coadministration of tenofovir and lamivudine resulted in decreased serum concentrations of lamivudine. Coadministration of tenofovir with indinavir, lopinavir, and ritonavir resulted in decreased serum concentrations of indinavir, lopinavir, and ritonavir. Coadministration of lopinavir/ritonavir with tenofovir resulted in increased serum concentrations of tenofovir. Redistribution and/or accumulation of body fat including central obesity, dorsocervical fat enlargement, peripheral wasting, facial wasting, breast enlargement, and cushingoid appearance have been observed in patients receiving antiretroviral therapy. Tenofovir may cause osteomalacia. Pregnancy Category B. No adequate and well-controlled studies in pregnant women. Use in pregnancy only if the potential benefit justifies the potential risks to the fetus. Excretion in human breast milk is unknown. Nursing mothers should be instructed not to breast-feed if they are receiving tenofovir. Safety and efficacy in pediatric patients have not been established. Most common adverse reactions observed in patients treated with tenofovir include nausea, diarrhea, asthenia, headache, vomiting, flatulence, abdominal pain, and anorexia. Increases in triglycerides, creatinine kinase, serum amylase, AST, urine glucose, ALT, and serum glucose have been observed in patients treated with tenofovir. Decreased neutrophil counts have also been reported.

Administration: Oral—once daily taken with food.

Patient Care Implications: Take with food. If coadministered with didanosine, tenofovir shoud be administered 2 hours before or 1 hour after administration of didanosine. Monitor for changes in serum creatinine and serum phosphorus levels in patients at risk or with a history of renal dysfunction. Women should be instructed not to breast-feed while taking tenofovir.

Preparations: Tablets, 300 mg (equivalent to 245 mg of tenofovir disoproxil).

TENORETIC®, Combination of Atenolol and Chlorthalidone

TENORMIN®, see Atenolol

TENSILON®, see Edrophonium

TENUATE®, see Diethylpropion

TEPANIL®, see Diethylpropion

TEQUIN®, see Gatifloxacin

TERAZOL 3®; TERAZOL 7®, see Terconazole

TERAZOSIN HYDROCHLORIDE—Hytrin®

Description/Actions: An alpha1 selective adrenergic receptor blocking agent that causes vasodilatation and a reduction in blood pressure. Indicated in the treatment of hypertension, and can be used alone or in combination with other antihypertensive agents. Also indicated for the treatment of benign prostatic hyperplasia.

Precautions/Adverse Reactions: May cause orthostatic hypotension, resulting in symptoms such as dizziness, lightheadedness, palpitations, and, in more severe cases, syncope. Syncope has occurred most often in association with the first dose or first few doses of therapy. To reduce the likelihood of syncope, treatment should be initiated with a 1 mg dose of terazosin, given at bedtime. Patients should be informed of the possibility of syncope and other orthostatic symptoms, and advised to avoid driving or other hazardous tasks for 12 hours after the first dose, after a dosage increase, and after interruption of therapy when treatment is resumed. They should also be advised to sit or lie down when symptoms associated with orthostatic hypotension occur, and to be cautious when rising from a sitting or lying position. Other adverse reactions include weakness, tiredness, fatigue, drowsiness, blurred vision, nasal congestion, nausea, peripheral edema, and weight gain.

Administration: Oral.

Preparations: Tablets 1, 2, 5, and 10 mg. Capsules, 1, 2, 5, and 10 mg.

TERBINAFINE HYDROCHLORIDE—Lamisil®

Description/Actions: An allylamine derivative that exhibits a fungicidal action by inhibiting squalene epoxidase, a key enzyme in sterol biosynthesis in fungi. Indicated for the topical treatment of interdigital tinea pedis, plantar tinea pedis, tinea cruris, and tinea corporis caused by *Epidermophyton floccosum, Trichophyton mentagrophytes,* or *Trichophyton rubrum.* Orally indicated in treatment of onychomycosis of the toenail and fingernail due to tinea unguium. Prior to initiating treatment for onychomycosis, nail specimens should be obtained to confirm the diagnosis of onychomycosis.

Precautions/Adverse Reactions: Adverse reactions include irritation and burning. Patients should be advised to avoid the use of occlusive dressings unless otherwise directed by the physician. Oral formulation contraindicated with preexisting hepatic disease or renal impairment (Cr Cl <50 ml/min). Discontinue if hepatobiliary dysfunction or progressive skin rash or severe neutropenia occurs. Rare cases of liver failure, some leading to death or liver transplant, have occurred with the use of terbinafine for the treatment of onychomycosis. Treatment with terbinafine should be discontinued if evidence of liver toxicity develops. Monitor CBC and liver functions.

Administration: Oral and topical.

Preparations: Tablets, 250 mg. Cream and topical solution, 1%. Spray pump solution, 1%.

TERBUTALINE SULFATE—Brethaire®, Brethine®, Bricanyl®

Description/Actions: Stimulates beta-adrenergic receptors. Indicated for bronchial asthma and for reversible bronchospasm that may occur in association with bronchitis and emphysema. Also used in management of preterm labor (tocolytic).

Precautions/Adverse Reactions: May cause increased heart rate and palpitations, and should be used cautiously in patients with cardiovascular disorders, especially those associated with arrhythmias. Other adverse reactions include nervousness, tremor, headache, nausea, vomiting, sweating, and muscle cramps. Other sympathomimetic agents should not be used concurrently. Beta-adrenergic-blocking agents and terbutaline may inhibit the effect of each other.

Administration: Oral, oral inhalation, and subcutaneous.

Preparations: Tablets, 2.5 and 5 mg. Metered dose inhaler (Brethaire). Ampules, 1 mg/ml.

TERCONAZOLE—Terazol 3®; Terazol 7®

Description/Actions: Antifungal agent indicated for the local treatment of vulvovaginal candidiasis.

Precautions/Adverse Reactions: Adverse reactions include headache, and vulvovaginal burning, itching, or irritation. Use during the first trimester of pregnancy should be avoided. Base contained in the vaginal suppository formulation may interact with certain rubber or latex products, such as those used in vaginal contraceptive diaphragms; therefore, concurrent use is not recommended.

Administration: Vaginal. Vaginal cream is administered for 7 consecutive days and the vaginal suppositories for 3 consecutive days.

Preparations: Vaginal cream (Terazol 7), 0.4%; vaginal suppository (Terazol 3), 80 mg.

TERIPARATIDE—Forteo™

Description/Actions: Teriparatide is a parathyroid hormone (PTH) analog manufactured by using a strain of *Escherichia coli* modified by recombinant DNA technology. Teriparatide is indicated in the treatment of osteoporosis, in postmenopausal women at high risk of fracture, and to increase bone mass in men with primary or hypogonadal osteoporosis who are at high risk for fracture.

Precautions/Adverse Reactions: Teriparatide is contraindicated in individuals hypersensitive to teriparatide or any of the formulation's components. **Warning**: In rats, teriparatide caused an increase in the incidence of osteosarcoma that was dependent on dose and treatment duration. Because of the uncertain relevance of the rat osteosarcoma finding to humans, teriparatide should be prescribed only to patients for whom the potential benefits are considered to outweigh the potential risk. Not to be prescribed for patients who are at increased baseline risk for osteosarcoma, including those with Paget's disease of bone or unexplained elevations of alkaline phosphatase, open epiphyses, or prior radiation therapy involving the skeleton. Patients with bone metastases or a history of skeletal malignancies and patients with metabolic bone diseases other than osteoporosis should be excluded from treatment with teriparatide. Use caution in patients at risk of orthostasis (including concurrent antihypertensive therapy) or in patients who may not tolerate transient hypotension. Because teriparatide increases serum calcium, it should be used with caution in patients taking digitalis; it has been suggested that hypercalcemia may predispose patients to digitalis toxicity. Pregnancy Category C. Most common adverse events were dizziness, leg cramps, and nausea.

Administration: Subcutaneous injection.

Preparations: Injection, solution: 250 mcg/ml (3 ml). Prefilled pen delivery device. Store under refrigeration at 2–8°C (36–46°F). Protect from light. Do not freeze.

TERPIN HYDRATE

Description/Actions: Expectorant most frequently used with codeine in an elixir formulation indicated for respiratory symptoms.

TERRAMYCIN®, see Oxytetracycline

TESLAC®, see Testolactone

TESSALON®, see Benzonatate

TESTODERM®, see Testosterone

TESTOLACTONE—Teslac®

Description/Actions: Antineoplastic agent indicated as adjunctive therapy in the treatment of advanced or disseminated breast cancer in post-menopausal women.

Preparations: Tablets, 50 mg.

TESTOSTERONE—Androderm®, Testoderm®

Description/Actions: Androgen indicated for use in male patients for replacement therapy for conditions associated with a deficiency or absence of endogenous testosterone. Transdermal system is indicated for primary hypogonadism and hypogonadotropic hypogonadism.

Preparations: Transdermal systems (Androderm), 2.5 and 5 mg, (Testoderm), 10 and 15 mg.

TESTOSTERONE CYPIONATE—Depo-Testosterone®

Description/Actions: Longer-acting ester of testosterone administered intramuscularly.

Preparations: Vials (in oil), 50 mg/ml 100 mg/ml, and 200 mg/ml.

TESTOSTERONE ENANTHATE—Delatestryl®

Description/Actions: Longer-acting ester of testosterone administered intramuscularly.

Preparations: Vials (in oil), 100 mg/ml, and 200 mg/ml.

TESTOSTERONE GEL—Androgel®

Description/Actions: Indicated for replacement therapy in males for conditions associated with a deficiency or absence of endogenous testosterone, such as primary hypogonadism and hypogonadotropic hypogonadism.

Precautions/Adverse Reactions: Adverse effects include acne, alopecia, application site reaction, depression, headache, hypertension, nervousness, breast pain, and decreased libido. Gynecomastia frequently develops, and sleep apnea may be potentiated. Edema with or without congestive heart failure may be a serious complication in patients with preexisting cardiac, renal, or hepatic disease. Androgens are contraindicated in men with carcinoma of the breast or known or suspected carcinoma of the prostate. Testosterone gel should not be used in women.

Administration: Topical. Do not apply to genitals. Hands should be washed with soap and water after application.

Preparations: Packets, 1%, 2.5 and 5 g. Pump, 1.25 g/depression.

TESTOSTERONE PROPIONATE

Description/Actions: Androgen indicated for intramuscular use in male patients for replacement therapy in conditions associated with a deficiency or absence of endogenous testosterone—primary hypogonadism, hypogonadotropic hypogonadism, and delayed puberty. Also used in women with advancing inoperable metastatic mammary cancer who are 1 to 5 years postmenopausal.

Preparations: Vials, 25 mg/ml, 50 mg/ml, and 100 mg/ml.

TETRACAINE HYDROCHLORIDE—Pontocaine®

Description/Actions: Local anesthetic indicated for spinal anesthesia, for anesthesia of the nose and throat, for ocular disorders, and skin conditions.

Preparations: Ampules (for spinal anesthesia), 0.2%, 0.3%, 1%, and powder. Solution (for anesthesia of the nose and throat), 2%. Ophthalmic solution and ointment (as base), 0.5%. Cream, 1%. Ointment (as base), 0.5%.

TETRACYCLINE HYDROCHLORIDE—Achromycin V®, Actisite®, Panmycin®, Sumycin®

Description/Actions: Tetracycline antibiotic active against many gram-positive and gram-negative bacteria, mycoplasmal, chlamydial, and rickettsial organisms, and certain spirochetes. Indicated in the treatment of respiratory and urinary tract infections and a number of other types of infections. Is useful as adjunctive therapy in the management of severe acne. Also indicated (for use as a periodontal fiber) as an adjunct to scaling and root planing for reduction of pocket depth and bleeding on probing in patients with adult periodontitis.

Precautions/Adverse Reactions: Use is best avoided during the last half of pregnancy and in childhood to the age of 8 years because of the risk of discoloration of the teeth. Adverse reactions include nausea, vomiting, diarrhea, rash, and fungal superinfections. May cause photosensitivity reactions, so patients should be cautioned to limit their exposure to sunlight and ultraviolet light. Must be used with caution in patients with impaired renal function. Absorption may be reduced by antacids, iron, calcium, and zinc salts, and other metal-containing formulations and foods; the administration of tetracycline and one of these agents should be separated by an interval of at least 1 hour.

Administration: Oral and topical.

Preparations: Capsules and tablets, 250 and 500 mg. Oral suspension, 125 mg/5 ml. Ointment, 3%. Topical solution. Periodontal fiber (Actisite), 12.7 mg.

TETRAHYDROZOLINE HYDROCHLORIDE—Tyzine®, Visine®

Description/Actions: Decongestant indicated for nasal use and for ophthalmic use to provide temporary relief of burning, irritation, and discomfort associated with certain ocular conditions.

Preparations: Nasal solution, 0.05% and 0.1%. Ophthalmic solution, 0.05%.

THALIDOMIDE—Thalomid®

Description/Actions: Thalidomide is an immunmmodulatory agent indicated in the treatment of erythema nodosum leprosum (ENL). Not indicated as monotherapy in patients with ENL with moderate to severe neuritis. Unlabeled uses include Behcet's syndrome, HIV-associated wasting syndrome, aphthous stomatitis (including HIV-associated), and Crohn's disease.

Precautions/Adverse Reactions: Contraindicated in pregnancy (Category X). Severe, life-threatening human birth defects can occur if thalidomide is taken during pregnancy. Prescribers must be registered in the STEPS program and understand the risk of teratogenicity if thalidomide is administered during pregnancy. There are strict government-mandated criteria that must be met prior to prescribing thalidomide for a woman or a man of childbearing potential. Because thalidomide is present in the semen of patients receiving the drug, males receiving thalidomide must always use a latex condom during any sexual contact with women of childbearing potential. Adverse reactions include somolence, peripheral neuropathy, dizziness, orthostatic hypotension, neutropenia, photosensitivity, hypersensitivity, bradycardia and an increase in HIV viral load. Serious dermatologic reactions, including Stevens-Johnson syndrome and toxic epidermal necrolysis, which may be fatal, have been reported. Seizures, including grand mal seizures, have also been reported during therapy with thalidomide. Patients with a history of seizures should be closely monitored.

Administration: Oral.

Patient Care Implications: Perform pregnancy testing 24 hours prior to the start of thalidomide and weekly thereafter for the duration of therapy. Instruct patients to safeguard access to this medication and not to share the drug with anyone else. Warn patients about the effects on the unborn fetus. Teach patients the symptoms of periperal neuropathies and to report them immediately to the prescriber. The medication should be discontinued if drug-induced neuropathy develops, to limit the potential for further nerve damage. Caution patients to avoid sun exposure because of the risk of photosensitivity. Advise patients to avoid alcohol during the course of treatment. Inform patients that dizziness and drowsiness may occur and to avoid medication that may increase either of these effects. Tell patients to avoid activities in which drowsiness may be potentially dangerous (e.g., driving a car, running machinery) until response is ascertained.

Preparations: Capsules, 50, 100, and 200 mg.

THALOMID®, see Thalidomide

THAM®, see Tromethamine with Electrolytes

THEELIN®, see Estrone

THEO-DUR®, see Theophylline

THEO-24®, see Theophylline

THEOPHYLLINE (see list of preparations below for trade names)

Description/Actions: A xanthine derivative indicated for the relief and/or prevention of symptoms of bronchial asthma and for reversible bronchospasm associated with chronic bronchitis and emphysema.

Precautions/Adverse Reactions: Adverse reactions include nausea, vomiting, diarrhea, headaches, irritability, restlessness, insomnia, palpitation, tachycardia, flushing, and hypotension.

Administration: Oral. Controlled-release formulations should not be chewed or crushed. A high-fat content meal may increase the rate and extent of absorption of theophylline from certain formulations (e.g., Theo-24); the labeling for individual formulations should be consulted for guidelines regarding administration in relationship to meals.

Preparations: Capsules and tablets (Elixophyllin®, Slo-Phyllin®), 50, 100, 125, 200, 225, 250, and 300 mg. Controlled-release capsules and tablets (Elixophyllin SR®, Slo-bid gyrocaps®, Theo-24®, Theo-Dur®, Theovent®, Uni-Dur®, Uniphyl®), 50, 100, 125, 200, 250, 300, 400, 450, 500, and 600 mg. Liquid (Elixophyllin®, Slo-Phyllin®), 80, 112.5, and 150 mg/15 ml.

THEOPHYLLINE CALCIUM SALICYLATE

Description/Actions: Bronchodilator used in combination with other agents in the treatment of asthma and other respiratory conditions.

THEOPHYLLINE ETHYLENEDIAMINE, see Aminophylline

THEOPHYLLINE SODIUM GLYCINATE

Description/Actions: Bronchodilator indicated for the relief of bronchial asthma and for reversible bronchospasm associated with chronic bronchitis and emphysema.

THEOVENT®, see Theophylline

THIABENDAZOLE—Mintezol®

Description/Actions: Anthelmintic indicated for the treatment of trichinosis, cutaneous larva migrans, visceral larva migrans, and strongyloidiasis. Is also effective in numerous other helmintic infestations.

Precautions/Adverse Reactions: Thiabendazole has been associated with abnormal sensations in eyes, xanthopsia, blurred vision, drying of mucous membranes, sicca syndrome, and abdominal pain.

Preparations: Chewable tablets, 500 mg. Suspension, 500 mg/5 ml.

THIAMINE HYDROCHLORIDE—Vitamin B₁

Description/Actions: Vitamin indicated for the treatment and prevention of thiamine deficiency and prevention of Wernicke's encephalopathy.

Preparations: Tablets, 5, 10, 25, 50, 100, 250, and 500 mg. Ampules and vials, 100 mg/ml and 200 mg/ml.

THIAMYLAL SODIUM

Description/Actions: Barbiturate anesthetic administered intravenously for induction of anesthesia, for supplementing other anesthetic agents, as anesthesia for short surgical procedures, and for inducing hypnotic states.

Preparations: Vials, 1, 5, and 10 g.

THIETHYLPERAZINE MALEATE—Norzine®, Torecan®

Description/Actions: Phenothiazine antiemetic indicated for the relief of nausea and vomiting.

Preparations: Tablets, 10 mg. Suppositories, 10 mg. Ampules, 10 mg/2 ml.

THIMEROSAL—Merthiolate®

Description/Actions: Antiseptic used for antisepsis of intact skin, treatment of contaminated wounds, and for preoperative and postoperative use.

Preparations: Solution and tincture, 1:1000. Aeropump tincture, 1:1000.

THIOGUANINE

Description/Actions: Antineoplastic agent indicated for the treatment of acute nonlymphocytic leukemias and chronic myelogenous leukemia.

Precautions/Adverse Reactions: Individuals with an inherited deficiency of the enzyme thiopurine methyltransferase (TPMT) may be unusually sensitive to the myelosuppressive effects of mercaptopurine and prone to developing rapid bone marrow suppression following initiation of treatment. This problem may be potentiated by coadministration of thioguanine with drugs that inhibit TPMT, such as olsalazine, mesalazine, and sulfasalazine. Use caution if these drugs must be coadministered.

Preparations: Tablets, 40 mg.

THIOLA®, see Tiopronin

THIOPENTAL SODIUM—Pentothal®

Description/Actions: Barbiturate anesthetic administered intravenously for induction of anesthesia, for supplementing other anesthetic agents, as anesthesia for short surgical procedures, for inducing hypnotic states, for control of convulsive seizures, in certain neurosurgical patients with increased intracranial pressure, and for narcoanalysis and narcosynthesis in psychiatric disorders. Has also been used in the form of a rectal suspension when preanesthetic sedation or basal narcosis by the rectal route is desired.

Preparations: Vials and syringes, 250, 400, and 500 mg; 1, 2.5, and 5 g. Rectal suspension, 400 mg/g.

THIOPLEX®, see Thiotepa

THIORIDAZINE HYDROCHLORIDE—Mellaril®

Description/Actions: Phenothiazine, antipsychotic agent. Mellaril® is now only indicated for the treatment of schizophrenic patients who fail to show an acceptable response to other antipsychotic agents.

Precautions/Adverse Reactions: Adverse reactions include drowsiness and other CNS effects; patients should be cautioned regarding activities such as driving and operating machinery, as well as interactions with other CNS-acting drugs including alcohol. Other adverse reactions include extrapyramidal symptoms, tardive dyskinesia, dry mouth, blurred vision, and dermatitis. Mellaril® has been shown to prolong the QTc interval and has been associated with torsades de pointes–type arrhythmias and sudden death. Mellaril® is contraindicated with fluvoxamine, propranolol, pindolol, and drugs that inhibit the cytochrome p450206 isozyme such as fluoxetine and paroxetine and agents known to prolong the QTc interval. Mellaril® is also contraindicated in patients known to have reduced levels of the cytochrome p450206 isozyme as well as in patients with congenital long QT syndrome or a history of cardiac arrhythmias. Baseline ECG and serum potassium levels should be monitored. Patients with a QTc interval greater than 450 msec should not receive Mellaril®. Mellaril® should be discontinued in patients who are found to have a QTc interval greater than 500 msec.

Administration: Oral.

Preparations: Tablets, 10, 15, 25, 50, 100, 150, and 200 mg. Oral solution (concentrate), 30 and 100 mg/ml. Oral suspension (as the base), 25 and 100 mg/5 ml.

THIOSULFIL FORTE®, see Sulfamethizole

THIOTEPA—Triethylenethiophosphoramide, Thioplex®

Description/Actions: Antineoplastic agent administered parenterally in the palliative treatment of adenocarcinoma of the breast, adenocarcinoma of the ovary, and for controlling intracavitary effusions secondary to diffuse or localized neoplastic disease of various serosal cavities, superficial papillary carcinoma of the bladder, lymphosarcoma, and Hodgkin's disease.

Preparations: Vials, 15 mg.

THIOTHIXENE—Navane®

Description/Actions: Antipsychotic agent indicated in the management of the manifestations of psychotic disorders.

Preparations: Capsules, 1, 2, 5, 10, and 20 mg. Concentrate (as the hydrochloride), 5 mg/ml.

THORAZINE®, see Chlorpromazine

3TC®, see Lamivudine

THROMBIN—Thrombinar®, Thrombostat®

Description/Actions: Hemostatic agent indicated for topical use whenever oozing blood and minor bleeding from capillaries and small venules is accessible. Also used in conjunction with absorbable gelatin sponge for hemostasis in various types of surgery.

Preparations: Vials, 1000, 5000, 10,000, 20,000, and 50,000 units.

THROMBINAR®, see Thrombin

THROMBOSTAT®, see Thrombin

THYLLINE®, see Dyphylline

THYMOL

Description/Actions: Anti-infective included in combination with other agents in certain topical formulations. Has also been included in mouthwash formulations for its aromatic and antiseptic properties.

THYROID

Description/Actions: Thyroid hormone and is indicated as replacement therapy in patients with hypothyroidism, and as a pituitary- and thyroid-stimulating hormone (TSH) suppressant in the treatment or prevention of various types of goiters.

Precautions/Adverse Reactions: Must be used cautiously in patients with cardiovascular disorders and endocrine disorders such as diabetes. Adverse reactions include headache, nervousness, palpitations, tachycardia, and nausea.

Administration: Oral.

Preparations: Tablets, 15, 30, 60, 90, 120, 180, 240, and 300 mg.

THYROTROPIN—Thyroid-stimulating Hormone (TSH), Thytropar®

Description/Actions: Used for diagnostic purposes.

Preparations: Vials, 10 IU of thyrotropic activity.

THYROXINE, see Levothyroxine

THYTROPAR®, see Thyrotropin

TIAGABINE HYDROCHLORIDE—Gabitril®

Description/Actions: Antiepileptic agent indicated as an adjunct in partial seizures.

Precautions/Adverse Reactions: Avoid abrupt cessation. Use cautiously in nursing mothers, hepatic impairment, and the elderly. Pregnancy Category C. Adverse reactions include dizziness, asthenia, somnolence, GI upset/pain, nervousness, tremor, abdominal pain, concentration difficulties, other CNS effects, serious rash, and possible long-term opthalmologic effects. Not recommended in children <12 years.

Administration: Oral. Take with food.

Preparations: Tablets, 2, 4, 12, 16 mg.

TIAZAC®, see Diltiazem

TICAR®, see Ticarcillin

TICARCILLIN DISODIUM—Ticar®

Description/Actions: Penicillin antibiotic that is bactericidal and active against many gram-positive and gram-negative bacteria, including *Pseudomonas aeruginosa.* Is usually used in conjunction with an aminoglycoside antibiotic in the treatment of *Pseudomonas* infections.

Precautions/Adverse Reactions: Contraindicated in patients with a history of allergic reaction to any of the penicillins. Adverse reactions include hypersensitivity reactions, gastrointestinal effects, bleeding manifestations, and hypokalemia. Disodium salt is utilized, and the administration of high doses may cause problems in patients in whom sodium intake must be closely monitored.

Administration: Intravenous and intramuscular.

Preparations: Vials, 1, 3, 6, 20, and 30 g.

TICARCILLIN DISODIUM/CLAVULANATE POTASSIUM—
Timentin®

Description/Actions: Penicillin antibiotic with beta-lactamase inhibitor. Clavulanic acid inhibits beta-lactamase enzymes and protects ticarcillin from degradation by these enzymes; the spectrum of action of ticarcillin is extended to include additional bacteria.

Preparations: Vials, 3.1 and 3.2 g (representing 3 g of ticarcillin and 0.1 and 0.2 g of clavulanic acid, respectively).

TICLID®, see Ticlopidine

TICLOPIDINE HYDROCHLORIDE—Ticlid®

Description/Actions: Is a platelet aggregation inhibitor that is thought to act primarily by inhibiting the adenosine diphosphate (ADP) pathway for platelet aggregation. Indicated to reduce the risk of thrombotic stroke in patients who have experienced stroke warning signs (e.g., transient ischemic attacks [TIAs]), and in patients who have had a complete thrombotic stroke. Use should be reserved for patients who are intolerant to aspirin therapy, or in situations in which there is a risk of stroke but aspirin is not indicated. Ticlopidine is also indicated as an adjunctive therapy with aspirin to reduce the incidence of subacute stent thrombosis in patients undergoing successful coronary stent implantation.

Precautions/Adverse Reactions: Contraindicated in the presence of hematopoietic disorders such as neutropenia and thrombocytopenia. Contraindicated in the presence of a hemostatic disorder or active pathologic bleeding and in patients with severe hepatic disease. Complete blood counts and white cell differentials should be performed every 2 weeks starting from the second week to at least the end of the third month of therapy. Causes a prolongation of bleeding time, and its use has been associated with bleeding complications (e.g., ecchymosis, epistaxis, hematuria, gastrointestinal bleeding). Should be used with caution in patients who may be at risk of increased bleeding from trauma, surgery, or pathological conditions, and in patients who have lesions with a propensity to bleed (e.g., ulcers). Medication may be discontinued 10–14 days prior to elective surgery. Patients should be advised that it may take them longer than usual to stop bleeding. The concomitant use of aspirin, an anticoagulant, or fibrinolytic agent with ticlopidine is best avoided. Other adverse reactions include diarrhea, nausea, dyspepsia, gastrointestinal pain, and rash. Signs and symptoms of jaundice have occurred infrequently, so patients should be advised to inform their physicians if they observe yellowing of the skin or whites of the eyes, or consistent darkening in the color of the urine, or lightening in the color of the stools. May cause severe hematologic reactions, including neutropenia, agranulocytosis, thrombotic thrombocytopenia purpura (TTP), and aplastic anemia.

Administration: Oral. Should be administered with food.

Preparations: Tablets, 250 mg.

TIGAN®, see Trimethobenzamide

TIKOSYN®, see Dofetilide

TILADE®, see Nedocromil Sodium

TILUDRONATE—Skelid®

Description/Actions: Indicated in the treatment of Paget's disease. In vitro studies indicated that tiludronate acts primarily on bone through a mechanism involving inhibition of osteoclastic activity, probably through a reduction in the enzymatic and transport process that leads to resorption of the mineralized matrix. Use in patients with severe renal failure (CrCl <30 ml/min) not recommended. Maintain adequate calcium and vitamin D intake. Use cautiously in patients with upper GI disease.

Precautions/Adverse Reactions: Adverse reactions include GI disorders (e.g., nausea, diarrhea, dyspepsia), chest pain, edema, paresthesia, hyperparathyroidism, arthrosis, rhinitis, sinusitis, cataract, conjunctivitis, and glaucoma.

Administration: Oral. Take with 6–8 oz of plain (not mineral) water at least 2 hours before or after any other beverages, food, or medication.

Preparations: Tablets, 240 mg (equivalent to 200 mg tiludronic acid).

TIMENTIN®, see Ticarcillin Disodium/Clavulanate Potassium

TIMOLOL MALEATE—Betimol®, Blocadren®, Timoptic®, Timoptic-XE®

Description/Actions: A nonselective beta-adrenergic blocking agent indicated in the treatment of hypertension and to reduce cardiovascular mortality and the risk of reinfarction in patients who have survived the acute phase of a myocardial infarction. Also indicated for migraine headache prophylaxis. Also indicated for ophthalmic administration in the treatment of chronic open-angle glaucoma, aphakic glaucoma, and secondary glaucoma.

Precautions/Adverse Reactions: Contraindicated in patients with bronchial asthma or severe chronic obstructive pulmonary disease, sinus bradycardia, second- and third-degree AV block, overt cardiac failure, and cardiogenic shock. Adverse reactions include fatigue, dizziness, bradycardia, cold hands and feet, and, when administered in the ophthalmic dosage form, ocular irritation. Adverse reactions also include anaphylaxis, angioedema, urticaria, and localized and generalized rash. Use is best avoided in patients with bronchospastic diseases, and therapy in diabetic patients must be closely monitored.

Administration: Oral and ophthalmic. Patients should be cautioned about the interruption or discontinuation of therapy; exacerbation of angina pectoris has occurred following the abrupt cessation of therapy, and, when therapy is to be discontinued, the dosage should be gradually reduced over a period of 1 to 2 weeks.

Preparations: Tablets, 5, 10, and 20 mg. Ophthalmic solution, 0.25% and 0.5%. Ophthalmic gel (Timoptic-XE®), 0.25% and 0.5%.

TIMOPTIC®, see Timolol Maleate

TIMOPTIC-XE®, see Timolol Maleate

TINACTIN®, see Tolnaftate

TINDAL®, see Acetophenazine

TINVER®, see Sodium Thiosulfate

TINZAPARIN—Innohep®

Description/Actions: Indicated for the treatment of acute symptomatic deep vein thrombosis, with or without pulmonary embolism, when administered in combination with warfarin sodium.

Precautions/Adverse Reactions: Tinzaparin is contraindicated in patients with a hypersensitivity to Tinzaparin or any component of the formulations, sulfites, benzyl alcohol, pork products, with major active bleeding, and current or history of heparin-induced thrombocytopenia. Patients with recent or anticipated neuraxial anesthesia (epidural or spinal anesthesia) are at risk of spinal or epidural hematoma and subsequent paralysis. This risk is increased by the use of indwelling epidural catheters and by the concomitant use of drugs affecting hemostasis (i.e., nonsteroidal anti-inflammatory drugs, as well as traumatic or repeated epidural or spinal puncture). Patients should be closely monitored for signs and symptoms of neurologic impairment. Health care providers should consider the potential benefit versus risk before neuraxial anesthesia intervention in patients anticoagulated or to be anticoagulated for thromboprophylaxis. Monitor patients for signs and symptoms of bleeding while on Innohep® therapy. Caution should be exercised in conditions where patients are at increased risk of hemorrhage. Risk factors for increased bleeding include bacterial endocarditis; severe or uncontrolled hypertension; congenital or acquired bleeding disorders; active ulceration or angiodysplastic GI diseases; recent GI bleed; hepatic failure, amyloidosis; gastrointestinal disease; shortly after brain, spinal, or ophthalmic surgery; in patients treated concomitantly with platelet inhibitors; hemorrhagic stroke; diabetic retinopathy; or in patients undergoing invasive procedures. Pregnancy Category B. No adequate and well-controlled studies in pregnant women. This drug should be used during pregnancy only if clearly needed. Innohep® multiple-dose vials contain benzyl alcohol as a preservative and benzyl alcohol administered to premature neonates has been associated with fatal gasping syndrome. Because benzyl alcohol may cross the placenta, Innohep® preserved with benzyl alcohol should be used with caution in pregnant women only if clearly needed. Excretion in breast milk is unknown; use caution. Safety and efficacy have not been established in pediatric patients. Use caution in the elderly. Thrombocytopenia can occur with Innohep® therapy; discontinue administration if platelets are <100,000/mm3. Administer subcutaneous injection only; do not mix with other injections or infusions. Due to the increased bleeding potential, use caution in patients receiving oral anticoagulants, platelet inhibitors, and thrombolytics. Some adverse effects are bleeding, injection site hematoma, increased ALT, thrombocytopenia, urinary tract infections, pulmonary embolism, angina pectoris, headache, epistaxis, nausea, and back pain.

Administration: SQ injection.

Patient Care Implications: Innohep® is administered by SC injection. It must not be administered by intramuscular or intravenous injection. SC injection technique: Patients should be lying or sitting, and Innohep® should be administered by deep SC injection. Alternate injection site daily between the left and right anterolateral and left and right posterolateral abdominal wall. The entire needle should be introduced into the skin fold formed by the thumb and forefinger. Hold the skin fold until injection is complete. To minimize bruising, do not rub the injection site. Lab monitoring should include CBC, including platelet count and hematocrit/hemoglobin. Inform patients to report immediately any unusual bleeding or bruising (i.e., mouth, nose, blood in urine, or stool) or any other adverse effects.

Preparations: Multidose 2 ml vial (20,000 anti-Xa IU per ml). Preparation contains metabisulfite and benzyl alcohol.

TIOCONAZOLE—Vagistat®

Description/Actions: An imidazole antifungal agent indicated for use as a local single-dose treatment of vulvovaginal candidiasis.

Precautions/Adverse Reactions: Adverse reactions include burning and itching.

Administration: Vaginal.

Preparations: Vaginal ointment, 6.5%.

TIOPRONIN—Thiola®

Description/Actions: Indicated for the prevention of cystine (kidney) stone formation in patients with severe homozygous cystinuria with urinary cystine greater than 500 mg/day, who are resistant to treatment with conservative measures of high fluid intake, alkali and diet modification, or who have had adverse reactions to penicillamine.

Precautions/Adverse Reactions: Contraindicated during pregnancy. Adverse reactions include rash, pruritus, drug fever, lupus erythematosus-like effects, reduction in taste perception, and wrinkling and friability of the skin. May cause gastrointestinal, pulmonary, neurologic, renal, and hematologic reactions.

Administration: Oral. Should be given in divided doses 3 times a day at least 1 hour before or 2 hours after meals.

Preparations: Tablets, 100 mg.

TIROFIBAN—Aggrastat®

Description/Actions: Platelet aggregation inhibitor indicated in combination with heparin for treating acute coronary syndrome.

Precautions/Adverse Reactions: Contraindicated in the following conditions within previous 30 days: active internal bleeding, bleeding diathesis, stroke, major surgery, or severe trauma. Contraindicated with a history of intracranial hemorrhage, intracranial neoplasm, arteriovenous malformation, aneurysm, hemorrhagic stroke, thrombocytopenia after previous tirofiban therapy, symptoms or findings suggestive of aortic dissection, severe hypertension, acute pericarditis, and concomitant parenteral GI 11b/111a inhibitor. Use cautiously in patients with platelet count <150,000/mm3, in patients with hemorrhagic retinopathy, and in chronic hemodialysis patients. Fatal bleeding events have been reported. Properly care for femoral artery access site to minimize bleeding. Minimize other arterial and venous punctures, IM injections, catheter use, and other invasive procedures to minimize bleeding risk. Avoid use of noncompressible IV access sites. Do baseline platelet counts, hemoglobin and hematocrit, and monitor during therapy. Discontinue tirofiban if confirmed thrombocytopenia occurs. Adjust heparin to maintain aPTT at two times control. Severe allergic reactions, including anaphylactic reactions, have occurred during the first day of tirofiban infusion, during initial treatment, and during readministration of tirofiban. Some cases have been associated with severe thrombocytopenia (platelet count <10,000/mm3). Adverse reactions include bleeding, decreased hemoglobin and/or hematocrit, reduced platelet counts, edema, vasovagal reaction, and others.

Administration: Intravenous.

Preparations: Premixed, 50 mcg/ml vials. Concentrate, 250 mcg/ml.

TISSUE PLASMINOGEN ACTIVATOR, see Alteplase, Recombinant

TITANIUM DIOXIDE

Description/Actions: Sunscreen used topically in cream, lotion, and ointment formulations.

TIZANIDINE—Zanaflex®

Description/Actions: Reduces muscle spasticity and is indicated in acute and intermittent management of increased skeletal muscle tone associated with spasticity.

Precautions/Adverse Reactions: Use cautiously in impaired hepatic or renal function, in cardiovascular disease, and in the elderly. Monitor ophthalmic and liver function (aminotransferases at baseline, 1, 3, and 6 months and periodically thereafter). Adverse reactions include sedation, dry mouth, somnolence, asthenia, dizziness, constipation, elevated liver enzymes, vomiting, speech disorders, blurred vision, dyskinesia, nervousness, pharyngitis, hypotension (including orthostatic), hallucinations, and psychosis.

Administration: Oral.

Preparations: Tablets, 2 and 4 mg (scored). Capsules, 2 mg, 4 mg, and 6 mg.

TMP-SMX, see Trimethoprim-sulfamethoxazole

TNKase™, see Tenecteplase

TOBRAMYCIN SULFATE—Nebcin®, Tobrex®

Description/Actions: Aminoglycoside antibiotic indicated for the parenteral treatment of serious infections caused by gram-negative bacteria including *Pseudomonas aeruginosa.* Is also effective in the treatment of staphylococcal infections. Has also been used topically in the treatment of ocular infections.

Precautions/Adverse Reactions: May cause nephrotoxicity, ototoxicity, and neurotoxicity, and the concurrent or serial use of other nephrotoxic or ototoxic agents should be avoided.

Administration: Intravenous, intramuscular, and ophthalmic.

Preparations: Vials and syringes, 20 mg/2 ml, 60 mg/1.5 ml, 80 mg/ 2 ml., and 1.2 g. Ophthalmic solution and ointment, 0.3%.

TOBREX®, see Tobramycin

TOCAINIDE HYDROCHLORIDE—Tonocard®

Description/Actions: Antiarrhythmic agent indicated for the suppression of symptomatic ventricular arrhythmias, including frequent premature ventricular contractions, unifocal or multifocal, couplets, and ventricular tachycardia.

Preparations: Tablets, 400 and 600 mg.

TOFRANIL®, see Imipramine

TOLAZAMIDE—Tolinase®

Description/Actions: Sulfonylurea hypoglycemic agent indicated as an adjunct to diet to lower the blood glucose in patients with noninsulin-dependent diabetes mellitus whose hyperglycemia cannot be controlled by diet alone.

Precautions/Adverse Reactions: May cause hypoglycemia, so patients should be advised to contact their physician if symptoms of hypoglycemia develop. Adverse reactions include nausea, heartburn, pruritus, and erythema. Oral hypoglycemic agents have been suggested to be associated with increased cardiovascular mortality as compared to treatment by diet alone or diet plus insulin.

Administration: Oral.

Preparations: Tablets, 100, 250, and 500 mg.

TOLAZOLINE HYDROCHLORIDE—Priscoline®

Description/Actions: Peripheral vasodilator indicated for intravenous use in the treatment of persistent pulmonary hypertension of the newborn when systemic arterial oxygenation cannot be satisfactorily maintained by usual supportive care.

Preparations: Ampules, 25 mg/ml.

TOLBUTAMIDE—Orinase®

Description/Actions: Sulfonylurea hypoglycemic agent indicated as an adjunct to diet to lower the blood glucose in patients with noninsulin-dependent diabetes whose hyperglycemia cannot be satisfactorily controlled by diet alone.

Preparations: Tablets, 250 and 500 mg.

TOLCAPONE—Tasmar®

Description/Actions: Anti-Parkinson agent indicated as an adjunct to carbidopa/levodopa in idiopathic Parkinson's disease.

Precautions/Adverse Reactions: Contraindicated in concomitant nonselective MAOIs (e.g., phenelzine), liver disease or a previous history of elevated liver function associated with the use of this agent, or a history of nontraumatic rhabdomyolysis, or fever or confusion possibly related to medication. Use cautiously in orthostatic hypertension/syncope, severe renal impairment (CrCl ≤25 ml/min), and severe hepatic impairment. Monitor transaminases every month for the first 3 months, then every 6 weeks for the next 3 months (more frequently if elevation occurs). Discontinue if enzyme elevations ≥5 times the upper limit of normal or jaundice occurs. Pregnancy Category C. Adverse reactions include dyskinesias, nausea, sleep disorders, dystonia, excessive dreaming, anorexia, muscle cramps, orthostatic complaints, somnolence, diarrhea, confusion, dizziness, headache, hallucinations, vomiting, constipation, fatigue, upper respiratory or urinary tract infection, falling, increased sweating, syncope, xerostomia, urine discoloration, and others.

Administration: Oral.

Preparations: Tablets, 100 and 200 mg.

TOLECTIN®, see Tolmetin

TOLINASE®, see Tolazamide

TOLMETIN SODIUM—Tolectin®, Tolectin DS®

Description/Actions: Nonsteroidal anti-inflammatory agent that inhibits prostaglandin synthesis and is indicated for the treatment of rheumatoid arthritis, juvenile rheumatoid arthritis, and osteoarthritis.

Precautions/Adverse Reactions: Should not be given to patients in whom aspirin or another NSAID causes asthma, rhinitis, urticaria, or other allergic-type reactions. May cause GI effects, so use should be avoided in patients with active GI tract disease and closely monitored in patients with a previous history of such disorders. Other adverse reactions include headache, weakness, edema, elevated blood pressure, weight changes, and skin irritation. Effect may be reduced by sodium bicarbonate.

Administration: Oral.

Preparations: Tablets and capsules, 200, 400, and 600 mg.

TOLNAFTATE—Tinactin®

Description/Actions: Antifungal agent used topically in the treatment of superficial fungal infections of the skin.

Preparations: Cream, powder, solution, gel, aerosol powder, and aerosol liquid, 1%.

TOLTERODINE TARTRATE—Detrol®, Detrol® LA

Description/Actions: A competitive muscarinic receptor antagonist indicated in treatment of patients with symptoms of urinary frequency, urgency, or urge incontinence.

Precautions/Adverse Reactions: Contraindicated in urinary retention, gastric retention, and uncontrolled narrow-angle glaucoma. Use cautiously in patients with bladder outflow obstruction, obstructive GI disease (e.g., pyloric stenosis), narrow-angle glaucoma, renal impairment, and hepatic dysfunction. Pregnancy Category C. Not recommended in nursing mothers. Adverse reactions include dry mouth, dyspepsia, headache, constipation, xerophthalmia, hypertension, dizziness, and other anticholinergic effects. May cause blurred vision. Anaphylactoid reactions, tachycardia, and peripheral edema have also been reported with the use of tolterodine.

Administration: Oral.

Preparations: Tablets, 1 and 2 mg. Extended-release capsules, 2 and 4 mg.

TONOCARD®, see Tocainide

TOPAMAX®, see Topiramate

TOPICORT®, see Desoximetasone

TOPIRAMATE—Topamax®

Description/Actions: Anticonvulsant indicated as adjunctive therapy for adult and pediatric patients ages 2–16 years with partial onset seizures, or primary generalized tonic-clonic seizures, and in patients 2 years of age and older with seizures associated with Lennox-Gastaut syndrome. Topiramate is also indicated for adults for the prophylaxis of migraine headaches.

Precautions/Adverse Reactions: Hyperchloremic, non-anion gap, metabolic acidosis (i.e., decreased serum bicarbonate below the normal reference range in the absence of chronic respiratory alkalosis) is associated with topiramate treatment. Conditions or therapies that predispose to acidosis (such as renal disease, severe respiratory disorders, status epilepticus, diarrhea, surgery, ketogenic diet, or drugs) may be additive to the bicarbonate-lowering effects of topiramate. Some manifestations of acute or chronic metabolic acidosis may include hyperventilation, nonspecific symptoms such as fatigue, and anorexia, or more severe sequelae including cardiac arrhythmias or stupor. Avoid abrupt cessation as this may precipitate seizures. Use cautiously in patients with hepatic or renal impairment. The risk of kidney stone formation is about 2–4 times that of the untreated population. This may be reduced by increasing fluid intake. Adverse reactions include somnolence, dizziness, ataxia, speech disorders, psychomotor slowing, nervousness, paresthesia, nystagmus, tremor, fatigue, confusion, decreased weight, language or mood problems, anorexia, and anxiety. A syndrome consisting of acute myopia associated with secondary angle-closure glaucoma has been reported in both adult and pediatric patients receiving topiramate. Symptoms include acute onset of decreased visual acuity and/or ocular pain. May be associated with supraciliary effusion resulting in anterior displacement of the lens and iris, with secondary angle-closure glaucoma. Topiramate should be discontinued if this occurs.

Administration: Oral.

Preparations: Tablets 25, 100, and 200 mg. Sprinkle capsules 15 and 25 mg.

TOPOTECAN HYDROCHLORIDE—Hycamtin®

Description/Actions: Antineoplastic agent used in the treatment of patients with metastatic ovarian cancer after failure of initial or subsequent chemotherapy.

Precautions/Adverse Reactions: Bone marrow suppression (primarily neutropenia) is the dose-limiting toxicity of topotecan. Administer only to patients with adequate bone marrow reserves (baseline neutrophil counts of at least 1500 cells/mm3 and platelet count of 100,000 mm3). Adverse effects include neutropenia, thrombocytopenia, and anemia.

Administration: Intravenous.

Preparations: Powder for injection, 4 mg.

TOPROL XL®, see Metoprolol Succinate

TORADOL®, see Ketorolac Tromethamine

TORECAN®, see Thiethylperazine

TOREMIFENE—Fareston®

Description/Actions: Indicated in metastatic breast cancer in postmenopausal women with estrogen-receptor positive or unknown tumors.

Precautions/Adverse Reactions: Contraindicated in pregnancy (Category D) and nursing mothers. Use not recommended in history of thromboembolic disorders, and long-term treatment not recommended in patients with preexisting endometrial hyperplasia. If bone metastases present, monitor for hypercalcemia for first few weeks. Discontinue if severe hypercalcemia occurs. Use cautiously with leukopenia and thrombocytopenia. Monitor blood counts, calcium levels, and liver function. Adverse reactions include hot flashes, sweating, GI upset, vaginal discharge/bleed, dizziness, edema, tumor flare, hypercalcemia, elevated liver tests, and cardiac, ocular, and thrombotic events. Instruct patients to report vaginal bleeding and symptoms of hypercalcemia.

Administration: Oral.

Preparations: Tablets, 60 mg.

TORNALATE®, see Bitolterol

TORSEMIDE—Demadex®

Description/Actions: Is a loop diuretic that is indicated for the treatment of edema associated with congestive heart failure, renal disease, or hepatic disease. Is also indicated for the treatment of hypertension and may be used alone or in combination with other antihypertensive agents.

Precautions/Adverse Reactions: Contraindicated in patients who are hypersensitive to any sulfonylurea derivative. Is also contraindicated in patients who are anuric. Adverse reactions include excessive urination, headache, dizziness, and rhinitis. May cause electrolyte imbalance and periodic monitoring of serum potassium and other electrolytes is advised.

Administration: Oral and intravenous. When given intravenously, should be administered slowly over a period of two minutes.

Preparations: Tablets, 5, 10, 20, and 100 mg. Ampules, 20 and 50 mg.

TOSITUMOMAB AND IODINE I 131—Bexxar®

Description/Actions: Bexxar® is a monoclonal antibody, antineoplastic, radiopharmaceutical. Tositumomab is a murine IgG2a lambda monoclonal antibody that binds to the CD20 antigen. This antigen is found on normal and malignant B lymphocytes. Iodine I 131 tositumomab is a radio-iodinated derivative of tositumomab covalently linked to iodine 131. Possible mechanisms of action of Bexxar® therapeutic regimen include induction of apoptosis, complement dependent cytotoxicity, and antibody-dependent cellular cytotoxicity mediated by the antibody. Cell death is associated with ionizing radiation from the radioisotope. Bexxar® is indicated for the treatment of relapsed or refractory (to rituximab) CD20 positive, follicular, non-Hodgkin's lymphoma. Bexxar® is not indicated for the initial treatment of patients with CD20 positive non-Hodgkin's lymphoma.

Precautions/Adverse Reactions: Bexxar® is contraindicated in patients hypersensitive to murine proteins or any component of the formulation, pregnancy, and breast-feeding. Hypersensitivity reactions, including anaphylaxis, have occurred. Patients who have received murine proteins should be screened for human anti-mouse antibodies (HAMA). Patients who are positive for HAMA may be at an increased risk of anaphylaxis and serious hypersensitivity reactions during administration. Pregnancy Category X. Can cause fetal harm when administered to a pregnant woman. Iodine 131 crosses the placenta and may cause severe and irreversible hypothyroidism in neonates. Secondary malignancies were reported. Treatment may lead to hypothyroidism;

patients should receive thyroid-blocking medications prior to the start of therapy and continue until 14 days after the therapeutic regimen. Iodine I 131 tositumomab and Iodine-131 are excreted primarily by the kidneys. Impaired renal function may decrease the rate of excretion of the radio-labeled iodine and increase patient exposure to the radioactive component. Safety and efficacy have not been established with impaired renal function or in pediatric patients. Most common adverse effects were neutropenia, thrombocytopenia, anemia, pneumonia, pleural effusion, and dehydration.

Administration: Intravenous.

Patient Care Implications: CBC with differential will be taken prior to therapy and at least weekly. Patients should be advised that they will have a radioactive material in their body for several days upon their release from the hospital or clinic. Should be provided with instructions for minimizing exposure of family members and the general public. Advise women of potential risks to fetus. Advise of potential risk of toxic effects on the male and female gonads, and instruct to use effective contraceptive methods during treatment and for 12 months following administration of Bexxar® therapeutic regimen. Inform of the risks of hypothyroidism and advise of the importance of compliance with thyroid-blocking agents and the need for lifelong monitoring. Thyroid stimulating hormone (TSH) level should be monitored before treatment and annually thereafter. Inform of risks of cytopenias and symptoms associated with cytopenia. Inform that secondary malignancies, secondary leukemia, and solid tumors have been observed. Report chills, persistent or acute headache, fever, rash, chest pain, muscle or back pain, upper respiratory symptoms, signs of infections, or other adverse reactions. Do not give blood during therapy or for 12 months following therapy. Do not breast-feed.

Preparations: Dosimetric package: Tositumomab 225 mg/16.1 mL (2 vials), tositumomab 35 mg/2.5 mL (1 vial), and Iodine I 131 tositumomab, within a lead pot, 0.1 mg/mL and 0.61 mCi/mL (20 mL vial). Therapeutic package: Tositumomab 225 mg/16/1 mL (2 vials), tositumomab 35 mg/2.5 mL (1 vial), and Iodine I 131 1.1 mg/mL and 5.6 mCi/mL (1 or 2 vials within a lead pot).

TOTACILLIN®, see Ampicillin

TPA, see Alteplase, Recombinant

TRACLEER™, see Bosentan

TRACRIUM®, see Atracurium Besylate

TRAMADOL HYDROCHLORIDE—Ultram®

Description/Actions: Analgesic indicated for the management of moderate to moderately severe pain.

Precautions/Adverse Reactions: Contraindicated in patients with alcohol, hypnotics, centrally acting analgesics, opioids, or psychotropic drugs. Do not give to opioid dependent patients. Adverse reactions include constipation, nausea, vomiting, dizziness, somnolence, central nervous system (CNS) stimulation, asthenia, and headache. Patients should be cautioned about driving or operating machinery. May increase the risk of seizures in patients with epilepsy. Unlikely to produce dependence and is not classified as a controlled substance.

Administration: Oral.

Preparations: Tablets, 50 mg.

TRAMADOL HYDROCHLORIDE/ACETAMINOPHEN— Ultracet™

Description/Actions: Ultracet™ is indicated for the short-term (5 days or less) management of acute pain.

Precautions/Adverse Reactions: Ultracet™ is contraindicated in any situation where opioids are contraindicated, including acute intoxication with any of the following: alcohol, hypnotics, narcotics, centrally acting analgesics, opioids, or psychotic drugs. It may worsen CNS and respiratory depression in these patients. Tramadol should not be used in opioid-dependent patients. Serious potential consequences of overdosage with tramadol are CNS depression, respiratory depression, and death. Administer Ultracet cautiously in patients at risk for respiratory depression. Seizures reported when taken within the recommended dosage. Risk is increased in patients taking selective serotonin reuptake inhibitors, tricyclic antidepressants, other tricyclic compounds, other opioids, monamine oxidate inhibitors (MAOIs), neuroleptics, or other drugs that reduce the seizure threshold. Use cautiously in patients with increased intracranial pressure or head injury. Not recommended in patients with liver disease. Do not coadminister with other tramadol- or acetaminophen-containing products. Safety and effectiveness have not been studied in the pediatric population. Use with caution in elderly patients, because there is a greater frequency of decreased hepatic, renal, or cardiac function, and concomitant disease, as well as multiple drug therapy. Most common side effects were somnolence, constipation, increased sweating, and dizziness. Pregnancy Category C. No well-controlled studies in pregnant women. Should not be used in pregnant women prior to or during labor. Chronic use during pregnancy may lead to physical dependence and postpartum withdrawal symptoms in the newborn.

Administration: Oral.

Patient Care Implications: May be taken with or without food. Advise patients they may be mentally impaired and to use caution when driving or engaging in tasks requiring alertness until response to drug is known. Patients should understand the 24-hour dose limit and the time interval between doses. Advise not to take with other tramadol- or acetaminophen-containing products.

Preparations: Tablets, acetaminophen, 325 mg, and tramadol hydrochloride, 37.5 mg.

TRANCOPAL®, see Chlormezanone

TRANDATE®, see Labetalol

TRANDOLAPRIL—Mavik®

Description/Actions: Inhibits angiotensin converting enzyme (ACE). Used in treatment of hypertension as monotherapy or as an adjunct to other antihypertensive agents. Also indicated in stabilized patients after MI who have LV systolic dysfunction or DHF symptoms.

Precautions/Adverse Reactions: Do not use in patients with a history of ACE inhibitor-associated angioedema. Monitor for neutropenia in collagen, vascular, and/or renal disease. Monitor for hyperkalemia in diabetes. Use cautiously in patients with renal impairment, cardiovascular or cerebrovascular disease, or salt/volume depletion. Adverse reactions include cough, dizziness, and diarrhea. Discontinue if laryngeal edema, angioedema, or jaundice occurs. (Black patients may have a higher risk of angioedema than non-Black patients.)

Administration: Oral.

Preparations: Tablets, 1 mg (scored), 2 and 4 mg.

TRANEXAMIC ACID—Cyklokapron®

Description/Actions: Antifibrinolytic agent indicated in patients with hemophilia for short-term use (2 to 8 days) to reduce or prevent hemorrhage and to reduce the need for replacement therapy during and following tooth extraction.

Precautions/Adverse Reactions: Contraindicated in (a) patients with acquired defective color vision, because this prohibits measuring one endpoint that should be followed as a measure of toxicity; and (b) patients with subarachnoid hemorrhage. Visual abnormalities have been experienced by some patients, and, for patients who are to be treated continually for longer than several days, an ophthalmological examination is advised before commencing and at regular intervals during the course of treatment. Other adverse reactions include nausea, vomiting, diarrhea, and giddiness. Hypotension has been observed when intravenous injection is too rapid, and the solution should not be injected more rapidly than 1 ml per minute.

Administration: Oral and intravenous.

Preparations: Tablets, 500 mg. Ampules, 100 mg/ml.

TRANSDERM-NITRO®, see Nitroglycerin

TRANSDERM-SCOP®, see Scopolamine

TRANXENE®, see Clorazepate

TRANYLCYPROMINE SULFATE—Parnate®

Description/Actions: Monoamine oxidase inhibitor antidepressant indicated for the treatment of major depressive episode without melancholia.

Precautions/Adverse Reactions: Hypertension or hypotension, coma, convulsions, and death may occur with opioids (avoid use of meperidine within 14–21 days of MAO inhibitor therapy; decrease initial dose of other agents to 25% of usual dose). Serious, potentially fatal, adverse reactions may occur with concurrent use of other antidepressants. Avoid using within two weeks of each other (wait 5 weeks from end of fluoxetine therapy).

Preparations: Tablets, 10 mg.

TRASTUZUMAB—Herceptin®

Description/Actions: Indicated in the treatment of patients with metastatic breast cancer with tumors overexpressing the human epidermal growth factor receptor2 (HER2) protein. It may be used as a single agent in patients who have received ≥1 chemotherapy regimens or in combination with placitaxel in patients who have not received chemotherapy for their metastatic disease. Use only in patients whose tumors have HER2 protein overexpression.

Precautions/Adverse Reactions: Trastuzumab administration can result in development of ventricular dysfunction and CHF. Evaluate the left ventricular function in all patients prior to and during treatment. Strongly consider discontinuing the trastuzumab in patients who develop a clinically significant decrease in the left ventricular function. Patients receiving trastuzumab in combination with anthracyclines and cyclophosphomide have demonstrated a particularly high incidence and severity of cardiac dysfunction. Adverse reactions include cardiotoxicity, anemia and leukopenia, diarrhea, infection, and infusion-related symptoms (During the first infusion 40% of the patients experienced chills and fever. Other infusional symptoms included nausea, vomiting, pain, rigors, headache, dizziness, dypsnea, hypotension, rash, and asthenia). Symptoms infrequently occurred with subsequent administrations of the drug.

Administration: Intravenous.

Patient Care Implications: Treat infusion-associated symptoms with acetaminophen, diphenhydramine, and meperidine as needed. Warn patients to avoid exposure to infectious sources. Teach patients to watch for early signs of an infection and to promptly report symptoms to the prescriber. Explain the need for ongoing cardiac function testing and the importance of adhering to the testing schedule.

Preparations: Powder for reconstitution, 400 mg (diluent contains benzyl alcohol).

TRASYLOL®, see Aprotinin

TRAVASE®, see Sutilains

TRAVATAN™, see Travoprost

TRAVERT®, see Invert Sugar

TRAVOPROST—Travatan™

Description/Actions: Travaprost is indicated for reduction of elevated intraocular pressure (IOP) in patients with open-angle glaucoma or ocular hypertension who are intolerant or unresponsive to other IOP-lowering medication.

Precautions/Adverse Reactions: Travoprost is contraindicated in individuals with a hypersensitivity to it, benzalkonium chloride, or any other ingredient in the product. Travoprost has been reported to cause changes to pigmented tissues. The most frequently reported changes have been increased pigmentation of the iris, eyelid, and eyelashes, and increase in growth of eyelashes. These changes may be permanent. Use caution in patients with intraocular inflammation, aphakic patients, pseudophakic patients with a torn posterior lens capsule, or patients with risk factors for macular edema. Pregnancy Category C. It may be teratogenic and may interfere with the maintenance of pregnancy and therefore should not be used by women during pregnancy or by women attempting to become pregnant. No adequate, well-controlled studies have been performed in pregnant women. The most common adverse effects were ocular hyperemia, conjunctival hyperemia, eyelash growth, decreased visual acuity, foreign body sensation, eye discomfort, pain, and itching.

Administration: Topical.

Patient Care Implications: Do not exceed once daily dosing; may decrease IOP-lowering effect. If used with other ophthalmic agents, separate administration by at least 5 minutes between each medication. Remove contacts prior to administration and wait 15 minutes before reinserting. Reduction of IOP starts approximately 2 hours after administration, and the maximum effect is reached after 12 hours. Patients should be informed of the possibility of iris color change. Patients should be instructed to avoid allowing the tip of the container to contact the eye or surrounding structures. This can cause tip to become contaminated. Serious damage to the eye and subsequent loss of vision may result from using contaminated solutions. Instruct patients to wash hands before instilling. Sit or lie down to instill. Discard container within 6 weeks of removing it from the sealed pouch.

Preparations: Solution, ophthalmic, 0.004% (2.5 ml and 5 ml).

TRAZODONE HYDROCHLORIDE—Desyrel®

Description/Actions: Antidepressant indicated for the treatment of depression.

Precautions/Adverse Reactions: Is not recommended for use during the initial recovery phase of myocardial infarction. Adverse reactions include drowsiness and other CNS effects. Patients should be cautioned regarding activities such as driving and operating machinery, as well as interactions with other CNS-acting drugs including alcohol. Trazodone is a substrate of the cytochrome P450 3A4 (CYP3A4) enzyme, and trazodone metabolism can be inhibited by the CYP3A4 inhibitors ketoconazole, ritonavir, and indinavir. Coadministration of trazodone and ritonavir resulted in nausea, hypotension, and syncope. Coadministration of trazodone and carbamazepine resulted in reduced plasma concentrations of trazodone. May cause priapism, and patients with prolonged or inappropriate penile erection should discontinue the drug and consult with the physician. Other adverse reactions include dry mouth, blurred vision, hypotension, nausea, and vomiting.

Administration: Oral.

Preparations: Tablets, 50, 100, 150, and 300 mg.

TRECATOR-SC®, see Ethionamide

TRELSTAR® Depot, see Triptorelin Pamoate

TRELSTAR™ LA, see Triptorelin Pamoate

TRENTAL®, see Pentoxifylline

TREPROSTINIL—Remodulin™

Description/Actions: Treprostinil is a tricyclic benzidene analog of prostacyclin (PGI_2). It produces direct vasodilation of pulmonary and systemic arterial vascular beds and inhibition of platelet aggregation. It is indicated as a continuous subcutaneous infusion for the treatment of pulmonary arterial hypertension (PAH) in patients with NYHA class II–IV symptoms to diminish symptoms associated with exercise.

Precautions/Adverse Reactions: Treprostinil is contraindicated in patients with a known hypersensitivity to it or to any component of the formulation. Adverse reactions include infusion site pain (85%); infusion site reaction—erythema, induration, and rash (83%); headache (27%); diarrhea (25%); nausea (22%); rash (14%); jaw pain (13%); vasodilation (11%); dizziness (9%); edema (9%); pruritus (8%); and hypotension (4%). Treprostinil does not appear to be an inhibitor of the cytochrome P450 enzyme system. Diuretics, antihypertensive agents, and/or vasodilators may enhance the hypotensive effects of treprostinil. Due to its inhibition of platelet aggregation, concomitant administration of treprostinil with anticoagulants may lead to an increased risk of bleeding.

Administration: Continuous subcutaneous infusion.

Preparations: Injection: solution 1 mg/mL (20 mL), 2.5 mg/mL (20 mL), 5 mg/mL (20 mL), and 10 mg/mL (20 mL).

TRETINOIN—Retinoic Acid, Vitamin A Acid, Avita®, Renova®, Retin-A®

Description/Actions: A vitamin A analog indicated for topical application in the treatment of acne.

Precautions/Adverse Reactions: Skin may become excessively red, edematous, blistered, or crusted in some patients. May increase susceptibility to sunlight, so patients should be advised to minimize exposure to sunlight, including sunlamps.

Administration: Topical.

Preparations: Cream, 0.02%, 0.025%, 0.05%, and 0.1%. Solution, 0.05%. Gel, 0.01% and 0.025%. Microspheres aqueous gel, 0.1%, 0.04%. Capsules, 10 and 25 mg.

TREXAN®, trade name formerly used for Naltrexone

TRIACETIN—Glyceryl Triacetate

Description/Actions: Antifungal agent indicated for topical use in the treatment of athlete's foot and other superficial fungal infections.

Preparations: Cream, 25%.

TRIAMCINOLONE—Aristocort®, Kenacort®

Description/Actions: Corticosteroid indicated in a wide range of endocrine, rheumatic, allergic, dermatologic, respiratory, hematologic, neoplastic, and other disorders.

Preparations: Tablets, 1, 2, 4, and 8 mg.

TRIAMCINOLONE ACETONIDE—Aristocort®, Azmacort®, Kenalog®, Nasacort®, Nasacort AQ®, Tri-Nasal®

Preparations: Vials (for intramuscular, intra-articular, intrabursal, and intradermal injection), 10 mg/ml and 40 mg/ml. Aerosol (for inhalation), 100 mcg/actuation (Azmacort®). Cream and ointment, 0.025%, 0.1%, and 0.5%. Lotion, 0.025% and 0.1%. Aerosol (for topical use). Nasal spray, 55 mcg/actuation (Nasacort®), 50 mcg/actuation (Tri-Nasal™).

TRIAMCINOLONE DIACETATE—Aristocort®, Kenacort®

Preparations: Syrup, 2 mg/5 ml and 4 mg/5 ml. Vials (for intramuscular, intra-articular, intrasynovial, and intralesional injection), 25 mg/ml and 40 mg/ml.

TRIAMCINOLONE HEXACETONIDE—Aristospan®

Preparations: Vials (for intra-articular, intralesional, and sublesional injection), 5 mg/ml and 20 mg/ml.

TRIAMTERENE—Dyrenium®

Description/Actions: A potassium-sparing diuretic indicated in the treatment of edema associated with congestive heart failure, cirrhosis of the liver, and the nephrotic syndrome; also used in steroid-induced edema, idiopathic edema, and edema due to secondary hyperaldosteronism.

Precautions/Adverse Reactions: Contraindicated in patients with anuria, severe hepatic or renal disease, or preexisting elevated serum potassium levels. Should not be used in patients receiving another potassium-sparing diuretic or potassium salts or supplements.

Administration: Oral.

Preparations: Capsules, 50 and 100 mg.

TRIAVIL®, Combination of Amitriptyline and Perphenazine

TRIAZOLAM—Halcion®

Description/Actions: Benzodiazepine indicated in the management of insomnia.

Precautions/Adverse Reactions: Contraindicated during pregnancy. Adverse reactions include residual sedation, amnesic effects, and other CNS effects upon awakening. Patients should be cautioned regarding activities such as driving and operating machinery, as well as interactions with other CNS-acting drugs including alcohol. Can cause dependence, and is included in Schedule IV.

Administration: Oral.

Preparations: Tablets, 0.125 and 0.25 mg.

TRICHLOROACETIC ACID

Description/Actions: Cauterizing agent applied topically to warts and to debride callus tissue.

TRICHLORMETHIAZIDE—Metahydrin®, Naqua®

Description/Actions: Thiazide diuretic indicated as adjunctive therapy in edema and in the management of hypertension.

Preparations: Tablets, 2 and 4 mg.

TRICOR®, see Fenofibrate

TRIDESILON®, see Desonide

TRIDIL®, see Nitroglycerin

TRIDIONE®, see Trimethadione

TRIENTINE HYDROCHLORIDE—Syprine®

Description/Actions: A chelating agent indicated in the treatment of patients with Wilson's disease who are intolerant of penicillamine.

Precautions/Adverse Reactions: Adverse reactions include fever, skin eruption, and iron deficiency anemia. Mineral supplements should usually not be administered concurrently because they may reduce the absorption of trientine. Should be administered at least 1 hour before or 2 hours after meals and at least 1 hour apart from any other drug, food, or milk.

Administration: Oral.

Preparations: Capsules, 250 mg.

TRIETHYLENETHIOPHOSPHORAMIDE, see Thiotepa

TRIFLUOPERAZINE HYDROCHLORIDE—Stelazine®

Description/Actions: Phenothiazine antipsychotic agent indicated for the manifestations of psychotic disorders.

Preparations: Tablets, 1, 2, 5, and 10 mg. Oral concentrate, 10 mg/ml. Vials, 2 mg/ml.

TRIFLUPROMAZINE HYDROCHLORIDE—Vesprin®

Description/Actions: Phenothiazine antipsychotic agent and antiemetic indicated for parenteral use for the manifestations of psychotic disorders, and for the control of severe nausea and vomiting.

Preparations: Vials, 10 mg/ml and 20 mg/ml.

TRIFLURIDINE—Viroptic®

Description/Actions: Antiviral agent indicated for ophthalmic use for the treatment of primary keratoconjunctivitis and recurrent epithelial keratitis due to *Herpes simplex* virus, types 1 and 2.

Preparations: Ophthalmic solution, 1%.

TRIHEXYPHENIDYL HYDROCHLORIDE—Artane®

Description/Actions: Antiparkinson agent indicated for the treatment of parkinsonism and the management of drug-induced extrapyramidal reactions.

Preparations: Tablets, 2 and 5 mg. Controlled-release capsules, 5 mg. Elixir, 2 mg/5 ml.

TRIIODOTHYRONINE, see Liothyronine

TRILAFON®, see Perphenazine

TRILEPTAL®, see Oxcarbazepine

TRILISATE®, see Choline Magnesium Trisalicylate

TRIMEPRAZINE TARTRATE—Temaril®

Description/Actions: Phenothiazine antihistamine indicated for the treatment of pruritic symptoms in a number of allergic and nonallergic conditions.

Preparations: Tablets, 2.5 mg. Controlled-release capsules, 5 mg. Syrup, 2.5 mg/5 ml.

TRIMETHADIONE—Tridione®

Description/Actions: Anticonvulsant indicated for the control of petit mal seizures that are refractory to treatment with other drugs.

Preparations: Tablets, 150 mg. Capsules, 300 mg.

TRIMETHOBENZAMIDE HYDROCHLORIDE—Tigan®

Description/Actions: Antiemetic indicated for the control of nausea and vomiting.

Preparations: Capsules, 100, 250, and 300 mg. Suppositories, 100 and 200 mg. Vials and syringes, 100 mg/ml.

TRIMETHOPRIM—Proloprim®, Trimpex®

Description/Actions: Antibacterial indicated in the treatment of urinary tract infections.

Preparations: Tablets, 100 and 200 mg. Oral solution, 50 mg/5 ml.

TRIMETHOPRIM—SULFAMETHOXAZOLE—TMP/SMX,
  Cotrimoxazole, Bactrim®, Septra®

Description/Actions: Combined actions of the 2 agents result in a synergistic action against many microorganisms. Is active against many gram-positive and gram-negative bacteria as well as certain other organisms. Indications include urinary tract infections, acute otitis media, acute exacerbations of chronic bronchitis, shigellosis, treatment and prophylaxis of *Pneumocystis carinii* pneumonitis, and the treatment of travelers' diarrhea in adults due to susceptible strains of enterotoxigenic *E. coli.* Is also useful in a number of other infections including prostatic infections.

Precautions/Adverse Reactions: Should not be used in pregnancy at term or during the nursing period. Adverse reactions include nausea, vomiting, rash, and urticaria. Because serious reactions such as the Stevens-Johnson syndrome have occurred in some individuals, therapy should be discontinued at the first appearance of skin rash or other adverse effects.

Administration: Oral and intravenous.

Preparations: Tablets, 80/400 and 160/800 mg. Suspension, 40/200 mg/5 ml. Ampules and vials, 16/80 mg/ml.

TRIMETREXATE GLUCURONATE—NeuTrexin®

Description/Actions: Is a structural analog of folic acid. Anti-infective agent that exhibits a folic acid antagonist (antifolate) action that leads to cell death of certain microorganisms such as *Pneumocystis carinii* that require folate metabolism for continued cell viability. Indicated with concurrent leucovorin administration (leucovorin protection) as alternative therapy for the treatment of moderate to severe *Pneumocystis carinii* pneumonia in immunocompromised patients, including patients with AIDS, who are intolerant of or are refractory to trimethoprim/sulfamethoxazole (TMP/SMX) therapy or for whom TMP/SMX is contraindicated.

Precautions/Adverse Reactions: Contraindicated in patients with a known hypersensitivity to trimetrexate or methotrexate. It is also contraindicated in patients with severe myelosuppression. It is essential that leucovorin be used concurrently to reduce the risk of bone marrow suppression, oral and gastrointestinal mucosal ulceration, and renal and hepatic dysfunction. It is recommended that blood tests be performed at least twice a week to assess absolute neutrophil counts and platelets, as well as renal function (serum creatinine) and hepatic function (AST, ALT, alkaline phosphatase). Adverse reactions include neutropenia, thrombocytopenia, anemia, increased AST and ALT, fever, rash, pruritus, nausea, and vomiting. It is recommended that zidovudine not be used during the period of trimetrexate therapy. May cause fetal harm if administered during pregnancy.

Administration: Intravenous. Administered once daily by IV infusion over 60–90 minutes. Leucovorin must be administered daily (every 6 hours) during treatment with trimetrexate and for 72 hours past the last dose of trimetrexate.

Prepartion: Vials, 25 mg trimetrexate.

TRIMIPRAMINE MALEATE—Surmontil®

Description/Actions: Tricyclic antidepressant indicated for the relief of symptoms of depression.

Preparations: Capsules, 25, 50, and 100 mg.

TRIMOX®, see Amoxicillin

TRIMPEX®, see Trimethoprim

TRINALIN®, Combination of Azatidine and Pseudoephedrine

TRI-NASAL®, see Triamcinolone Acetonide

TRIOSTAT®, see Liothyronine

TRIOXSALEN—Trisoralen®

Description/Actions: Photoactive agent indicated for repigmentation of idiopathic vitiligo, enhancing pigmentation, and increasing tolerance to sunlight in blond persons and those with fair complexions who suffer painful reactions when exposed to sunlight.

Preparations: Tablets, 5 mg.

TRIPELENNAMINE—PBZ®

Description/Actions: Antihistamine indicated for the management of allergic disorders.

Preparations: Tablets (as the hydrochloride), 25 and 50 mg. Controlled-release tablets (as the hydrochloride), 100 mg. Elixir (as the citrate), equivalent to 25 mg of the hydrochloride/5 ml.

TRIPLE SULFAS, see Trisulfapyrimidines

TRIPROLIDINE HYDROCHLORIDE

Description/Actions: Antihistamine used in combination with pseudo-ephedrine

TRIPTORELIN PAMOATE—Trelstar® Depot, Trelstar™ LA

Description/Actions: Indicated in the palliative treatment of advanced prostate cancer. It offers an alternative to orchiectomy or estrogen therapy.

Precautions/Adverse Reactions: Triptorelin is contraindicated in patients with hypersensitivity to triptorelin or to any other component of the product, other LH-RH agonists, or LH-RH. Initial increase in testosterone levels may lead to the temporary worsening of symptoms of prostate cancer. Cases of spinal cord compression have been reported. Cases of anaphylactic shock and angioedema have been reported. Chronic administration of triptorelin results in suppression of the pituitary-gonadal axis. Diagnostic tests to access pituitary function performed during therapy or up to 8 weeks after discontinuation of therapy may be misleading. No formal drug interaction studies have been conducted.

Coadministration with hyperprolactinemic drugs is not recommended because hyperprolactinemia decreases the number of pituitary gonadotropin releasing hormone receptors. Pregnancy Category X. Triptorelin is contraindicated in pregnancy. Triptorelin may cause fetal harm when administered to pregnant women. Excretion in human breast milk is unknown. It should not be used by nursing mothers. Safety and efficacy in children have not been established. Most common adverse reactions observed in patients treated with triptorelin include hot flashes (59%), bone pain (12%), impotence (7.1%), headache (5%), injection site pain (3.6%), and hypertension (3.6%).

Administration: IM injection.

Patient Care Implications: Worsening of symptoms may occur during the first few weeks of therapy. Reconstitute each vial with 2 ml of sterile water for injection. Do not use any other diluent. Shake well and withdraw the entire reconstituted suspension into the syringe, and use immediately.

Preparations: Powder for injection, Trelstar®Depot 3.75 mg single-dose vials. Trelstar™ LA 11.25 mg single-dose vials.

TRISENOX®, see Arsenic Trioxide

TRISORALEN®, see Trioxsalen

TRISULFAPYRIMIDINES—Triple Sulfas

Description/Actions: Anti-infective agents (sulfadiazine, sulfamerazine, sulfamethazine) indicated in the treatment of infections caused by susceptible organisms.

Preparations: Tablets, 500 mg. Suspension, 500 mg/5 ml.

TRITEC®—Combination of Ranitidine and Bismuth Citrate

TRIVAGIZOLE 3™, see Clotrimazole

TRIZIVIR™, see Abacavir, Lamivudine, and Zidovudine

TROBICIN®, see Spectinomycin

TROLAMINE SALICYLATE—Aspercreme®, Myoflex®

Description/Actions: Salicylate analgesic indicated for topical use for the temporary relief of minor aches and pains of muscles and joints. Also used as a topical adjunct in arthritis.

Preparations: Cream, 10%.

TROLEANDOMYCIN—Tao®

Description/Actions: Antibiotic indicated for infections caused by susceptible gram-positive bacteria.

Preparations: Capsules, 250 mg.

TROMETHAMINE—Tham®

Description/Actions: Alkalinizing agent indicated for parenteral use for the prevention and correction of systemic acidosis in selected patients.

Preparations: Bottles, 18 g/500 ml.

TRONOLANE®, see Pramoxine

TRONOTHANE®, see Pramoxine

TROPICAMIDE—Mydriacyl®

Description/Actions: Anticholinergic agent indicated for ophthalmic use to provide mydriasis and cycloplegia for diagnostic purposes.

Preparations: Ophthalmic solutions, 0.5% and 1%.

TRUSOPT®, see Dorzolamide Hydrochloride

TRYPSIN

Description/Actions: Proteolytic enzyme used in combination with other agents for enzymatic debridement and to promote normal healing.

TUBOCURARINE CHLORIDE—Curare

Description/Actions: Nondepolarizing neuromuscular blocking agent indicated as an adjunct to anesthesia to induce skeletal muscle relaxation.

Preparations: Vials, 3 mg/ml.

TUMS®, see Calcium Carbonate

TUSSI-ORGANIDIN®NR, Combination of Codeine and Guaifenesin

TYLENOL®, see Acetaminophen

TYLOX®, Combination of Oxycodone and Acetaminophen

TYZINE®, see Tetrahydrozoline

U

UCEPHAN®, see Sodium Benzoate and Sodium Phenylacetate

ULTANE®, see Sevoflurane

ULTRACET™, see Tramadol Hydrochloride/Acetaminophen

ULTRA-LENTE INSULIN, see Insulin

ULTRAM®, see Tramadol Hydrochloride

ULTRAVATE®, see Halobetasol Propionate

UNASYN®, see Ampicillin Sodium/Sulbactam Sodium

UNDECYLENIC ACID AND SALTS—Desenex®
Description/Actions: Antifungal agent applied topically in the management of superficial fungal infections.
Preparations: Powder, cream, ointment, liquid, foam, and soap.

UNI-DUR®, see Theophylline

UNIPEN®, see Nafcillin

UNIPHYL®, see Theophylline

UNIRETIC®, Combination agent of Moexipril HCl and Hydrochlorothiazide (ACE Inhibitor and Diuretic)

UNISOM®, see Doxylamine

UNIVASC®, see Moexipril Hydrochloride

UNOPROSTONE—Rescula®

Description/Actions: Unoprostone is indicated for the lowering of intraocular pressure in patients with open-angle glaucoma or ocular hypertension. Unoprostone should be used in patients who are intolerant of other intraocular pressure (IOP) medications or failed therapy on other IOP-lowering medications.

Precautions/Adverse Reactions: Utilization is contraindicated in patients with known hypersensitivity to unoprostone isopropyl, benzalkonium chloride, or any other formulation components. Permanent changes in eye pigmentation have been reported with usage; long-term effects and consequences from the changes in eye coloration for potential injury to the eye are currently not known. Bacterial keratitis has been reported and associated with the inadvertent contamination of multiple-dose ophthalmic solutions. Safety and efficacy have not been established in patients with active intraocular inflammation, angle closure, inflammatory or neovascular glaucoma, hepatic or renal impairment, and pediatrics. Rescula® contains benzalkonium chloride, which may be adsorbed by contact lenses; contact lenses should be removed prior to instillation, and lenses may be reinserted 15 minutes following administration. Pregnancy Category C. Unoprostone should be used during pregnancy only if the potential benefit justifies the potential risk to the fetus. Excretion into the breast milk is unknown; use with caution if administering to a nursing woman. Because the drug acts locally in the eye, it has limited systemic side effects. Some adverse effects are burning/stinging (upon instillation), dry/itching eyes, increased length of eyelashes, abnormal vision, eyelid disorder, foreign body sensation, and lacrimation disorder.

Administration: Ophthalmic.

Patient Care Implications: Inform patients to avoid allowing the tip of the dispensing container to contact the eye or surrounding structures because this could cause the tip to become contaminated by bacteria. If more than one ophthalmic drug is being used, the drugs should be administered at least 5 minutes apart. Patients should be informed of the warnings regarding the possibility of eye color changes and to remove contact lenses before instilling the solution (see precautions).

Preparations: Solution, ophthalmic: 0.15% (5 ml).

URACIL MUSTARD

Description/Actions: Antineoplastic agent indicated for the treatment of chronic lymphocytic leukemia, non-Hodgkin's lymphomas, chronic myelogenous leukemia, polycythemia vera, and mycosis fungoides.

Preparations: Capsules, 1 mg.

UREA—Carbamide, Aquacare®, Ureaphil®

Description/Actions: Osmotic agent administered intravenously to reduce intraocular pressure and to reduce intracranial pressure in the control of cerebral edema. Also used topically to promote hydration and removal of excess keratin in dry skin and hyperkeratotic conditions.

Preparations: Bottles (for intravenous use), 40 g. Cream, 2%, 10%, 20%, 30%, and 40%. Lotion, 2%, 10%, 15%, and 25%.

UREA PEROXIDE, see Carbamide Peroxide

UREAPHIL®, see Urea

URECHOLINE®, see Bethanechol

URISPAS®, see Flavoxate

UROCIT-K®, see Potassium Citrate

UROFOLLITROPIN—Metrodin®

Description/Actions: Gonadotropin administered intramuscularly and given sequentially with human chorionic gonadotropin for the induction of ovulation in selected patients with polycystic ovarian disease.

Preparations: Ampules, 0.83 mg.

UROKINASE—Abbokinase®

Description/Actions: Thrombolytic enzyme indicated for parenteral use in the management of pulmonary embolism and coronary artery thrombosis. Also used for the restoration of patency to intravenous catheters.

Preparations: Vials, 250,000 IU.

URSO FORTE™, see Ursodiol

URSODIOL—Actigall®, URSO®, Urso Forte™

Description/Actions: A bile acid that decreases hepatic synthesis and secretion of cholesterol. Used for dissolving gallstones and is indicated for patients with radiolucent, noncalcified gallbladder stones less than 20 mm in greatest diameter in whom elective cholecystectomy would be undertaken except for the presence of increased surgical risk due to systemic disease, advanced age, idiosyncratic reaction to general anesthesia, or for patients who refuse surgery. Prevention of gallstone formation in obese patients experiencing rapid weight loss.

Precautions/Adverse Reactions: Contraindicated in patients with a history of allergy to bile acids, chronic liver disease, or with gallstones of a type (e.g., calcified) against which ursodiol is not active. Adverse reactions include diarrhea. May cause hepatotoxicity, so patients should have liver function tests performed. Cholestyramine, colestipol, and aluminum-containing antacids may reduce the absorption and efficacy of ursodiol; therefore, doses should be separated from doses of these other medications by as long an interval as possible.

Administration: Oral.

Preparations: Tablets, 250 mg, 500 mg. Capsules, 300 mg.

UTICORT®, see Betamethasone Benzoate

V

VAGIFEM®, see Estradiol

VAGISTAT®, see Tioconazole

VALACYCLOVIR—Valtrex®

Description/Actions: Antiviral agent indicated for the treatment of herpes zoster (shingles). It is also indicated for the treatment or suppression of genital herpes in immunocompetent individuals and for the suppression of recurrent genital herpes in HIV-infected individuals.

Precautions/Adverse Reactions: Thrombotic thrombocytopenic purpura (TTP)/hemolytic uremic syndrome (HUS) has been reported in patients with advanced human immunodeficiency virus (HIV) disease as well as in bone marrow transplant and in renal transplant recipients; this reaction has not been reported in immunocompetent patients, and valacyclovir is not indicated for the treatment of immunocompromised patients. Other adverse reactions include headache and nausea.

Administration: Oral.

Preparations: Capsules, 500 mg.

VALCYTE™, see Valganciclovir

VALGANCICLOVIR—Valcyte™

Description/Actions: Valganciclovir is indicated in the treatment of cytomegalovirus retinitis in patients with acquired immunodeficiency syndrome (AIDS). Valcyte™ is indicated for the prevention of cytomegalovirus (CMV) disease in kidney, heart, and kidney-pancreas transplant patients at high risk for CMV disease. Valganciclovir is not indicated for use in liver transplant patients. The safety and efficacy of valganciclovir for the prevention of CMV disease in other solid organ transplant patients such as lung transplant patients have not been established.

Precautions/Adverse Reactions: Valganciclovir is contraindicated in anyone with a known hypersensitivity to valganciclovir, ganciclovir, or any component of the formulation. Valganciclovir should not be administered if the absolute neutrophil count is less than 500 cells/l, the platelet count is less than 25,000/l, or the hemoglobin is less than 8 g/dl. Severe leukopenia, neutropenia, anemia, thrombocytopenia, pancytopenia, bone marrow depression, and aplastic anemia have occurred with the use of valganciclovir. Use with caution in patients with preexisting cytopenias, prior or current use of myelosuppressive drugs, or irradiation. The clinical toxicity of valganciclovir includes granulocytopenia, anemia, and thrombocytopenia. It is considered probable that in humans, valganciclovir at the recommended doses may cause temporary or permanent inhibition of spermatogenesis. Suppression of fertility in females may also occur. Pregnancy Category C. No adequate and well-controlled studies in pregnant women. Use during pregnancy only if the potential benefit justifies the potential risk to the fetus. Women of childbearing age are advised to use effective contraception during treatment with valganciclovir. Men should also be advised to practice barrier contraception during and for at least 90 days following treatment with valganciclovir. Excretion in human breast milk is unknown. Women should be instructed not to breast-feed while receiving valganciclovir. Safety and efficacy in pediatric patients have not been established. Strict adherence to dosage recommendations is necessary to avoid overdose. Valganciclovir tablets cannot be substituted for ganciclovir capsules on a one-to-one basis. Zidovudine and ganciclovir each have the potential to cause neutropenia and anemia, and some patients may not tolerate concomitant therapy at full dosage. Coadministration of ganciclovir and probenecid resulted in increased ganciclovir blood levels and decreased clearance of ganciclovir. Patients with renal impairment should be monitored carefully when ganciclovir and mycophenolate are coadministered, as levels of metabolites of both drugs may increase. Major adverse effects associated with valganciclovir include diarrhea, nausea, fever, neutropenia, anemia, headache, vomiting, insomnia, abdominal pain, retinal detachment, peripheral neuropathy, paresthesia, and thrombocytopenia. Adverse effects occurring in less than 5% of patients treated with valganciclovir include pancytopenia, bone marrow depression, aplastic anemia, decreased creatinine clearance, local and systemic infections, and sepsis; potentially life-threatening bleeding associated with thrombocytopenia; convulsions, psychosis, hallucinations, confusion, and agitation.

Administration: Oral. Valganciclovir should not be prescribed to patients receiving hemodialysis. For patients on hemodialysis (creatinine clearance <10 ml/minute), it is recommended that ganciclovir be used with dosage adjustments as recommended in ganciclovir product labeling.

Patient Care Implications: Complete blood counts, platelet counts, and renal function should be monitored. Patients should be instructed to take valganciclovir with food. Patients should be informed that ganciclovir has caused decreased sperm production in animals and may cause decreased fertility in humans. Women of childbearing potential should be instructed to use effective contraception during treatment. Men should be advised to practice barrier contraception during and for at least 90 days following treatment with valganciclovir. Patients should be told that valganciclovir is not a cure for cytomegalovirus retinitis and that progression of the disease may occur. Patients should be informed to have ophthalmogic examinations every 4–6 weeks while receiving treatment. Patients should be instructed to observe caution when driving, operating machinery, or performing tasks requiring alertness, due to the potential for valganciclovir to cause convulsions, sedation, dizziness, ataxia, and/or confusion. Valganciclovir tablets should be handled and disposed of properly. Tablets should not be broken or crushed. Avoid direct contact of broken or crushed tablets with skin or mucous membranes. If contact occurs, wash thoroughly wih soap and water, and rinse eyes thoroughly with plain water.

Preparations: Tablets, 450 mg (496.3 mg of valganciclovir HCL corresponding to 450 mg of valganciclovir).

VALISONE®, see Betamethasone Valerate

VALIUM®, see Diazepam

VALPROIC ACID—Depacon®, Depakene®

Description/Actions: Anticonvulsant indicated for use in the treatment of simple (petit mal) and complex absence seizures. Also used adjunctively in patients with multiple seizure types, including absence seizures. Also indicated for the treatment of manic episodes associated with bipolar disorder and prophylaxis against migraine headaches. Contraindicated in patients with a known hypersensitivity to divalproex sodium or to any component of the formulation. Contraindicated in patients with hepatic disease or significant hepatic dysfunction. Hepatic failure resulting in fatalities has occurred in patients receiving valproic acid and its derivatives. Children under 2 years of age are at an increased risk of developing hepatotoxicity. Use with extreme caution in these individuals. Cases of life-threatening pancreatitis have been reported in both children and adults. Contraindicated in patients with urea cycle disorders. Hyperammonemic encephalopathy, sometimes fatal, has been reported following initiation of valproate therapy in patients with urea cycle disorders. Pregnancy Category D. Valproic acid and its derivatives have been shown to produce teratogenic effects such as neural tube defects. Use only if the benefits outweigh the potential risk of injury to the fetus. Excreted in breast milk. Nursing is not recommended.

Preparations: Capsules (as valproic acid), 250 mg. Syrup (as sodium valproate), 250 mg/5 ml. Enteric-coated tablets (divalproex sodium—representing a stable coordination compound composed of sodium valproate and valproic acid in a 1:1 molar relationship), 125, 250, and 500 mg. Extended-release tablets, 250 and 500 mg. Sprinkle capsules (divalproex sodium), 125 mg, 100 mg/ml solution for IV infusion.

VALRELEASE®, see Diazepam

VALRUBICIN—Valstar®

Description/Actions: Indicated for intravesical therapy of BCG refractory carcinoma in situ (CIS) of the urinary bladder in patients for whom immediate cystectomy would be associated with unacceptable morbidity or mortality.

Precautions/Adverse Reactions: Valrubicin is contraindicated with a known hypersensitivity to this agent or Cremophor EI (polypoxyethyleneglycol tricinoleate), concurrent urinary tract infection, and small bladder capacity. Inform patients that valrubicin includes complete response in only about 1 out of 5 patients and that delaying cystectomy could lead to development of metastatic bladder cancer, which is lethal. If there is not a complete response to valrubicin, or CIS recurs within 3 months, reconsider cystectomy. Do not administer to patients with a perforated bladder or to those in whom the integrity of the bladder mucosa has been compromised. Adverse reactions include irritable bladder symptoms. These reactions usually occur during or shortly after installation and resolve within 1–7 days post instillation.

Administration: 800 mg intravesically once a week for 6 weeks. Empty the bladder, instill the medication via catheter under aseptic conditions, withdraw the catheter, and have patient retain the medication for 2 hours before voiding.

Patient Care Implications: Instruct patients to void at the end of the 2-hour period. Patients should be told to maintain adequate hydration postadministration of the medication. Use appropriate cytotoxic precautions when handling the agent for administration. May not be administered via IV/IM route.

Preparations: Solution for intravesical administration, 40 mg/ml.

VALSARTAN—Diovan®

Description/Actions: Angiotensin II receptor antagonist indicated in the treatment of hypertension either as monotherapy or in combination with other antihypertensives for the treatment of heart failure in patients who are intolerant of angiotensin-converting enzyme inhibitors.

Precautions/Adverse Reactions: Contraindicated in pregnancy, hyperaldosteronism, and biliary cirrhosis. Correct hypovolemia before beginning therapy or monitor closely. Use cautiously in severe CHF, renal artery stenosis, hepatic dysfunction, or severe renal impairment. Adverse reactions include viral infection, fatigue, and abdominal pain. In clinical studies comparing valsartan to ACE inhibitors, the incidence of dry cough was significantly greater in the ACE inhibitor group.

Administration: Oral.

Preparations: Tablets, 40, 80, 160, and 320 mg.

VALTREX®, see Valacyclovir

VANCENASE®, see Beclomethasone Dipropionate

VANCENASE AQ®, see Beclomethasone Dipropionate

VANCERIL®, see Beclomethasone Dipropionate

VANCOCIN®, see Vancomycin

VANCOLED®, see Vancomycin

VANCOMYCIN HYDROCHLORIDE—Lyphocin®, Vancocin®, Vancoled®

Description/Actions: Antibiotic used primarily for the intravenous treatment of staphylococcal infections. Also used orally for the treatment of staphylococcal enterocolitis and antibiotic-associated pseudomembranous colitis produced by *Clostridium difficile*.

Preparations: Vials, 500 mg. Capsules, 125 and 250 mg. Powder for oral solution, 1 and 10 g when reconstituted.

VANIQA™, see Eflornithine (topical)

VANOS®, see Fluocinonide

VANSIL®, see Oxamniquine

VANTIN®, see Cefpodoxime Proxetil

VARDENAFIL—Levitra®

Description/Actions: Vardenafil is a phosphodiesterase-5 enzyme (PDE5) inhibitor; it is used in the treatment of erectile dysfunction. It does not directly cause penile erection, but affects the response to sexual stimulation. Penile erection is a process initiated by the relaxation of smooth muscle in the corpus cavernosum. During sexual stimulation, nitric oxide (NO) is released in the corpus cavernosum. NO activates the enzyme, guanylate cyclase, resulting in increased synthesis of cyclic guanosine monophosphate (cGMP) in the smooth muscle cells of the corpus cavernosum. The cGMP in turn triggers smooth muscle relaxation allowing increased blood flow into the penis, resulting in erection. Vardenil enhances the effect of NO by inhibiting PDE5, which is responsible for degradation of cGMP in the corpus cavernosum.

Precautions/Adverse Reactions: Vardenafil is contraindicated in patients hypersensitive to vardenafil or any component of the formulation, concurrent use of organic nitrates (scheduled or as needed), and concomitant use of alpha blockers. Vardenafil is not recommended for use in patients with congenital QT prolongation or those taking Class Ia or III antiarrhythmics. Use caution with effective CYP3A4 inhibitors, the elderly, or those with hepatic impairment. Safety and efficacy have not been studied in patients with the following conditions: hypotension, uncontrolled hypertension, unstable angina, severe cardiac failure; a life-threatening arrhythmia, myocardial infarction, or stroke within the last 6 months; severe hepatic impairment; end-stage renal disease requiring dialysis; retinitis pigmentosa or other degenerative retinal disorders. Therefore, use in these patients is not recommended at this time. There is a degree of cardiac risk associated with sexual activity. In men for whom sexual activity is not recommended because of their underlying cardiovascular status, any treatment for erectile dysfunction generally should not be used. Patients with left ventricular outflow obstruction can be sensitive to the action of vasodilators. Vardenafil has systemic vasodilatory properties that have resulted in transient decreases in supine blood pressure. Use caution in patients with anatomical deformation of the penis and in patients who have conditions that may predispose them to priapism (sickle cell anemia, multiple myeloma, leukemia). Most common adverse reactions are headache, flushing, rhinitis, dyspepsia, and flu syndrome.

Administration: Oral.

Patient Care Implications: May experience headache, flushing, or blurred vision; use caution when driving until response to drug is known. Report immediately chest pain, acute headache, respiratory difficulty, genital swelling, or other adverse reactions. Counsel patients that use of vardenafil with nitrates could cause drop in blood pressure to an unsafe level, resulting in dizziness, syncope, or even heart attack or stroke. Inform patients that there have been rare reports of prolonged erections greater than 4 hours and priapism (painful erections greater than 6 hours in duration). If an erection lasts longer than 4 hours, the patient should seek immediate assistance. If priapism is not treated immediately, penile tissue damage and permanent loss of potency may result.

Preparation: Tablet, film coated: 2.5 mg, 5 mg, 10 mg, and 20 mg.

VASCOR®, see Bepridil Hydrochloride

VASERETIC®, see Enalapril/Hydrocholorothiazide

VASODILAN®, see Isoxsuprine

VASOPRESSIN—Pitressin®

Description/Actions: Hormone indicated for parenteral use in the prevention and treatment of postoperative abdominal distention, in abdominal roentgenography to dispel interfering gas shadows, and in diabetes insipidus.

Preparations: Ampules, 10 and 20 units.

VASOTEC®, see Enalapril

VASOXYL®, see Methoxamine

V-CILLIN K®, see Penicillin V Potassium

VECURONIUM BROMIDE—Norcuron®

Description/Actions: Nondepolarizing neuromuscular blocking agent indicated as an adjunct to general anesthesia, to facilitate endotracheal intubation, and to provide skeletal muscle relaxation during surgery or mechanical ventilation.

Preparations: Vials, 10 mg.

VEETIDS®, see Penicillin V Potassium

VELBAN®, see Vinblastine

VELOSEF®, see Cephradine

VELOSULIN®, see Insulin

VENLAFAXINE HYDROCHLORIDE—Effexor®, Effexor XR®

Description/Actions: Is extensively metabolized, and one of its metabolites, odesmethylvenlafaxine (ODV), is also pharmacologically active. Inhibits the neuronal reuptake of both serotonin and norepinephrine. Indicated for the treatment of depression, generalized anxiety disorder, and the prevention of recurrence of depression and relapse of depression. Effexor XR® is also indicated for the short-term treatment of social anxiety disorder.

Precautions/Adverse Reactions: Antidepressants increased the risk of suicidal thinking and behavior (suicidality) in short-term studies in children and adolescents with Major Depressive Disorder (MDD) and other psychiatric disorders. Anyone considering the use of venlafaxine or any other antidepressant in a child or adolescent must balance this risk with the clinical need. Patients who are started on therapy should be observed closely for clinical worsening, suicidality, or unusual changes in behavior. Venlafaxine is not approved for use in pediatric patients. Adverse reactions include somnolence, dizziness, insomnia, nervousness, anxiety, tremor, dry mouth, nausea, constipation, anorexia, weight loss, vomiting, asthenia, sweating, blurred vision, and, in men, abnormal ejaculation and impotence. Patients should be advised to avoid the consumption of alcoholic beverages and cautioned about driving or operating machinery until they are certain that the drug does not adversely affect their ability to engage in such activities. May cause sustained increases in blood pressure, and blood pressure should be monitored regularly. It is recommended that it not be used in combination with a monoamine oxidase inhibitor (MAOI) or within 14 days of discontinuing treatment with an MAOI. There should be at least a 7-day interval after stopping venlafaxine before starting therapy with an MAOI.

Administration: Oral. Administered with food for the purpose of reducing the occurrence of gastrointestinal side effects.

Preparations: Tablets, 25, 37.5, 50, 75, and 100 mg. Release capsules, 37.5, 75, and 150 mg.

VENTOLIN®, see Albuterol

VEPESID, see Etoposide

VERAPAMIL HYDROCHLORIDE—Calan®, Calan SR®, Covera HS®, Isoptin®, Isoptin SR®, Verelan®

Description/Actions: Is a calcium channel-blocking agent that is indicated in the treatment of (a) hypertension, (b) vasospastic and unstable angina, (c) chronic stable angina, (d) in association with digitalis for the control of the ventricular rate at rest and during stress in patients with chronic atrial flutter and/or atrial fibrillation, and (e) prophylaxis of repetitive paroxysmal supraventricular tachycardia. Also indicated for intravenous use in the treatment of supraventricular tachycardia.

Precautions/Adverse Reactions: Contraindicated in patients with hypotension or cardiogenic shock, sick sinus syndrome, second- or third-degree AV block, and certain other cardiovascular disorders. Adverse reactions include constipation, dizziness, headache, and edema. May increase serum digoxin levels. Should not be administered IV to a patient also receiving a beta-adrenergic blocking agent IV; the concurrent oral administration of these agents may be beneficial in some patients, but therapy must be closely monitored. Concomitant use with disopyramide is not recommended. Coadministration of verapamil with aspirin has led to increased bleeding times greater than that observed with aspirin alone. Coadministration of verapamil and grapefruit juice may lead to increased levels of verapamil.

Administration: Oral and intravenous.

Preparations: Tablets, 40, 80, and 120 mg. Sustained-release tablets 120, 180, and 240 mg. Sustained-release capsules 120, 180, 240, and 360 mg. Ampules, vials, and syringes, 5 mg/2 ml.

VERCYTE®, see Pipobroman

VERELAN®, see Verapamil

VERMOX®, see Mebendazole

VERSED®, see Midazolam

VERSENATE CALCIUM DISODIUM®, see Edetate Calcium Disodium

VERTEPORFIN—Visudyne®

Description/Actions: Verteporfin is a light-activated drug used in photodynamic therapy. It is indicated for the treatment of age-related macular degeneration in patients with predominantly classic subfoveal choroidal neovascularization. It is also indicated for the treatment of predominantly classic subfoveal choroidal neovascularization secondary to either pathologic myopia or presumed ocular histoplasmosis.

Precautions/Adverse Reactions: Verteporfin is contraindicated in patients with porphyria. Avoid exposure of skin or eyes to direct sunlight or bright indoor light for 5 days following injection with verteporfin. Avoid extravasation. If extravasation occurs, stop the infusion immediately and apply cold compresses. The extravasation area must be protected from direct sunlight until the swelling and discoloration have faded in order to prevent a burn that could be severe. It is recommended that the largest arm vein possible, preferably the antecubital, be used for the injection. If surgery is required within 48 hours after verteporfin therapy, as much of the internal tissue as possible should be protected from intense light. Patients who experience a severe decrease of vision of 4 lines or more within 1 week after treatment should not be retreated until their vision returns to pretreatment levels and the potential benefits and risks of future treatments are carefully considered by the physician. Use only approved lasers. Use of incompatible lasers may cause undertreatment, overtreatment, or damage to the surrounding normal tissue. Calcium channel blockers, polymixin B, or radiation therapy may enhance the rate of verteporfin uptake by the vascular endothelium. Photosensitizing drugs such as tetracyclines, sulfonamides, phenothiazines, sulfonylurea hypoglycemic agents, thiazide diuretics, and griseofulvin could increase the potential for skin photosensitivity reactions. Drugs or compounds that quench active oxygen species or scavenge radicals, such as dimethyl sulfoxide, betacarotene, ethanol, formate, and mannitol, may decrease verteporfin's efficacy. Drugs that decrease clotting, vasoconstriction, or platelet aggregation, such as thromboxane A2 inhibitors, could also decrease the efficacy of verteporfin therapy. Pregnancy Category C. Verteporfin has been shown to be embryotoxic in animals. There are no adequate and well-controlled studies in pregnant women. Verteporfin should be used in pregnancy only if the benefit justifies the potential risk to the fetus. Excretion in human breast milk is unknown. Safety and efficacy in pediatric patients have not been established. Most common adverse reactions include headache, injection site reactions, and visual disturbances. These occur in 10–20% of patients. Adverse reactions occurring in 1–10% of patients include ocular treatment site (cataracts, conjunctivitis/conjunctival injection, dry eyes, itching, severe vision loss, subconjunctival, subretinal, or vitreous hemorrhage), asthenia, back pain during infusion, fever, flu-like syndrome, photosensitivity reactions in the form of sunburn following exposure to sunlight, atrial fibrillation, hypertension, peripheral vascular disorder, varicose veins, eczema, constipation, gastrointestinal cancers, nausea, anemia, decreased or increased white blood cell count, increased liver function tests, albuminuria, increased creatinine, arthralgias, hypesthesia, sleep disorder, vertigo, pharyngitis, pneumonia, decreased hearing, diplopia, lacrimation disorder, and prostatic disorder. Severe vision decrease equivalent to 4 lines or more within 7 days after treatment has been reported in 1–4% of patients. Partial recovery of vision was observed in many patients.

Administration: IV with light activation via laser.

Patient Care Implications: Avoid extravasation. Use the largest vein possible, preferably the antecubital. Avoid small veins. Avoid contact with the eyes and skin during the preparation and administration of verteporfin. Any exposed person must be protected from bright light. Use of rubber gloves and eye protection is recommended. Wipe any spills with a damp cloth, and dispose of properly. Reconstituted vials must be protected from light and used within 4 hours. Patients should be instructed to avoid direct sunlight or bright light such as tanning salons, bright halogen lights, and high-power lighting during the first 5 days after treatment. If direct sunlight or bright light cannot be avoided, patients should be instructed to protect all parts of their skin and eyes by wearing protective clothing and sunglasses. Ultraviolet sunscreens are not effective in protecting against photosensitivity reactions. Ambient light is encouraged to help inactivate the drug.

Preparations: Injection, single-use glass vial containing 15 mg of verteporfin.

VESPRIN®, see Triflupromazine

VFEND®, see Voriconazole

VIACTIV®—Combination Drug of Calcium Carbonate 500 mg with Vitamin D 100 units, Vitamin K 400 mcg in soft chewable tablets

VIADUR™, see Leuprolide Acetate

VIAGRA®, see Sidenafil Citrate

VIBRAMYCIN®, see Doxycycline

VIBRA-TABS®, see Doxycycline

VICODIN®, Combination of Hydrocodone and Acetaminophen

VICOPROFEN®, Combination Agent of Hydrocodone Bitartate and Ibuprofen (Opioid and NSAID)

VIDARABINE—Vira-A®

Description/Actions: Antiviral agent indicated for ophthalmic use for the treatment of acute keratoconjunctivitis and recurrent epithelial keratitis due to herpes simplex virus types 1 and 2.

Preparations: Ophthalmic ointment, 3%.

VIDEX®, see Didanosine

VIDEX® EC, see Didanosine

VINBLASTINE SULFATE—Velban®

Description/Actions: Antineoplastic agent administered intravenously in the treatment of Hodgkin's disease, lymphocytic lymphoma, histiocytic lymphoma, mycosis fungoides, advanced carcinoma of the testes, Kaposi's sarcoma, choriocarcinoma resistant to other agents, and carcinoma of the breast that is not responsive to other therapy.

Preparations: Vials, 10 mg.

VINCASAR PFS®, see Vincristine

VINCRISTINE SULFATE—Oncovin®, Vincasar PFS®

Description/Actions: Antineoplastic agent administered intravenously in the treatment of acute leukemia, Hodgkin's disease, lymphosarcoma, reticulum cell sarcoma, rhabdomyosarcoma, neuroblastoma, and Wilms' tumor.

Preparations: Vials and syringes, 1, 2, and 5 mg.

VINORELBINE TARTRATE—Navelbine®

Description/Actions: Antineoplastic agent indicated as monotherapy or in combination with cisplatin for the first-line treatment of ambulatory patients with unresectable advanced nonsmall-cell lung cancer.

Precautions/Adverse Reactions: Contraindicated in patients with pretreatment granulocyte counts of less than 1000 cells/mm3. Cautious use is recommended in patients with previous irradiation or chemotherapy because of increased risk of myelosuppression. Granulocytopenia is the major dose-limiting toxicity. Sepsis has occurred and patients should be taught to immediately report the occurrence of fever or chills. Adverse reactions include fatigue, peripheral neuropathy, alopecia, constipation, diarrhea, nausea and vomiting, chest pain, shortness of breath, and elevation of liver enzymes. Observe vesicant precautions.

Administration: Intravenous.

Preparations: Vials, 10 mg/ml.

VIOFORM®, see Clioquinol

VIOKASE®, see Pancrelipase

VIRA-A®, see Vidarabine

VIRACEPT®, see Nelfinavir

VIRAMUNE®, see Nevirapine

VIRAZOLE®, see Ribavirin

VIREAD™, see Tenofovir Disoproxil Fumarate

VIROPTIC®, see Trifluridine

VISICOL™, see Sodium Phosphates

VISINE®, see Tetrahydrozoline

VISKEN®, see Pindolol

VISTARIL®, see Hydroxyzine

VISTIDE®, see Cidofovir

VISUDYNE®, see Verteporfin

VITACARN®, see L-carnitine

VITAMIN A—Aquasol A®

Description/Actions: Vitamin indicated for the treatment of vitamin A deficiency.

Preparations: Capsules, 10,000, 25,000, 50,000 IU. Drops, 5000 IU/0.1 ml. Vials, 50,000 IU/ml.

VITAMIN A ACID, see Tretinoin

VITAMIN B₁, see Thiamine

VITAMIN B₂, see Riboflavin

VITAMIN B₃, see Nicotinic Acid

VITAMIN B₆, see Pyridoxine

VITAMIN B₁₂, see Cyanocobalamin

VITAMIN B COMPLEX

Description/Actions: Vitamin mixture usually including thiamine, riboflavin, niacin, pantothenic acid, pyridoxine, and cyanocobalamin.

VITAMIN C—Ascorbic acid, Sodium Ascorbate, Cevalin®

Description/Actions: Vitamin indicated in the prevention and treatment of scurvy. Has been suggested to be of benefit in high doses in the prevention and treatment of colds. Has been used as a urinary acidifier.

Preparations: Tablets, 25, 50, 100, 250, and 500 mg. Chewable, controlled-release, and effervescent tablets. Solution, syrup, powder, and crystals. Ampules and vials, 100 mg/ml, 250 mg/ml, and 500 mg/ml.

VITAMIN D, see Cholecalciferol and Ergocalciferol

VITAMIN D₂, see Ergocalciferol

VITAMIN D₃, see Cholecalciferol

VITAMIN E—Aquasol E®

Description/Actions: Vitamin indicated for the treatment and prevention of vitamin E deficiency. Has been used in certain premature infants to reduce the toxic effects of oxygen therapy on the lung parenchyma and to decrease the severity of hemolytic anemia in infants.

Preparations: Capsules, 50, 100, 200, 400, 500, 600, and 1000 IU. Drops, 15 IU/0.3 ml.

VITAMIN K, see Menadiol Sodium Diphosphate

VITAMIN K₁, see Phytonadione

VIVACTIL®, see Protriptyline

VIVELLE®, see Estradiol

VLEMASQUE®, see Sulfurated Lime

VOLMAX®, see Albuterol Sulfate

VOLTAREN®, see Diclofenac

VONTROL®, see Diphenidol

VORICONAZOLE—Vfend®

Description/Actions: Voriconazole is a triazole antifungal agent. Its antifungal activity is due to the loss of ergosterol in the fungal cell wall. Voriconazole has shown activity against *Aspergillus fumigatus, Aspergillus flavus, Aspergillus niger, Aspergillus terreus, Scedosporium apiospermum,* and *Fusarium* species, including *Fusarium solani.* It is indicated for use in the treatment of serious fungal infections caused by *Scedosporium apiospermum* and *Fusarium* species, including *Fusarium solani,* in patients intolerant of, or refractory to, other therapy.

Precautions/Adverse Reactions: Voriconazole is contraindicated in patients with a known hypersensitivity to voriconazole or to any component of the formulation. Coadministration of voriconazole and terfenadine, astemizole, cisapride, pimozide, or quinidine is contraindicated because increased plasma concentrations of these drugs can lead to QT interval prolongation and rare occurrences of torsade de pointes. Coadministration of voriconazole with sirolimus is contraindicated because voriconazole significantly increases sirolimus concentrations. Coadministration of voriconazole with rifampin, carbamazepine, and long-acting barbiturates (phenobarbital, mephobarbital) is contraindicated because these drugs are likely to significantly decrease plasma levels of voriconazole. Coadministration of voriconazole with rifabutin is contraindicated because voriconazole significantly increases rifabutin plasma concentrations, and rifabutin significantly decreases voriconazole plasma concentrations. Coadministration of voriconazole with ergot alkaloids (ergotamine, dihydroergotamine) is contraindicated because voriconazole may increase the plasma concentration of the ergot alkaloid, which may lead to ergotism. Voriconazole causes visual disturbances, including altered/enhanced visual perception, blurred vision, color vision change, and/or photophobia. Serious hepatic reactions, including clinical hepatitis, cholestasis, and fulminant hepatic failure (including fatalities) have occurred during therapy with voriconazole. Voriconazole tablets contain lactose and should not be given to patients with rare hereditary problems of galactose intolerance, Lapp lactase deficiency, or glucose-galactose malabsorption. Voriconazole should be administered with caution to patients with potentially proarrhythmic conditions. Electrolyte abnormalities (hypokalemia, hypomagnesemia, and hypocalcemia) should be corrected prior to starting voriconazole. Anaphylactoid-type reactions, including flushing, fever, sweating, tachycardia, chest tightness, dyspnea, faintness, nausea, pruritus, and rash, have occurred during infusion of the intravenous formulation of voriconazole. Infusion should be stopped if this occurs. Accumulation of the intravenous vehicle sulfobutyl ether beta-cyclodextrin sodium (SBECD) occurs in patients with moderate to severe renal impairment (creatinine clearance <50 mL/min). Serum creatinine should be monitored in these patients and oral voriconazole should be administered to these patients, unless the benefits/risk to the patient justifies the use of the intravenous formulation. Pregnancy Category D. Voriconazole is metabolized by the cytochrome P450 enzyme system CYP2C19, CYP2C9, and CYP3A4. Inhibitors or inducers of these enzymes may increase or decrease voriconazole plasma concentrations. Coadministration of voriconazole and cyclosporine resulted in increased serum concentrations of cyclosporine. When initiating therapy with voriconazole in patients already receiving cyclosporine, decrease cyclosporine dosage by 50%. Monitor levels and when voriconazole is discontinued, readjust the dose as warranted. Coadministration of voriconazole and tacrolimus resulted in increased serum levels of tacrolimus. When initiating therapy with voriconazole in patients already receiving tacrolimus, decrease tacrolimus dosage to one-third of the original dose. Monitor levels and readjust dose as necessary once voriconazole is discontinued. Coadministration of voriconazole and warfarin resulted in increased prothrombin time. Prothrombin time and INR should be monitored. Coadministration of voriconazole and statins (HMG-CoA reductase inhibitors) is likely to result in increased serum levels of the statin. Increased levels of statins have been associated with myopathy/rhabdomyolysis. Coadministration of voriconazole and benzodiazepines (midazolam, triazolam, and alprazolam) resulted in increased plasma levels of the benzodiazepine and a prolonged sedative effect. Dosage adjustment of the benzodiazepine may be warranted. Coadministration of voriconazole and dihydropyridine calcium channel blockers may result in increased serum concentrations of the calcium channel blocker. Monitor patient for adverse effects and toxicity related to the calcium channel blocker. Dosage adjustment of the calcium channel blocker may be needed. Voriconazole may increase plasma levels of sulfonylureas (tolbutamide, glyburide, and glipizide) and lead to hypoglycemia. Blood glucose levels should be monitored and the dose of the sulfonylurea adjusted accordingly. Voriconazole may increase the plasma concentration of vinca alkaloids (vincristine and vinblastine) and lead to neurotoxicity. Consider dosage adjustment of the vinca alkaloid. Coadministration of voriconazole and phenytoin has resulted in decreased plasma levels of voriconazole. Dosage of voriconazole should be increased. Monitor phenytoin levels and adjust dose as needed. Coadministration of voriconazole and omeprazole (>40 mg/day) resulted in increased serum concentrations of omeprazole. When coadministering with voriconazole, decrease the dose of omeprazole by 50%. Metabolism of other proton pump inhibitors may also be affected. Voriconazole may inhibit the metabolism of HIV protease inhibitors (saquinavir, ritonavir, and amprenavir), and the metabolism of voriconazole may also be inhibited by HIV protease inhibitors. Patients should be monitored for drug toxicity when these agents are coadministered. The metabolism of voriconazole may be inhibited when coadministered with Non-Nucleoside Reverse Transcriptase Inhibitors (delavirdine and effavirenz), resulting in increased serum concentrations of voriconazole. The metabolism of voriconazole may be induced by effavirenz or nevirapine, resulting in decreased serum levels of voriconazole. Voriconazole may also inhibit the metabolism of delavirdine. Patients should be monitored for drug toxicity. Most common adverse reactions observed in patients treated with voriconazole include visual disturbances, fever, rash, vomiting, nausea, diarrhea, headache, sepsis, peripheral edema, abdominal pain, and respiratory disorder.

Administration: Intravenous, oral on empty stomach.

Preparations: Lyophilized powder for injection, 200 mg voriconazole and 3200 mg SBECD. Tablets, 50 and 200 mg. Powder for oral suspension, 45 g.

VOSOL®, see Acetic Acid

VP-16®, see Etoposide

VUMON®, see Teniposide

W

WARFARIN SODIUM—Coumadin®

Description/Actions: Indicated for (a) the prophylaxis and treatment of venous thrombosis and its extension, (b) the treatment of atrial fibrillation with embolization, (c) the prophylaxis and treatment of pulmonary embolism, (d) as an adjunct in the treatment of coronary occlusion, (e) for the prevention and treatment of thromboembolic complications associated with cardiac valve replacements, and (f) to reduce the risk of death, recurrent myocardial infarction, and thromboembolic events such as stroke or systemic embolization after myocardial infarction.

Precautions/Adverse Reactions: Contraindicated during pregnancy in patients with bleeding tendencies associated with active ulceration, hemorrhagic tendencies, or blood dyscrasias or in patients who have recently undergone or are to undergo surgery of the CNS or eye, or other surgery that has resulted in large, open surfaces. Adverse reactions include hemorrhage, and therapy must be closely monitored. Effect may be increased by the concurrent administration of allopurinol, antibiotics, cimetidine, erythromycin, monoamine oxidase inhibitors, phenylbutazone, quinidine, salicylates, sulfonylurea hypoglycemic agents, and trimethoprim-sulfamethoxazole, as well as by other agents. Effect may be reduced by barbiturates, carbamazepine, griseofulvin, and other agents.

Administration: Oral, intravenous, and intramuscular.

Preparations: Scored tablets, 1, 2, 2.5, 3, 4, 5, 6, 7.5, and 10 mg. Vials, 2 mg/ml, 5 mg/ml.

WELCHOL™, see Colesevelam

WELLBUTRIN®, see Bupropion

WELLBUTRIN® SR, see Bupropion

WELLBUTRIN® XL, see Bupropion

WELLCOVORIN®, see Leucovorin

WHITFIELD'S OINTMENT, see Benzoic Acid

WINSTROL®, see Stanozolol

WINTERGREEN OIL, see Methyl Salicylate

WOOL FAT, see Lanolin

WYAMINE®, see Mephentermine

WYCILLIN®, see Procaine Penicillin G

WYDASE®, see Hyaluronidase

WYMOX®, see Amoxicillin

WYTENSIN®, see Guanabenz

X

XALATAN®, see Latanoprost

XANAX®, see Alprazolam

XANAX® XR, see Alprazolam

XELODA®, see Capecitabine

XIGRIS™, see Drotrecogin Alfa

XOPENEX HFA™, see Levalbuterol

XYLOCAINE®, see Lidocaine

XYLOMETAZOLINE HYDROCHLORIDE—Otrivin®
Description/Actions: Decongestant used topically for the relief of nasal congestion.
Preparations: Nose drops, 0.05% and 0.1%. Nose spray, 0.1%.

XYREM®, see Sodium Oxybate

Y

YASMIN®, see Ethinyl Estradiol and Drospirenone

YODOXIN®, see Iodoquinol

YOHIMBINE HYDROCHLORIDE
Description/Actions: Has been suggested to have an aphrodisiac effect.
Preparations: Tablets, 5 mg.

YUTOPAR®, see Ritodrine

Z

ZADITOR®, see Ketotifen

ZAFIRLUKAST—Accolate®

Description/Actions: Antiasthmatic (leukotriene receptor antagonist) indicated for the prophylaxis and chronic treatment of asthma in adults and children 5 years of age and older.

Precautions/Adverse Reactions: Not for primary treatment of acute asthma attacks. Cases of life-threatening hepatic failure have been reported in patients treated with zafirlukast. In rare cases, patients have either presented with fulminant hepatitis or progressed to hepatic failure, liver transplantation, or death. Adverse reactions include headache, infection (respiratory tract), and nausea. Remind patients that this drug should be taken regularly as prescribed and not to make changes in dosing on their own. This drug is not a bronchodilator. Although it may be used during an acute episode, it is not indicated for the reversal of acute bronchospasm.

Administration: Oral, on empty stomach.

Preparations: Tablets, 20 mg.

ZAGAM®, see Sparfloxacin

ZALCITABINE—Hivid®

Description/Actions: Also known as dideoxycytidine or ddC. Antiviral agent that inhibits the replication of the human immunodeficiency virus (HIV). Is converted by cellular enzymes to the active antiviral metabolite that inhibits viral replication, in part, by interfering with reverse transcriptase. Indicated for use in combination with zidovudine for the treatment of adult patients (i.e., 13 years of age and older) with advanced HIV infection (CD4 cell count less than or equal to 300 cells/mm3) who have demonstrated significant clinical or immunologic deterioration. Also indicated for second-line monotherapy in HIV-infected patients who experience disease progression with zidovudine or are intolerant of zidovudine.

Precautions/Adverse Reactions: May cause peripheral neuropathy, which may become severe and potentially irreversible if the drug is not stopped promptly. Patients should be advised to report symptoms such as tingling, burning, pain, or numbness in the hands or feet. Use should be avoided in patients with moderate or severe peripheral neuropathy, and the concurrent use with other drugs that have the potential to cause peripheral neuropathy (e.g., didanosine) should be avoided where possible. May cause pancreatitis and, if a patient develops abdominal pain and nausea, vomiting, or elevated amylase levels, the use of the drug should be interrupted until the possibility of pancreatitis is excluded. Other adverse reactions include esophageal ulcers, cardiomyopathy, congestive heart failure, anaphylactoid reactions, oral ulcers, nausea, dysphagia, anorexia, abdominal pain, vomiting, rash, pruritus, headache, dizziness, myalgia, fatigue, pharyngitis, anemia, leukopenia, and elevation of hepatic enzymes. May cause fetal harm and women of childbearing potential should not receive the drug unless they are using effective contraception.

Administration: Oral.

Preparations: Tablets, 0.375 and 0.75 mg.

ZALEPLON—Sonata®

Description/Actions: Zaleplon is used in the treatment of insomnia.

Precautions/Adverse Reactions: Zaleplon dosage should be reduced in patients with mild hepatic impairment and not given to patients with severe hepatic disease. The drug should not be administered to pregnant women, breast-feeding women, or children. Some adverse effects are anorexia, colitis, constipation, dyspepsia, nausea, vomiting, abdominal pain, back pain, fever, headache, malaise, conjunctivitis, hyperacusis, otalgia, pruritus, migraine, angina, hypertension, syncope, anxiety, depression, dizziness, hallucination, vertigo, bronchitis, epistaxis, and myalgia.

Administration: Oral.

Patient Care Implications: The drug should be administered in reduced doses to patients with mild hepatic impairment and not given to patients with severe hepatic disease.

Preparations: Capsules, 5 and 10 mg.

ZANAFLEX®, see Tizanidine

ZANAMIVIR—Relenza®

Description/Actions: Zanamivir is an inhaler that is used in the treatment of influenza A and B.

Precautions/Adverse Reactions: Zanamivir should be used with caution in patients with COPD, asthma, pregnant women, and breast-feeding women. The drug should not be administered to children <7 years of age. Some side effects are bronchospasm, headache, diarrhea, nausea, vomiting, sinusitis, bronchitis, cough, nasal congestion, and dizziness.

Administration: Oral inhalation.

Patient Care Implications: Patients with respiratory disease should be careful using the inhaler, and the drug should not be administered to children <12 years of age. If patient is on a bronchodilator, then it should be administered before zanamivir.

Preparations: Diskhaler, 5 mg (4 blister pack).

ZANTAC®, see Ranitidine

ZANTAC® 150 EFFERDOSE®, see Ranitidine Effervescent

ZARONTIN®, see Ethosuximide

ZAROXOLYN®, see Metolazone

ZEBETA®, see Bisoprolol Fumarate

ZEGERID™, see Omeprazole

ZELNORM™, see Tegaserod Maleate

ZEMURON®, see Rocuronium Bromide

ZEPHIRAN®, see Benzalkonium Chloride

ZERIT®, see Stavudine

ZESTORETIC®, Combination of Lisinopril and Hydrochlorothiazide

ZESTRIL®, see Lisinopril

ZETIA™, see Ezetimibe

ZEVALIN™, see Ibritumomab Tiuxetan

ZIAC®, Combination of Bisoprolol and Hydrochlorothiazide

ZIDOVUDINE—AZT, Retrovir®

Description/Actions: Also known as azidothymidine (AZT), it inhibits the replication of certain retroviruses, including human immunodeficiency virus (HIV), which causes acquired immunodeficiency syndrome (AIDS). Antiviral agent indicated for the management of adult patients with symptomatic HIV infection (AIDS and advanced AIDS-related complex [ARC]) who have a history of cytologically confirmed pneumonia (PCP) or an absolute CD4 (T4 helper/inducer) lymphocyte count of less than 200/mm3 in the peripheral blood before therapy is begun. Also indicated for the management of patients with HIV infection who have evidence of impaired immunity, and for HIV-infected children who have HIV-related symptoms or who are asymptomatic with abnormal laboratory values indicating significant HIV-related immunosuppression. Also indicated for the prevention of maternal-fetal HIV transmission.

Precautions/Adverse Reactions: Hematologic toxicity (e.g., granulocytopenia, anemia) is the adverse event reported most frequently and may require dose adjustment, discontinuation of the drug, and/or blood transfusions. Frequent (at least every 2 weeks) blood counts are strongly recommended in patients taking the medication. Lactic acidosis and severe hepatomegaly with steatosis, including fatal cases, have been reported with the use of nucleoside analogs alone or in combination. Other adverse reactions include headache, nausea, insomnia, and myalgia. Caution must be exercised in patients taking other medications that are nephrotoxic, cytotoxic, or that interfere with the number or function of red blood cells and/or white blood cells, because the risk of toxicity may be increased. Probenecid may increase the activity of zidovudine.

Administration: Oral and intravenous.

Preparations: Capsules, 100 mg. Tablets, 300 mg. Syrup, 50 mg/5 ml. Vials, 10 mg/ml.

ZILABRACE®, see Benzocaine

ZILADENT®, see Benzocaine

ZILEUTON—Zyflo®

Description/Actions: Antiasthmatic indicated in the prophylaxis and chronic treatment of asthma.

Precautions/Adverse Reactions: Contraindicated in acute liver disease. Do not administer if transaminase levels are greater than or equal to 3 times the upper limit of normal. Evaluate liver function before initiation of and during therapy (discontinue if signs of liver disease occur). Use cautiously in patients with a history of liver disease or alcohol consumption. Adverse reactions include dyspepsia, pain, nausea, asthenia, headache, and myalgia. Documented drug interactions require a full drug profile review and adjustment of the regimen accordingly.

Administration: Oral.

Preparations: Tablets, 600 mg (scored).

ZINACEF®, see Cefuroxime Sodium

ZINC CHLORIDE

Description/Actions: Trace metal supplement added to intravenous solutions given for total parenteral nutrition.

ZINC GLUCONATE

Description/Actions: Dietary supplement to prevent or treat deficiencies of zinc.

Preparations: Tablets, 35, 50, and 105 mg.

ZINC OXIDE

Description/Actions: Protectant and antiseptic applied topically in the treatment of various dermatologic conditions.

Preparations: Ointment, 25%. Paste, 25% with 25% starch.

ZINC SULFATE

Description/Actions: Trace metal supplement added to intravenous solutions given for total parenteral nutrition. Also used as a dietary supplement to prevent or treat deficiencies of zinc. Has been investigated in dermatologic and arthritic disorders and in situations in which there is delayed wound healing associated with zinc deficiency. Also used in an ophthalmic solution for the relief of minor eye irritation.

Preparations: Vials, 1 mg/ml and 5 mg/ml. Capsules and tablets, 110 and 220 mg. Ophthalmic solution, 0.25%.

ZINECARD®, see Dexrazoxane

ZIPRASIDONE—Geodon™

Description/Actions: Antipsychotic agent indicated for the treatment of acute manic or mixed episodes associated with bipolar disorder with or without psychotic features. Ziprasidone intramuscular is indicated for the treatment of acute agitation in schizophrenic patients for whom treatment with ziprasidone is appropriate and who need intramuscular antipsychotic medication for rapid control of the agitation.

Precautions/Adverse Reactions: Usage is contraindicated in patients with a hypersensitivity to ziprasidone or any component of the formulation, history of (or current) QT prolongation, congenital long QT interval, recent acute myocardial infarction, or uncompensated heart failure. Ziprasidone is contraindicated with concurrent use of other QTc–prolonging agents, including amiodarone, dofetilide, class A antiarrythmics, cisapride, pimozide, moxifloxacin, sparfloxacin, chlorpromazine, droperidol, halofantrine, levomethadyl acetate, dolasetron mesylate, probucol, or tacrolimus. Ziprasidone usage may result in a dose-related prolongation QTc, which has been associated with the development of malignant ventricular arrhythmias (torsades de pointes) and sudden death. The observed QTc prolongation was greater than with other atypical antipsychotic agents. Elderly patients with dementia-related psychosis treated with atypical antipsychotic drugs are at an increased risk of death compared to placebo. Most deaths appeared to be either cardiovascular (e.g., heart failure, sudden death) or infectious (e.g., pneumonia) in nature. Ziprasidone is not approved for the treatment of patients with dementia-related psychosis. Avoid hypokalemia and hypomagnesemia, and use caution in patients with bradycardia; these circumstances may increase the risk of the occurrence of torsades de pointes. Discontinue therapy in patients found to have persistent QTc intervals >500 msec. Patients who exhibit symptoms of dizziness, palpitations, or syncope should receive further cardiac evaluation. Antipsychotic therapy may cause extrapyramidal reactions and neuroleptic malignant syndrome (NMS). Use with caution in patients with a history of seizures or with conditions that lower the seizure threshold. May induce orthostatic hypotension; use with caution in patients at risk for this effect. May cause cognitive and motor impairment. Use with caution in patients with Parkinson's disease, Alzheimer's disease, breast cancer, or other prolactin-dependent tumors. Ziprasidone is associated with high incidence of rash; discontinue if alternative etiology is not identified. Safety and efficacy have not been established in pediatric patents. Pregnancy Category C. Use only if potential benefit justifies risk to the fetus. Excretion in breast milk is unknown; breast-feeding is not recommended. Some adverse effects are somnolence, QTc prolongation, tachycardia, postural hypotension, dizziness, akathisia, extrapyramidal symptoms, dystonia, rash, nausea, constipation, dyspepsia, diarrhea, weight gain, dry mouth, respiratory disorders, and abnormal vision.

Administration: Intravenous and oral.

Patient Care Implications: Inform patients that they may experience drowsiness, lightheadedness, impaired coordination, dizziness, or blurred vision. Patients should use caution when driving or engaging in hazardous tasks until response to the drug is known. Patients should report to their physician any signs of cardiac arrhythmias (fainting or loss of consciousness, or palpitations).

Preparations: Capsule, 20, 40, 60, and 80 mg. Injection, 20 mg.

ZITHROMAX®, see Azithromycin

ZITHROMAX® TRI-PAK, see Azithromycin

ZOCOR®, see Simvastatin

ZOFRAN®, see Ondansetron

ZOLADEX®, see Goserelin Acetate

ZOLEDRONIC ACID—Zometa®

Description/Actions: Zoledronic acid is indicated for hypercalcemia of malignancy (HCM), a common life-threatening metabolic complication of cancer, multiple myeloma, and bone metastases of solid tumors. It is also indicated for the treatment of patients with multiple myeloma and patients with bone metastasis from solid tumors along with standard antineoplastic agents.

Precautions/Adverse Reactions: Renal function should be assessed prior to and after treatment; additional treatments should be held until renal function returns to baseline. Because of risk of significant deterioration in renal function, which may progress to renal failure, single doses should not exceed 4 mg, and the duration of infusion should not be less than 15 minutes. Use is not recommended in patients with severe renal impairment (serum creatinine >3.0 mg/dl). Use caution when bisphosphonates are administered with aminoglycosides, because these agents may have an additive effect of lowering serum calcium level for prolonged periods. Exercise caution when zoledronic acid is used in combination with loop diuretics because of the increased risk of hypocalcemia. In multiple myeloma patients, the risk of renal dysfunction may be increased when zoledronic acid is used with thalidomide. Pregnancy Category D. May cause fetal harm. Excretion in human breast milk is unknown; breast-feeding not recommended. Adverse reactions are usually mild and similar to some seen with other bisphosphonates, such as conjunctivitis and hypomagnesemia. Fever is common, and occasionally a flu-like syndrome (chills, fever, bone pain, arthralgia, and myalgia) occurs. Osteonecrosis of the jaw (ONJ) has been reported in patients with cancer who are receiving zoledronic acid. A dental examination with appropriate preventive dentistry should be considered prior to treatment with zoledronic acid in patients with concomitant risk factors (e.g., cancer, chemotherapy, corticosteroids, poor oral hygiene). Invasive dental procedures should be avoided during treatment with zoledronic acid.

Administration: Intravenous.

Patient Care Implications: Vigorous saline hydration should be initiated. Urine output should be about 2 L per day throughout treatment. Reconstitute 4 mg vial with 5 ml sterile water for injection. Zoledronic acid must not be mixed with calcium-containing solutions, such as lactated Ringer's solution. Patients with diagnosis of multiple myeloma or metastatic bone lesions from solid tumors should take a daily calcium (500 mg) and daily multivitamin (with 400 IU vitamin D). However, patients should avoid taking vitamins during infusion or for 2–3 hours after completion of zoledronic acid.

Preparations: Injection, powder for reconstitution, 4 mg (as monohydrate 4.264 mg).

ZOLICEF®, see Cefazolin

ZOLMITRIPTAN—Zomig®, Zomig-ZMT®

Description/Actions: Indicated in the acute treatment of migraine headache with or without auras.

Precautions/Adverse Reactions: Use not recommended in children. Contraindicated in ischemic heart disease, coronary artery vasospasm, uncontrolled hypertension, other significant cardiovascular disease, or basilar or hemiplegic migraine, within 24 hours of other 5-HT1 agonists or ergot-type drugs, during or within 2 weeks after discontinuing MAOIs. Serious cardiovascular events have been reported in association with the use of zolmitriptan and in very rare cases, these events have occurred in the absence of known cardiovascular disease. 5–HT1 agonists may cause vasospastic reactions other than coronary artery vasospasm, such as peripheral and gastrointestinal vascular ischemia. Confirm diagnosis and exclude underlying cardiovascular disease. Supervise first dose and consider monitoring ECG in patients with likelihood of unrecognized coronary disease (e.g., postmenopausal women, men over age 40), hypertension, hyperocholesterolemia, obesity, diabetes, smokers, strong family history). Monitor cardiovascular function in longer-term intermittent use. Use not recommended in Wolff-Parkinson-White syndrome or arrhythmias associated with other cardiac accessory conduction pathway disorders. Use cautiously in hepatic dysfunction, elderly, and nursing mothers. Pregnancy Category C. Adverse reactions include paresthesia, asthenia, nausea, dizziness, pain, chest or neck tightness/heaviness, somnolence, anaphylaxis or anaphylactoid reactions, and warm feeling.

Administration: Oral.

Preparations: Tablets, 2.5 mg and 5 mg. Orally disintegrating tablet, 2.5 and 5 mg. Nasal spray, 5 mg.

ZOLOFT®, see Sertraline

ZOLPIDEM TARTRATE—Ambien®

Description/Actions: Is an imidazopyridine derivative that is indicated for the short-term treatment of insomnia.

Precautions/Adverse Reactions: Adverse reactions include drowsiness, dizziness, drugged feelings, and diarrhea. Patients should be cautioned against engaging in activities requiring complete mental alertness or motor coordination, including potential impairment of the performance of such activities the following day. Patients should also be warned about the risk of additive depressant effects when other agents with central nervous system depressant activity (including alcohol) are used concurrently. Has a potential for causing problems of dependence and abuse, and is classified in Schedule IV.

Administration: Oral.

Preparations: Tablets, 5 and 10 mg.

ZOMETA®, see Zoledronic Acid

ZOMIG®, see Zolmitriptan

ZONALON®, see Doxepin Hydrochloride

ZONASAR®, see Streptozocin

ZONEGRAN®, see Zonisamide

ZONISAMIDE—Zonegran®

Description/Actions: Indicated as adjunctive treatment of partial and tonic-clonic seizures.

Precautions/Adverse Reactions: Major adverse reactions include nephrolithiasis, impaired memory, drowsiness, ataxia, nystagmus, diplopia, tremors, psychosis, Stevens-Johnson syndrome, and leukopenia. Zonegram is contraindicated in patients who have demonstrated hypersensitivity to sulfonamides or zonisamide. Pediatric patients appear to be at an increased risk for zonisamide-associated oligohydrosis and hyperthermia. Monitor patients closely for evidence of decreased sweating and increased body temperature, especially in warm/hot weather. Safety and efficacy in pediatric patients have not been established.

Administration: Oral.

Preparations: Capsules, 25, 50, and 100 mg.

ZORPRIN®, see Aspirin

ZOSTRIX®, see Capsaicin

ZOSTRIX—HP®, see Capsaicin

ZOSYN®, see Piperacillin Sodium/Tazobactam Sodium

ZOVIRAX®, see Acyclovir

Z-PAK®, see Azithromycin

ZYBAN®, see Bupropion

ZYFLO®, see Zileuton

ZYLOPRIM®, see Allopurinol

ZYMASE®, see Pancrelipase

ZYPREXA®, see Olanzapine

ZYPREXA® IM, see Olanzapine

ZYPREXA ZYDIS®, see Olanzapine

ZYRTEC®, see Cetirizine Hydrochloride

ZYRTEC-D 12 HOUR™, see Cetirizine and Pseudophedrine

ZYVOX®, see Linezolid

PART III

Glossary of Side Effects

Agranulocytosis—Severe acute shortage of certain types of blood cells (neutrophils) as a result of damage to the bone marrow by toxic drugs or chemicals.

Akathesia—A syndrome characterized by an inability to remain in a sitting posture with motor restlessness and a feeling of muscular quivering. May appear as a side effect of antipsychotic and neuroleptic medication.

Akinesia—Loss of normal muscle tonicity or responsiveness.

Allergic reactions—A response caused by sensitization to a particular antigen that provokes the release of histamine. Symptoms present as local or systemic effects, ranging from local rash to respiratory wheezing.

Alopecia—Absence of hair from where it normally grows; baldness.

Amenorrhea—Stopping of menstrual flow.

Anaphylactic shock—An extreme and generalized allergic reaction in which widespread release of histamine causes swelling (edema), constriction of the bronchioles, heart failure, circulatory collapse, and sometimes death.

Anaphylaxis—An abnormal reaction to a particular antigen in which histamine is released from the tissues and causes either local or widespread symptoms typical of an allergic response. This response may be characterized by hives, itching, nasal congestion, abdominal cramping, diarrhea, dyspnea, hypotension, fainting, and choking sensation.

Angioedema (Angioneurotic edema)—An allergic condition producing transient or persistent swelling of areas of the skin accompanied by itching, which may be severe.

Anorexia—Loss of appetite.

Anticholinergic effects—Dry mouth, blurred vision, urinary retention, constipation.

Aphakic—Absence of the crystalline lens.

Apnea—Temporary cessation of breathing.

Arrhythmias—Any alteration from the normal sinus rhythm of the heart.

Arthralgia—Joint pain.

Asthenia—Weakness or loss of strength.

Atony—A state in which the muscles are floppy or lacking in normal tone.

AV block—Atrial-ventricular heart block.

Blepharitis—Inflammation of the eyelids.

Blepharospasm—Involuntary contraction of the eyelid.

Blood dyscrasias—Abnormal state found in the blood cells.

Bradycardia—Slowing of the heart beat to less than 50 beats per minute.

Cardiogenic shock—Shock that originates from a cardiac source.

Catabolism—The breaking down in the body of complex chemical compounds into simpler ones.

Cataplexy—A transient attack of extreme generalized muscle weakness.

Chemosis—Swelling (edema) of the conjunctiva of the eye.

Chloasm—Patchy brown discoloration of the skin, mainly on the forehead, temples, and cheeks. Usually associated with pregnancy or use of birth control pills (oral contraceptives).

Conjunctivitis—Inflammation of the conjunctiva (delicate mucous membrane that covers the front of the eyes and lines the inside of the eyelids) that becomes red and swollen and produces a watery or pus-containing discharge.

Constipation—A condition in which bowel evacuation occurs irregularly or in which the feces are hard and small or where passage of feces is difficult or painful.

Diarrhea—Frequent bowel evacuation or the passage of abnormally soft or liquid feces.

Diplopia—Double vision.

Disulfiram-like reactions—Disulfiram is a drug used in treatment of alcoholism, which, when taken in combination with alcohol, produces unpleasant reactions such as flushing, difficulty breathing, headache, palpitations, nausea, and vomiting. Drugs that produce these same unpleasant effects are classified as disulfiram-like reactions.

Dyesthesia—A condition in which a disagreeable sensation is produced by ordinary stimuli.

Dysgeusia—Taste perversion; bad taste in the mouth.

Dysmenorrhea—Painful menstruation.

Dyspepsia—Refers to pain or discomfort in the lower chest or abdomen after eating; may sometimes be accompanied by nausea and vomiting.

Dyspnea—Labored or difficult breathing.

Dystonia—A postural disorder caused by an effect on the basal ganglia of the brain characterized by muscle spasms of the shoulder, neck, and trunk.

Dysuria—Difficult or painful urination.

Ecchymosis—A bruise ("black-and-blue mark") resulting from release of blood into the tissues.

Edema—Excessive accumulation of fluid in the body tissue.

Emotional lability—Emotional instability.

Eosinophilia—An increase in the number of eosinophils (a variety of white blood cells) in the blood stream.

Epiphyses—Part of a long bone developed from a center of ossification distinct from that of the shaft and separated at first from the latter by a layer of cartilage.

Epistaxis—Severe nosebleed.

Erythema—Abnormal flushing of the skin caused by dilation of the blood capillaries.

Erythema multiforme—An acute inflammatory skin disease caused by an adverse reaction to medication(s) and characterized by lesions consisting of concentric circles of erythema, usually appearing on the neck, face, and legs. Occasionally blisters are observed. Often accompanied by fever, malaise, arthralagia, and gastric distress.

Extrapyramidal side effects—Reactions seen when the nerve tracts and pathways connecting the cerebral cortex, basal ganglia, thalmus, cerebellum reticular function, and spinal neurons are affected by a drug. Reactions are characterized by akinesia, fixed positioning of the limbs (rigidity), sudden violent movement of the arms and head (dystonias), akathesia, and rhythmic, clonic muscular activity (tremor).

Gynecomastia—Enlargement of the breasts in males.

Heart block—A condition in which the normal electrical conduction of the heart is disrupted so that the pumping action of the heart slows down.

Hematuria—Presence of blood in the urine.

Hepatomegaly—Enlargement of the liver so that it can be felt below the margin of the rib.

Hyperbilirubinemia—Presence in the blood of an abnormally high amount of bilirubin.

Hyperemia—Excess blood in vessels supplying a part of the body (e. g., hyperemia of the eye presents as redness of the white of the eye).

Hyperkalemia—Presence in the blood of an abnormally high amount of potassium.

Hypernatremia—Presence in the blood of an abnormally high amount of sodium.

Hypersalivation—Presence in the mouth of an abnormally high amount of saliva; excessive salivation.

Hypersensitivity reactions—Abnormal response to a particular antigen that may cause a variety of tissue reactions such as serum sickness and allergy (including anaphylaxis).

Hypertension—Elevation of the blood pressure above the normal range (high blood pressure).

Hypertonia—Exceptionally high tension in the muscles.

Hypertrophy—Increase in the size of a tissue or an organ by enlargement of the cells as opposed to an increase in the number of cells.

Hyperuricemia—Presence in the blood of an abnormally high amount of uric acid.

Hypoesthesia—Diminished sensitivity to stimulation.

Hypoglycemia—A deficiency of glucose in the blood stream that causes muscular weakness, incoordination, mental confusion, and sweating.

Hypokalemia—Presence in the blood of an abnormally low amount of potassium.

Hyponatremia—Presence in the blood of an abnormally low amount of sodium.

Hypotension—Reduction in the blood pressure below the normal range (low blood pressure).

Ichthyosis—Skin condition characterized by dry, rough, scaly appearance.

Impotence—Inability of a man to have intercourse.

Insomnia—Inability to fall asleep or stay asleep for an adequate duration of time.

Keratitis—Inflammation of the cornea of the eye.

Kyphoscoliosis—Lateral and posterior curvature of the spine.

Lactic acidosis—Lactic acid is the end product of glucose metabolism in the absence of oxygen. Lactic acidosis is the buildup of these products to an excessive level that results in the pH of the bloodstream becoming more acidic.

Laryngospasm—Involuntary closure of the larynx, obstructing the flow of the air to the lungs.

Lupus-like syndrome—Symptoms characteristic of lupus caused by an adverse drug reaction.

LV hypertrophy—Left ventricular hypertrophy of the heart.

Lymphopenia—A decrease in the number of lymphocytes in the blood.

Malignant hyperthermia—Rare condition most commonly precipitated by exposure to anesthetic or neuromuscular blocking agents. It is characterized by excessive muscle contraction, severe skeletal muscle rigidity, lactic acidosis, sharply elevated body temperature, tachycardia, tachypnea, and cyanosis.

Miosis—Constriction of the pupil.

Myalgia—Muscle pain.

Mydriasis—Widening of the pupil.

Myelosuppression—A reduction in the blood cell production by the bone marrow.

Nausea—A feeling that one is about to vomit.

Neuropathy—Disease of the peripheral nerves causing weakness and numbness.

Neutropenia—A decrease in the number of neutrophils in the blood.

Nystagmus—Rapid involuntary movement of the eyes that may be from side to side, up and down, or rotary.

Orthostatic hypotension—Abrupt lowering of the blood pressure in response to a position change from lying to sitting or standing.

Paresthesia—An abnormal sensation, such as burning, pricking, tickling, or tingling, described as "pins and needles."

Peripheral neuropathy—See Neuropathy.

Petechiae—Small, round dark spots caused by bleeding into the skin.

Pharyngitis—Inflammation of the part of the throat behind the pharynx.

Phlebitis—Inflammation of the wall of the vein, most commonly seen in the legs. A segment of the vein becomes swollen and tender, and the surrounding skin becomes reddened and warm to the touch.

Photophobia—Abnormal intolerance to light in which exposure to light causes intense discomfort to the eyes.

Photosensitivity—Abnormal and severe reaction of the skin when exposed to sunlight.

Polyuria—Production of large amounts of urine, which is dilute and pale in color.

Postprandial—Occurring after eating.

Postural hypotension—See Orthostatic hypotension.

Priapism—Sustained erection.

Proteinuria—Presence of protein in the urine.

Pruritus—Itching caused by skin irritation.

Pseudomembranous colitis—Inflammation of the colon caused by use of antibiotics. It is characterized by severe foul-smelling diarrhea, sometimes accompanied by blood, mucous, and abdominal pain.

Pseudophakic—An eye in which a natural lens is replaced with an intraocular lens.

Psychosis—Mental disorder in which the patient loses contact with reality.

Psychotomimetic effects—Reactions that mimic the effects seen with psychoactive drugs.

Ptosis—Drooping of the upper eyelid.

Punctate keratitis—Puncture injury of the cornea that causes inflammation.

Purpura—Skin rash that results from bleeding of the small blood vessels (capillaries) into the skin.

Pyuria—Presence of pus in the urine.

QT interval prolongation—QT interval on an electrocardiogram represents ventricular contraction. Prolongation indicates the ventricle is taking a longer time contracting.

Rhinitis—Inflammation of the mucous membranes of the nose. Frequently presents as a runny nose.

Serum sickness—A delayed hypersensitivity reaction that sometimes occurs 7–12 days after ingesting a drug. The usual symptoms are rash, fever, joint pain, and enlargement of the lymph nodes. The reaction is due to the presence of antigenic material still circulating at the time the body is forming antibodies against it.

SIADH (syndrome of inappropriate antidiuretic hormone)—The stimulation of production of antidiuretic hormone, which results in water retention and water intoxication.

Somnolence—Sleepiness.

Steatosis—Fatty degeneration.

Stevens-Johnson syndrome—The most severe form of erythema multiforme characterized by high fever, headache, and inflammatory lesions of the mouth, eyes, and genitalia. Frequently the bronchial and visceral mucosa are involved. Death may occur from renal failure.

Stomatitis—Inflammation of the mucous lining of the mouth.

Superinfection—An infection arising in the course of treatment of another infection, caused by a different organism and which is usually resistant to the drug used to treat the primary infection.

Syncope—Loss of consciousness caused by temporary decrease in blood flow to the brain (fainting).

Tachycardia—An above-normal increase in the heart rate.

Thrombocytopenia—A reduction in the number of platelets in the blood.

Thrombophlebitis—See Phlebitis.

Turbinate edema—Swelling of the bones that form the nasal cavity.

Urticaria—An allergic reaction on which round red wheals form on the skin, ranging in size from very small spots to several inches in diameter.

Uveitis—Inflammation of any part of the uveal tract of the eye.

Vertigo—A disabling sensation in which the affected individual feels the ground is swirling or the surroundings are in constant motion. Most commonly associated with disorders of the inner ear.

Vitreitis—Inflammation involving the vitreous humor of the eye.

PART IV

REFERENCES

1. Forest Pharmaceuticals. Package literature for Campral®. July 2004.
2. Mylan Bertek Pharmaceuticals, Inc. Package literature for Apokyn™. April 2004.
3. Bristol-Myers Squibb Company. Package literature for Abilify®. April 2005.
4. Pharmion Pharmaceuticals. Package literature for Vidaza™. August 2004.
5. Genentech Pharmaceuticals. Package literature for Avastin™ December 2004.
6. Imclone Pharmaceuticals. Package literature for Erbitux™. June 2004.
7. Amgen Inc. Package literature for Sensipar™. March 2004.
8. Genzyme Corporation. Package literature for Clolar™. December 2004.
9. Novartis Pharmaceuticals. Package literature for Enablex®. December 2004.
10. Hameln Pharmaceuticals. Package literature for Pentetate Calcium Trisodium. August 2004.
11. Hameln Pharmaceuticals. Package literature for Pentetate Zinc Trisodium. August 2004.
12. Eli Lilly and Co. Package literature for Cymbalta®. Revised January 2005.
13. OSI Pharmaceuticals, Inc. Package literature for Tarceva™. November 2004.
14. Sepracor, Inc. Package literature for Lunesta™. December 2004.
15. Amphastar Pharmaceuticals, Inc. Package literature for Amphadase™. October 2004.
16. Ista Pharmaceuticals, Inc. Package literature for Vitrase®. May 2004.
17. Cotherix, Inc. Package literature for Ventavis®. February 2005.

18. Octapharma Pharmaceuticals. Package literature for Octagam®. March 2004.
19. Shire US, Inc. Package literature for Fosrenol™. October 2004.
20. Amgen, Inc. Package literature for Kepivance™. December 2004.
21. Pfizer, Inc. Package literature for Macugen®. December 2004.
22. Eli Lilly and Co. Package literature for Alimta®. August 2004
23. Salix Pharmaceuticals, Inc. Package literature for Xifaxan™. June 2004.
24. GlaxoSmithKline. Package literature for Vesicare®. November 2004.
25. Aventis Pharmaceutical, Inc. Package literature for Ketek®. October 2004.
26. Presutti Laboratories. Package literature for Tindamax™. May 2004.
27. Pfizer. Package literature for Spiriva®. September 2004.
28. Odyssey Pharmaceuticals, Inc. Package literature for Sanctura™. July 2004.
29. Elan Pharmaceuticals. Package literature for Prialt®. December 2004.
30. www.lexi.com (Lexi-comp 1978–2004).
31. www.fda.gov